Additional contributions by

G.M. Hall
MB BS, PhD, FIBiol, FRCA
Professor of Anaesthetics,
St George's Hospital Medical School,
University of London

Professor K.J. Broadley
BPharm, PhD, DSc, MIBiol, FRPharmS
Welsh School of Pharmacy,
University of Cardiff

Dr G. Taylor
BSc, PhD, MRPharmS
Welsh School of Pharmacy,
University of Cardiff

Dr D. John
BPharm, PhD, MRPharmS
Welsh School of Pharmacy,
University of Cardiff

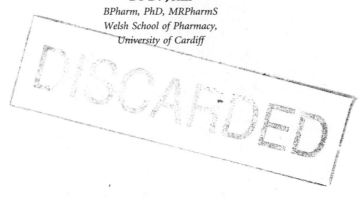

Contents

Preface to the eighth edition

Rapid advances in pharmacology and the continuing flow of new drugs make a new edition of a book such as this essential at relatively short intervals. In fact, the gap between editions on this occasion has been too long: a lot of revision and updating of existing material has been necessary, even before any consideration of adding new material. At the same time, our publishers expressed the hope that this edition could be about 10 per cent shorter than the previous edition, to comply with which would clearly involve pruning of much of the previous contents.

At the same time there was a good case for continuity. A book which reaches eight editions, which has been distributed widely in parts of the developing world through cheap editions and which has been 'pirated' in others, is clearly doing something right. It is obviously meeting a need.

The authors of previous editions have always visualized two audiences. Firstly, there are the trainee anaesthetists, getting to grips not only with the drugs which they use but those which, increasingly, their patients are receiving before surgery for intercurrent medical conditions. They need to understand a good deal of the pharmacological theory involved if they are to react intelligently to new or unforeseen interactions. We hope it is also an aid to their teachers, not only for examination purposes but for consultation when unusual situations arise. The second purpose which the book seeks to serve is therefore as a reference source for specific problems. Both functions are identifiable in the traditional layout of the chapters, with a detailed review of the pharmacological basis of a group of drugs or a therapeutic area followed by monographs on important or prototypical drugs and notes on similar compounds which exhibit minor variations. The index, of course, is the key to easy use.

One of the changes we have introduced makes this separation more explicit. In the previous edition, in long chapters a monograph on (for example) diazepam followed the section on benzodiazepines while a monograph on chlorpromazine would have followed a section on phenothiazine derivatives. In this edition, in all chapters which contain discussion of individual drugs (all except Chapters 1 and 16) the separation is absolute: pharmacology and any other necessary basic science are in the first part and all the monographs are together in the second part.

The most obvious change, however, is in the title. With experience in intensive care medicine now a clear requirement for trainees in anaesthesia, and with evidence that the great majority of intensive care units in the United Kingdom are managed and generally staffed by anaesthetists, the traditional title implies too narrow a focus which we hope to change by altering it to *Drugs in Anaesthetic and Intensive Care Practice*. To give substance to the change we have recruited Dr Martyn Read, a consultant with specific ITU clinical commitments, to make sure that any special applications to intensive care of any drug are included in the text. He has been invaluable in revising particularly Chapters 12, 13 and 19 which have a lot of intensive care connotations.

This edition coincides with an important change in the international nomenclature of drugs which the Medicines Control Agency has signalled as imminent. By means of a European Directive, an international agreement on approved official names is soon to apply in the United Kingdom. There are some major changes for some drugs which are commonly used in this field and discussed extensively in this book. Some fourteen are deemed to pose such a risk of confusion that both the old and the new name will have to appear on labels and in information leaflets. This list includes adrenaline and noradrenaline which from now on will adopt the US names of epinephrine and norepinephrine, respectively, and tetracaine, furosemide and alimemazine which are the recommended International Non-proprietary Names (rINNs) for amethocaine, frusemide and trimeprazine, respectively. This situation will last for at least five years until everyone is thoroughly familiar with the new names. Throughout the text, therefore, for drugs in this list we have used the new approved name, giving the old name in parenthesis the first time it is used within any section which a reader might choose to read in isolation.

A second list of about 200 drugs contains those with 'minor' changes which should be adopted immediately. This includes the US ending for barbiturates (thiopental for thiopentone) and several others which will initially 'look wrong' such as amfetamine, chromoglicate, clomethiazole and etacrynic acid. These are all designated as rINNs which should be adopted immediately. Both lists, as published by the Medicines Control Agency, are given in full in the Appendix, but we have taken the liberty of highlighting those which are of particular importance to readers of this textbook.

We have deleted most of the drugs which are no longer available in the United Kingdom, but mindful of the overseas readership have retained some which are still widely used in developing countries, notably ether and tubocurarine. We have also retained some drugs which are of particular historical interest, generally in a much abbreviated form. It has also been necessary to include details of newer modes of administration, particularly continuous infusions.

Any text of this type faces irreconcilable conflicts between various ways of grouping the material. In some cases logic suggests the grouping together of drugs according to a particular therapeutic strategy such as bronchodilatation. In other cases, drugs acting on a system which has great powers of reaction to imposed changes need to be considered together, such as drugs acting on the heart and circulation or on the endocrine glands. In yet other cases, a common receptor group (β-adrenoceptor agonists and antagonists) or common chemical features (benzodiazepines) seem more appropriate. We have looked very hard at the previous edition and in the end concluded that we could not improve very much on the existing arrangement. In particular, although much of the material could be distributed to different chapters according to therapeutic use, we have even retained, and indeed enlarged, Chapter 16 on Chemical Transmitters and Enzymes as the only way of ensuring adequate coverage of a rapidly expanding field of research. We have, however, axed that part of Chapter 20 which dealt with acid-base and physical chemistry and the associated discussions on infusion fluids which could not be classed as having drug actions, while retaining some, such as dextrans and oxygen-carrying solutions, which clearly are used for therapeutic objectives.

We are grateful to Professor George Hall for revising his chapter on Hormones and to Professor Broadley, Dr Taylor and Dr John, for invaluable help in various specialist fields, and hope that the contents overall will meet the needs of anaesthetists for the next few years at least.

M.D. Vickers
M. Morgan
P.S.J. Spencer
M.S. Read

Preface to the first edition

The modern practice of anaesthesia necessitates a considerable knowledge of physiology and pharmacology. Not only should the anaesthetist know about the action and side effects of those drugs that he uses himself, but also about those employed by his surgical and medical colleagues on the patients he is called upon to anaesthetize, as they may have a marked influence on the course of anaesthesia.

We have therefore included not only those drugs which produce anaesthesia and analgesia and those controlling their complications, but also others which may have some influence on their course. Some drugs have been included because of their historic interest or because they have become the yardstick by which other drugs are measured: even though they are not now used in clinical practice they may still be of experimental interest.

We hope that the book will be of assistance to students studying for higher examinations in anaesthesia and to practising anaesthetists who require a book of reference. We think surgical students will also find it useful as their ever increasing curriculum requires a knowledge of many of the drugs and problems discussed.

The classification of the drugs described has caused some difficulty. As far as possible they have been grouped according to their main actions and the purposes for which they are used. There have had to be some exceptions, as if a drug could be placed in one of several groups an arbitrary decision had to be made. Much of the information given is well known and references are not needed: where, however, recent research has brought new facts to light, or when well summarized accounts of certain problems have been quoted, appropriate references are included.

Each section is preceded by a general article on the drugs concerned, and this is followed by monographs on individual drugs. Other articles have been included to link up various sections, especially where the drugs concerned are described in other groups. It is suggested that whenever a monograph on an individual drug is consulted it should be read, if possible, in conjunction with the general article on the group. In the text, BP, BPC or approved names of drugs are used throughout; chemical names, synonyms and trade names are given under the headings of individual drugs.

Although new drugs are continually being produced by pharmaceutical firms, few prove of sufficient value to pass the test of time. Older drugs, thought to be of therapeutic benefit on empirical grounds, may eventually prove to be ineffective, some even harmful. We have tried to keep up to date, and much of the script written earlier has been revised recently. We are, however, conscious of the fact that in the course of time reconsideration of the value of certain drugs, especially the newer ones, will be necessary.

We would like to extend our special thanks to Dr C. L. Cope for writing for us the section on Corticosteroids, and to Dr P. J. Horsey for that on Electrolytes and Infusion Fluids. Our thanks are also due to Dr J. B. E. Baker for his advice and assistance during the early stages of the book, and to Mr C. R. Day of May and Baker Ltd, whose help with the preparation of drafts, advice on pharmaceutical aspects of drugs and the production of facts and figures has been of great value.

It is with considerable pleasure that we also acknowledge the helpful criticism and advice of our many colleagues whom we have consulted, and the patience of Butterworths, our publishers, during the time that the book has been in preparation. Finally we want to thank Joan Wood-Smith for much secretarial help and for looking after us so patiently during our many meetings.

Geoffrey Wood-Smith
H. C. Stewart

1

General pharmacology

Dictionaries define a drug as a 'medicinal substance', implying that drugs are used for therapeutic or prophylactic purposes. Drugs are also used in research, as aids to diagnosis and for quasi-social reasons, for example female sex steroids in contraception, or ethyl alcohol, caffeine and nicotine as social aids.

Others have described drugs as agents which modify living processes, a much wider definition which would include environmental pollutants and poisons and perhaps also some food additives. People also refer misleadingly to the pharmacological actions of drugs, when in fact it is the special structures or receptors in a living tissue or organ that determine that tissue's response to the presence of any natural or foreign substance. For example, the pharmacological effects elicited by an agent such as norepinephrine (noradrenaline) are very much determined by the target tissue and its receptors. It must be emphasized that drugs do not usually elicit wholly new or unique responses from a tissue: on the contrary, drug effects are usually expressed as increases or decreases of normal physiological responses from the target organs or tissues. Furthermore, these effects are frequently due to the tissues or organs mistaking a foreign substance or drug as an endogenous physiological agent, and further investigation often shows dramatic similarities in structure between the endogenous (physiological) and exogenous (pharmacological) substances.

Pharmacology is not simply a study of what responses a drug elicits from some living tissue since, from the moment the drug is administered, the body starts to apply a range of processes that will dispose of the drug, either chemically or physically. The response of the whole body to the drug is therefore determined by the balance between these phenomena: the influence of the drug on the physiological activities of the body's various tissues and organs (pharmacodynamics) and the body's response in determining distribution, chemical change and eventual elimination from the body (pharmacokinetics).

The early part of this chapter is devoted to a description of the principal subcellular mechanisms by which drugs can quantitatively alter the physiological processes of the human body, from which pharmacological responses are observed and potential useful (or harmful) effects are elicited. Following this, a pharmacokinetic consideration is given to the many ways the human body relocates or redistributes this foreign material (drug) to sites where it can chemically modify and ultimately eliminate it. It should be understood how important is this control by the body of the drug's location and chemical integrity in determining the potency, duration and breadth of action.

Mechanisms of action of drugs

There are numerous ways in which drugs may produce their therapeutic or harmful effects. They may act directly upon specific sites or receptors, inducing or enhancing, or conversely impeding, the normal physiological response of that tissue. Drugs can also raise or lower the concentration of a neuronal transmitter or modulator, for example by acting as a competitive substrate for an inactivating enzyme. Some drugs have very specific effects upon just a few cells, whereas others may exert their effects quite indiscriminately on a wide range of cell or tissue types, perhaps on the basis of a physical rather than a chemical property. General anaesthetics were thought once to possess CNS depressant activity on the basis of their lipophilicity. While this remains important in determining their rapid access to the brain, there is emerging evidence to show that specific sites on neurones are the basis of their actions.

Where a drug possesses a dramatic and clearly defined therapeutic effect, this can usually be attributed to a single major action upon just one group of cells or target tissue. When this 'useful' effect is extended to a range of tissues, or if the drug possesses a second or third property within its main target tissue, then the desirable or useful effects will be accompanied by additional or 'side effects' which may be deemed to be adverse to the patient (adverse effects). Even with the most singular drug action aimed at the most concise biological target, adverse effects may arise if this action is too great or of too long a duration. Even natural physiological events may be the basis of illness if those events are exaggerated. In practice, most drugs exert their primary and secondary properties on a range of tissues or organs, and careful clinical management will be required to optimize the desirable while minimizing the adverse effects.

The response to a drug often varies significantly between different patients. The predicted effect may not be observed or conversely it may occur more vigorously than anticipated; or it may be unduly long lasting. Many of these differences can be explained by the existence of quantitative differences in the way that two patients handle the same drug in the body: these may be small differences in the rate and degree of absorption from the site of administration, small differences in the rate of metabolic transformation of the drug by the liver; perhaps differences in the volume of distribution. These factors working together may yield very substantial differences in pharmacological (clinical) response following the same dose of drug to different patients. Patients' compliance also differs markedly: it is a factor consistently difficult to estimate accurately, or convincingly eradicate as an explanation of inter-patient variation.

Patients may also experience qualitatively different responses to the same drug, although these are rarer. One individual may have a genetically determined absence of some enzyme pathway responsible for the inactivation (or activation) of the foreign chemical in the body; or in a few people, a first exposure to the drug may induce antibodies, so that an allergic response may accompany second and subsequent exposures to the drug. Evidence is also emerging to suggest that qualitative differences may exist in the structures of some receptors, for example genetically-determined differences in $GABA_A$ and benzodiazepine receptors, which render some patients more prone to drug tolerance and the subsequent development of drug dependence. Fortunately, major differences in patients' qualitative responses to drugs are infrequent, but biological variation – whatever its cause – does occur throughout the human population, and startling differences can occur to the same dose of the same drug in different patients. Differences in age, sex, diet and ethnic origins may be important factors as a basis for these variations in drug response.

Minor chemical differences between two drugs may result in totally different pharmacological properties. For example, replacing the N-methyl group in the piperidine ring of morphine with a N-allyl group yields the agent 'nalorphine' which is a potent mixed agonist/antagonist – this simple chemical substitution has retained occupation or 'affinity'

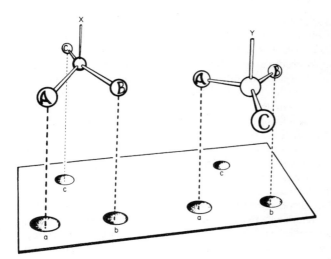

Figure 1.1 Diagrammatic representation of goodness of fit. The conformation of drug X ideally fits that of its receptor, whereas Y, the optical isomer of X, is a poor fit

for the opioid receptor but significantly reduced the intrinsic activity. In a second example, replacing the sulphur bridge of the phenothiazine neuroleptic 'promazine' with a twin methylene bridge yields the antidepressant imipramine. The importance of the three-dimensional aspects of a drug's structure is epitomized by the many quantitative and qualitative differences between two isomeric forms of the same drug. Thus (+)-amfetamine, widely called dexamfetamine, possesses central stimulant effects, whereas its isomer (−)-amfetamine does not. This three-dimensional aspect of a drug's structure, and the critical way in which it may determine that an agent is, or is not, pharmacologically active is a major factor underlying our concept of specific 'receptors' found on the membranes of cells. In the past decade, pharmaceutical companies have paid increased attention to this phenomenon, so that it is increasingly likely that only single isomer drugs or medicines are made available for clinical use. Even where the stereochemistry of two drugs is closely similar, very small changes in chemical structure (for example substituting a fluorine for a chlorine atom in some ring system) can significantly alter the affinity of a drug for the target receptor, and therefore its clinical potency. *Figure 1.1* illustrates in a simple diagrammatic way how two stereoisomers with the same chemical constitution will fit differently onto a receptor.

Patients generally have an expectation of beneficial effects from drug treatment, and will respond to 'therapeutic suggestion' – the expectation varies considerably between patients, according to their mood, their recent history, hopes or expectations built up by physicians and other healthcare workers, and their own psychological make-up. This is the 'placebo' effect: it can convert a genuine but modestly acting drug into a substantial one, or it may insinuate therapeutic response where there is no underlying pharmacological intervention from the drug. For these reasons, the proper clinical study of new or experimental treatments should wherever possible, and whenever ethically justifiable, be conducted in a manner which allows a proper comparison between the new test drug and a control or placebo preparation. However, it may be unethical to withhold existing effective medication from the control group, so that increasingly the objective clinical evaluation of a new drug or new treatment schedule involves comparisons with existing effective therapy.

Reference has already been made to the body's capacity to metabolize drugs into inactive forms, and it is important to emphasize that the interaction between drug and body is a dynamic contest. Onset and maintenance of drug effect is balanced by the body's capacity to chemically alter and finally eliminate the drug and its metabolites from the body. Typically, the absorption of a drug from the gastrointestinal tract and its progressive entry into the systemic circulation may produce peak blood levels 2–3 h after ingestion; by contrast, intravenous administration or administration via the lungs will achieve peak blood levels of the drug almost instantaneously. Thereafter, blood levels will decline, through a combination of the drug's deposition in the tissues (which is usually reversible) and its progressive breakdown and elimination from the body. The so-called duration of drug effect is a difficult matter to estimate or calculate. What tissue concentration produces the desirable effect? What is the relationship between blood and tissue concentrations? To what extent is the drug protein bound within the blood – a feature that on the one hand dramatically reduces the effective concentration gradient between blood and tissues, yet delays the drug's metabolism and elimination from the body? Thus, how much in excess of the required tissue concentrations will be the peak blood concentration? In practice, a study of a drug's pharmacokinetic profile reveals only the relation between a drug's blood concentration and time after administration, not the drug's effect and time. A drug's 'half-life' is the time in hours it takes for the blood concentration to be reduced by half (following a single dose, or discontinuation of an infusion or successive doses). A drug with a half-life ($t_{1/2}$) of say 2 h is short-lasting, whereas a drug with a $t_{1/2}$ of say 30 h (such as diazepam) is clearly long lasting. Indeed, given a typical exponential decline in blood levels, measurable amounts of a long-lasting drug can be detected in the blood for several days after a single dose. At what stage its tissue concentration falls below a pharmacologically effective level is simply not known.

Context-sensitive half-time (half-life) is a concept which is restricted to concentrations in plasma. When a drug is given by continuous intravenous infusion, its half-life (time for plasma concentration to be reduced by 50 per cent) is not constant, but depends on the duration of the infusion (the context). Thus the half-life of fentanyl increases significantly as the duration of infusion increases, whereas the context-sensitive half-time of alfentanil increases very slowly, making it much more suitable for use by continuous infusion. A very rapidly metabolised drug such as remifentanil is the ideal for such use as its half-life remains around three minutes irrespective of the duration of administration.

Plasma half-lives therefore can only be a guide to the duration of a drug's effect. Distribution of the drug into other tissues, notably adipose tissue, can ensure a drug's continuing presence for a considerably longer period. The onset of drug action is also an important issue, and a knowledge of the rates of absorption are also important: for example, in anaesthesia, this knowledge helps to predict duration of drug effect and the potential for drug–drug interactions; in another example, the continuing prevention of pain is very much linked to onset and duration of action, and determining the dose and frequency of administration of analgesics. Or again, the switching of analgesic provision from a partial agonist (such as pentazocine) to a full agonist (such as pethidine or morphine) is influenced by making allowances for the elimination of the partial agonist whose continuing presence in the body may attenuate the effects of the 'replacement' full agonist.

Concept of a receptor

The concept of a drug interacting with a specific, selective area on or in a cell, the so-called 'drug receptor', was introduced by the British physiologist Langley (1852–1925), following work by Ehrlich (1854–1915) on histological dyes and staining methods at the beginning of the twentieth century. That these receptors might exist for physiological purposes, namely for their interaction with endogenous chemicals such as might be released from a nerve ending, was the conclusion developed and confirmed by pioneering pharmacologists such as Dale and Loewi. More recent discoveries of previously unidentified highly sensitive drug receptors have led to the successful identification of endogenous analgesic agents, the endorphins, and has stimulated an as yet unsuccessful search for endogenous anxiolytic and antidepressant agents. Thus, the majority of drugs exert their pharmacological effects by interacting with the receptors that exist on the cells of tissues for producing the effects of the naturally occurring neurotransmitters and hormones. For example, the neurotransmitters released from the terminals of autonomic nerves and mediating the responses to nerve activation of smooth and cardiac muscle and glandular tissue are acetylcholine (parasympathetic nerves) and norepinephrine (noradrenaline) (sympathetic nerves). These neurotransmitters cross the synapse with the muscle cell, bind to muscarinic receptors or adrenoceptors, respectively and this triggers a cascade of events that culminate in the tissue response.

There is a wide range of other biogenic substances that serve as mediators of physiological and pathological processes and which are not neurotransmitters. Examples include histamine released from mast cells, angiotensin, the inflammatory products of arachidonic acid metabolism such as prostaglandins and leukotrienes, and adenosine, all of which produce their effects by a selective interaction with an appropriate receptor. The various phenomena which follow receptor activation will be briefly considered later.

Many drugs produce their pharmacological responses by interacting with the same receptor and thus mimic the endogenous transmitters and hormones. These are known as agonists. Other drugs selectively bind to the receptor, but do not activate the secondary cascade and in so doing prevent the binding of the endogenous substance and its consequent physiological activity; these are the receptor antagonists. There are, of course, many drugs whose mechanism of action is independent of receptor interactions. These include drugs which interfere with enzyme activity, such as the monoamine oxidase inhibitors and phosphodiesterase inhibitors, drugs that affect the transport of endogenous amines, such as the norepinephrine and serotonin uptake inhibitors, and drugs that open or close ion channels, such as the ATP-sensitive K^+ channel inhibitor and antidiabetic agent, glibenclamide. The following sections deal with drug actions that involve interactions with a target receptor.

Characterization and classification of receptors

The concept of a physiological or pharmacological response being the result of an interaction between the neurotransmitter or drug molecule and a receptor was developed with little knowledge of the nature of these receptors or that they even existed. The first steps towards confirming the existence of receptors and their identification was the development of radioligand binding technology. These techniques demonstrated the presence in tissue homogenates of specific binding sites for radioactively labelled neurotransmitters, hormones or their analogues, known as ligands. These binding sites displayed the same characteristics of selectivity and binding potency as determined for the functional response of the tissue and are therefore deemed to be the same as the receptors reponsible for the pharmacological response.

Receptor characterization by radioligand binding

Radiolabelled antagonists (or, less commonly, agonists) are incubated with membrane fractions of tissue homogenates and their binding to the receptors is determined after separation of the membrane fraction from the free unbound radioligand by centrifugation or filtration. The total binding to the membranes is determined by scintillation or gamma counting depending on the radiolabel (e.g. ^{3}H or ^{125}I, respectively). There will also be some non-specific binding to non-receptor components of the tissue and materials used in the assay. This is measured after displacing the radioligand from the receptor under study with a relatively high concentration of unlabelled agonist or antagonist that has high affinity and specificity for that receptor. The receptor-specific binding is therefore always the difference between the total tissue binding and the non-specific binding.

Radioligand binding can be used to identify the presence of particular receptors and their density in a tissue and the affinity of binding of the radioligand. This is achieved by generating a saturation curve of total binding at increasing concentrations of ligand which is usually quite linear with no apparent saturation as concentration increases. Receptor-specific binding, however, should characteristically be saturable, the plateau indicating that there are a finite number of binding sites (B_{max}). From these saturation binding graphs, the affinity of the radioligand for its binding site (K_D) can be determined as the molar concentration required for 50 per cent occupancy. The binding of an agonist (A) or radioligand (L) to its receptor (R) to form a complex (RL), like any drug–receptor interaction, obeys the law of mass action. The affinity of the interaction is the equilibrium dissociation constant (K_D), where:

$$K_D = \frac{(R)(L)}{(RL)} \tag{1}$$

The total receptor population $R_t = (R) + (RL)$ where R_t is equivalent to B_{max}, (R) is the number of free unbound receptors and (RL) is the concentration of bound ligand. Therefore:

$$K_D = \frac{(R_t - RL)(L)}{(RL)} \tag{2}$$

Rearrangement gives

$$\frac{RL}{R_t} = \text{Fractional receptor occupancy} = \frac{(L)}{K_D + (L)} \tag{3}$$

This is the equation representing the saturation curve for specific binding, from which the affinity (equilibrium dissociation constant, K_D) is the concentration (L) at 50 per cent receptor occupancy [$(RL)/(R_t) = 0.5$]. Reading off the K_D and B_{max} from saturation curves is unreliable, since it is essential to achieve saturation which involves the use of very high concentrations of radioligand where binding may become atypical and non-specific binding dominates. This is avoided by conversion to a Scatchard plot of bound/free ligand against bound ligand. This is a linear relationship which can be more accurately fitted and does not require determination of saturation. B_{max} can be obtained by extrapolation to the intercept on the bound ligand axis and K_D derived from the slope. The equation for the Scatchard plot of bound/free [$(RL)/(L)$] against bound ligand (RL) is derived by rearranging equation (3) above:

$$\frac{(RL)}{(L)} = \frac{(R_t)}{K_D} - \frac{(RL)}{K_D} \tag{4}$$

where B_{max} (R_t) is obtained from the intercept on the bound ligand axis and K_D is $-1/\text{slope}$.

The affinity of a radioligand for a receptor is a fundamental property of that ligand. Ligands and drugs do not have absolute selectivity for one receptor and will bind to some degree to other receptors, but the affinity will be substantially less than for the receptor for which it is selective. The K_D of binding to the tissue homogenate will therefore provide evidence for the presence of those receptors in the tissue. The B_{max} will provide a measure of the number of receptors (per mg of protein). This has been used to detect changes that occur in disease or after chronic drug treatments. For example, a fall in β-adreno-ceptor density has been found in the hearts of patients with advanced heart failure due to idiopathic dilated cardiomyopathy or end-stage ischaemic cardiomyopathy. Also, chronic treatment with β-adrenoceptor agonists has been shown to cause a down-regula-tion of β-adrenoceptor number in the airways and on circulating lymphocytes. Both of these phenomena have implications in the use of β-adrenoceptor agonists which may display a loss of activity or tolerance.

As we will see later, many receptors for the naturally occurring ligands have now been subdivided into two or more subtypes. The adrenoceptors, for example, were first divided into α- and β-subtypes, and with the introduction of more selective agonist and antag-onist ligands it has become apparent that these in turn require subdivision into α_1-, α_2-, β_1-, β_2- and β_3-subtypes. Radioligand binding techniques have assisted in this sub-classi-fication and have enabled the distribution of these receptors in tissues to be determined. It is clear from radioligand binding that most tissues contain a mixed or heterogeneous population of the various receptor subtypes. For example, homogenates from the heart contain predominantly β_1-adrenoceptors but also β_2-adrenoceptor binding sites. Yet it is generally accepted that the increases in rate and force of contraction of the heart to sympathetic nerve stimulation or to sympathomimetic amines such as epinephrine (adrenaline) are mediated via β_1-adrenoceptors. The question remains as to the roles of minor populations of receptors. Could they mediate other responses not normally monitored, such as metabolic responses? Could they be non-functional binding sites not coupled to an end response? This remains one major limitation of radioligand binding data; it does not tell us the functional role of the binding sites detected.

Another major application of radioligand binding techniques is for the rapid screen-ing of novel chemical entities for their ability to bind to selected receptors. The affinity of binding of unlabelled compounds to the receptor can be determined from their ability to displace a radioligand. Increasing concentrations of the unlabelled compound are incubated with a single low concentration (L) of the radioligand close to its K_D to minimize non-specific binding. From the displacement curve of percentage inhibition of specific binding against concentration, the affinity or dissociation constant (K_I) is deter-mined from the equation:

$$K_I = \frac{IC_{50}}{1 + [(L)/K_D]} \tag{5}$$

where K_D is the dissociation constant of the radioligand and IC_{50} is the molar concen-tration of compound which inhibits binding by 50 per cent.

The rank order of affinities of a series of agonists should be similar to that for their potency in producing the pharmacological response of the tissue from which the homogenate was prepared. This rank order characterizes the receptor type present. Where compounds have an asymmetric centre and exist as more than one optical isomer, the displacement must display stereoselectivity. At adrenoceptors, the $R(-)$-isomers of sympa-thomimetic amines show greater potency. The ability of a compound to selectively displace a radioligand does not predict whether that agent will possess agonist or antagonistic properties in functional tests; it merely shows that the compound selectively binds to the receptor under study. The screening of novel compounds for binding to a wide range of receptors has been greatly improved in recent years by the availability of cloned human receptors. This avoids the possibility of erroneous conclusions regarding binding to receptors of animal origin which may have slightly different binding characteristics. For example, β-adrenoceptors and A_3 purine receptors of rats are different from the human versions. Cloned cDNA from human gene libraries has been introduced into mammalian cell lines such as Chinese hamster oocytes or the bacterium *Escherichia coli* which do not usually express mammalian receptors. These cells then express the receptor that the cDNA encodes. Verification of the presence of the receptor is achieved by radioligand binding, which displays the characteristics of the natural receptor in terms of rank order of potency of displacing agents and stereoselectivity.

Receptor characterization from functional pharmacological responses

Radioligand binding data only provides information on the ability of a drug to interact with a receptor and its affinity for the receptor. The selectivity for a particular receptor is indicated by high affinity binding with that receptor compared with other receptors. This is determined by the goodness of fit of the three-dimensional structure of the ligand with the receptor configuration (see *Figure 1.1*). The forces of attraction between drug/ligand and receptor are:

- *Ionic bonds.* Drug molecules may contain cationic and anionic groups which may be electrostatically attracted to oppositely charged groups on or around the receptor. These ionic bonds dissociate readily and the drug–receptor interaction is reversible.
- *Hydrogen bonds.* Hydrogen atoms on or near the surface of a large molecule such as the receptor protein possess a partial positive charge and can form ionic bonds with negatively charged atoms of the drug molecule (e.g. oxygen and nitrogen). Hydrogen bonds are usually weaker than ionic bonds and these too should be reversible.
- *Van der Waals' forces.* These are formed by a weak attraction that exists between dipoles or induced dipoles generated from orbital distortion of outer shells of electrons that are in close proximity to each other. Again they are weak and easily reversed.
- *Covalent bonds.* These are generated when an atom of the drug molecule and one of the receptor share a pair of electrons. These bonds impart strong binding of the drug with the receptor which is slowly reversible or even irreversible. The effects are usually antagonistic. Such interactions occur between the alkylating antagonist phenoxybenzamine and α-adrenoceptors.

Agonists and partial agonists

The dose–response curve for a tissue response to an agonist is the basis of characterization of the drug–receptor interaction and the classification of receptors. The dose–response curve can be described from its position with regard to the concentration of agonist, the slope and the maximum. The position of the curve is the most widely used and is a measure of the potency of the agonist. The most used index of potency is the EC_{50}, the molar concentration for 50 per cent of maximum response. The slope of the curve should comply with that predicted by the law of mass action for the drug–receptor interaction. The form of the mass action equation is the same as used for radioligand binding (equation 3):

$$\text{Fractional receptor occupancy} = \frac{RA}{R_t} = \frac{(A)}{K_A + (A)} \tag{6}$$

where (A) is the concentration of agonist and K_A is the equilibrium dissociation constant or affinity of the agonist (which is the reciprocal of the binding constant).

The response to an agonist is related to its affinity and a scaling factor which describes the ability of the combination of one drug molecule with one receptor to produce a response. Ariens (1954) introduced the term intrinsic activity $(\propto)$ to define this drug-related scaling factor, so that

$$\frac{E_A}{E_{max}} = \text{Functional response} = \propto \frac{(A)}{K_A + (_A)} \tag{7}$$

According to this relationship, agonists producing a maximum response of the tissue have intrinsic activities $= 1$ and are referred to as full agonists. Antagonists have zero intrinsic activity, whereas partial agonists have intrinsic activities ranging between zero and unity. According to the above equation, the affinity or K_A is given by the EC_{50}. However, this is only the case when the maximum response is achieved with precisely 100 per cent receptor occupancy. It is apparent that this is rarely the case with potent full agonists, which can produce a maximum response with only a fraction of the receptors occupied. Thus, at the maximum response there are said to be 'spare receptors' or the existence of a 'receptor reserve'. The relationship between response and receptor occupancy is therefore non-linear and occupancy–response curves are typically hyperbolic, with a steep slope indicating efficient coupling. To explain this non-linear relationship, Stephenson (1956) introduced the term *stimulus* (S). The response of a tissue is some undefined function of the stimulus; two agonists producing the same stimulus would generate the same response irrespective of the receptor occupancy:

$$\frac{E}{E_{max}} = f(S) \tag{8}$$

The relationship between receptor occupancy (RA/R_t) and stimulus (S) is defined as the *efficacy* (e):

$$S = e(RA/R_t) \tag{9}$$

From the mass action equation (6):

$$S = e \frac{(A)}{K_A + (A)} \tag{10}$$

and from equation (8):

$$\frac{E}{E_{max}} = f\left[\frac{e(A)}{K_A + (A)}\right] \tag{11}$$

Efficacy is both a drug- and receptor-related factor since it depends upon R_t. Furchgott

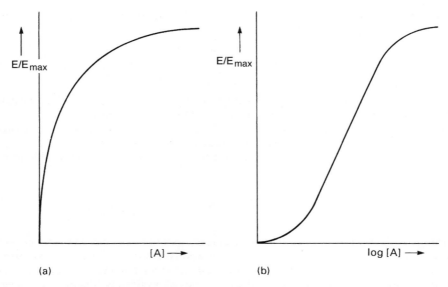

Figure 1.2 Dose–response curves for an agonist. The graph of response, expressed as a fraction of the maximum response [E/E_{max}] against concentration [A] is exponential (a), but becomes sigmoid when log of [A] is substituted (b). A straight-line relationship exists over most of the range between 16 per cent and 84 per cent of the maximum or ceiling effect [E_{max}]

(1966), however, introduced the strictly receptor-related term, intrinsic efficacy (ϵ) to define the occupancy–stimulus relationship for one receptor ($e = \epsilon. R_t$).

The currently used equation for the occupancy model of drug–receptor interactions to describe the agonist dose–response curve is therefore

$$\frac{E}{E_{max}} = f\left[\frac{\epsilon(R_t)\ (A)}{K_A + (A)}\right] \tag{12}$$

The tissue-related factors are the total receptor population (R_t) and the relationship between stimulus and response (f), while the drug-related factors are its dissociation constant (affinity, K_A), intrinsic efficacy and the concentration (A).

When response (E/E_{max}) is plotted against drug concentration (A), an exponential curve is obtained. If the concentration is plotted on a logarithmic scale, then a sigmoidal relationship is observed (*Figure 1.2*). This relationship is linear between 16 per cent and 84 per cent of the maximum response and indicates a fundamental property of drug action – responses increase as the concentration increases logarithmically not arithmetically. Dose–response curves plotted in this way are the basis for measurement of a drug's potency, usually as the EC_{50}. The potency of an agonist is determined by both its affinity (K_A) and intrinsic efficacy (ϵ) and ideally these two independent factors should be determined. However, this is not always possible because of the unknown nature of the relationship between stimulus and response. With full agonists, the EC_{50} occurs at a lower concentration than the K_A because of amplification of the signal; the EC_{50} is therefore a poor estimate of the affinity of a full agonist. In the case of partial agonists, where there is no receptor reserve, the EC_{50} is a closer approximation of the affinity (*Figure 1.3*).

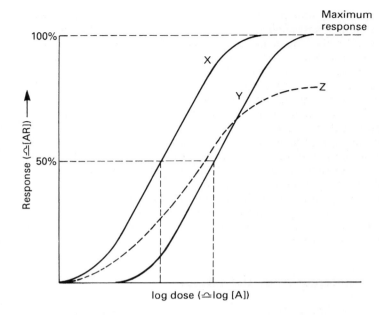

Figure 1.3 Curve X illustrates the relationship between log dose against tissue response for an agonist presumed to have an efficacy equal to or greater than unity (a full agonist). Curve Y illustrates the response to the same agonist (now at higher doses) because of the presence of a competitive antagonist. Note that the ceiling or maximum effect is unchanged but potency is reduced. Curve Z illustrates the effect of a partial agonist (efficacy less than unity) at the same receptors

Antagonists

Competitive antagonists have proved to be far more accurate and useful in the classification of receptors. The affinity of an antagonist can be measured more accurately than for agonists because the activity is not influenced by the stimulus–response relationship. In the presence of a competitive antagonist, the dose–response curve for an agonist is displaced to the right in a parallel manner with no depression of the maximum response (*Figure 1.3*). The degree of shift is measured as the dose ratio (DR), which is the ratio of EC_{50} values in the absence and presence of antagonist. The dose ratio is related to the concentration of antagonist (B) and its affinity (K_B) according to the following equation:

$$\log(DR{-}1) = \log[B] - \log K_B \qquad (13)$$

This is derived from the mass action equations for the agonist in the absence and presence of antagonist, in which the agonist affinity and efficacy cancel because they are the same at the 50 per cent response in the absence and presence of antagonist (i.e. this is known as a null method). This is the equation for the Schild regression of $\log(DR{-}1)$ against log molar concentration of antagonist $[B]$. It is usual practice to examine at least three concentrations of antagonist to produce a Schild plot of $\log(DR{-}1)$ against $\log[B]$. If the antagonism is competitive and the assay is performed under equilibrium conditions, the Schild plot will be linear and have unity slope. The affinity of the antagonist (K_D) is obtained from the intercept on the concentration axis ($-\log K_B$) which is known as the pA_2 value ($pA_2 = -\log K_D$). Provided that the antagonism is competitive and there is a slope of unity, then the pA_2 is the affinity and may be regarded as a constant for the antagonist at the receptor under study.

The pA_2 value is independent of the agonist used, provided that it acts upon the receptor in question. For example, atropine is an antagonist of the muscarinic receptors for acetylcholine and will produce similar pA_2 values against acetylcholine and other muscarinic agonists including methacholine and pilocarpine. At other receptors, an antagonist may have a weaker blocking action, such as atropine at histamine receptors, and will generate a substantially lower pA_2 value. The pA_2 value is also useful for characterizing the receptors in different tissues. These will yield similar pA_2 values if the receptors mediating the pharmacological responses are identical. If the pA_2 values differ significantly, it suggests that different receptors or subtypes are involved.

Irreversible antagonists form covalent bonds with the receptor and effectively remove a proportion of the receptors that are available for agonist occupation. Unlike the competitive antagonists, they do not produce progressive parallel shifts of the agonist dose–response curve. Instead, the shift of the agonist dose–response curve may be parallel initially as spare receptor capacity is used up, but with higher concentrations there is a depression of the maximum response. This is the type of antagonism produced by the alkylating α-adrenoceptor antagonist, phenoxybenzamine. The action of such antagonists is prolonged and recovery is usually dependent upon the synthesis of new receptor protein. These drugs are very useful in receptor characterization studies since they can remove receptor populations and permit the measurement of agonist affinities.

Receptor types and subtypes

As a result of radioligand binding studies and analysis of the functional responses of agonist and antagonists, the receptors involved in most tissue responses have now been identified. The receptors for the common neurotransmitters and endogenous biogenic amines are shown in *Table 1.1*. It can be seen that most of these endogenous substances exert their effects through the activation of more than one receptor subtype. Which receptor subtype is involved in the response has been identified from potency orders of agonists and the actions of selective antagonists.

It is beyond the scope of this book to describe the criteria for classifying all of the major receptor subtypes. However, to illustrate this point a couple of examples are provided. β_1-adrenoceptors are classified by a potency order for a simple range of agonists of isoprenaline > norepinephrine (noradrenaline) > epinephrine (adrenaline) > phenylephrine, whereas β_2–adrenoceptors have the potency order isoprenaline > epinephrine > norepinephrine > phenylephrine. β_1-adrenoceptor-mediated responses are preferentially antagonized by β-blockers such as atenolol and acebutolol, which have weak activity against β_2-adrenoceptor-mediated effects such as bronchodilatation. The type of response produced by an agonist in a tissue or organ will therefore depend upon the distribution of functional receptors and the selectivity of the agonist for those receptors. Thus, in the heart β_1-adrenoceptors predominate and in the lungs β_2-adrenoceptors predominate. Salbutamol is a β_2-adrenoceptor selective agonist and will therefore exert mainly bronchodilator actions in the lungs with minimal cardiac stimulation.

The structures of the major receptors have now been identified. Most of the receptors have been cloned and their amino acid sequences determined. As can be seen from *Table 1.1*, with few exceptions they belong to a G-protein superfamily which display common features. The G-protein-coupled receptors consist of single polypeptide chains having from 300 to 500 amino acid units and their properties will be considered in the next section. A few receptors are not coupled to G-proteins but are linked directly to or form an integral part of an ion channel. These include the acetylcholine nicotinic receptors (N_N and N_M) which have been crystallized from the electric organ of the electric ray (*Torpedo californica*) and shown to consist of a pentamer of five subunits arranged around the Na^+

Table 1.1 Receptors mediating responses to neurotransmitters and other biogenic amines

Transmitter/ amine	Receptor and subtypes		Response	Second messenger	Ion channel direct coupling
Norepinephrine	α	α_1	Smooth muscle contractions	$IP_3/DAG\uparrow$	
		α_2	Prejunctional – inhibits transmitter release	$cAMP\downarrow$	
	β	β_1	Cardiac +ve inotropy and chronotropy	$cAMP\uparrow$	
			Gut relaxation	$cAMP\uparrow$	
		β_2	Smooth muscle relaxation	$cAMP\uparrow$	
		β_3	Lipolysis	$cAMP\uparrow$	
Acetylcholine	Nicotinic	N_N	Ganglion transmission Release of epinephrine		Na^+ channel
		N_M	Skeletal muscle contraction		Na^+ channel
	Muscarinic				
		M_1	Ganglion transmission Gastric acid secretion	$IP_3/DAG\uparrow$	
		M_2	Heart – –ve inotropy and chronotropy Prejunctional – inhibits transmitter release	$cAMP\downarrow$	
		M_3	Smooth muscle contraction	$IP_3/DAG\uparrow$	
Histamine		H_1	Smooth muscle contraction	$IP_3/DAG\uparrow$	
		H_2	Gastric acid secretion Cardiac stimulation	$cAMP\uparrow$	
		H_3	Prejunctional – inhibits transmitter release		
Adenosine	P_1	A_1	Cardiac inhibition Prejunctional – inhibits transmitter release	$cAMP\downarrow$	
		A_2	Smooth muscle relaxation	$cAMP\uparrow$	
		A_3	Mast cell degranulation	$IP_3/DAG\uparrow$	
	P_2	P_{2x}	Smooth muscle contraction		Cation channel
		P_{2y}	Smooth muscle relaxation	$IP_3/DAG\uparrow$	
Dopamine		D_1	Vasodilatation	$cAMP\uparrow$	
		D_2	Prejunctional – inhibits transmitter release	$cAMP\downarrow$	

ion channel. Each unit of the nicotinic receptor spans the cell membrane of a ganglionic cell (N_N) four times, and from X-ray diffraction studies, these membrane-spanning sections have an α-helical arrangement. Another example of a receptor coupled to an ion channel is the GABA$_A$ receptor for γ-aminobutyric acid which also consists of a pentameric arrangement associated with Cl⁻ channels on postjunctional membranes of neurones in the brain. GABA exerts an inhibitory action on central neurotransmisssion by increasing Cl⁻ permeability and thereby reducing the depolarization due to excitatory transmitters.

G-Protein-coupled receptors

Structural features

The G-protein receptors have as yet not been successfully crystallized and their three-dimensional structure is still not known for certain. However, their amino acid sequences are known and seven stretches of 20–30 hydrophobic amino acids can be identified. Bacteriorhodopsin, a membrane pigment from *Halicobacterium halobium*, has been crystallized, making X-ray crystallography possible. High-resolution electron microscopy has shown this protein to be arranged into seven hydrophobic membrane-spanning α-helices extending perpendicular to the membrane (*Figure 1.4*). This has therefore formed the model for all of the G-protein-coupled receptors which are presumed also to consist of seven membrane-spanning hydrophobic domains arranged as α-helices. The amino terminal of the peptide chain lies extracellularly and the carboxy terminal lies intracellularly. There are three intracellular loops and three extracellular loops joining the α-helices. The α-helices are probably arranged around a central pocket that serves as the point of entry of the ligands which are then attached to specific amino acid residues. These essential amino acids have been identified by cloning receptors in which they are replaced, such receptors showing reduced binding capacity.

Post-receptor signal transduction

The cell surface receptors are coupled to the intracellular processes involved in the tissue response via guanine nucleotide binding proteins or G-proteins. These heterotrimeric proteins have three individual protein units of separate genetic origin, known as α-, β- and γ-subunits (*Figure 1.4*). The receptor is linked to the G-protein via the intracellular loops and the carboxyl terminus, but mainly through the third intracellular loop. The binding of an agonist to the receptor catalyses the substitution of GDP bound to the α-subunit of the G-protein with GTP. The α-subunit is thereby activated and cleaved from the β- and γ-subunits and then stimulates or inhibits enzymes to alter intracellular levels of second messengers involved in the tissue response.

There are several types of G-protein in which it is the α-subunits that vary. G-proteins linked to adenylyl cyclase are either stimulatory (G_s) or inhibitory (G_i). G-proteins (G_q) are also linked to phosphoinositide hydrolysis. These and other G-protein types are distinguished by their susceptibility to biological toxins, including cholera toxin and pertussis toxin.

Second messengers

The two principal second messenger systems are cyclic adenosine 3',5'-monophosphate (cAMP) and an increased turnover of phosphoinositide to generate inositol triphosphate (IP_3) and diacylglycerol (DAG).

cAMP   Receptors mediating their effects through cAMP are subdivided into two types: those where G-protein activation (G_s) causes stimulation of adenylyl cyclase and an increase in intracellular cAMP levels and those which decrease cAMP levels by inhibition of adenylyl cyclase through coupling to an inhibitory G-protein (G_i). Receptors positively linked to cAMP via G_s include β-adrenoceptors (*Figure 1.4*), dopamine D_1-receptors, histamine H_2-receptors and adenosine A_2-purinoceptors. In contrast, $α_2$-adrenoceptors,

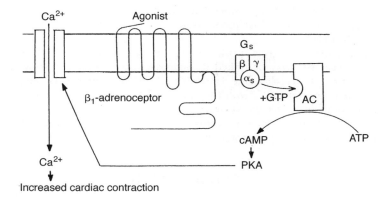

Figure 1.4 Diagram of the coupling of a cardiac β_1-adrenoceptor through the G-protein (G_s) to adenylyl cyclase (AC) and the subsequent conversion of ATP to cyclic AMP (cAMP). The agonist interacts with the receptor which consists of seven transmembrane spanning α-helices. The increased levels of cAMP activates cAMP-dependent protein kinase (PKA) which phosphorylates effector proteins on the L-type Ca^{2+} channel. This allows influx of calcium and the generation of a positive inotropic response

dopamine D_2-receptors, muscarinic M_2-receptors, opioid receptors and adenosine A_1-purinoceptors are coupled to G_i and inhibit cAMP production when agonists interact (see *Table 1.1*).

Increases in cAMP levels activate PKA which in turn phosphorylates a wide range of substrates to produce different responses depending on the tissue. In cardiac muscle, where cAMP levels rise after β-adrenoceptor stimulation, the activated PKA phosphorylates effector proteins on the L-type Ca^{2+} channel. This allows influx of Ca^{2+} and the increase in cardiac contraction produced by epinephrine and other sympathomimetic amines (*Figure 1.4*). In smooth muscle of blood vessels and the airways, for example, increases in cAMP due to stimulation of β-adrenoceptors or adenosine A_2-receptors, cause relaxation. The mechanisms involved in this are still incompletely understood, and several sites of phosphorylation by the activated PKA have been proposed. Most likely is a restriction of cytoplasmic Ca^{2+} levels due to enhanced uptake into the sarcoplasmic reticulum or prevention of its influx through L-type channels.

Inhibition of cAMP levels due to α_2-adrenoceptor and adenosine A_1-receptor stimulation causes a range of effects, many of which have yet to be explained. One response is a reduction of transmitter release from peripheral autonomic nerve endings where the fall in cAMP is associated with reduced intracellular Ca^{2+} levels.

IP$_3$/DAG Stimulation of histamine H_1-, muscarinic M_1- and M_3-receptors, α_1-adrenoceptors and several other receptor types causes activation of the G-protein G_q which stimulates the enzyme phospholipase C (PLC). This enzyme promotes the hydrolysis of phosphoinositides, principally phosphatidylinositol 4,5–bisphosphate (PIP_2) to inositol triphoshate (IP_3) and diacylglycerol (DAG). IP_3 interacts with an IP_3 receptor located on the intracellular sarcoplasmic reticulum storage site for Ca^{2+}. This causes the intracellular release of Ca^{2+} which in smooth muscle initiates a contractile response and in exocrine glands release of secretions (e.g. saliva). The other product of PIP_2 hydrolysis is DAG, which activates another enzyme, protein kinase C (PKC). PKC causes the phosphorylation of a range of cellular proteins, but the role of DAG in the responses to these agonists is less certain than for IP_3. It is possible that PKC phosphorylates proteins associated with the L-type Ca^{2+} channel and thus allows influx of Ca^{2+} which contributes to the contraction of smooth muscle.

Some pharmacological effects appear to be produced independent of a second messenger pathway. Receptors may be linked through a G-protein directly to an ion channel. For example, the M_2-acetylcholine (muscarinic) receptor in cardiac tissue is directly coupled via the G protein (GK) with the outward K^+ channel. Stimulation of this receptor by acetylcholine increases the outward movement of K^+ which reduces action potential duration. This decreases the time available for Ca^{2+} influx into cardiac and pacemaker tissues and force and rate of contraction are reduced.

Drug interactions

Drug interactions are common, but clinically important interactions should be infrequent. The anaesthetist should be aware of the mechanisms by which drug interactions can occur. Patients obtain drugs in three ways. They may be prescribed by a doctor; patients in hospital often receive 10–12 different drugs. They may indulge in self-medication, for example by purchasing vitamins, cold and cough mixtures, or antacids from their local pharmacist. Thirdly, unbeknown to themselves, they may be absorbing drugs from their environment, for instance penicillin which is often present in low concentrations in the milk of cows treated with penicillin for bovine mastitis. The theoretical size of the problem is enormous but fortunately only a few of these interactions are therapeutically important, although it is likely that many more drug interactions will be described in the future as techniques for measuring drug plasma levels become more widely used.

When the effect of one drug is inhibited by another drug, antagonism has occurred. If the effect of one drug is enhanced by another and the effect is greater than the sum of their individual active effects, potentiation (or synergy) has resulted. Addition is the term used when the combined effect is equal to the sum of their individual effects. The reduced anaesthetic requirement for volatile agents when given together with nitrous oxide is an example of a therapeutically useful drug interaction, nitrous oxide having an additive effect with the volatile agent to produce deeper anaesthesia.

Drug interactions can occur at different stages of drug action. In general, interactions may occur before absorption occurs, by interfering with the binding, during biotransformation or excretion of a drug, or by an effect at receptors. An example of the first stage is the mixing of thiopental and suxamethonium before administration. Likewise, antacids can bind tetracyclines and digoxin in the stomach and reduce the amount available for absorption.

Plasma protein binding

Binding to plasma proteins occurs to a greater or lesser extent with most drugs. Only the unbound form of the drug is available to diffuse through membranes and interact with receptors. Hence only the free (unbound) drug is active. Competition between two drugs for the binding sites on plasma proteins may cause a reduction in drug binding and the concomitant increase in free drug concentration could potentiate drug action. While many such interactions have been reported *in vitro*, very few are therapeutically important. Plasma protein binding interactions occurring *in vivo* will only be of clinical significance under specific conditions. Firstly, most of the drug in plasma has to be

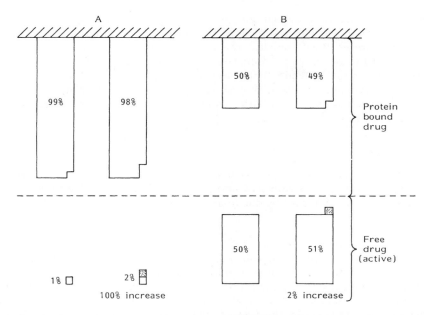

Figure 1.5 Diagrammatic representation of two drugs: drug A is 99 per cent bound to plasma protein, drug B is 50 per cent bound. A displacement of 1 per cent of drug bound will result for drug A in a 100 per cent increase in free (active) drug concentration but only a 2 per cent increase in free drug concentration for drug B

protein-bound, as illustrated in *Figure 1.5*. Secondly, the drug which is acting as the displacer has to be present in plasma in similar molar concentrations to those of the binding protein. Even when these conditions do occur and result in a higher fraction of drug in a free form in plasma, the actual free concentration may only be elevated transiently, if at all. Unless the drug has a small volume of distribution, any increase in the free concentration in plasma will be largely compensated by a redistribution to the tissues. Furthermore, even for drugs with small volumes of distribution, the increase in free concentration may only be transient because a decrease in binding is often accompanied by an increase in drug elimination. As a result, the free drug concentration returns to its previous value. Many of the serious drug interactions which were previously believed to result from a change in plasma protein binding, such as that between phenylbutazone and warfarin, are now recognized to be largely due to interference with drug elimination.

Extensive binding to tissue proteins also occurs with some drugs and offers a potential source for interaction. An interaction between quinidine and digoxin is believed to result from a change in the tissue binding of digoxin.

Drug metabolism

Drug metabolism occurs mainly in the liver, the microsomal cytochrome P-450 enzymes being responsible for the transformation of drugs to more polar substances. Many drugs are capable of stimulating the activity of these microsomal enzymes. There is no clear relationship between their ability to stimulate enzymes and their chemical structures or pharmacological effects. Among commonly used drugs, barbiturates, inhalation anaesthetics, analgesics, insecticides and nicotine (from cigarette smoking) are well known to stimulate cytochrome P-450 activity. The effects of coumarin anticoagulants can be greatly reduced by concomitant administration of phenobarbital. Clinically important interactions can occur if phenobarbital therapy is stopped or started in a patient stabilized on a coumarin anticoagulant. Women taking oral contraceptives have been known to become pregnant when treated with rifampicin, an antituberculosis drug which is a powerful enzyme inducer.

Enzyme induction

Repeated administration of a drug may cause induction of the enzymes responsible for its metabolism; this process is known as auto-induction. Tolerance to barbiturates following chronic administration may be due to auto-induction.

Enzyme inhibition

Enzyme inhibition can also occur, reducing the metabolism and therefore the elimination of drugs. Many monoamine oxidase inhibitors (MAOIs) elevate levels of catecholamines and can enhance the effects of indirectly acting sympathomimetic amines such as ephedrine and amfetamine. Foods such as cheese and meat extracts, which have a high tyramine content, can cause severe hypertension in patients receiving MAOI therapy. Many MAOIs also inhibit hepatic microsomes, which may explain the prolonged effects of pethidine and related narcotic analgesics in patients who are receiving MAOIs.

Enzyme inhibition can also be used in therapeutics. For example, about 95 per cent of an oral dose of levodopa (an anti-Parkinsonian agent) is metabolized to dopamine systemically by L-amino acid decarboxylase. This reduces the amount of the amino acid available for penetration of the brain as well as causing systemic side effects. Concurrent administration of carbidopa, an inhibitor of this enzyme in the periphery, reduces by 75 per cent the dose of levodopa necessary to produce the required central effect, as well as reducing the systemic effects. The reversal of non-depolarizing relaxants by anticholinesterases is an everyday example.

Drug excretion

Renal excretion is the most important method of excretion of drugs. Drug effects can be modified by alterations of active tubular secretion or of tubular reabsorption. Probenecid, by blocking tubular secretion, potentiates the actions of penicillin. Substances that affect urinary pH may profoundly affect reabsorption of drugs. This is made use of in the treatment of aspirin overdose by forced alkaline diuresis. In alkaline urine, aspirin is more ionized and less lipid soluble and thus its excretion is promoted.

Interactions at receptors

The actions of a drug at receptors may be altered in many ways. Competition for receptors is often used for therapeutic purposes, and the treatment of morphine overdose with naloxone is an example of competitive antagonism at a receptor level. Receptor responses can be modified such as when digitalis is given to a patient who is hypokalaemic following diuretic therapy. The concentration of a drug at receptors may be modified by other drugs. Tricyclic antidepressants may affect the actions of some antihypertensive drugs:

Table 1.2 Drug interactions

Primary drug	Secondary drug	Effect
Tetracyclines	Methoxyflurane	Nephrotoxicity
	Antacids	Reduced antibiotic absorption
Aminoglycosides (gentamicin, streptomycin)	Competitive neuromuscular blocking agents	Enhanced neuromuscular block
	Cephalosporins	Nephrotoxicity
	furosemide, ethacrynic acid	Ototoxicity
MAOIs	Indirectly acting sympathomimetic amines, food with high tyramine content	Excessive pressor response
	Oral hypoglycaemic agents	Prolonged hypoglycaemia
	Pethidine	Hypotension and coma
	Tricyclic antidepressants	Excitation
Suxamethonium	Ecothiopate, cytotoxic drugs	Prolonged neuromuscular block
Benzodiazepines	Antithyroid drugs	Increased antithyroid activity
Coumarin anticoagulants	Oral antibiotics, salicylates	Enhanced anticoagulant effect
	barbiturates, phenytoin, cigarette smoking, insecticides	Reduced anticoagulant effect
Tricyclic antidepressants	Epinephrine, ephedrine, amfetamine	Increased pressor effect

they block re-uptake of norepinephrine at presynaptic adrenergic nerve endings and also prevent uptake of the antihypertensive agent into the nerve terminal.

The table of drug interactions (*Table 1.2*) is in no way exhaustive.

Tolerance

Tolerance to a drug can be said to occur when the dose administered has to be increased to produce the same pharmacological effect; for instance, if the dose of morphine given to a patient has to be increased from 10 mg to 20 mg to obtain the same degree of pain relief, tolerance to morphine has occurred.

Different mechanisms, however, may produce tolerance. Tolerance can be produced if there is a change in the pharmacokinetics of the drug; for example, it may be metabolized faster. Tolerance to phenobarbital can occur in this way. Receptor tolerance is another entity; changes in the number (and possibly sensitivity, often now called down-regulation) of receptors may occur during chronic treatment. Morphine is believed to produce tolerance by this poorly understood mechanism following long-term treatment. Physiological tolerance depends on the presence of physiological control loops; for instance, in the intact animal the failure of an α_1-adrenoceptor blocking agent to maintain its initial drop in blood pressure when given chronically is due to cardiovascular reflexes coming into play, resulting in an increase in cardiac output which counteracts the fall in blood pressure.

Cross-tolerance is said to occur when, tolerance having been established to one drug, it is found necessary to give higher doses than were previously necessary of pharmacologically related drugs.

Tachyphylaxis is a physiological tolerance or desensitization, when tissue responses are reduced over a period of time due to progressive reductions in receptor sensitivity or the availability of an endogenous ligand. For example, pressor responses to successive injections of indirectly acting pressor amines are smaller due to the progressive depletion of sympathetic nerve-ending stores or norepinephrine.

Resistance

This is a term often used in relation to antimicrobial agents. For instance, strains of bacteria that were once sensitive to an antimicrobial agent become resistant to the drug. Bacteria can become resistant because of differential survival of sub-strains that produce enzymes which render them resistant to the drug. Penicillinase production by staphylococci is a well-known example; or the strain may switch its metabolic pathway to one less prone to interference by the antibiotic agent.

Transfer of drugs across membranes

In order to produce their pharmacological effects, drugs must attain an adequate concentration in the tissues upon which they act. Pharmacologists talk of biophase concentration; that is, the concentration of a drug in the immediate vicinity of the receptor. In only a few cases are drugs applied directly; most drugs are administered at a point remote from their eventual sites of action and are transported to receptors at their site of action via the plasma and extracellular space. Drugs injected directly into the bloodstream reach tissues rapidly. When given by intramuscular or subcutaneous injection a drug is readily able to traverse the endothelium of capillaries or lymphatics to reach the plasma. Drugs given by other routes have to circumvent other barriers before reaching the plasma.

Membranes in the body, whether surrounding individual cells or subcellular structures within those cells, generally consist of a bimolecular lipid layer covered on both sides with a monomolecular layer of protein. Body membranes are about 10 nm thick and are thought to be discontinuous, being interspersed with pores of about 0.4 nm radius. As a consequence, four mechanisms may be involved in the transport of a drug across a membrane.

Simple diffusion

Drugs will naturally flow down a concentration gradient. Other factors which influence the rate of transfer include molecular size or protein binding. Lipophilic drugs will dissolve in the lipid portion of a membrane and diffuse down the concentration gradient to the aqueous phase on the other side of the membrane.

Aqueous diffusion

Lipid-insoluble hydrophilic substances may cross membranes by passing through the pores in the membrane. Such passage is assisted by a hydrostatic or osmotic pressure difference across the membrane, when water transport may drag dissolved drugs across. This form of passage is limited by the molecular size of the drug. Most drugs have molecular radii considerably in excess of 0.4 nm and cannot cross membranes in this fashion. The vascular endothelium differs from other membranes. Capillary endothelial cells have large channels of up to 4.0 nm radius, and molecules as large as albumin can pass through these pores from plasma to the extracellular fluid.

Active transport

This consists of the movement of a substance against a concentration or electrochemical gradient. Active transport systems, such as the sodium pump, are widely distributed in the body. Drugs chemically resembling actively transported naturally occurring substances may be transported by the same mechanisms. Thus α-methyldopa, which resembles phenylalanine, is absorbed from the intestine by an amino acid transporting mechanism.

Phagocytosis and pinocytosis

Drugs of high molecular weight or which exist as molecular aggregates may be transported by being engulfed as small droplets by cells.

Physical properties affecting transfer

Water and lipid solubility

In order to cross a membrane, a drug must first enter into solution in the aqueous phase in contact with that membrane. Thus the rate of absorption of a drug will be a function of its water solubility. Having come into contact with the membrane, most drugs partition from the aqueous solution and enter the lipid component of the membrane. Lipid uptake will depend on the drug's lipophilicity, usually assessed by its partition coefficient, which is the concentration ratio at equilibrium of the drug between lipid and aqueous phases of the membrane environment. A high lipid/water partition coefficient will promote uptake into the lipid membrane. For most drugs, however, aqueous solubility will tend to decrease with higher lipid/water partition coefficients. Thus rapid absorption, which involves fast transfer from aqueous to lipid to aqueous environments, is associated with an optimum partition coefficient. This optimum partition coefficient varies for different membranes throughout the body.

Measurement of partition coefficients is most frequently performed *in vitro* using octanol as the lipid substitute and thus an octanol/water partition coefficient ($P_{o/w}$) is frequently quoted, often as $\log P$, for a drug.

Ionization and absorption

Most drugs are weak electrolytes, containing acidic or basic groups (or both) and are capable of being ionized in aqueous solution. The cell membrane is relatively impermeable to the ionized form of any drug, unless the ionized species is small enough to pass through the aqueous pores as is the case with lithium. Thus it is the non-ionized drug species which is most rapidly absorbed across membranes. An equilibrium will exist between the non-ionized and ionized drug species, with the proportion ionized being determined by the drug's ionization constant (or dissociation constant) K_a and the pH

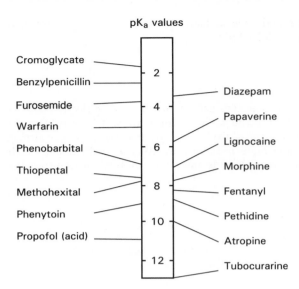

pK$_a$ values

Figure 1.6 The pK$_a$ values of some commonly used drugs

of the environment surrounding the drug. For an acidic drug, AH, the ionization constant $K_a = [A^-][H^+]/[AH]$. By analogy with pH notation, $pK_a = -\log_{10} K_a$. pK$_a$ is thus defined as the negative logarithm of the dissociation constant, just as pH is the negative logarithm of the hydrogen ion concentration. Put simply, pK$_a$ is the pH at which a drug is 50 per cent ionized.

The ionization constant of a basic drug, B, with water, can similarly be expressed in terms of an ionization constant, $K_b = [BH^+][OH^-]/[B]$, although by international convention the dissociation of both acidic and basic drugs is expressed on the same Ka scale. For a base, $K_a = [B][H^+]/[BH^+]$. The pK$_a$ for a basic drug is equal to $14 - pK_b$. The pK$_a$ values of some commonly used drugs are given in *Figure 1.6*.

The degree of ionization of drugs in different pH environments can be calculated from the Henderson–Hasselbalch equations:

For a weak acid:
$$pK_a - pH = \log_{10}[(\text{non-ionized concentration})/(\text{ionized concentration})]$$

For a weak base:
$$pH - pK_a = \log_{10}[(\text{non-ionized concentration})/(\text{ionized concentration})/]$$

When $pH = pK_a$, the non-ionized and ionized concentrations are equal. Increasing the pH of the local environment will increase the non-ionized proportion for acidic drugs but decrease the non-ionized proportion for basic drugs. Small changes in pH can make large differences to the extent of ionization, particularly if the pH and pK$_a$ values are similar. Equally, drugs with similar pK$_a$ values may ionize to different extents in biological fluids. For example, in blood at a pH of 7.4, about 60 per cent of any thiopental (pK$_a$ of 7.6) is non-ionized. Methohexital has a pK$_a$ of 8.3 and almost 90 per cent of this drug is non-ionized at pH 7.4. This may partially explain the transiently faster onset of central nervous system (CNS) effects with methohexital compared with thiopental. Thus the degree of ionization is important in determining passage across cell membranes, which affects absorption, transfer to active sites and excretion of drug via the kidneys.

Transfer across special membranes

Blood–brain barrier

The concept of a blood–brain barrier arose from the observation that many aniline dyes, when given intravenously to animals, stained all tissues except the cerebrospinal fluid (CSF) and brain. The barrier is formed by the close investment of cerebral capillaries by glial cells. These capillaries have permeability characteristics closely resembling those of cellular lipid membranes, and are less permeable than normal capillary endothelial cells. Penetration of the barrier by a drug depends upon the degree of ionization, lipid solubility, and the degree of binding on each side of the barrier. Highly ionized substances such as vecuronium cannot cross the boundary. The naturally occurring anticholinesterase, physostigmine, is a tertiary amine which can readily enter the brain; neostigmine closely resembles physostigmine but, being a quaternary compound and highly ionized at plasma pH, is without actions on the CNS.

Brain penetration by non-ionized molecules is a function of lipid solubility and partitioning. Thiopental, which is about 60 per cent non-ionized at plasma pH and has a high partition coefficient, readily enters the brain. The corresponding oxybarbiturate, pentobarbital, even though 80 per cent is non-ionized at plasma pH, penetrates the brain slowly because its partition coefficient is some 50–fold lower than thiopental.

Chemotherapeutic agents for the treatment of brain infections must be able to penetrate this barrier. Penicillin penetrates the normal barrier slightly, but passes through more readily in the presence of inflammation. Chloramphenicol, streptomycin and isoniazid pass into the brain in amounts sufficient to give adequate chemotherapeutic concentrations; tetracyclines and p-aminosalicylic acid do not.

Placental barrier

The placenta is best regarded as a modified lipid membrane across which drug passage is chiefly governed by lipid solubility. Besides lipid solubility and ionization, other factors that affect placental transport are the degree of binding of the drug to plasma proteins and the placental blood flow. Highly ionized drugs of low lipid solubility, such as non-depolarizing relaxants and suxamethonium, penetrate the placenta only slowly. Inhalational anaesthetics and thiopental rapidly attain equilibrium with fetal blood. Morphine, pethidine and other narcotic analgesics also readily pass to the fetus. Depressant drugs given to the mother during labour may have untoward or enhanced effects on the fetus because of the immature drug-metabolizing and excretory systems of the newborn.

Routes of drug administration

Drugs are administered by many different routes, including, oral, intravenous, intramuscular, subcutaneous, transdermal, pulmonary, nasal, buccal, ocular, rectal and vaginal routes. The choice of route depends upon a number of factors, including site of drug action, required duration of action, the nature of the biological barrier along the different routes, and practicability.

Oral

This is the most common route of administration and normally the most convenient and effective way of giving drugs. They are given in a variety of different dosage forms, most commonly tablets, capsules, solutions, suspensions and emulsions. Tablets are most frequently used, primarily because of their convenience and versatility. A number of different types of tablet formulation are available which are designed to control drug absorption, or protect the drug from gastric juices. A formulation may also be designed to protect the gastric mucosa from the drug, or mask the taste of the drug. One type, the 'dispersible' tablet, uses an effervescent base which readily disperses in water, thus providing the drug in a rapidly absorbable form.

Gastro-intestinal absorption of many drugs is efficient; for other drugs, however, it may be slow, incomplete and sometimes irregular. Some dosage forms may stick in the oesophagus, giving local release of the drug, and cause damage. Slow-release potassium chloride tablets and doxycycline have been reported to cause oesophageal damage. Patients at special risk are those who have oesophageal obstruction, for example due to enlargement of the left atrium. The drug's dosage form is important and, in general, capsules are more likely than tablets to stick or dissolve in the oesophagus. Drugs known to be mucosal irritants should normally be taken with a glass of water to reduce the risk of oesophageal damage. Indeed, most drugs are best given with a glass of water to aid oesophageal transit and promote intestinal absorption.

Irritant drugs should be well diluted and given with or after meals to reduce their tendency to cause nausea and vomiting. Drugs that are subject to acid hydrolysis or other instability in the gastric juices and those causing stomach irritation may be formulated as enteric-coated tablets or capsules which only liberate the drug after reaching the small intestine.

Some substances taken orally (e.g. ethanol) are absorbed from the stomach, but the majority of drugs administered by the oral route are absorbed from the small intestine. The acidity of the gastro-intestinal tract varies from about pH2 in the stomach to about pH7 in the small intestine. Thus the absorption of acidic drugs might be expected to occur primarily from the stomach rather than the intestine, due to a greater degree of non-ionization in the acidic environment of the stomach. However, the overriding factor controlling the absorption of most drugs is the surface area available for absorption. Thus most drugs, regardless of their chemical nature, are absorbed predominantly from the small intestine, with its very large surface area (approximately 100 m^2).

Drugs absorbed from the stomach and the gastro-intestinal tract are carried to the liver in the portal vein. Here they may be metabolized and their activity reduced (the so-called 'first-pass' effect). The liver may also secrete drugs and their metabolites into the bile and thence back into the intestine. This 'enterohepatic recycling' can prolong the duration of action of a drug.

Some drugs are given by mouth to act locally in the gastro-intestinal tract rather than by absorption. Examples of these agents are: antacids and absorbents such as aluminium hydroxide and magnesium trisilicate, which neutralize gastric acid; inhibitors of gastric acid secretion such as ranitidine and omeprazole; anti-reflux agents such as the alginates and drugs for treating infections of the gastro-intestinal tract such as streptomycin, neomycin and some sulphonamides.

Sublingual

Tablets may be specially formulated to disintegrate slowly and be resistant to chewing, thus assisting their retention in the mouth. Drugs such as glyceryl trinitrate and buprenorphine may then be absorbed from the buccal cavity into the general circulation, enhancing their onset of action and protecting them from first-pass metabolism.

Parenteral injection routes

Parenteral injection routes include intravenous, intramuscular and subcutaneous, and injection formulations may be solutions, suspensions or emulsions. The pH and the strength of parenteral injection fluids need to be considered. Injections which are too acidic or alkaline or those which are not isotonic may cause irritation and even tissue damage at the site of injection. Intrathecal injections of chemotherapeutic agents or local anaesthetics require special care and must be non-irritant. Clearly, absorption is not involved if the drug is given by intravenous or intra-arterial injection but absorption, involving diffusion across tissues into lymph and capillaries, does occur after intramuscular and subcutaneous injection. The rate of absorption by these routes is faster than by the oral route for most drugs. The rate of absorption is decreased if the drug – or mixture of drugs – causes vasoconstriction, and may be increased by increasing the blood supply to the injection site, for example by exercise or rubbing.

Intravenous injection

As the drug in this case is introduced directly into the circulation, its onset of action will be more rapid but its duration of action shorter than when given by any other route (*Figure 1.7*). The use of this route is not without risk: in cases of overdose or idiosyncrasy the effects are immediate and it may not be possible to antagonize them before serious toxic symptoms or even death have intervened. The effects of a drug given intravenously can be greatly modified by the rate of administration. Complete mixing of a drug with the circulating blood volume takes several circulation times. With rapid intravenous injection, tissues can be exposed to high concentrations of drug poorly diluted with blood and travelling as a bolus. The rapid onset of sleep when intravenous anaesthetic induction agents are given over a period of 30 s or less is related to this 'slug' effect. Subsequent rapid recovery is more dependent upon a fall in effective blood concentration due to mixing than to a rapid initial redistribution to lipid depots.

If a drug causes cardiovascular or respiratory depression, these effects are particularly likely to be seen after intravenous injection, as high concentrations of the drug rapidly reach the vital centres in the medulla.

Substances too irritant for subcutaneous or intramuscular injection can often be given intravenously. However, an irritant drug may give a risk of venous thrombosis, but this may be minimized by giving a well-diluted solution as a slow infusion. A sustained blood level of a drug can also be maintained by giving a continuous intravenous infusion at a controlled rate.

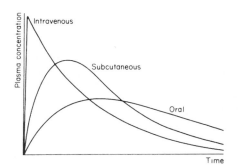

Figure 1.7 Time course of a hypothetical drug given by three different routes. Note the high initial plasma concentration after intravenous injection followed by a rapid fall. After oral administration there is a slow rise and the peak plasma concentration is low.
Subcutaneous injection results in a curve with a higher and earlier peak than after the oral route

Intramuscular injection

Absorption by this route is usually faster than by subcutaneous injection, especially when the drug is water soluble. Absorption can be slowed if the drug is in an oily solution or emulsified, when the active drug will be slowly released to pass to the tissues. Water-soluble drugs may be converted into less soluble compounds. The procaine salts of penicillin and the insulin–zinc complexes are examples of the therapeutic advantages of reduced water solubility: prolonged effects can be attained, smoother and more sustained blood levels achieved, and fewer injections needed than if the highly water-soluble parent compounds are used.

Subcutaneous injection

Subcutaneous administration may be more painful than other forms of injection because of the rich sensory innervation of the skin, and the injection volume which can be tolerated is much smaller than with the other routes. Irritant drugs such as digoxin should not be given subcutaneously as they may cause local sloughing of the skin or abscess formation.

Inhalation

Absorption of drugs from the lung is more rapid than from the oral route. Additionally, drugs which are poorly absorbed orally may be well absorbed after inhalation. Consequently the pulmonary route is being investigated for the systemic delivery of drugs, including narcotic analgesics and polypetides and proteins such as insulin, which are either poorly absorbed or slowly absorbed after oral administration. Lipophilic drugs are very rapidly absorbed from the lung since the alveoli offer a large surface area, thin membrane barrier and an abundant blood supply. The effect produced by this route is almost as quick as when a similar drug is given by intravenous injection. The factors which govern the absorption of inhaled volatile anaesthetics are discussed in Chapter 4. Aerosols of sympathomimetics, steroids and other anti-inflammatory drugs are commonly used in the treatment of asthma. Absorption of these drugs limits their duration by removing them from the site of action. Their absorption may also give rise to systemic side effects. A hazard in our society is the indiscriminate sniffing of volatile agents, especially by young adolescents, for pleasure. Deaths have occurred due to rapid absorption of toxic substances.

Transdermal route

The use of transdermal patches which give controlled drug release at a constant zero-order rate to maintain plateau blood concentrations is well established for a few drugs including nitroglycerin, estradiol, fentanyl and nicotine. A limiting factor in the suitability of a drug for this route is the dose necessary to achieve a therapeutic effect and in practice needs to be less than 10 mg per 24 h. It is important to note, however, that contrary to experience with inhalation anaesthetics, maintaining a constant blood level is not synonymous with a constant effect. Tolerance may develop quite quickly. The objective of the method is to maintain a constant therapeutic effect without the side effects which are presumed to be due to the transient peak concentrations associated with other routes of administration. However, the improvement over other routes has generally not been marked. Transcutaneous nitroglycerin and fentanyl 20–30 minutes before induction are effective in attenuating the hypertensive response to intubation.

Other routes

Drugs are applied to mucous membranes of the mouth, nose, eye, rectum and vagina primarily for their local effects. However, significant drug absorption into the systemic circulation can occur from these sites. Indeed there are a number of circumstances in which drugs are administered via these routes to exert a systemic action. Glyceryl trinitrate, for example, exerts its pharmacological action within a few minutes of sublingual administration but is inactivated by the liver when given orally. The rectal route is useful for the administration of drugs which cause gastric irritation or nausea and for morphine premedication in children. The nasal route is frequently used to achieve systemic effects from peptide drugs such as oxytocin and vasopressin analogues. When local anaesthetics are applied to mucous surfaces they can readily give rise to systemic effects; these can be minimized by the use of a vasoconstrictor such as epinephrine.

Drugs are also absorbed through the peritoneum. This was a cause of re-curarization in neonates when neomycin was applied to the peritoneum before wound closure. It is not a route which is used therapeutically.

Antibiotics may be given intrathecally for the treatment of meningitis. Both the CSF and the epidural space are utilized for local anaesthesia.

Factors affecting drug dosage

The required dose of a drug depends mainly on its effect at a given tissue concentration, on its toxicity, and on the duration of its effect, which is governed by its rate of inactivation. When a new drug is produced, initial animal experiments involving different species can give an approximate idea of its toxicity. If its actions and toxicity do not vary much from one species to another, the chances are that man will behave similarly when exposed to the drug. Initial studies in man are always performed on volunteers to determine by trial what is a reasonable dose to give the desired effect, and the duration of this effect can be studied and correlated with the rate of drug excretion. Gradually information is built up that will enable a reasonable estimate to be made of the dose required in patients. The manufacturers' recommended doses for new drugs are determined in this manner. The doses of older drugs were determined empirically in a much more haphazard way by trial and error, and it was rare for animal experiments to be employed.

The maximum dose for the majority of drugs depends on the dose level that is effective therapeutically, relative to the toxic effects produced. Some drugs, such as insulin, penicillin and various antisera, are given in a dose that depends on the severity of the condition, so that a severely ill child may receive more than an adult.

Some drugs are used for one purpose at one dose level and for a completely different purpose at another. Aspirin is an example: it is widely used for certain types of pain in doses of 0.3–1.0 g, whereas in rheumatic fever ten times the dose may be given for its other actions.

The amount of a drug necessary to produce and maintain a given effect depends on several factors, as governed by the drug's pharmacokinetics and pharmacodynamics. This is discussed in more detail later in this chapter. The frequency of dosing is determined by the need to maintain a therapeutic blood level; this is especially important with chemotherapeutic agents or in the use of opioids to maintain prolonged analgesia. When a drug is given, a peak blood level is reached which subsides as the drug is eliminated from the body. The time taken for blood levels to decline by one half is the 'half-life' ($t_{1/2}$) of the drug. The frequency and magnitude of doses will obviously vary considerably with different drugs. The elimination of benzylpenicillin is rapid, associated with a half-life of less than 1 h, whereas that of thyroxine is much slower, with a half-life of 1 week. Consequently benzylpenicillin needs to be given more frequently than thyroxine.

In some cases the duration of action of a drug and its cumulation follow certain simple general principles related to its half-life. Drugs obeying these principles have a duration of action that varies as the logarithm of the dose, and doubling the dose will increase the duration of action by one half-life. It is often unwise to give large doses of a drug on a logarithmic scale to increase the duration of action, especially with short-acting drugs as the blood concentration necessary may cause toxic effects. A longer acting preparation can be substituted if available, smaller doses can be given at more frequent intervals, or the drug may be given by intravenous infusion.

The dose of a drug may have to be decreased after a few days, as in the case of digoxin, because of accumulation. Tolerance or tachyphylaxis may require the dose to be increased. Iodine in thyrotoxicosis and morphine or pethidine given to drug addicts may have to be administered at continually increasing dose levels to evoke the same response.

Paediatric doses

Many equations have been devised for estimating the requirements of children; some are based on age, but the majority on weight. These equations tend to produce inappropriate doses at the extremes of the scale and, to accommodate this, two or three different ranges have to be included.

Many physiological requirements and metabolic processes are more related to surface area than age or weight, and Catzel (1963) has worked out a single schedule covering the range from 1 month to the young adult in which the percentage of the adult dose required is derived from the equation:

$$\text{Percentage of adult dose} = \frac{\text{Surface area of child}}{\text{Surface area of adult}} \times 100 \qquad (14)$$

It can be seen that even should *Table 1.3* not be available, the four reference points at which the dose is one-eighth, one-quarter, a half, and three-quarters of the adult dose can be simply memorized as approximately 1 month, 1 year, 7 years and 12 years, respectively. Predicting the requirements of premature infants or normal babies during the first two weeks of life, when detoxicating and excretory mechanisms are immature, is much more difficult.

Timing of administration

When a drug is given by mouth it is usually administered in divided doses over the day, thus obviating the higher blood concentrations associated with single large doses and reducing the tendency for toxic effects to occur.

Table 1.3 Estimation of doses for children as a percentage of the adult dose

Approximate age	Weight (kg)	(lb)	Percentage of adult dose	Fraction of adult dose
1 month	3.2	7	12.5	1/8
2 months	4.5	10	15	
4 months	6.5	14	20	
12 months	10	22	25*	1/4
18 months	11	24	30	
5 years	18	40	40	
7 years	23	50	50	1/2
10 years	30	66	60	
11 years	36	80	70	
12 years	40	88	75	3/4
14 years	45	100	80	
16 years	54	120	90	
Adult	65	145	100	1

* In the original table from Butler and Ritchie (1960), an infant weighing 22 lb receives 28 per cent of the adult dose. This has been reduced to 25 per cent for the convenience of remembering that an infant at 1 year requires about one-quarter of the adult dose (Catzel, 1963a). Reproduced from *Paediatric Prescriber*, by P. Catzel (1963b), by courtesy of Blackwell Science, Oxford.

The exact time of administration of a drug depends on a number of factors. For example, if a drug is given in order to stimulate appetite, it must be given before food, while gastric irritants such as NSAIDs should never be given on an empty stomach. Drugs that depress the CNS, such as antihistamines, should as a rule be given at night, whereas some CNS stimulants are best given in the early part of the day so as not to interfere with sleep.

The duration of action of a drug governs the spacing of doses. It is essential to maintain adequate drug tissue concentrations if effects are to be maintained in an unbroken manner. This is important to the patient and reduces the tendency for tolerance and addiction to develop.

Binding of drugs

A variable proportion of a drug present in the intravascular compartment is reversibly bound to plasma proteins, chiefly albumin and α_1-acid glycoprotein. The physicochemical forces involved in the combination of a drug and protein are the same as those involved in the drug–receptor complex (see page 8). Only the unbound portion of a drug is pharmacologically active; the bound drug cannot diffuse from the vascular space and is pharmacologically inert, except that the drug–protein complex acts as a reservoir and can be antigenic.

The degree of binding of a drug may thus greatly influence its rate of metabolism. Tricyclic antidepressants such as imipramine may be plasma protein bound to 90 per cent, so less than 10 per cent may be available for pharmacological action. Although tricyclic antidepressants have long plasma half-lives, this extensive protein binding keeps the drug in circulation and exposed to major organs of elimination. On the other hand, the low unbound plasma levels may be responsible for the significant delay in response to these drugs.

The greater solubility of volatile anaesthetics in plasma and whole blood than can be accounted for by their water or lipid solubility is due to binding of these agents. Ultimately, the binding of anaesthetic agents to receptor proteins may play an important part in their mechanisms of anaesthesia at a molecular level.

Other body constituents besides plasma may bind drugs. Thiobarbiturates, which have a high lipid/water partition coefficient, tend to accumulate in fat. Tetracyclines and heavy metals are stored in bone. Carbon monoxide can readily penetrate the red cell membrane and is so firmly bound to haemoglobin that negligible concentrations are present in the plasma. The accumulation of drugs at specific sites may be of great therapeutic significance. The selective affinity of iodine for the thyroid gland is utilized in the diagnosis of thyroid disorders and the treatment of hyperthyroidism with radioactive iodine isotopes. When iodine isotopes are used for investigations not involving the thyroid it is usually necessary to pretreat the patient with a large dose of non-labelled iodine which will saturate thyroid-binding sites and diminish thyroid uptake of the subsequently administered radioactive isotope.

Distribution of drugs in the body

At equilibrium the freely diffusible portion of a drug is in equal concentration in all accessible tissues. Because variable fractions of the drug cannot penetrate membranes due to binding or ionization, different total amounts of drug may be present in different tissues. The total concentration of a drug in a tissue will increase as binding within that tissue increases. Similarly, tissues in which ionization is high will contain a greater amount of a drug than those compartments in which the drug exists mainly in the non-ionized form. This implies that acidic drugs will tend to accumulate in areas of high pH, while basic drugs will accumulate in regions of low pH. As the intracellular pH is lower than the blood pH, bases thus tend to be concentrated intracellularly.

Drug metabolism

A knowledge of drug metabolism is essential for good therapeutic practice for the following reasons:

- The metabolites formed may have pharmacological activity; for example, paracetamol, used extensively as a mild analgesic agent, is in fact the active metabolite of a previously widely used analgesic, phenacetin.
- The metabolite may have toxic properties; for example, fluoride ions produced by the metabolism of methoxyflurane caused kidney damage and led to its abandonment. Paracetamol's toxicity is due to its metabolite.
- It may be possible to inhibit the metabolism of a drug, thereby prolonging its action. A classic example is the use of an anticholinesterase to prolong the duration of action of acetylcholine.
- The metabolism of a drug can be increased, thereby shortening its duration of action; for example, barbiturates can decrease the duration of action of oral anticoagulants.

Fish can excrete lipophilic drugs through their structured gills into the sea. Frogs can similarly excrete lipophilic substances through their skins. Man, however, is largely devoid of such mechanisms. Lipophilic substances easily pass through the kidney glomeruli into the tubular lumen, but as water is reabsorbed the resulting high concentration gradient results in efficient reabsorption of lipophilic drugs into the circulation through the lipid barrier of the tubular cell. A closed system would therefore exist if there was no mechanism for making such compounds more water soluble (less lipophilic).

Fortunately there are such mechanisms, otherwise the duration of action of lipophilic drugs would be very long. One of the most important is found in the human liver, which contains a system of microsomal enzymes that can modify the chemical structure of such highly lipophilic compounds so that the lipid/water partition coefficient of the metabolite is lower than that of the parent drug.

Liver cells contain a network of lipoprotein tubules distributed throughout the cytoplasm. Part of this reticulum is studded with ribonucleic acid globules, called ribosomes, the 'rough' endoplasmic reticulum; the other is smoother in surface and called 'smooth' endoplasmic reticulum. Associated with the smooth endoplasmic reticulum are a number of enzymes involved in the metabolism of drugs. These are called microsomal enzymes as they can be found on ultracentrifugation in the microsomal fraction. Features of their action are that substances with high lipid solubility usually serve as substrates, and that they are relatively non-specific and will therefore metabolize a wide variety of substances. Smooth endoplasmic reticulum occurs in other cells but most studies have concentrated on hepatic cells.

Liver microsomes (as well as microsomes of other cells) contain a pigment – P-450 – that is important in the metabolism of drugs. It is unusual in that its reduced form has virtually the same spectrum as the oxidized form. The name originates from the observation that the reduced enzyme can form a complex with carbon monoxide which has an absorption maximum at 450 nm. Cytochrome P-450 is not a single enzyme but encompasses a whole family of similar microsomal enzymes. Microsomal enzyme activity can be modified by pathological processes such as liver damage. Malnutrition can depress it. Drugs may enhance or inhibit specific microsomal enzyme activities.

The majority of drugs undergo some form of metabolism in the body. The metabolic products usually have less pharmacological activity than the unmetabolized drug. Sometimes pharmacologically active metabolites are formed from inactive precursors; such precursors are called pro-drugs. For example, chloral is inactive until converted into trichloroethanol. In other cases the metabolites may have different pharmacological actions to the drugs from which they are derived.

There are four principal pathways of drug metabolism: oxidation, reduction, hydrolysis and conjugation. Although some drugs are metabolized by a single process, the majority are metabolized by at least two processes. For example, pethidine can be hydrolysed, or alternatively, N-demethylated. Phase 1 consists of transformation by oxidation, reduction or hydrolysis. In phase 2 the transformed product or parent drug is conjugated with another substance to produce a pharmacologically inactive, water-soluble, rapidly excreted product.

Oxidation

The majority of oxidative transformations involve the microsomal enzymes of the liver and include aromatic and aliphatic hydroxylation; N-, O- and S-dealkylation; epoxidation; N- and S-oxidation; deamination; and dehalogenation. Thus aromatic substances such as phenobarbital and pethidine, and polycyclic compounds such as steroids, undergo aromatic hydroxylation. Dealkylation is responsible for the conversion of pethidine to norpethidine (N-dealkylation) and codeine to morphine (O-dealkylation). Thioethers such as the phenothiazines undergo sulphoxidation to form sulphoxides. Desulphurization of thiopental converts it into pentobarbital.

Not all oxidative transformations involve microsomal enzymes. Caffeine and alcohol utilize non-microsomal enzymes. Alcohols are metabolized by the enzyme alcohol dehydrogenase. Ethanol is completely converted into water and carbon dioxide:

$$CH_3CH_2OH \rightarrow CH_3CHO \rightarrow CH_3COOH \rightarrow CH_3CO{:}CoA \rightarrow H_2O + CO_2$$
$$\text{ACETYLCOENZYME A}$$

Monoamine oxidase (MAO) is a mitochondrial enzyme responsible for the conversion of catecholamines into the corresponding aldehydes. MAO is also responsible for the conversion of 5–hydroxytryptamine (5–HT) into 5–hydroxyindoleacetic acid.

Reduction

Reduction is a less common form of drug transformation than oxidation. Again microsomal enzymes of the liver are mainly responsible. Examples of reduction occurring in the liver are the reduction of chloral hydrate to trichloroethanol.

Cleavage

A number of drugs contain the ester linkage -O-C=O. Examples are esters of choline such as suxamethonium, local anaesthetics such as cocaine and narcotic analgesics such as remifentanil and pethidine. Ester linkages are hydrolysed in the body by specific or non-specific esterases. These are widely distributed in tissues or in the blood. Hydrolysis is an important mechanism for the metabolism of esters and amides. The best known examples of hydrolysing enzymes are the cholinesterases, which are widely distributed in mammalian tissue and are responsible for the hydrolysis of many ester drugs, including suxamethonium and procaine. Pethidine is similarly hydrolysed by a hepatic microsomal enzyme. Atracurium undergoes spontaneous hydrolysis, called Hofmann elimination.

Conjugation

In conjugation reactions, drugs or their metabolic products combine with endogenous substrates. Conjugation plays a major role in the disposition of many products of normal metabolism. Thus the methylation of catecholamines and the glucuronic conjugation of bile salts and steroid hormones are important for normal metabolism.

The endogenous substrate taking part in conjugation reactions is usually a product of carbohydrate or amino acid metabolism. The following conjugation reactions are of importance in man.

Methylation

In these reactions the methyl donor is methionine. A methyl group is transferred from *S*-adenosylmethionine to phenols, amines and some thiols. *N*-methylation of histamine produces the pharmacologically inactive 4–methylhistamine. Catechol-*O*-methyltransferases are involved in the transfer of methyl groups to the *O*-hydroxyl groups of catechol; these reactions are important in both the synthesis and the degradation of catecholamines.

Acetylation

Acetylcoenzyme A is the acetyl donor. Many alkyl- and arylamines are acetylated by various transferases, including *p*-aminobenzoic acid and sulphonamides.

Glucuronidation

This occurs with a wide range of compounds. The glucuronyl residue from uridine diphosphate glucuronic acid (UDPGA) is transferred to the acceptor molecule. The UDP glucuronosyl transferases which catalyse the reaction are located in the liver microsomes. The general reaction is:

$$\text{R-OH} + \text{UDPGA} \rightarrow \text{R-O-C}_6\text{H}_6\text{OG} + \text{UDP}$$
$$\text{ACCEPTOR DRUG} \qquad \text{GLUCURONIDE}$$

Among the many drugs that are conjugated with glucuronic acid are morphine, *p*-aminosalicylic acid and chloramphenicol. Glucuronic acid conjugates are secreted into the bile and enter the small intestine, where they may be hydrolysed back to the parent drug by an enzyme, β-glucuronidase. This is a mechanism whereby the drug can undergo enterohepatic recycling. Chloramphenicol, morphine, certain steroids and phenolphthalein form glucuronides which are hydrolysed in the intestine by this enzyme; the released active drugs are reabsorbed and carried back to the circulation and reconjugation by the liver.

Amino acid conjugations

Glycine and glutamine form peptide conjugates with acids. The reaction involves the formation of the acetylcoenzyme A derivative of the acceptor molecule, which then reacts with the amino acid:

$$\overset{\text{Glycine}}{\text{R-COOH} + \text{CoA} + \text{ATP-R·CO-CoA} \longrightarrow \text{R·CO-NH-CH}_2\text{-COOH}}$$
$$\text{ACID} \qquad \text{COENZYME A} \qquad \text{GLYCINE CONJUGATE}$$
$$\text{COMPLEX}$$

Glycine combines with isoniazid, salicylic acid and nicotinic acid. Salicylic acid also conjugates with glutamine.

Ethereal sulphate conjugation

Aromatic and aliphatic hydroxyl groups may be converted into a sulphanilic acid, ROH-ROSO$_3$H. Sulphate is transferred from the coenzyme adenosine-3-phosphate-5-phosphosulphate (PAPS). Paracetamol, isoprenaline and oestrone undergo sulphate conjugation by three separate cytosolic sulphotransferases.

Drug excretion

The kidney and gastro-intestinal tract are the major routes of drug excretion. Inhalational anaesthetics because of their volatility are, however, excreted mainly by the lungs, and a few drugs are secreted by the salivary glands. Drugs excreted in milk may have an effect on a breast-fed child.

Drugs may be excreted either in an unchanged form or after they have been modified by metabolic processes. Metabolic changes that increase the polarity and reduce the lipid solubility of a substance will facilitate excretion.

Renal excretion

Elimination of drugs in the urine is governed by three factors: glomerular filtration, tubular secretion and tubular reabsorption. The glomerular filtration of any substance depends on its molecular weight and the blood concentration of unbound drug. The glomerular capillaries permit the passage of most solutes, but drug bound to plasma protein is retained in the circulation. In the nephron the fate of a drug is largely dependent on its lipid solubility. Molecules that have a high lipid/water partition coefficient and are non-ionized will readily diffuse back from glomerular filtrates across the tubular epithelium. Large ionic species, however, are unable to traverse this lipid boundary.

The cells of the proximal convoluted tubule possess two separate mechanisms for the active transport of organic acids and bases. These systems transport ionized molecules into the filtrate. Ions compete for these relatively non-specific transport systems. The prolongation of duration of action of penicillin by probenecid is due to a competitive inhibition of renal tubular acid-transporting systems by this acid. As glomerular filtrate passes down the nephron, water reabsorption increases the concentration of any drugs present and promotes reabsorption of lipid-soluble species.

Most drugs are subject to some degree of ionization. The relative proportions of ionized and non-ionized molecules depends upon pK_a and the environmental pH (as discussed on page 22). Urinary pH varies from about 5 to 8, dependent upon dietary and other factors. In alkaline urine, weak acids are predominantly ionized and thus little reabsorption occurs and they remain in the urine to be excreted. Similarly, weak bases are more ionized and rapidly excreted in acidic urine. Advantage is taken of pH-dependent excretion in the management of salicylate and phenobarbital overdose. These drugs are weak acids with relatively low pK_a values; alkalinization of the urine by the systemic administration of bicarbonate significantly hastens their rate of renal elimination.

Intestinal excretion

The physicochemical factors involved in the absorption of drugs from the gastro-intestinal tract (water solubility and lipid/water partition) also influence the elimination of drugs and their metabolites into the gut and their removal in faeces. The biliary system acts as a specialized transport mechanism for the intestinal excretion of drugs, especially drugs of high molecular weight or those capable of being metabolically transformed and conjugated. Specialized mechanisms also exist for the active transport of acids and bases from blood to bile. These transport mechanisms closely resemble those of the kidney.

Factors determining biophase concentration

Principle

Size of drug effect (E) is a function of the concentration of drug (C) at the site of action (the biophase) where the effect sequence is initiated:

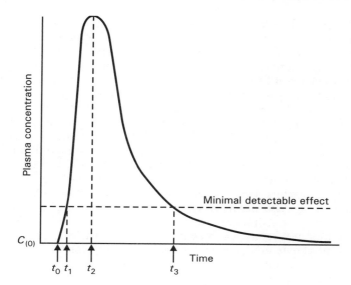

Figure 1.8 Magnitude of drug concentration as a function of time. Drug administered at time $t0$; latency $= t_1, - t_0$; time to peak effect $= t_2 - t_0$; duration of action $= t_3 - t_1$

$$E = f(C) \tag{15}$$

Pharmacokinetics is a term used to describe the factors influencing the amount of drug at various body sites as a function of time. Pharmacodynamics is concerned with the relationships between concentrations at the site of action and drug effects. It is usual to divide the time course of drug action into three parts: firstly, the latency (time for onset of action); secondly, the time to peak effect; and thirdly, the duration of action. An idealized view of these is presented in *Figure 1.8*. It is often assumed that blood (or plasma) concentration correlates positively with the intensity of drug effect. This assumption is probably valid if rapid equilibrium occurs between blood and biophase and the drug exerts a direct, rapidly reversible effect. If the time to equilibrium is long, however, then the relationship between blood concentration and effect is likely to be complex.

Drug absorption

Absorption is the process which describes transfer of drug from the site of administration into the systemic circulation. In most instances, if concentrations at the absorption site are below saturation, then first-order kinetics will apply. Thus, the rate is proportional to the concentration of drug (and the amount remaining) at the absorption site. At higher concentrations, or where solubility restricts the amount of drug in solution then zero-order kinetics may apply. Under such conditions the rate is constant.

Drug elimination

Elimination is the term used to describe the processes by which a drug is removed from the circulation by excretion and metabolism. For any particular drug, more than one process may be involved; for example, a drug can be partially metabolized and also excreted unchanged in the urine or bile and, if a volatile anaesthetic, by exhalation. The elimination of most drugs follows first-order kinetics: the rate of elimination is dependent on the blood concentration (*Figure 1.9*). High blood concentrations result in a large elimination rate and as the blood concentration declines so the elimination rate is proportionally decreased. One consequence of first-order kinetics is that the time required for the blood concentration to decrease by one-half is a constant, the half-life, $t_{1/2}$.

Where drug elimination is by metabolism, the factors determining the enzyme reaction rate are important. At low substrate concentrations, there will be an abundance of active sites on the enzyme available for occupation by the drug, and thus first-order kinetics will apply since the rate of reaction will be determined by the drug concentration. If the drug concentration rises to a level where the active sites become fully occupied, then zero-order kinetics will apply. It should be remembered that the 'enzyme complex' contains not only the enzyme but often cofactors. If the demand on these cofactors exceeds the supply then zero-order kinetics can also occur. Alcohol is a good example of a drug where, at blood levels produced by social drinking, zero-order kinetics apply (*Figure 1.9*). Where zero-order metabolism occurs, saturation of some part of the metabolic process results in a constant rate of metabolite production, independent of drug concentration. As a consequence the drug's half-life will not be a constant but will be dependent upon blood concentration, with higher concentrations resulting in a longer time to eliminate half of the drug. For example (*Figure 1.10*) it takes over 3 h for the plasma concentration to decrease from 1 to 0.5 mg/ml, but less than 1 h to decrease from 0.2 to 0.1 mg/ml.

Compartment models

From the point of view of practical drug administration, the user wants guidance on the size of dose required to produce the necessary concentration at the site of action, and the length of time for which it will be effective. To estimate these, pharmacokineticists often start by making assumptions about how the body is likely to handle a drug and use mathematical models and 'compartment analysis' (see below) to calculate indices which will provide this practical information.

To obtain useful indicators of drug action, the most commonly calculated parameters are the volume of distribution and the rate of elimination (or clearance) from the body. To make these calculations, assumptions have to be made as to whether the body behaves as a single compartment, as two compartments or as more than two compartments. The assumption chosen depends on fitting successive values of plasma concentration of the drug over time to predictions of what they would be using assumptions as to the number of compartments. In practice, most drugs behave as though the body were one, two or three compartments.

Volume of distribution

The volume of distribution (V) is a proportionality constant which relates plasma concentration (C) to the total amount of drug in the body (A):

$$A = V \times C \tag{16}$$

It is important to note that V does not represent an actual physiological volume such as the extracellular space; consequently V is sometimes referred to as the 'apparent volume

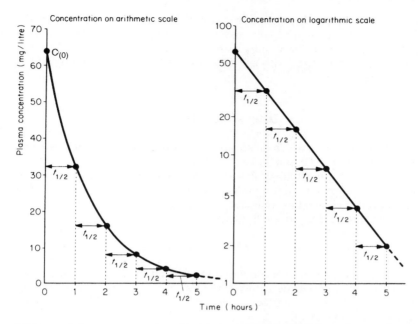

Figure 1.9 Decay of plasma concentration with time for a drug given intravenously whose initial plasma concentration was 64 mg/l; $t_{1/2}$ (indicated by double arrows) is 1 h. Note: plasma level has fallen to 32 mg/l in the first hour, and to 16, 8, 4 and 2 mg/l respectively at 2, 3, 4 and 5 h. Logarithmic conversion of concentration (right-hand graph) will produce a straight line

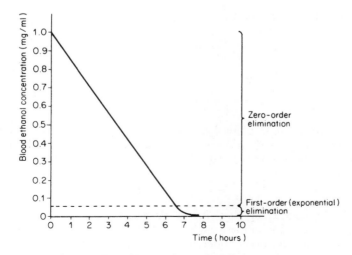

Figure 1.10 Zero-order elimination of ethanol over the concentration range 0.05–1 mg/ml. First-order kinetics apply only at concentrations of ethanol below 0.05 mg/ml

of distribution'. Factors which influence the size of V include: drug characteristics such as lipophilicity and binding to plasma and tissue proteins, and patient characteristics including body size, composition and plasma protein concentration. V_D varies widely between drugs such as warfarin with a V of about 5 litres to chloroquine with a V_D of about 15 000 litres.

Drug elimination

In *Figure 1.9* the only factors which determine the plasma concentration at time zero $C_{(0)}$ are the dose administered (D) and V, i.e. $C_{(0)} = D/V$.

Elimination of most drugs follows first-order kinetics, that is, the rate of elimination is dependent upon the amount of drug remaining in the body. Mathematically we express this as the first-order elimination rate constant (k). This relates the rate of elimination ($-dA/dt$) and amount of drug in the body (A):

$$-dA/dt = KA \text{ or } dA/dt = -kA \tag{17}$$

The negative sign indicates decreasing amounts of drug in the body with time. From equation (16) it is possible to derive by a process of integration and substitution the following equation which can be used to calculate the amount of drug remaining in the body after a specific time ($A_{(t)}$):

$$A_{(t)} = A_{(0)}e^{-kt} = De^{-kt} \tag{18}$$

where $A_{(0)}$ is the amount of drug present at time zero, which is equal to the dose administered after an intravenous injection (D), and e is the base of natural logarithms.

The amount of drug eliminated in time $0-t$ is given by

$$A_{(0)} - A_{(t)} = D - De^{-kt} = D(1 - e^{-kt}) \tag{19}$$

Substituting for A from equation (16) in (18) it is apparent that

$$C_{(t)}V = C_{(0)}Ve^{-kt} = De^{-kt}$$

hence

$$C_{(t)} = C_{(0)}e^{-kt} \text{ and } C_{(t)} = (D/V_D)e^{-kt} \tag{20}$$

Equation (20) is much more useful than equation (17) since the plasma concentration, rather than the amount of drug in the body, is of greater importance in determining drug action. If equation (20) is transformed using natural logarithms, then

$$\log_e C_{(t)} = \log_e C_{(0)}^{-kt} \tag{21}$$

Hence plotting the natural log ($\log_e$, ln) of plasma concentration against time would produce a straight line with an intercept equal to $\log C_{(0)}$ and a slope of $-k$. In *Figure 1.9* plasma concentrations have been plotted with the y axis on a logarithmic scale. However, for clarity this axis is labelled with actual plasma concentrations, rather than the log transform, hence the intercept appears as $C_{(0)}$, not $\log_e C_{(0)}$.

As discussed earlier in this chapter, the half-life of a drug is the time taken for its plasma concentration to decline by one-half (e.g. $C_{(t)} = 1/2C_{(0)}$). Hence substituting $t_{1/2}$ for t in equation (21) and rearranging gives

$$1/2C_{(0)} = C_{(0)}e^{-kt_{1/2}}$$

and by taking logs and solving for $t_{1/2}$ then,

$$t_{1/2} = 0.693/k \qquad (22)$$

Clearance

Although $t_{1/2}$ and k are indicators of drug elimination, a precise measure of the body's potential to eliminate drugs is given by clearance (CL). Clearance relates the rate of drug elimination ($-dA/dt$) to plasma concentration (C):

$$-dA/dt = CL \times C \qquad (23)$$

By comparison of equations (16), (17) and (22) with (23):

$$CL.C = kA = kVC, \text{ hence:}$$

$$CL = kV = (0.693/t_{1/2})V \text{ and}$$

$$t_{1/2} = 0.693V/CL \qquad (24)$$

It is important to appreciate that $t_{1/2}$ is dependent upon V_D and CL but not vice versa. For example, the liver and kidney may very efficiently remove drug from the plasma, but if that drug has a large V, then only a small fraction of drug in the body will reside in the plasma. As a result, its $t_{1/2}$ will be long. Hence $t_{1/2}$ is not a good measure of drug elimination, but is a good indicator of the decline in plasma concentrations and is thus used to calculate the frequency with which drugs are dosed. Conversely, CL is an accurate measure of elimination and is very useful in calculating the amount of drug to be administered each day, during multiple dosing, dosing by non-intravenous routes and dosing in patients with various disease states.

Pharmacokinetic compartment models

These are entirely theoretical constructs which have no equality with any anatomical space in the body such as the extracellular fluid compartment. As well as providing the starting point for calculation of effective dose and duration of action, the models can also be used to predict blood and plasma concentrations resulting from different dosage regimens, disease conditions and changes resulting from drug interactions.

One-compartment model

The simplest model is a one-compartment model. The body is considered to be a single compartment into which a drug, once administered, distributes and instantaneously

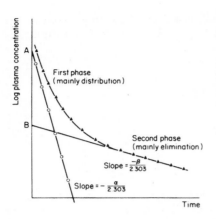

Figure 1.11 Biphasic curve of log plasma concentration-time. Two-compartment analysis can be applied by which A, B, α and β can be obtained by the method of residuals ('curve peeling'). The line of best fit through the terminal points of the second phase yields a slope from which β can be calculated. Subtraction of this line from the original data points (▲) yields a series of points (○) to which the 'residual' line can be fitted, giving A and α

equilibrates. Few, if any, drugs actually behave in this way but, although simplistic, this model can adequately predict the plasma concentration–time profiles of many drugs which rapidly distribute between plasma and tissue after administration. This model does not assume that plasma and tissue concentrations are the same, but does assume that there is a constant relationship between concentrations in plasma and in all of the tissues into which the drug distributes. The distribution of drug throughout the body is quantified by the term, volume of distribution (V).

Two-compartment model

A fundamental assumption of the one-compartment model is that drug is instantaneously distributed to various tissues in the body. This assumption is not valid for most drugs. As a consequence of a slower distribution, a biphasic log plasma concentration curve, as exemplified in *Figure 1.11* is seen, rather than the straight line of *Figure 1.9*. In the two-compartment model, the body is considered to consist of two compartments between which transfer of drug can occur (*Figure 1.12*). The compartments need have no physiological or anatomical basis; however, it is usual to conceive of compartment 1 as containing the blood and all of the eliminating organs; hence drug administration and removal only occur from this compartment. The first phase of the curve in *Figure 1.11* is primarily a reflection of drug transfer from compartment 1 to 2, that is, distribution in the body. The second phase represents elimination and occurs after a pseudo-equilibrium between concentrations in the two compartments has been reached. The equation

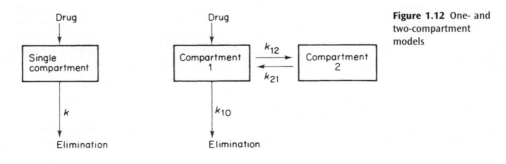

Figure 1.12 One- and two-compartment models

describing plasma concentrations is the sum of two exponential functions – one reflecting distribution, the other reflecting elimination:

$$C = Ae^{-\alpha t} + Be^{-\beta t} \tag{25}$$

where α and β are the first-order rate constants for distribution and elimination; A and B are the theoretical concentrations at time zero associated with the two exponentials such that $C_{(0)} = A + B$; α and β are complex functions of the rate constants k_{10}, k_{12}, k_{21} in *Figure 1.12*.

The distribution half-life ($t_{1/2,\alpha}$) and elimination half-life ($t_{1/2,\beta}$) are given by:

$$t_{1/2,\alpha} = 0.693/\alpha$$

and

$$t_{1/2,\beta} = 0.693/\beta \tag{26}$$

A drug is not instantaneously distributed in the body in the two-compartment model and as a consequence the volume of distribution increases during the distribution phase. Immediately after intravenous injection, the whole of the drug dose is located in compartment 1 and the initial volume of distribution (V_1) is equal to the volume of compartment 1, hence:

$$V_1 = D/C_{(0)} = D/(A + B) \tag{27}$$

After the distribution phase is complete the volume of distribution (V) remains constant:

$$V = CL/\beta \tag{28}$$

Clearance has the same definition in both the one- and two-compartment models. This 'model-independence' is another favourable quality of clearance.

Multi-compartment models

It is possible to construct multi-compartment models, for example three-compartment models. Such models are required to describe the pharmacokinetics of drugs such as intravenous anaesthetics and opioids. Readers interested in multi-compartment models are referred to an excellent text on this subject (Gibaldi and Perrier, 1982).

Multiple dosing

The aim is to maintain plasma concentration of the drug in what has been aptly called 'the therapeutic window', that is, above the minimum effective and below the minimum toxic concentrations. Failure to consider the drug pharmacokinetics for each individual patient can result in a plasma concentration profile, as exemplified in *Figure 1.13*.

If a drug is administered at a constant rate (R_0), e.g. by intravenous infusion, then plasma concentrations will increase until a steady-state concentration (C_{ss}) is reached, where the rate of drug elimination (CLC_{ss}; see (eqn 22) equals the rate of administration thus:

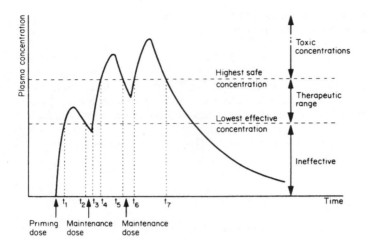

Figure 1.13 Between t_1, and t_2, t_3 and t_4, and t_5 and t_6, the plasma concentration of the drug falls in the 'therapeutic window'. Because the maintenance dose is too large, between t_4 and t_5, and t_6 and t_7, the plasma concentration is high enough to produce dose–dependent toxicity

$$CLC_{ss} = R_0 \qquad (29)$$

Thus if the clearance (CL) of the drug is known then the infusion rate (R_0) required to produce a target concentration (C_{ss}) can be readily calculated. It will, however, take time to reach the steady-state concentration. The time taken will be dependent solely upon the drug's half-life; for example it takes 3.3 drug half-lives to reach 90 per cent of the steady-state concentration. Thus since most drugs have half-lives of several hours it could take a considerable time to achieve effective plasma concentrations if the drug was solely given by a single infusion rate. To rapidly achieve a plasma concentration in the therapeutic window, a loading (or priming) dose of drug may be given. This dose can be calculated from:

$$\text{IV loading dose} = VC_{ss} \qquad (30)$$

where C_{ss} is the target concentration required and V is the volume of distribution. If the drug shows two-compartment pharmacokinetics, then V_1 should be used in this equation.

If equal doses of a drug are given at regular intervals, rather than by infusion, then once again plasma concentrations will increase until a steady-state situation is reached where the average rate of elimination equals the average rate of drug administration. Under these conditions a constant steady-state concentration will not exist, but concentrations at steady-state will rise and fall around an 'average' steady-state concentration ($C_{ss,av}$).

To maintain the average steady-state concentration it is necessary to administer maintenance doses of drug at a rate equal to the average rate of drug elimination.

$$FD/\tau = CLC_{ss,av} \qquad (31)$$

where D is the maintenance dose, F is the bioavailable fraction and τ is the dosing interval.

Thus the dosing rate (maintenance dose/dosing interval FD/τ) required to produce the target concentration can be calculated if the drug's CL and F are known. The bioavailable fraction is the proportion of the administered dose which reaches the systemic circulation intact. For intravenous dosing, F is usually equal to 1 but will be less than one for most other routes. This is discussed in more detail on page 44. Clearly a particular dosing rate can given by choosing a number of different combinations of D and τ. The choice of these is determined by the drug's half-life and to some extent by convenience and strength of the available dosage forms.

As with infusion dosing, steady-state concentrations will take some time to achieve and a loading dose may be used to rapidly produce effective concentrations. The loading dose is calculated in accord with eqn (30); where a non-intravenous route is used, then

$$FD = VC_{ss,av} \qquad (32)$$

A commonly used dosing regimen of an initial two tablets, followed by one tablet three times daily, will rapidly achieve and maintain concentrations which rise and fall about the average steady-state concentration for a drug with an 8-hour half-life. In this regimen the loading dose is one tablet and the dosing interval is equal to the half-life. Clearly the average steady-state concentration will be determined by the amount of drug in the tablet and the patient's clearance of this drug and these need to be carefully considered in order to achieve effective levels while avoiding toxicity.

Pharmacokinetics of inhalation anaesthetics

For volatile anaesthetics the required pharmacological response is a function of the partial pressure of the anaesthetic (the tension) in the brain. At equilibrium, 'brain tension' equals arterial blood tension, which in turn equals the partial pressure of the anaesthetic in alveolar air. In practice this is not obtained. In a gas mixture the fractional concentration of the anaesthetic agent in the mixture is equal to its pressure divided by the total pressure, that is, concentration is proportional to partial pressure. To obtain the necessary brain tension quickly, inhalation anaesthetics are given initially at concentrations higher than for maintenance concentration; priming dose followed by a lower maintenance dose is the usual rule.

Four factors determine brain tension. These are the partial pressure of the anaesthetic in the inspired gas mixture; the respiratory rate and depth of respiration; the transfer of anaesthetic through the alveolar wall to the blood flowing through the lung; and the elimination of the anaesthetic from the arterial blood to other tissues.

In the absence of ventilation–perfusion problems, the factors that determine how rapidly anaesthetics pass from the alveolar space into the blood are the anaesthetic's solubility in blood, the rate of blood flow through the lung, and the partial pressures of the anaesthetic in arterial and mixed venous blood. The blood/gas partition coefficient (λ) represents the ratio of anaesthetic concentration in blood to anaesthetic concentration in a gas phase when the two are in equilibrium. Partial pressures will then be equal in both phases. Anaesthetic agents that are very soluble in blood have a high λ (compare methoxyflurane 12.1 with nitrous oxide 0.47). The blood tension rises slowly with soluble agents. The factors that determine the loss of an anaesthetic agent from the blood to the tissues (for example, the brain) are the solubility of the agent in the tissue (that is, its tissue/blood partition coefficient), the blood flow to the particular tissue, and the partial pressures of the agent in the tissue and in the blood.

Potency of anaesthetics can be quantitatively compared by determining their minimum alveolar concentration (MAC) values. The MAC of an anaesthetic is defined as the concentration at one atmosphere that produces immobility in 50 per cent of patients or animals exposed to noxious stimuli (Eger, Saidman and Brandstater, 1965). The MAC value for halothane is approximately 0.8 per cent, while that for nitrous oxide is >100 per cent. Halothane is therefore much more potent than nitrous oxide. For further discussion on uptake, distribution and elimination of anaesthetics see Chapter 4.

Bioavailability

While pharmacists have known for many years that the amount of active agent available for absorption depends on its formulation, it is only relatively recently that the therapeutic importance of this phenomenon has become widely appreciated. Different preparations of the same drug can contain the same amount of active ingredient but produce different therapeutic responses due to their different bioavailabilities (*Figure 1.14*). Formulation can dramatically influence the bioavailability of a drug: particle size, physicochemical form, the presence of excipients and manufacturing variables, may all be important. Equally the same dose of drug administered by different routes is likely to reach the circulation at different rates and amounts, as discussed on page 45.

Bioavailability is defined as the rate and relative amount of drug reaching the systemic circulation as intact drug: dosage forms having equivalent bioavailabilities are said to be bioequivalent. As illustrated in *Figure 1.14*, the rate of absorption can be important in determining therapeutic effect. The extent of absorption is, however, usually of greater importance than the rate. The bioavailable fraction (F) is the fraction of the administered dose reaching the circulation as intact drug. It is usually determined by measuring the area under the plasma concentration–time curve (AUC) and has the following relationship:

$$F = CL \text{ } AUC/D \tag{33}$$

The clearance of a drug is usually determined after intravenous administration, since by convention, $F = 1$ for this route. Administration by other routes is likely to produce F values of less than 1 due to incomplete absorption or first-pass metabolism. Where two dosage forms are to be directly compared, then a relative bioavailable fraction (F_{rel}) is calculated (from $F_{rel} = F_{test}/F_{std}$). Bioequivalence is usually accepted if F_{rel} lies in the range of 0.8–1.2.

With drugs that have a low therapeutic ratio, slight changes in bioavailability may produce therapeutically important sequelae. For instance, different formulations of digoxin containing the same chemical equivalent of digoxin can yield up to seven-fold differences in plasma digoxin levels.

First-pass effect

The majority of drugs when given orally are absorbed through the gastro-intestinal tract into the portal circulation and hence pass into the liver. If the liver metabolizes the drug, then the bioavailable fraction will be less than 1. This 'first-pass' effect is important for a number of drugs, including salicylates, β-adrenoceptor blocking drugs such as propranolol, and tricyclic antidepressants such as nortriptyline. Lidocaine also exhibits a high first-pass effect, as does morphine. Drugs which show a large first-pass effect will have a low value of F when given orally and for the examples quoted only 5–30 per cent of the

(a)

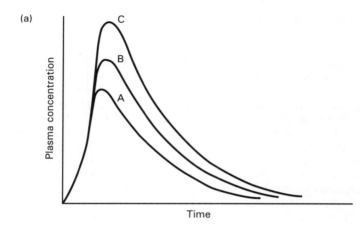

(b)

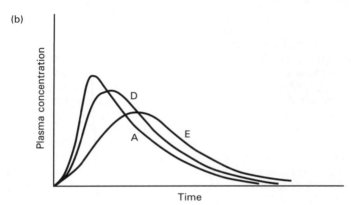

Figure 1.14 Variation of plasma concentration with time; following oral administration of different dosage forms. In the upper figure (a), formulations A, B and C have the *same* absorption rate constants but different amounts are delivered to the circulation (i.e. C>B>A), producing different peaks. In the lower figure (b), formulations A, D and E deliver the same amounts of drug (as shown by the areas under the curves) but exhibit *different* absorption rate constants (i.e. A>D>F)

administered doses will reach the systemic circulation as intact drug. The oral bioavailable fraction is determined by the efficiency of the liver to metabolize (eliminate) the drug. As discussed previously, clearance is a measure of drug elimination and hepatic metabolic clearance, that is drug elimination by liver metabolism, (CL_H), can be used to predict F as follows:

$$F = 1 - CL_H/Q_H \tag{34}$$

where Q_H is liver blood flow.

Hence, drugs with high hepatic clearances will have low oral bioavailable fractions. It follows that a knowledge of hepatic clearance can be useful in deciding the oral dose needed for a patient already stabilized on an intravenous dosage regimen. If the orally administered drug is incompletely absorbed from the intestine into the portal vein, or is broken down by the gastric or intestinal contents, then equation (34) will overestimate the value of F.

Some drugs are designed as pro-drugs which have favourable absorption characteristics in the intestine. First-pass metabolism in the liver converts these agents to the active drug.

Automated drug delivery systems

Continuous infusions

A constant rate of infusion has been a rare mode of administration in mainstream therapeutics because of the delay in reaching a steady state with most drugs and the difficulty in
calculating the correct loading dose to overcome this problem. However, within anaesthetic
practice, very short-acting drugs have led to the development of continuous intravenous
infusions as a more logical method than the traditional administration of intermittent
boluses. It usually results in lower dosage overall. Successful use depends on a sensitive
means of measuring the effect so that, for example, continuous infusion of a muscle relaxant requires regular assessment of neuromuscular block or the use of a powerful vasodilator requires continuous (or very frequent) measurement of blood pressure. The drugs have
been given in high concentrations but small volumes by specially designed syringe drivers.
These need to be designed with safety in mind, to prevent inadvertent overdose.

It was soon realized that to produce a constant effect, the rate of infusion would have to
be modelled on the pharmacokinetic properties of the drug in order to produce a constant
plasma level. Initially, propofol was administered for total intravenous anaesthesia (TIVA)
using a dosage system which provided a good approximation to the phamacokinetic model.
This involved an initial bolus based on body weight, followed by a simplified infusion regimen
designed to give a good approximation to the constantly decreasing rate theoretically required.
This was achieved with a 10-minute infusion at one rate, based on mg/kg/h, followed by a
10-minute infusion at 80 per cent of the initial infusion rate. This in turn was followed by
an infusion at 60 per cent of the initial rate for as long as required. This produced near steady-
state conditions, although strictly speaking they were 'pseudo-steady' states. The later development of these ideas are considered under Target Controlled Infusions, below.

In the particular case of providing analgesia in conscious patients, inhalational agents
have provided a convenient alternative route of administration and the use of 'gas and
air', later replaced by nitrous oxide and oxygen mixtures and by low concentrations of
volatile agents, has a long history of satisfactory use in obstetric practice, particularly for
the first stage of labour. This 'closes the loop' because the patient only takes the drug
when pain is experienced and stops when the pain eases. The safety feature is the need
for the patient to be able to hold the mask on the face and close the air-hole, motor skills
which are lost if anaesthesia supervenes.

For some years, enthusiasts have attempted to 'close the loop' for intravenously administered drugs, so that a measured variable (neuromuscular block, blood pressure, etc.)
itself controlled the rate of administration. This gets round the main difficulty with most
such drugs which, in general, do not have such a low volume of distribution and rapid
metabolism or excretion that the rate of administration can remain constant over time
and whose pharmacokinetics are less consistent at predicting how to produce a constant
drug concentration at the effect site.

However, when it comes to controlling the rate of drug administration to maintain
adequate anaesthesia, there has been difficulty in defining a suitable measured variable.
Derivatives of the EEG, oesophageal contractions, evoked cortical potentials and heart
rate variability are among those which have undergone evaluation and some are still the
subject of investigation.

Patient controlled analgesia (PCA)

From the use of patient controlled inhalation of nitrous oxide or a low concentration of
a volatile agent, it was a short step conceptually to trying to design a patient controlled

system for the use of systemic analgesics in labour, and from thence for other severe pain, notably after major surgery. The safety feature mimicking the finger over the air-hole was a demand button which needed to be pressed twice within 0.5 s, difficult for the heavily sedated patient. In practice, this precaution was found to be unnecessary. To take account of the very great pharmacokinetic differences between an insoluble gas and a lipid soluble parenteral drug, a further safety feature was the introduction of a 'lock-out' time, following a successful demand, so that the full CNS effects of the bolus would be experienced before another dose could be obtained.

The system was first used with pethidine, because of its development and introduction in the field of obstetric pain relief, but in the relief of postoperative pain, morphine was preferred by many. The method has also been of value in establishing equi-analgesic effectiveness of different drugs. Bolus doses are typically 10–20 mg of pethidine or 1–2 mg of morphine. Lock-out times have been of the order of 5–10 minutes.

One perceived weakness of the system is that when a series of boluses has produced satisfactory analgesia, the patient may fall asleep for a while and awake in pain, which then takes several more boluses to relieve. Sleep is thus disturbed. To deal with this, some clinicians have introduced background infusions, aimed at being only just insufficient and therefore requiring much less frequent top-up demand boluses. The retention of the feedback stimulus of pain is an important safety feature of PCA and while this practice is a theoretical advance, it usually results in more complications. The principal reason is that insufficient allowance is made for the progressive reduction in the need for analgesia postoperatively, not matched by adequate reductions in background administration, with consequent relative overdose.

The system has been extended to epidural use (PCEA) and the same considerations of safety apply. This mode of administration is inherently more hazardous so that it is highly desirable for it to be restricted to high nursing dependency areas. Hospitals with well developed pain teams and good protocols may use PCEA in general surgical wards, but it is not recommended.

Target controlled infusions (TCI)

Using at first two-compartment and then later three-compartment models, algorithms have been developed to control infusion devices so that the user does not need to decide on the rate of infusion of the drug, merely on the desired plasma concentration, a concept known as target controlled infusion (TCI). For an anaesthetic drug, choosing the desired plasma concentration would be analogous to choosing the setting on the vaporizer during inhalational anaesthesia.

In anaesthesia using TCI, a slow bolus is given initially to achieve the desired concentration rapidly in the central compartment, after which there is a decreasing infusion rate calculated to compensate for losses into other compartments and for elimination. An instruction from the user to increase the target plasma concentration would result in another bolus followed by a higher rate of infusion. An instruction to decrease the target plasma concentration would result in the infusion being stopped for a short time and then restarted with a lower rate of infusion. The infusion can be controlled by a computer or by a dedicated microprocessor-driven device, and one such device is marketed for the TCI of propofol under the trade name of Diprifusor.

To use this system, it is necessary to have some knowledge of the required blood levels of propofol to meet the differing demands of surgery and anaesthesia. Anaesthetists are used to working with blood levels of inhalational agents, as these are indicated by the end-tidal concentrations, but there is no on-line system of measurement for intravenous anaesthetics. The range of blood concentrations found in different individuals is quite wide – perhaps as much as 100 per cent variation. Thus it is essential to adjust the target level according to the patient's response. TCI is nevertheless much easier to use than manual infusion schemes and gives a closer match between the desired and the measured plasma levels. This is discussed further in the monograph on propofol in Chapter 3.

Just emerging is the application of this system to conscious sedation, thus allowing the introduction of feedback control by the patient. This is potentially a considerable improvement on what has been called 'monitored sedation', in which the desired level of sedation has been manipulated on the patient's behalf.

The logical next step in the automation of anaesthetic drug delivery systems is to couple the TCI device to a another device which is able to measure a surrogate for the level of consciousness and thereby produce so-called closed loop control of anaesthesia (CLAN). The final system would then alter the administration of anaesthetic agent to ensure that the patient remains at a satisfactory level of unconsciousness for the entire procedure. At present there is only one measurable physiological variable that can be used satisfactorily to measure depth of anaesthesia, the mid-latency auditory evoked potential. This is derived by averaging the EEG response to a repeated auditory stimulus. Greater sensitivity and specificity have been obtained by deriving the so-called auditory evoked potential index (AEPI). Even with this, certain caveats must be observed: it can only be used to measure anaesthesia caused by drugs with which it has been validated; auditory and electrical interference must be at acceptably low levels; the patient must not be deaf or in status epilepticus.

Automation of infusions of muscle relaxant drugs has been comparatively easy to produce, with the input of the control system being the output of a 'muscle relaxation monitor' such as the Datex Relaxograph. Automation of infusions of powerful antihypertensive drugs such as nitroprusside has also been described, with the input of the control system being the output of a direct arterial blood pressure monitor. One major problem has been recognition and rejection of artefacts such as the arterial catheter being flushed or becoming blocked.

Idiosyncrasy

This term is used to describe a qualitatively abnormal reaction to a drug. An example is primaquine anaemia (see page 51) which is due to a genetic deficiency.

Allergic reactions (anaphylactic reactions)

These are mediated by an antigen–antibody reaction. Those occurring at induction of anaesthesia can be extremely severe, though fortunately rare. The Association of Anaesthetists of Great Britain and Ireland (AAGBI) has produced guidelines for handling the problem.

Management

An anaphylactic reaction is an exaggerated response to a substance to which an individual has become sensitized, and is mediated by IgE antibodies; it may be precipitated by a very small dose of a drug. Histamine, serotonin (5-HT) and other vasoactive substances are released from mast cells and basophils and a variety of symptoms may result: pruritus, erythema, flushing, urticaria, angio-oedema, nausea, vomiting, diarrhoea, laryngeal oedema, bronchospasm, hypotension, cardiovascular collapse and death. Anaphylactoid reactions are clinically identical to the above but not mediated via IgE antibodies and may occur on *first exposure* to a precipitating agent.

The AAGBI recommended treatment in a patient with suspected anaphylaxis is shown in *Table 1.4*. No attempt should be made to discover a cause for the problem until the

Table 1.4 Management of a patient with suspected anaphylaxis as suggested by the Association of Anaesthetists of Great Britain and Ireland. (Reproduced by kind permission of the AAGBI)

Initial therapy
1. Stop administration of drugs(s) likely to have caused the anaphylaxis.
2. Call for help.
3. Maintain airway: give 100 per cent oxygen.
4. Lay patient flat with feet elevated.
5. Give **epinephrine (adrenaline)**. This may be given *intramuscularly* in a dose of 0.5–1 mg (0.5–1.0 ml of 1:1000) and may be repeated every 10 minutes according to the arterial pressure and pulse until improvement occurs.
   Alternatively, 50–100 µg *intravenously* over 1 minute has been recommended (0.5–1 ml of 1:10 000) for hypotension, with titration of further doses as required.
   In a patient with cardiovascular collapse, 0.5–1 mg (5 to 10 ml of 1:10 000) may be required intravenously, in divided doses, by titration. This should be given at a rate of 0.1 mg/minute, stopping when a response has been obtained.
6. Start intravascular volume expansion with suitable crystalloid or colloid.

Secondary therapy
1. Antihistamines   **Chlorpheniramine** 10–20 mg by slow iv infusion
                     Consider H_2-antagonists
2. Corticosteroids   **Cortisol (hydrocortisone)** 100–300 mg i.v.
3. Catecholamine infusions – starting doses:
   Epinephrine 0.05–0.1 µg/kg/min (approx 4–8 µg/min).
   (5 mg epinephrine in 500 ml saline gives 10 µg/ml)
   Norepinephrine 0.05–0.1 µg/kg/min (approx. 4–8 µg/min)
   (4 mg norepinephrine in 500 ml dextrose gives 8 µg/ml)
4. Perform arterial blood gas analysis.
   Consider bicarbonate (0.5–1 mmol/kg i.v.) for acidosis
   (equivalent to 0.5–1 ml of an 8.4 per cent solution of bicarbonate).
5. Airway evaluation (before extubation).
6. Bronchodilators may be required for persistent bronchospasm.

Investigations
1. Do not attempt any investigation until the immediate treatment of the emergency has been completed.
2. Diagnosis is made on clinical grounds. It is important to make a detailed written record of events, including time of administration of all drugs (and doses) in relation to the onset of the reaction.
3. Approximately 1 h after the beginning of the reaction, take 10 ml venous blood into a plain glass tube. Separate serum and store at –20°C until the sample can be sent to a reference laboratory for estimation of serum tryptase concentration.
4. The patient and his/her general practitioner should be made aware of the reaction and its implication.

acute phase is over. A 10 ml sample of blood should be taken about 1 h after a suspected reaction (and certainly before 6 h) for measurement of serum tryptase levels. This is the main protein in mast cell granules and is released in an anaphylactic or anaphylactoid reaction. It is not present in red or white cells and hence levels are not affected by haemolysis. A raised serum tryptase confirms that an anaphylactic or anaphylactoid reaction has occurred, but gives no indication as to the cause.

Following a reaction, attempts should be made by skin prick tests to identify the causative agent. The patient must be informed of the findings and carry the appropriate information at all times.

Blood dyscrasias

Many drugs can produce blood dyscrasias; among the most notable is chloramphenicol. In the United Kingdom, the Committee on Safety of Drugs considered that this drug should never be used for the treatment of trivial infections but recognized that it was a highly effective agent in the treatment of *Haemophilus influenzae* meningitis and in typhoid fever. The drug might interfere with the bone marrow by affecting phenylalanine metabolism or, alternatively, by inhibiting the incorporation of iron into the red cell. An allergic basis has also been postulated and genetic factors might influence the sensitivity of patients to chloramphenicol-induced aplastic anaemia. There are a number of other drugs that can produce blood dyscrasias. These include gold salts and thiouracil derivatives.

Pharmacogenetics

This term originally covered the study of genetically determined variants that are revealed solely by the effect of drugs. Some investigators now include within the sphere of pharmacogenetics those hereditary disorders which may be revealed spontaneously but are often precipitated or aggravated by drugs. There is a considerable variation in the way different individuals handle and respond to drugs. The population variability can be continuous or discontinuous. In continuous variation, results form a bell shape or unimodal distribution, but in discontinuous variation yield bimodal or trimodal curves. A unimodal distribution implies that metabolism of the drug in question is under the control of many genes (multifactorial) and analysis of genetic factors in such cases is usually not possible.

Genetic variations revealed solely by drugs

Isoniazid

This drug is acetylated and there are slow, intermediate and fast inactivators. Slow inactivators are homozygous for an autosomal (non-sex-linked) recessive gene. In the USA and Europe about 50 per cent of the population are slow inactivators. Polyneuritis (a toxic effect of isoniazid) is commoner in slow inactivators. Similarly, there are slow and fast inactivators of hydralazine, phenelzine and sulphadimidine. Acetylation is not the only metabolic process whose rate may be genetically determined: for instance phenytoin, which is hydroxylated, also demonstrates fast and slow inactivation.

The hepatic enzyme CPY2D6 is involved in the breakdown of codeine and tramadol. In its absence, codeine is less effective because none is transformed into morphine. In the case of tramadol, the metabolite makes no significant contribution to the analgesia but there is a suggestion that opioid-like side effects are less common when the enzyme is missing. This genetic variation is not constant in all communities. The enzyme is absent in about 8 per cent of Caucasians but not as frequently missing in the Japanese population.

Suxamethonium

This drug is short acting (2–4 minutes) because it is broken down by plasma cholinesterase. However, about 1 in 3000 patients given suxamethonium have apnoea which may last for an hour or more, and this is due to an abnormal form of plasma cholinesterase. Four allelomorphic variants of plasma cholinesterase have been described: the usual, the atypical, the fluoride-resistant, and the 'silent' types (see Chapter 16). The atypical variant is the commonest abnormal plasma cholinesterase and is characterized by a relative lack of the inhibition of the hydrolysis of benzoylcholine by the local anaesthetic cinchocaine (Dibucaine).

Malignant hyperthermia

There is a genetic basis for this condition: a dominant gene with reduced penetrance and variable expressivity is responsible. The syndrome occurs during anaesthesia and there are a number of triggering agents: it is liable to be seen especially if suxamethonium and/or halothane are used. Muscle rigidity occurs, there is a rapid rise in temperature, hyperkalaemia and acidosis.

Primaquine

Following administration of this drug some people, after a few days of treatment, begin to pass very dark, often black, urine; jaundice develops and the red cell count falls. The cause is a deficiency of glucose-6-phosphate dehydrogenase (G-6-PD). People with this deficiency are not only sensitive to primaquine but also to phenacetin, sulphonamides, nitrofurantoin and salicylates. G-6-PD is inherited as an X-linked recessive trait and deficiency is much commoner in Afro-Caribbeans than Caucasians.

Nitrites

Lack of methaemoglobin reductase (NADH ferrihaemoglobin reductase) in erythrocytes causes persistence of methaemoglobin after intake of nitrites, amidopyrine, or other drugs that cause methaemoglobin formation.

Hereditary disorders with altered drug responses

These are not strictly within the original definition of pharmacogenetics.

Acute intermittent porphyria

This disease is genetically determined by an autosomal dominant trait. Some individuals have skin lesions, particularly on exposed surfaces. Others may have mental disturbances or severe abdominal pain. An acute attack can be precipitated by barbiturates. In parts of South Africa as many as 1 per cent of the population may have porphyria. There are a number of drugs outside the barbiturate group which can induce porphyria in man. These include griseofulvin, sex steroids and oral hypoglycaemic agents.

Thiazide diuretics

These drugs can precipitate gout in patients genetically predisposed to it. Thiazides also aggravate symptoms of diabetic patients and in the future it may be possible to use chlorothiazide to recognize persons predisposed to diabetes in the population.

Chemotherapeutic index

It is difficult to compare the therapeutic efficiency of drugs as it involves taking into account both their pharmacological activity, their duration of action and their toxicity. However effective its actions, a drug is of no clinical use if it does not have a sufficient margin of safety. This problem was appreciated by Ehrlich, who took the minimum curative dose as a measure of a drug's efficacy and compared that with the maximum tolerated dose. The therapeutic index of the drug was the ratio of the maximum tolerated dose to the minimum curative dose, and where extremes are concerned, as with penicillin and some of the early arsenicals, it is obvious that with the former the ratio is very high (safe) and with the latter low (unsafe).

Maximum and minimum doses are very difficult to determine, and the minimum lethal dose of a drug was therefore discarded as a measurement in favour of the doses that kill 50 per cent of a group of animals (LD_{50}) and cure 50 per cent (ED_{50}). These are known as the median lethal and median effective doses, respectively. The ratio (LD_{50}/ED_{50}) has, therefore, replaced the earlier ratio, and the index this provides is much more reliable and is now widely used.

Approved names

At the time of writing, a major change is proposed by the Medicines Control Agency (United Kingdom) to conform with European Directives arising from negotiations within the WHO, to produce approved names which are acceptable world-wide. It is expected that the necessary changes will be in force by the time this book is published. The 'recommended International Nonproprietary Name' (rINN) will be required in all leaflets, data sheets and labels from a date to be announced.

However, some changes which are believed to create potentially dangerous confusion will be handled by requiring both the rINN and the existing British Approved Name (BAN) to be shown together, the rINN first. This will continue for at least five years. As far as anaesthetists and intensivists are concerned, the most obvious are the replacement of adrenaline and noradrenaline by epinephrine and norepinephrine. Frusemide will be replaced by furosemide, amethocaine by tetracaine, bendrofluazide by bendroflumethiazide and trimeprazine by alimemazine.

A second list of less dramatic changes affecting some 200 drugs will be implemented from the appointed date. This includes changing *-one* to *-al* for barbiturates and lignocaine to lidocaine. The other changes involve re-spellings such as 'i' for 'y', 'f' for 'ph', 'c' for 'ch' and 't' for 'th'. The new names are used throughout this edition.

Trade names are names given by manufacturers to their formulated products. There are advantages besides cost to the patient or health service in prescribing by approved names. Drugs with similar pharmacological actions have similar stems. For instance, propranolol, sotalol and timolol have the stem '-ol', which indicates that they are β-adrenoceptor blocking agents of the propranolol group. The importance of formulation in relation to the bioavailability, which can vary between manufacturers as well as by a specific manufacturer, is noted in the section on bioavailability (page 44).

Clinical trials

Clinical trials are frequently performed in anaesthetic practice. They may take many forms, but the commonest is to compare the efficacy of two drugs. Before using a new drug in patients, it would have undergone exhaustive toxicology testing in animals and also have been given to volunteers. Before entering into clinical trials, permission has to be sought from the Medicines Control Agency who maintain rigorous control over the introduction of new drugs.

Ethics

All studies on humans, including volunteers, must receive the approval of a properly constituted ethics committee. The latter will ensure that the study conforms with the principles of the Declaration of Helsinki and will at all stages ensure that the rights of the individual are protected. The patient should be fully informed of the purpose of the trial and of any risks involved. It should be made clear to them that they are free to withdraw from the study at any stage and that this will not in any way affect their treatment. It should be remembered that patients entering a study involving anaesthesia would not be able to withdraw once consciousness is lost. Ethics committees will be particularly rigorous in assessing protocols concerning non-therapeutic research. Each patient must sign a consent form after having due time to consider the study, which must be explained in writing in layman's language. If any change is made to a protocol during the course of a study, the ethics committee must be informed and their permission given before the changes are implemented.

Many drugs in anaesthesia are frequently used outwith their product licence, e.g. epidural and spinal opioids and the use of drugs in children. In this litigious age, it is prudent to obtain a Doctors and Dentists Exemption Certificate from the MCA before proceeding with such a trial. Informed consent should also be obtained. Trials in children raise special problems and parental consent is always mandatory.

Planning

The object of the trial must be specified. This will take the form of testing a hypothesis (i.e. a drug does or does not have a certain action) or more commonly forming an estimate of the quantitative effects of a drug on the body. If a new drug is being tested, it is important to remember that there is no point in having it unless it is in some respect better than drugs that already exist. It should therefore be tested against a standard drug in that group (e.g. thiopental for intravenous anaesthetics) and the study designed to show in what aspect it is superior. The question of using a placebo comparator is controversial, but in general if a drug already exists that is known to be therapeutically efficacious, use of a placebo is unethical. This particularly applies to investigations of analgesics.

Selection of subjects

The types of patients used must be defined in terms of age, sex and racial characteristics. The investigators must take into account concurrent disease and whether this might interfere with the trial drugs, e.g. renal failure. Drug therapy must also be taken into account. Exclusion criteria must be defined in the protocol presented to the ethics committee.

Trial design

Most anaesthetic studies are between two or more groups of patients who have received different drugs and under these circumstances it is essential that there are no differences between the groups, e.g. preponderance of females in one group. One way of avoiding this problem is to use a crossover design, where each patient receives each treatment. This is not often possible in anaesthetic-based studies, although it can be used in patients with chronic pain and in volunteer studies. When subjects act as their own control, it is possible that the effects of the first drug administered may modify the response to the subsequent drug, e.g. due to slow excretion or an effect on metabolic enzymes. Thus an adequate 'washout' time must be allowed between drug treatments.

Another method of study is sequential analysis. This requires strict matching of one patient with another and then plotting the outcome (A is better than B, B is better than A, or no difference detected) on a specially designed chart. This technique will then produce a result, if one treatment is better than another, without having to calculate in advance the size of the sample and removes concerns of a negative result being due to an inadequate sample size.

Sample size

It is incumbent on all investigators to ensure that they study a sufficient number of patients to produce a scientifically meaningful result and yet at the same time keep this number to the minimum necessary. The main concern is where a study has shown no difference between two treatments but where there might have been a significant difference if a larger number had been studied, i.e. a type II error. Gore and Altman (1982) have described a simplified method of calculating the number of cases required, using a nomogram. This is the power of the study: an 80 per cent power at least should be aimed for to detect a useful difference and preferably 90 per cent. In order to calculate the power, it is necessary to have some idea of the standard deviation that is required to show a statistical difference between groups. This can be obtained from previously published work, although if none is available it may be necessary to perform a pilot study. It is up to the investigators to decide at what level an event becomes significant, e.g. reduction in blood pressure of 20 per cent of control.

Randomization

This is the underlying principle in sampling populations for a clinical trial. It is imperative that, at the end of the trial, there must be no important difference in the characteristics between the patient groups. It can be shown mathematically that a sample of adequate size taken at random from a population will tend to be representative of the population.

The method of random allocation to a group must be acceptable and such that a patient must have an equal opportunity of being in any of the groups. One of the best methods is to use a table of random numbers; if only two groups are involved, the patient is placed in one group if the number is odd and the other if even. Tossing a coin is also an acceptable method of randomization into two groups. Apparently random criteria such as alternation of patients on an operating list should not be used, as the order may have been decided by events unknown to the investigator which may affect the results of treatment. Use of the hospital number is also unacceptable, as it may be affected by matters of which the investigator is unaware, for example an outpatient clerk giving even numbers to all female patients.

Blinding

'The advent of randomised, controlled, double-blind trials has unquestionably enabled medicine to emerge from the dark ages into the sunlight of the scientific era' (Editorial, 1994).

It is a basic requirement of any clinical investigation that observer and subject bias be removed as far as possible. Both can be influenced by knowledge of the treatment. The best way of doing this is the double-blind trial, where neither the investigator nor the patient knows the treatment group. This is perfectly feasible in the majority of trials in anaesthetic practice, although on occasion it can be difficult and raise ethical issues, e.g. injecting a placebo into the intrathecal or epidural space.

If the outcome of a study is objective and completely independent of the judgement of the investigator, e.g. death, then blinding is probably not important. However, where the end-point is a 'soft' one involving subjective observations of patients and observer, then double-blinding becomes crucial. This is particularly important in studies involving analgesic drugs.

Data collection

Well-designed data collection forms are essential for any clinical study, as is a method of converting to electronic storage. To reduce variables to a minimum, the number of investigators collecting data should be kept to a minimum.

Statistics

All studies will require statistical evaluation when completed. Sophisticated statistical analysis can never compensate for a poorly designed study. Involvement of a statistician from the point of study design is therefore imperative, especially to calculate sample size and advise on the correct statistical tests when all data have been collected. It is essential to avoid the common error of applying parametric tests, e.g. Student's t test, to non-parametric data (i.e. not normally distributed). If in doubt, a non-parametric test should always be chosen.

Legal aspects of medicines

Statutory controls of medicines in the United Kingdom that mainly concern the medical profession are the Medicines Act 1968 and the Misuse of Drugs Act 1971 and the numerous Statutory Instruments (SIs) made under them. Many Statutory Instruments have been introduced as a result of European Directives, resulting in harmonisation of legislation throughout the European Community.

Medicines Act 1968

The Medicines Act 1968 regulates the manufacture, distribution, importation, promotion, labelling and supply of medicinal products. The Act does so by licensing medicinal products via a Marketing Authorisation, or MA (formerly a Product Licence) and via licences for manufacture and wholesale dealing. The licensing system regarding new products in Europe comprises three procedures, namely a centralized system, a decentralized system and a national system. For the centralized system, one application for a Marketing Authorisation is made to the European Medicines Evaluation Agency (EMEA), this being compulsory for biotechnology products. The decentralized system permits a pharmaceutical company to submit an application to the Licensing Authority in one member state (for example, the Medicines Control Agency in the United Kingdom). Once approved by the regulatory body in this member state the decision must be accepted by other member states unless refusal is made on the grounds of public health. For the centralized and decentralized procedures, the Committee for Proprietary Medicinal Products (CPMP), consisting of representatives of the European Commission and member states, provides the expertise for assessing the application for a Marketing Authorisation.

If a company wishes to submit an application for a product intended only for its own domestic market, then the application is made to the national licensing authority, for example, the MCA, and the expertise is provided by an expert national body, not the CPMP. For the United Kingdom this body is the Committee on Safety of Medicines. Prior to application for a Marketing Authorisation, clinical trials with patients must be undertaken in accordance with a system of good clinical practice and in the United Kingdom require the granting of a Clinical Trials Certificate (CTC) or an exemption certificate (CTX) before a trial may commence. A doctor or dentist must apply for a certificate (a DDX) in order to administer a product to one or more patients as part of a clinical trial, but must not receive sponsorship from a company to undertake such a study. The Medicines Control Agency grants such certificates, which are not required where the drug is administered for a non-therapeutic purpose (that is, usually to healthy volunteers).

Following the marketing of medicinal products the Committee on Safety of Medicines (CSM) monitors certain adverse reactions to drugs. All suspected reactions, including minor ones, that could conceivably be attributable to a recently introduced product which are identified by a black triangle (▲) in the British National Formulary (BNF), all reactions to vaccines and serious or unusual suspected reactions to all agents including reactions that are fatal, life-threatening, disabling, incapacitating, or which result in prolonged hospitalisation should be reported. Reports are made on Yellow Cards which are available at the back of the BNF and a number of other sources.

The Medicines Act 1968 also controls the registration of community pharmacies and lays down the legal class of medicines, namely whether they are prescription only (POM), general sales list (GSL) which may be sold from any retail premises, or pharmacy only

(P) which may be sold only from a registered pharmacy by, or under, the supervision of a pharmacist. A prescription for a POM for a human must contain the following particulars: the name and address of the patient (and age if under 12 years), the name and address of the prescriber and an indication of whether the prescriber is a doctor, dentist or nurse prescriber, and must be signed by the prescriber. The prescription must also bear a date, as an NHS prescription for a POM is valid only for six months.

The legislation allows a hospital to supply a POM in the course of its business, against a 'written direction' of a doctor, instead of a prescription. The direction does not need to comply with the requirements specified for prescriptions, the intention being to supply medicines against the patient's bed card or patient notes. In April 1998 a Review of Prescribing, Supply and Administration of Medicines under group protocols was published (see References). A group protocol is defined as a specific written instruction for the supply or administration of named medicines in an identified clinical situation. It is drawn up locally by doctors, pharmacists and other appropriate professionals, and approved by the employer, advised by the relevant professional advisory committees. It applies to groups of patients or other service users who may not be individually identified before presentation for treatment. They should specify clear arrangements for professional responsibility and accountability, and contribute to the effective use of resources.

The following should not normally be included in group protocols: new drugs under intensive monitoring and subject to special adverse reaction reporting to the CSM (the black triangle scheme); unlicensed medicines, and medicines used outside their licensed indications; and medicines being used in clinical trials.

There are a number of exemptions with regard to the supply and administration of a POM. For example, ophthalmic opticians and chiropodists may supply and administer certain POMs to their patients, and certificated ambulance paramedics may administer certain named parenteral products, such as glucose and naloxone, for the immediate, necessary treatment of sick or injured persons. For the purpose of saving a life in an emergency, anyone may administer by injection certain products such as epinephrine (adrenaline) and hydrocortisone in the absence of directions from a practitioner.

Certain practice nurses, health visitors and community nurses working in some United Kingdom Health Authorities are able to prescribe a limited number of POMs such as co-danthrusate capsules or nystatin pastilles, such medicines being listed in the Nurse Prescribers' Formulary. It is hoped that the scheme will become nation-wide in the United Kingdom, but the training of all appropriate nurses may mean that it could be a matter of many months before all eligible nurses will be in a position to prescribe.

Certified practising midwives may supply any P or GSL medicines in the course of their professional practice and also a limited number of POMs, namely chloral hydrate, dichlorphenazone, ergometrine maleate (but not for parenteral use), pentazocine hyrochloride and triclofos sodium. Certified midwives may also administer parenterally in the course of their professional practice the following: ergometrine maleate, levallorphan tartrate, lidocaine and its hydrochloride, naloxone hydrochloride, oxytocins (natural and synthetic), pentazocine lactate, pethidine and its hydrochloride, phytomenadione and promazine. In the case of lidocaine and its hydrochloride and promazine hydrochloride these may only be administered while attending on a woman in childbirth.

Misuse of Drugs Act 1971

The 1971 Act, and Statutory Instruments made under it, control the export, import, production, supply and possession of dangerous or otherwise harmful drugs, hereafter referred to as controlled drugs, as well as the control and treatment of addicts and the promotion of education and research relating to drug dependence. The general effect of this legislation is to make unlawful all activities involving the drugs which are controlled under the 1971 Act, except as provided in the Misuse of Drugs Regulations 1985. These regulations relax the restrictions such to allow practitioners to prescribe and pharmacists to possess and supply such substances, but only when acting in the course of their professional practice.

Legislation classifies the drugs into five schedules according to different levels of control.

- *Schedule 1* includes cannabis and the hallucinogenic drugs such as lysergic acid diethylamide, as they are considered by the authorities to have virtually no therapeutic use. A licence from the Home Office is required to produce, possess or supply, and the legitimate uses are restricted to research or 'other special purposes'.
- *Schedule 2* includes the opiates (such as diamorphine, methadone), many amphetamines and quinalbarbital. A pharmacist may supply them to a patient only on a prescription issued by an appropriate practitioner in the prescribed manner. In addition to the requirements for a prescription for a POM, prescriptions for Schedule 2 (and Schedule 3) drugs must:

1. Be in ink or otherwise indelible;
2. Be signed by the prescriber with his/her usual signature and be dated by him/her;
3. Bear in the practitioner's own handwriting the name and address of the person for whom the treatment is prescribed;
4. Specify in the prescriber's own handwriting the dose to be taken. 'Take as directed' and 'take when needed' are not sufficient: the dose needs to be written such as 'take one as directed' or 'take two when needed';
5. When prescribed as a preparation, state the form, e.g. tablets, solution, ampoules, etc., even if available only as one form;
6. Where there is more than one strength available, state the strength of the preparation;
7. Specify the total amount of each controlled drug or the total number of tablets or volume of liquid to be supplied. These total amounts must be stated both in words and in figures;
8. In the case of prescription for a total amount to be supplied in instalments, give a direction specifying the intervals to be observed when dispensing;
9. Be written by a prescriber whose address is in the United Kingdom;
10. When written by a dental practitioner, state the words 'For dental treatment only'.

It is a criminal offence to issue or dispense a prescription that does not comply with the above requirements, and is an offence to dispense such a prescription before the date on the prescription or more than 13 weeks after the date on the prescription. Also, a product may only be dispensed if the supplier is either acquainted with the prescriber's signature and has no reason to suppose that it is not genuine, or has taken reasonably sufficient steps to satisfy himself/herself that it is genuine.

Schedule 2 controlled drugs may be administered by a doctor or dentist, or in accordance with their directions. Written records must be made in the Controlled Drugs register regarding the receipt and supply of these drugs on the day of supply or the next day. They must be kept for two years following the last entry in the register. Schedule 2 controlled drugs (plus temazepam and buprenorphine) must be stored in a locked receptacle and the key is held by a person authorized to hold the drugs.

Operating theatre department assistants or practitioners are not authorized to requisition controlled drugs, but may hold the keys to the locked receptacle containing controlled drugs, under the supervision of the sister or acting sister. Under such circumstances, it is the sister or acting sister who is responsible for all supplies from such locked receptacles. There are also controls over the destruction of Schedule 2 drugs.

- *Schedule 3* drugs include buprenorphine, benzphetamine and most barbiturates. Similar restrictions to those drugs in Schedule 2 apply, including prescription requirements, except that records in a register of Controlled Drugs need not be kept and requirements regarding destruction do not apply. Temazepam is a Schedule 3 drug but is exempt from the prescription requirements for Schedule 2 and 3 drugs (see above).
- *Schedule 4* drugs are divided into two parts. Part I contains most of the anabolic and androgenic steroids, clembuterol and growth hormones, and Part II contains most of the benzodiazepines. For practitioners and pharmacists while acting in the course of their professional practice these may be treated as any other POM. An import or export licence is required from the Home Office if the substance is listed in Part I and is not solely for the administration of the drug to the person himself/herself.
- *Schedule 5* contains preparations of certain controlled drugs, for example, codeine, morphine and pholcodine (and their salts) which are exempt from full control when present in medicinal products of low strength. Examples include co-codamol, codeine linctus, pholcodine linctus and kaolin and morphine mixture.

There is an Advisory Council on the Misuse of Drugs that keeps under review the situation in the United Kingdom with respect to drugs that are or appear likely to be misused. A recent example is flunitrazepam (Rohypnol®) which has become known as the 'date rape' drug, as it was being used to sedate women. The need to tighten statutory control on the storage, import, export and unauthorized possession has resulted in its reclassification from a Schedule 4 drug to one in Schedule 3.

Medical practitioners may not prescribe or administer cocaine, diamorphine or dipipanone or their salts, to an addicted person, except for the purpose of treating organic disease or injury, unless the practitioner is licensed to do so by the Secretary of State. Repeatable prescriptions and emergency supplies are allowable for drugs in Schedules 4 and 5 but not for other controlled drugs. The Secretary of State has power to direct that a practitioner or pharmacist who has been convicted of an offence under the Misuse of Drugs legislation may not possess, administer, manufacture, prescribe or supply certain controlled drugs for a specified period. The Minister may also give such a direction without a conviction where the practitioner has been prescribing controlled drugs in an irresponsible manner.

References and further reading

Ariens, E.J. (1956) Affinity and intrinsic activity in the theory of competitive inhibition. *Archives Internationale de Pharmacodynamie et Therapie*, **99**, 32–49

Benet, L.Z., Massoud, N. and Gambertoglio, J.G. (1984) *Pharmacokinetics of Drug Treatment.* New York: Raven Press

Benet, L.Z., Kroetz, D.L. and Sheiner, L.B. (1996) Pharmacokinetics: the dynamics of drug absorption, distribution and elimination. In *Goodman and Gilman's 'The Pharmacological Basis of Therapeutics'*, 9th edn, Chapter 1, pp. 3–27 (Eds: Hardman, J.G., Limbird, L.E. and Gilman, A.G.). New York: McGraw-Hill

Brodie, B.B. (1965) Displacement of one drug by another from carrier or receptor sites. *Proceedings of the Royal Society of Medicine*, **58**, 946

Butler, A.M. and Richie, R.H. (1960) Prescribing for children. *New England Journal of Medicine*, **262**, 903

Catzel, P. (1963a) The estimation of doses for infants and children. A review and a proposed standardized method. *Medical Proceedings*, **9**, 20

Catzel, P. (1963b) *Paediatric Prescriber*. Oxford: Blackwell

Chaudhri, S., Colvin, J.R., Todd, J.G. and Kenny, G.N. (1992) Evaluation of closed loop control of arterial pressure during hypotensive anaesthesia for local resection of intraocular melanoma. *British Journal of Anaesthesia*, **69**, 607–10

Colvin, J.R. and Kenny, G.N. (1989) Microcomputer-controlled administration of vasodilators following cardiac surgery: technical considerations. *Journal of Cardiothoracic Anesthesia*, **3**, 10–15

Conney, A.H. (1967) Pharmacological implications of microsomal enzyme induction. *Pharmacological Reviews*, **19**, 317

Crown, J. (1988) Review of prescribing, supply and administration of medicines. *A Report on the Supply & Administration of Medicines Under Group Protocols* (Department of Health, April, 1988)

Dekker Herxheimer, A. and Lionel, N.D.W. (1970) Assessing reports of therapeutic trials. *British Journal of Pharmacology*, **39**, 204P

Editorial (1994) Blinded by science. *Lancet* **343**, 553–4

Eger, E.I., Saidman, L.G. and Brandstater, B. (1965) Minimum alveolar anaesthetic concentration; a standard of anaesthetic potency. *Anesthesiology*, **26**, 756

Furchgott, R.F. (1966) The use of β-haloalkylamines in the differentiation of receptors, and in the determination of dissociation constants of receptor-agonist complexes. In *Advances in Drug Research*, vol 3 pp 21–55. (Eds: Harper, N.J. and Simmonds, A.B.). London: Academic Press

Gibaldi, R. and Perrier, D. (1982) *Pharmacokinetics*. New York: Marcel Dekker.

Gore, S.M. and Altman, D.G. (1982) *Statistics in Practice*. London: British Medical Association

Herxheimer, A. and Lionel, N.D.W. (1970) Assessing reports of clinical trials. *British Journal of Pharmacology*, **39**, 204P

Hughes, M.A., Glass, P.S., Jacobs, J.R. (1992) Context-sensitive half-time in multicompartment pharmacokenetic models for intravenous anesthetic drugs. *Anesthesiology*, **76**, 334–341

Ross, E. (1996) Pharmacodynamics: mechanisms of drug action and the relationship between drug concentration and effect. In *Goodman and Gilman's 'The Pharmacological Basis of Therapeutics'*, 9th edn, Chapter 2, pp. 29–41 (Eds: Hardman, J.G., Limbird, L.E. and Gilman, A.G.). New York: McGraw-Hill

Stephenson, R.P. (1956) A modification of receptor theory. *British Journal of Pharmacology and Chemotherapy*, **11**, 379–393

2

Perioperative therapy

The anaesthetist has a responsibility for the patient both before and after operation. After surgery this may just involve recovery room care but may extend to the high dependency and intensive care units. This is particularly the case when complex modes of pain relief are initiated.

At the preoperative visit, the anaesthetist may find that the patient is already receiving drugs for conditions related or unrelated to the proposed surgery. Medical conditions as different as hypertension, angina, heart failure, chronic obstructive airways disease, arthritis, diabetes, peptic ulcer or mental disorders may be being successfully managed and depend on the continuation of optimum therapy during the preoperative period. The anaesthetist must decide whether to modify the dosage, or the route of administration, stop the drug or change to another one. In many cases the withdrawal of the drug will be contraindicated.

In addition, the anaesthetist may think it appropriate to prescribe other therapy in relation to the proposed procedure. The most commonly prescribed drugs are those intended to relieve preoperative anxiety, to ensure sleep, to prevent nausea and vomiting, to relieve pain, to minimize the hypertensive response to laryngoscopy and intubation, and to minimize the possibility of regurgitation of stomach contents or their effect on the lungs if inhaled. When so doing, the anaesthetist must consider the possibility and clinical significance of interaction between existing medication and any therapy that he/she initiates.

Anxiety

The commonest reason for prescribing premedicant drugs is for the relief of anxiety. It is not just the induction of anaesthesia which patients fear, but loss of control, and pain or discomfort on waking; there is also an unspoken and often unadmitted fear that consciousness will not return or may return during the surgical procedure while they are paralysed.

Much can be done to allay anxiety by explanation and reassurance and some believe that few patients either need, or benefit from, preoperative sedation. On the other hand, there are many patients who are grateful to receive some relief from anxiety.

The sedative drugs most commonly employed prior to operation are the benzodiazepines. In the starved patient oral premedication with a lipid-soluble drug is reliable, and many hypnotics and tranquillizers are effective if given 1–2 h preoperatively. The phenothiazines also retain some popularity, particularly alimemazine (trimeprazine) for children.

All of the phenothiazines have an anti-emetic action which is particularly important in patients prone to post-anaesthetic vomiting. However, they may add to the gastro-intestinal inhibitory effects of anaesthetics and other drugs and produce long-lasting somnolence. As a consequence, there has been increasing use of specific anti-emetics which lack side effects. The first of these was ondansetron, but similar drugs such as granisetron and tropisetron, are emerging.

Where patients are in pain, as is often the case before emergency surgery, powerful analgesics such as morphine and pethidine or their derivatives will be required. Sedatives with only hypnotic activity should then be avoided as they cause restlessness and confusion in the presence of pain.

Many premedicant drugs cause anterograde amnesia or potentiate the amnesic effects of anaesthetic agents. The most potent amnesic drugs of those commonly used as premedicants are hyoscine, lorazepam and diazepam. Intravenous administration of premedicants 15–30 minutes before operation markedly potentiates the anterograde amnesic properties of such drugs and intravenous midazolam is used when this is thought to be desirable.

Unwanted autonomic responses to anaesthesia

The most common unwanted side effect of many anaesthetic techniques is vagal preponderance, which often occurs with halothane and powerful opioids such as alfentanil and remifentanil and may cause bradycardia, hypotension and even cardiac arrest. This effect can be prevented by the prior administration of atropine or glycopyrrolate given intravenously just prior to induction. This has the advantage of ensuring that the vagus is adequately blocked during induction, while the patient avoids the discomfort of a dry mouth while waiting for operation. Even if not administered prophylactically, it is important to have a suitable dose drawn up ready at induction.

All patients, but particularly those with inadequately controlled hypertension, are prone to develop arrhythmias and hypertension during laryngoscopy and intubation. These adverse autonomic effects can be attenuated by the prior administration of a variety of agents. Short-acting, powerful analgesics such as alfentanil and remifentanil are commonly used, but other agents have their adherents, including intravenous lidocaine (lignocaine), glyceryltrinitrin transdermal patches, angiotensin-converting enzyme (ACE) inhibitors, sublingual nifedipine and β-blockers.

Diethyl ether causes an increase in bronchial and salivary secretions which needs to be blocked by the prior administraion of an anti-sialogogue.

Induction movements

Premedicant drugs, as well as influencing the drug requirements for anaesthesia, also modify the characteristics of induction. Induction with some induction agents, particularly etomidate and methohexital, and to a lesser extent with propofol, may be associated with spontaneous involuntary muscle movements. Premedication with analgesic drugs diminishes this response.

Regurgitation, vomiting and pulmonary aspiration

Many drugs affect gut function in ways that influence the likelihood of regurgitation or vomiting, and the chemical nature of such material. Some drugs directly block or enhance secretion of gastric acid, bile salts and pancreatic enzymes, while other drugs have marked effects on various aspects of gut function. They may, for example, affect the tone of the lower oesophageal sphincter, delay or promote gastric emptying, induce vomiting, increase or decrease gut transit time, relieve smooth muscle spasm, or act as constipating agents. Many of these effects are also unwanted side effects of drugs given for other therapeutic purposes: the effect of opiates in delaying gastric emptying is an obvious example. The reduction of lower oesophageal barrier pressure by atropine is another. Anaesthetists thus need to consider giving drugs preoperatively which can modify gut function and they are also likely to meet patients on chronic therapy already affecting gut function. For instance, patients who previously presented for surgery for peptic ulcer now present for other conditions but are taking drugs regularly to reduce gastric acidity.

Preoperatively, the anaesthetist is most concerned with affecting the pH and volume of gastric contents, the rate of stomach emptying and lower oesophageal barrier pressure. Many of the drugs that are used are discussed in other chapters. Drugs that affect gut smooth muscle tone are considered in Chapters 10 and 11. The H_2-receptor blockers, which are effective in reducing gastric acid secretion are considered in Chapter 8. Others are considered below.

Nausea and vomiting

Nausea and vomiting can be induced by a variety of mechanisms, which are mainly either central or affecting primarily the gut. Central mechanisms include raised intracranial pressure, motion sickness, anxiety, biochemical upsets and the action of emetic drugs. These act either on the chemoreceptor trigger zone or on the vomiting centre itself. Some drugs affect the gut to initiate vomiting via vagal afferents to the vomiting centre.

The receptors involved include dopamine (D_2) and serotonin (5-HT_3) in the case of the chemoreceptor trigger zone, histamine (H_2) and cholinergic receptors (muscarinic M_3) in the case of the vomiting centre and 5-HT_3 and 5-HT_4 in the case of the gut. The drugs mainly used to control postoperative nausea and vomiting are metoclopramide (D_2) and ondansetron (5-HT_3), although many anaesthetists still use droperidol and non-selective antihistamines.

One of the main causes of postoperative nausea is the administration of opiates before, during or after the operation and metoclopramide is probably the most specific agent to combat this, and may be given prophylactically. Ondansetron is increasingly being used for postoperative nausea and vomiting. Although 5-HT_3 receptors are found both in the gut and in the chemoreceptor trigger zone, which of these is the important site of action is not known.

Control of gastric acidity

Acid is produced by the parietal cells of the stomach. There are receptors on the cell surface in the stomach for acetylcholine, histamine and gastrin, all of which stimulate acid secretion. Acetylcholine acts by opening calcium channels. Histamine and gastrin stimulate the production of cyclic AMP and this mechanism can be inhibited by prostaglandin $E_{2\alpha}$ thus preventing histamine-stimulated gastric acid secretion. The final common pathway for the production of acid in the parietal cells is thought to be a H^+/K^+ ATP-ase driven 'proton pump' which takes up K^+ from the cell and pumps H^+ into the acid-containing canaliculi. Since this pump is unique to parietal cells, agents which specifically inhibit this system combine a blockade of gastric acid secretion to any extent required with minimal other pharmacodynamic properties. This enzyme system can be inhibited by a new class of compounds (the benzimidazoles), of which omeprazole was the first example.

Antacids

A large number of proprietary preparations are available to neutralize gastric acidity. In anaesthetic practice, magnesium trisilicate mixture was extensively used in doses of 15 ml every 2 h during labour. Its effectiveness is not in doubt, but pathological studies have shown that it can itself cause lung damage if particles of the suspension are inhaled. This mixture also contains peppermint oil flavouring which lowers the tone of the lower oesophageal sphincter.

As a consequence, 0.3 molar sodium citrate is now recommended. It contains no particles and mixes better within the stomach, although it is less palatable. A single dose of 30 ml will raise the gastric pH above 2.5 (which is thought to be the critical level for triggering the acid aspiration syndrome) if given 10 minutes before induction. During labour it needs to be given every 2 h, and 30 ml seems to be the minimum effective dose. Unfortunately, these quantities increase the volume of the gastric contents. The effectiveness of antacids is influenced by the rate of gastric emptying. If acid production is not suppressed, rapid emptying will remove the antacid and the pH will fall again.

H_2-receptor blockade

The agents cimetidine and ranitidine are considered in Chapter 8. These agents are widely used in the treatment of peptic ulceration, reflux oesophagitis and the Zollinger–Ellison syndrome. They can markedly diminish gastric acid production if given 90–150 minutes before induction of anaesthesia. They are effective if given intravenously 45–60 minutes before induction. However, they cannot influence acid already present in the stomach. This depends on gastric emptying. There has been a vogue for their use in patients receiving artificial ventilation in intensive care units to diminish the risk of acid aspiration into the lungs, but it is now believed that there is a concomitant increase in 'ventilator pneumonia' and the practice has fallen out of favour.

Proton pump inhibitors

Chemically, omeprazole and lansoprazole possess substituted benzimidazole and pyridine rings linked by a bridge containing a sulphinyl group (see *Figure 8.1*, page 247). In their administered form, both are in actually 'pro-drugs': at neutral pH, they are devoid of activity, but after absorption into the bloodstream and reaching the stomach's parietal cells, both agents are protonated and rearrange to form a sulfenic acid and a sulfenamide. This latter agent combines covalently with the membrane-spanning H^+/K^+ ATP-ase system, providing a long-lasting suppression of gastric acid secretion.

The therapeutic indications for proton pump inhibitors are similar to those of the H_2-antagonists, and include the treatment of reflux oesophagitis and the healing of peptic ulcers resistant to standard therapy with H_2-antagonists. They are valuable in the preoperative preparation of patients who are particularly at risk of acid aspiration, including those scheduled for Caesarean section. The proton pump inhibitors' ability to provide a long-lasting and complete suppression of both basal and stimulated gastric acid secretion is important, for example, in patients resistant to the usual clinical doses of H_2-receptor antagonists and also when treating the more resistant Zollinger–Ellison syndrome.

A dose of 40 mg of omeprazole causes the median 24-h intragastric pH to rise from 1.4 to 5.3. This prolonged effect is in contrast to the drug's rapid disappearance from the circulation because the drug is trapped within the cell by its covalent binding to receptors.

Omeprazole and lansoprazole both have a potential to interact with microsomal cytochrome P-450 enzymes, slowing the hepatic metabolism and thus enhancing the effects of other drugs (see the monograph, page 68).

Reducing the volume of gastric contents

Although a 4-h fast before anaesthesia is traditional, the rate of gastric emptying is extremely unpredictable and much delayed by trauma, pain, anxiety and opioids. A wide-bore stomach tube will remove most of the stomach contents; equally effective is apomorphine (10 mg) which stimulates the chemoreceptor trigger zone and induces vomiting. Both procedures are unpleasant and may not be well tolerated in the very ill, so attention has focused on drugs which stimulate peristalsis (prokinetic drugs). In this category are metoclopramide and domperidone which, in addition to reducing vomiting by an action on the chemoreceptor trigger zone, stimulate peristalsis, increase gastric emptying rate and decrease small bowel transit time. Metoclopramide has been shown to be effective by any route, but its onset is quickest if given intravenously. Neither drug empties the stomach completely, but if combined with an H_2-receptor blocker there is an increase in pH and reduction in volume which is more effective than that of either class of drug given alone.

Cisapride, a 5-HT_4 receptor agonist, is another example of a prokinetic drug. It enhances lower oesophageal sphincter tone and hastens gastric emptying, but has lesser effects on the remainder of the gut. The side effects include abdominal cramps, borborygmi and diarrhoea. Because of its favourable combination of properties, it is promoted for the relief of gastro-oesophageal reflux: doses are 10 mg 3 times a day, 15 minutes before food. Because its effects are ultimately produced by enhancing parasympathetic activity in the gut, its actions are reversed by atropine. Drugs such as this may find a place in the preoperative preparation of patients for emergency surgery.

Cisapride diminishes the absorption of drugs from the stomach, but enhances the uptake of drugs which are absorbed from the intestine. This may be a problem with oral anticoagulants and prothrombin time may be prolonged. It must not be taken with fluconazole, erythromycin or clarithromycin: the combination has occasionally resulted in serious arrythmias including Torsade de Pointes and QT prolongation.

Lower oesophageal sphincter tone

This is thought to be the most important factor in inhibiting gastro-oesophageal reflux. It is influenced by many drugs (*Table 2.1*). It tends to increase when there are rises in intragastric or intra-abdominal pressure, thus preventing any reflux which might otherwise occur. Thus it is really the difference between lower oesophageal sphincter pressure and intragastric pressure – the so-called barrier pressure – which matters. This is low in patients with hiatus hernia who have symptoms of reflux and in pregnant patients with symptoms of regurgitation. It is important to bear in mind that the case for avoiding or using agents because of their effect on lower oesophageal sphincter tone is largely theoretical: there has been little direct evidence of a reduced or an increased incidence of actual regurgitation and aspiration. However, as *Table 2.1* shows, many drugs used for premedication decrease lower oesophageal sphincter tone, although, fortunately, suxamethonium increases it during fasciculation.

Table 2.1 Effect of drugs on lower oesophageal sphincter tone

Increase	Decrease
Metoclopramide	Glycopyrrolate
Cisapride	Atropine
Domperidone	
Cyclizine	
Neostigmine	Nitroprusside
Edrophonium	β-adrenergic stimulants
	Dopamine
Suxamethonium	Opioids
Pancuronium	Anaesthetic vapours
	Thiopental
Histamine	
α-adrenergic stimulants	
Antacids	Peppermint oil
Ergometrine	

Anaesthetic sparing

Dexmedetomide, a centrally acting selective α_2-adrenoceptor agonist, is undergoing clinical trials as a premedicant which reduces the requirement for both sedative and analgesic agents during and after surgery. It is also being investigated as an anxiolytic and sedative for patients in intensive care. Whilst it appears to be highly effective in both roles, it causes bradycardia and a fall in both systolic and diastolic blood pressure, as well as prolonged sedation, any of which may be undesirable. It is also an effective analgesic when administered epidurally.

Premedication in children

The avoidance of injections by the use of oral or rectal premedication in children is a widespread practice, and many drugs and dose regimens have been tried. None is completely satisfactory and drugs that produce a satisfactory condition in the anaesthetic room may be associated with postoperative restlessness or prolonged somnolence. As with adults, good rapport achieved at a preoperative visit can do much to reduce the need for chemical premedication.

Rectal thiopental, 5 per cent solution in a dose of 40–50 mg/kg, almost always produces narcosis. It is now relatively unpopular, requiring supervision of the patient from the time of administration until the child is handed over to the anaesthetist. The use of the sedative H_1-receptor antagonist alimemazine syrup (6 mg/ml) is widespread, in doses of 1–2 mg/kg. Note, however, that it has minimal analgesic activity and if given alone may give rise to postoperative restlessness in the presence of pain as well as prolonged somnolence. It also causes amnesia and pallor if given in doses at the upper end of the range.

Diazepam (0.22 mg/kg) is more satisfactory than alimemazine in the anaesthetic room, but has poor drying properties. The chloral hydrate derivative Triclofos (75 mg/kg; maximum dose 1.6 g) is also satisfactory in 80 per cent of cases. Adequate drying can be achieved with oral atropine (0.05 mg/kg; maximum dose 1.2 mg).

In unprepared patients, in small babies, in the presence of pain, and where certainty of action is required, standard adult premedicating regimens can be employed with suitable reduction of dose.

MONOGRAPHS

METOCLOPRAMIDE

Metoclopramide hydrochloride (rINN)

Pharmacology

Metoclopramide is a specific anti-emetic. In normal therapeutic doses it has no narcotic or sedative action. It is a dopamine (D_2) receptor antagonist, and its actions are elicited at two levels: it is effective centrally at the chemoreceptor trigger zone, and also has a peripheral action, diminishing the sensitivity of the visceral nerves to local emetics. In addition, it hastens gastric emptying, possibly by a central action on brain stem nuclei controlling gastric motility, and increases the tone of the lower oesophageal sphincter. These peripheral effects are antagonized by atropine.

Indications

Metoclopramide may be used to control nausea and vomiting associated with peptic ulcer and epidemic viral gastroenteritis, X-ray therapy, malignant disease and uraemia. It is effective in the control of post-anaesthetic vomiting and shortens the duration of postoperative ileus. However, the delay in gastric emptying which is caused by narcotic analgesics is not significantly influenced by metoclopramide. It has been employed as an agent for hastening the emptying of the full stomach when general anaesthesia is required after an accident.

Dosage and administration

Metoclopramide may be given orally or by intramuscular or intravenous injection. The usual dose is 10 mg, which can be repeated 3 times a day. It is not recommended for children under 5 years, but older children may be given proportionate doses.

Precautions

It may produce drowsiness and restlessness: dystonic muscle movements and other extrapyramidal side effects are produced if the dosage exceeds 0.5 mg/kg. Constipation may occur. Atropine antagonizes its action on gastric motility. It slightly prolongs the recovery time of suxamethonium.

OMEPRAZOLE

Omeprazole (rINN)

Pharmacology

Omeprazole is a substituted benzimidazole (see *Figure 8.1*). In the administered form, it is in fact a 'pro-drug': at neutral pH, omeprazole is devoid of activity, but after absorption into the bloodstream and reaching the stomach's parietal cells, it is rearranged to form a sulfenic acid and a sulfenamide. This latter agent combines covalently with the membrane-spanning H^+/K^+ATP-ase system, providing a long-lasting suppression of gastric acid secretion. The drug may be described as a 'hit and run' drug, since suppression of acid secretion lasts well beyond the individual drug's removal from the body. Omeprazole, by acting on the final common pathway of acid secretion, inhibits both basal and stimulated acid secretion.

Indications

The therapeutic indications for proton-pump inhibitors are similar to those of the H_2-antagonists and they are valuable in the preoperative preparation of patients who are particularly at risk of acid aspiration, including those scheduled for Caesarean section, for which it is claimed to be more effective than H_2-antagonists. Omeprazole is also effective in the treatment of reflux oesophagitis and the healing of peptic ulcers resistant to standard therapy with H_2 receptor antagonists. The proton pump inhibitors' ability to provide a long-lasting and complete suppression of gastric acid secretion is particularly valuable in patients resistant to the usual clinical doses of H_2-receptor antagonists, and also when treating the more resistant Zollinger–Ellison syndrome.

Dosage and administration

A dose of 40 mg causes the median 24-h intragastric pH to rise from 1.4 to 5.3. This prolonged effect is probably because the drug is trapped within the cell by its covalent binding to receptors. For prophylaxis against acid aspiration at induction of anaesthesia, the recommended regimen is 40 mg the evening before surgery and another 40 mg 2–6 h before surgery.

Precautions

Like cimetidine (but unlike ranitidine, famotidine and nazitidine), omeprazole has the potential to interact with microsomal cytochrome P-450 enzymes, slowing the hepatic metabolism and thus enhancing the effects of other drugs. Thus interactions with phenytoin, certain benzodiazepines and warfarin should be anticipated and doses of these agents adjusted as appropriate.

Lansoprazole and **pantoprazole** have very similar pharmacological profiles differing from omeprazole in the site of binding to the proton pump. Pantoprazole may have a lower potential for drug interactions (*Drug and Therapeutics Bulletin*, 1997).

Pantoprazole – a third proton pump inhibitor (1997) *Drug and Therapeutic Bulletin*, **35**, 93–4

ONDANSETRON

Ondansetron (rINN)

Pharmacology

Ondansetron is a potent and highly selective 5-HT$_3$ receptor antagonist. Its precise mode of action in the control of nausea and vomiting is not known. 5-HT$_3$ receptor antagonists block a reflex initiated in the gut by many chemicals which release 5-HT and also the release of 5-HT in the chemoreceptor trigger zone as a response to this reflex. Which of these two sites is crucial for the action of such a specific blocking agent is not clear. It does not cause sedation or, indeed, any other CNS effect.

Fate in the body   Ondansetron is metabolized in the liver. Clearance is significantly reduced in the presence of hepatic impairment and the plasma half-life consequently prolonged.

Indications

Ondansetron was introduced for the treatment of nausea and vomiting caused by radio-therapy and chemotherapeutic agents, for which it is still used. It is, however, now licensed for the prevention and treatment of postoperative nausea and vomiting.

Dosage and administration

For the prevention of postoperative nausea and vomiting, ondansetron 8 mg can be given orally, 1 h before anaesthesia or 4 mg by slow intravenous injection just prior to induction. For the treatment of established symptoms, 4 mg can be given slowly by intravenous injection or intramuscularly.

Precautions

Ondansetron increases transit time in the large intestine and may cause constipation. There have been occasional reports of hypersensitivity reactions. It should be used with caution in cases of hepatic impairment.

Granisetron has a very similar pharmacological profile but hepatic impairment is not associated with any evidence of reduced clearance. It is only available as an intravenous injection. It is not licensed in the United Kingdom for the treatment of postoperative nausea and vomiting but has been used for this indication. The minimum effective dose has been estimated to be 40 µg/kg (Fujii *et al.*, 1998).

Tropisetron has broadly similar pharmacological characteristics to ondansetron, hepatic cirrhosis and impaired kidney function leading to higher plasma concentrations. Its actions are prolonged in poor debrisoquine metabolizers. It is claimed to block the excitation of the pre-synaptic 5-HT receptors on neurones in the visceral mucosa, and may exert additional direct actions within the CNS. It is not yet licenced for the treatment or prevention of postoperative nausea and vomiting.

Fujii, Y., Saitoh, Y., Tanaka, H. and Toyooka, H. (1998) Effective dose of granisetron for the prevention of post-operative nausea and vomiting in patients undergoing laparoscopic cholecystectomy. *European Journal of Anaesthesiology*, **15**, 287–91

3

Central nervous system depressants

Narcotics, hypnotics, anxiolytic sedatives, neuroleptics and general anaesthetics

'**Narcosis**' is a term once used widely to describe a progressive and reversible widespread depression of the central nervous system (CNS). The word is derived from the Greek for 'stupor', and its successive stages are well recognized: sedation, sleep and general anaesthesia – a progressive and deepening, unselective series of phenomena which, if pursued unremittingly, are eventually overtaken by coma and death. At one time, any chemical agent that induced narcosis would be called a '*narcotic*', but in recent years '*narcotics regulations*' around the world have covered both depressant and stimulant drugs of abuse, and the terms 'narcosis' and 'narcotic' are thus infrequently used, to avoid confusion.

Agents of a very diverse range of chemical structures are able to enter the CNS and exert depressant effects. For many of these agents their only obvious chemical similarity (which was thus linked to their possible mechanism of action) was their abundant lipid solubility, and for many years this property (*lipophilicity*) was thought to be the primary basis of their pharmacological actions, whether it was simple sedation or profound general anaesthesia. In some cases, different doses and/or different routes of administration of the same agent could be used to exert clinically different effects: thus the now redundant amylobarbital was sedative at 30 mg orally, hypnotic at 200 mg orally, or a general anaesthetic if 1.0 g was given intravenously. Perhaps more relevantly, between the 1930s and 1960s, one or other of the barbiturates would find a clinical use in epilepsy, anxiety, insomnia and anaesthesia, only their pharmacokinetic properties (namely short-, medium- or long-acting) determining their exact clinical purpose.

Whether or not the term is seldom used, anaesthetists continue to induce narcosis, a condition of insensibility or stupor from which only partial arousal can be achieved with simple physical stimuli such as noise, shaking or slapping, and the consequent 'arousal' is not sustained. Analeptic agents such as nikethamide can produce a type of arousal (or reversal) from the drug-induced narcosis because certain vital centres in the medulla may be stimulated; but unwanted adverse effects such as convulsions are an attendant danger with such reversal.

The discovery of the phenothiazine antihistamines in the late 1930s (H_1-antagonists as they are more precisely described today) raised the possibility of producing drug-induced partial or selective depression of CNS function. The sedation accompanying these antihistamines was atypical and did not develop to a full sleep or anaesthesia at higher doses and the term 'tranquillization' was coined to describe this new phenomenon. This 'selective' CNS depressant effect was thought to have a potential value in the treatment of mental illness, and prompted further development and the discovery of the phenothiazine 'major tranquillizers' (neuroleptics, antipsychotics) in the 1950s.

The benzodiazepine anxiolytics and sedatives (the 'minor tranquillizers') were discovered in the 1960s. Here was another group of agents which exerted profound CNS depressant effects which fell short of a genuine hypnotic or general anaesthetic action, until the introduction of diazepam, later superseded by midazolam, produced benzodiazepines capable of inducing anaesthesia. The clinical use of these agents over the last 30 years has informed and markedly changed our approach to the treatment of anxiety and sleep disorders.

'**Hypnotics**' is an older term used to describe drugs used primarily to promote sleep or to make people sleep more soundly when wakefulness is not due to cough or severe pain; in other words, they should induce a condition indistinguishable from natural sleep. In fact, even though the physiological state may resemble sleep, the EEG shows characteristic changes with most hypnotics. They are a class of depressant within the larger category of narcotics and some act mainly upon the reticular activating system. The difference in action between sedatives and hypnotics is mainly one of degree, the same groups of drugs being used to produce either effect, larger doses being necessary to ensure a hypnotic effect. Typical examples were the barbiturates, chosen according to the duration of action desired. Some antihistamine drugs, such as promethazine, are now principally employed for their sedative and hypnogenic actions, as are many benzodiazepines of short duration of action, such as temazepam, or the longer acting lorazepam and nitrazepam. Other drugs of widely differing chemical composition which are employed as hypnotics include chlormezanone and chloral.

Many drugs have various degrees of hypnogenic action, but their most powerful effect may be some other type of CNS depression, and this determines their classification. It is then correct to speak of the hypnotic effects of such drugs, but not of the drugs themselves as hypnotics. Morphine, for instance, can produce in a normal pain-free person a feeling of well-being, comfort and remoteness from the outside world that tempts sleep. It promotes sleep in a patient kept awake by pain even more so, but its main use is, of course, as an analgesic.

Conversely, true hypnotics given to a patient in slight pain, for example with a mild headache, can induce sleep, and in sleep the pain threshold is always raised. But when severe pain is present, hypnotics cannot induce sleep for they are not analgesics unless the dose is raised to an anaesthetic level. The same is true with regard to wakefulness due to cough, and sleep in the presence of severe pain or cough should therefore be induced by analgesics or cough suppressants primarily, combined with a hypnotic if necessary.

Overdose with hypnotics will lead to depression of the vasomotor and respiratory centres of the medulla. Anaesthesia can be produced with some benzodiazepines, but coma can be reversed with specific antagonists. Conversely, ketamine produces a condition in which the patient makes no response to the environment, while medullary centres are relatively undepressed even with large doses.

Distinction should be clear between the pharmacological use of the term hypnosis, meaning drug-induced sleep, and that of 'hypnosis' (originally called neurohypnosis), meaning the sleep-like state inducible in most people by suitable conditions of concentration and suggestion.

Anxiolytic sedatives (minor tranquillizers)

Before the introduction of the benzodiazepines in 1961, anxiety-related illness was treated with a variety of sedatives, usually involving the administration of small doses of agents (such as phenobarbital or amobarbital) which at higher doses would induce sleep. These were dangerous in overdose, a property not entirely desirable considering some of the mental states for which they were prescribed. A number of alternatives were available: traditional agents such as ethyl alcohol or chloral had a number of well-recognized problems, and had largely been replaced by some barbiturate derivatives such as glutethimide, thalidomide and chlomethiazole. Thalidomide, for example, contrasted strongly with the barbiturates, having a high therapeutic index and remaining safe in acute overdose. (Its more profound effects on the fetus, of course, have since been well recognized as well as its anti-tumour properties.)

Today, one still talks of the sedative effects of drugs, and they are certainly prescribed for their hypnotic effects. They are no longer classified as 'sedatives' or 'hypnotics' however, but as a class together – the 'anxiolytic sedatives' – a classification now promoted by the World Health Organization. Insomnia today is considered to be a manifestation of anxiety, and ostensibly is treated with the same anti-anxiety benzodiazepines, although the speed of onset and duration of action of some benzodiazepines make then better fitted than others for treating insomnia. Anxiolytic sedatives (*Figure 3.1*)

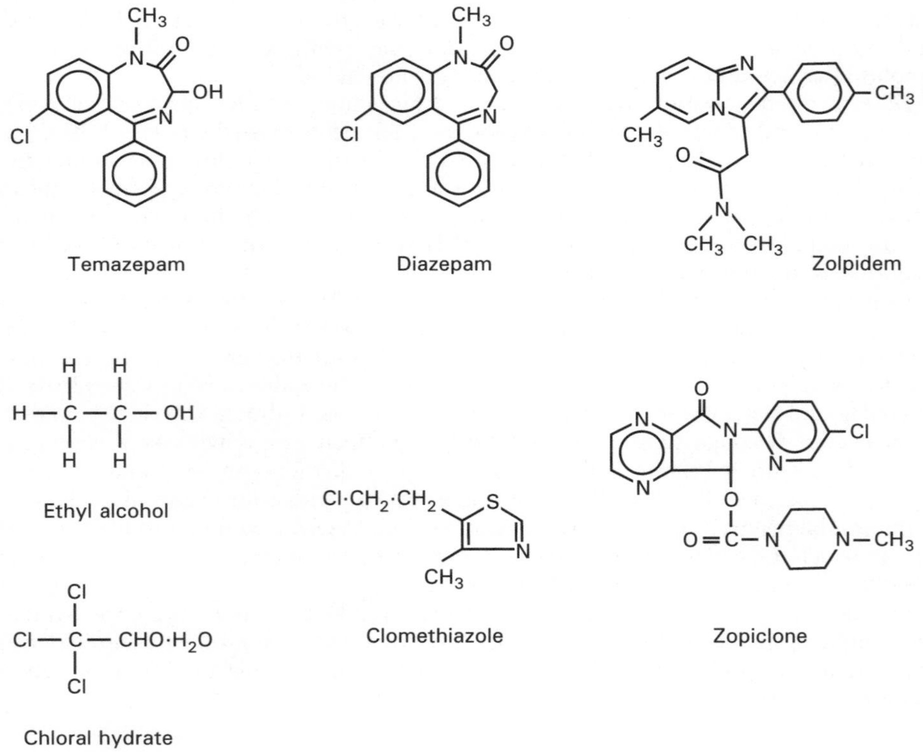

Figure 3.1 Structural formulae of some principal anxiolytic sedatives. Temazepam (benzodiazepine), zolpidem and zopiclone are short-acting anxiolytic sedatives used to induce sleep (treat insomnia). Diazepam is much longer acting and provides prolonged anxiolytic activity. Ethyl alcohol, chloral hydrate (and its derivatives) and clomethiazole are older alternatives

are drugs that reduce anxiety and may thus permit or promote sleep, and the term has largely replaced those of sedative, hypnotic or minor tranquillizer.

As with the earlier barbiturates, the sensible clinical use of individual benzodiazepines is closely linked to their pharmacokinetic properties. The benzodiazepines may be 'short acting' or 'long acting'. Drugs with a rapid onset and relatively short duration of action (such as triazolam, temazepam, oxazepam) are useful in the treatment of insomnia, usually at somewhat higher doses than those which can be used for intermittent or 'on demand' alleviation of anxiety. In contrast, longer acting benzodiazepines (for example, diazepam, chlordiazepoxide, nitrazepam, flunitrazepam) are used to promote sleep where continuing sedation is desirable the next day. Smaller doses of these same agents may be used in sustained or continuous treatment of anxiety.

Benzodiazepines

Pharmacological actions

Benzodiazepines act at specific receptors in the central nervous system which were first described by Mohler and Okada in 1977. The receptors are most dense in the cerebral cortex, hypothalamus, cerebellum, corpus striatum and medulla. This regional distribution closely parallels that of the receptors of the inhibitory neurotransmitter γ-aminobutyric acid (GABA). The receptors are not identical because the substances do not show competitive binding to the respective receptor sites. There are also high-affinity benzodiazepine binding sites in peripheral organs and in non-neural tissue in the CNS, whose function is unknown, and on plasma proteins.

Benzodiazepines differ from barbiturates in that they are not general neuronal depressants, but more selectively promote the actions of GABA. Herein may lie an explanation of their safety in overdose, their sparing of respiration at all but the highest doses, and their inability to produce surgical anaesthesia or coma. Electrophysiological studies show that the enhancement of GABA-induced inward chloride ion currents, which produce neuronal inhibition through membrane hyperpolarization and resistance to the propagation of nerve potentials, can be induced by benzodiazepines throughout the CNS. Of the two GABA-receptor sub-types presently recognized, benzodiazepines promote the function of $GABA_A$ receptors, the drug binding closely to a stereospecific receptor complex closely associated with the $GABA_A$ receptor. Benzodiazepines thus require intact $GABA_A$ receptors and GABA function to exert their effects, but the actual identity of the endogenous or natural ligand for this 'benzodiazepine receptor' remains unknown.

The interaction of different ligands at the benzodiazepine receptors is shown in *Figure 3.2*. Both GABA and benzodiazepine receptors are found on the cell surface. Benzodiazepines combine with the receptor and as a result change the effect of GABA on chloride channels, thus allowing chloride ions to enter the cell. This causes an increase in the neurone's resting membrane potential making it refractory to any excitatory impulse. By enhancing the effects of GABA in this way, benzodiazepines will inhibit certain pathways in the CNS.

The natural ligand for the benzodiazepine receptor is not known. Recently the concept of a central physiological anxiety system involved in arousal has been suggested, which would involve a central anxiogenic neurotransmitter. Drugs mimicking such a substance and binding to these receptors would cause anxiety and convulsions, and would be antagonized by benzodiazepines; such substances are known as inverse agonists. Partial agonists have been described for both the inhibitory and stimulatory aspects of benzodiazepine

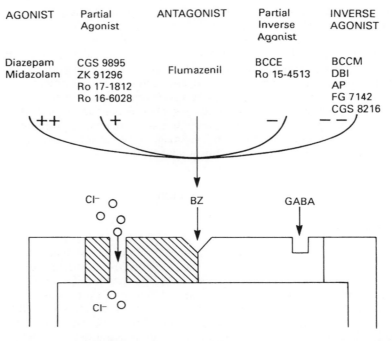

Figure 3.2 Interaction of ligands at the benzodiazepine receptor. The combination of a benzodiazepine with the receptor enhances the effects of GABA and allows chloride ions to enter the cells with resultant inhibition of certain pathways in the CNS. Substances binding with the system to cause anxiety are called inverse agonists. Like the opioids, there are also partial agonists. Partial inverse agonists also exist. These latter two are unable to exert a full effect at the receptor. BCCE and BCCM are β-carbolines; DBI, diazepam binding inhibitor; AP, anxiety peptide; CGS 9895, ZK 91296, Ro 17–1812, Ro 16–6028 and Ro 15–413 are chemical compounds that have not yet been named by the manufacturers. Flumazenil is an antagonist at the receptor which will reverse the effects of the agonist, partial agonist, inverse agonist and partial inverse agonist (Reproduced by courtesy of Professor J.G. Whitwam)

receptor functions as well as an antagonist, i.e. flumazenil. There are thus five groups of ligands for the benzodiazepine receptors, namely agonists (benzodiazepines), partial agonists, inverse agonists, partial inverse agonists and antagonists (flumazenil). Flumazenil will antagonize all the other four groups of ligands (Whitwam, 1987).

All benzodiazepines exert qualitatively the same depressant effects at every level of the neuraxis, although small differences in drug distribution or the pharmacodynamic sensitivities of individual parts of the CNS can yield subtle quantitative variations in clinical response. These differences can be magnified by the host of biologically active metabolites that are produced and which considerably enhance the overall duration of clinical effect.

The success of the benzodiazepines as therapeutic agents, accompanied by the virtual disappearance of the barbiturates, is due to their efficacy as anxiolytics, hypnotics and anticonvulsants, together with their flat log dose–effect curve (*Figure 3.3*) which gives a much greater safety margin. Thus their therapeutic index (ratio of effective to lethal dose) is high and even very large overdoses rarely result in serious side effects or death unless combined with alcohol. In fact, potentiation by most other CNS depressants is impor-

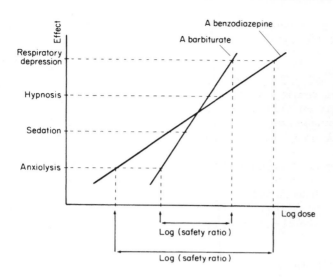

Figure 3.3 Diagrammatic representation of the high margin of safety of the benzodiazepines. Because of the flat dose–effect curves characteristic of the benzodiazepines, the ratio between the lethal dose and the therapeutically useful dose (for example, for anxiolysis) is very high compared with drugs like the barbiturates

tant. All the benzodiazepines have the full spectrum of activity depending on dose. They have five basic properties.

The most marked and predictable central effects are sedation, decreased anxiety, muscle relaxation, anticonvulsant activity, sleep and anterograde amnesia. Although higher dose levels increase the likelihood of sleep and even induction of 'light' anaesthesia when administered intravenously, none of the benzodiazepines produces a deep stupor or surgical anaesthesia typical of the sustained administration of a volatile anaesthetic. Their inhibition of the arousal system is of considerable use in anaesthesia because they potentiate the effects of other hypnotic drugs.

Anti-anxiety   Anxiolytic effects are seen with the lowest doses, but in severe anxiety and panic attacks, sedative or even hypnotic doses may have to be used.

Sedation   There is a decreased responsiveness to a constant level of stimulation, with a decrease in spontaneous activity. Increasing dosage will eventually produce sleep and the drugs have gained considerable popularity as hypnotics. Intravenously, benzodiazepines are used extensively to produce 'conscious sedation' during unpleasant procedures such as upper gastrointestinal endoscopy, bronchoscopy and dental treatment under local anaesthesia; they are also used during more major surgery under regional anaesthesia. As rapid recovery is required after these procedures, it is important that a drug with appropriate pharmacokinetic parameters is chosen, and hence midazolam has virtually replaced diazepam for this purpose.

Diazepam and midazolam have also been used as intravenous induction agents. Cardiovascular stability is a feature of such use, but the drugs are not as reliable and predictable as thiopental for induction and there is a wide variation between patients in the dose required to produce the desired effect. Midazolam, however, potentiates propofol in the techniques of co-induction (see page 110).

Anticonvulsant   Like most classes of sedative-hypnotics, benzodiazepines are capable of preventing and terminating convulsive activity. Clonazepam and diazepam are effective in status epilepticus, while the former is also of use in petit mal epilepsy.

Muscle relaxation Benzodiazepines reduce muscle tone and this is mediated via an action on interneurones in the spinal cord.

Amnesia
Intravenous benzodiazepines will reliably produce anterograde amnesia. Following diazepam and midazolam this is very intense for 20–30 minutes and hence a very useful property when performing short unpleasant endoscopic procedures. Longer amnesia, up to 6 h, has been reported following lorazepam. The amnesic effects of the benzodiazepines when given intramuscularly or orally is much more variable. The mechanism of the amnesic action is not known.

It is important to note that benzodiazepines are not analgesic or antidepressant. Small falls in blood pressure and cardiac output are most likely the consequences of a reduction in pre-existing centrally mediated anxiety. In very high plasma concentrations, such

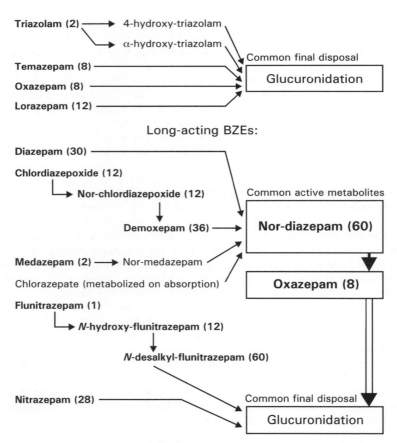

Figure 3.4 The important role of metabolism of benzodiazepines via active metabolites in determining the overall duration of activity as anxiolytic sedatives. Names in bold type followed by a numeral indicate a biologically active agent and its approximate half-life

as might follow intravenous administration, transient coronary dilatation has been attributed to a direct action on coronary vessels.

Pharmacokinetics

The clinical use of individual benzodiazepines is almost entirely determined by their pharmacokinetics. Some agents are rapidly absorbed by mouth and produce their effects within a few minutes, whereas others may induce their full pharmacological effects only after several hours. Further, some agents have only a relatively short duration of action before they are inactivated by hepatic metabolism and excreted by the kidneys. In marked contrast, the longer acting benzodiazepines are first metabolized via a series of pharmacologically-active intermediates before their glucuronidation, so that a single dose may exert significant pharmacological activity for several days. This is illustrated in *Figure 3.4.*

Short-acting benzodiazepines such as midazolam may be given intravenously or intramuscularly as an induction agent: the onset of action is rapid but the drug is quickly cleared from the body under most clinical circumstances. Other relatively short-acting benzodiazepines, such as temazepam or oxazepam, are used to relieve insomnia. They are rapidly absorbed following oral medication and are intended to provide a drug-induced sleep for the first few hours, the patient then continuing to sleep and awake refreshed and 'drug free', without hangover effects. Short-acting benzodiazepines, at lower doses, may also be used to provide 'on demand' relief of acute symptoms of anxiety, such as panic attacks and phobias.

Long-acting benzodiazepines, such as diazepam or chlordiazepoxide, have a slower onset of action following oral administration and, subsequently, a prolonged pharmacological action. At modest doses, administered just once or twice daily, they provide sustained relief from persistent symptoms of anxiety, the expectation being that such treatment may be required continuously over several days or weeks. Sedation and sleep may ensue – sleep particularly, if this has been denied by anxiety or concurrent illness and particularly if higher doses are administered. Because of their persistent pharmacological action, the long-acting benzodiazepines may also be used in some forms of epilepsy; and (rarely) will find a use in preventing the increased muscle tone of tetanus infection. Longer acting benzodiazepines are also used to treat resistant or recurrent insomnia (where the patient may awake in the middle of the night, notwithstanding treatment with a short-acting drug), and also where daytime sedation the following day may be desirable.

Not only do pharmacokinetic factors produce remarkable clinical differences between individual drugs, but inter-patient variation, particularly in the elderly, may also result in unpredictable quantitative variations in clinical response.

Distribution

With one or two exceptions, all benzodiazepines are completely absorbed following oral administration, and are subsequently rapidly and widely distributed throughout the body. Lipid solubility of individual agents varies between 'good' and 'very substantial'. After initially high levels in the brain and other well-perfused organs, benzodiazepines are redistributed into all compartments of the body, which means other major organs, across the placenta into the fetus, and into the human milk and the feeding infant. They are also substantially bound to plasma proteins. Thus, their widespread distribution, plasma protein binding and, for some, their metabolism via pharmacologically active intermediates, all contribute to a picture of a group of compounds, many of which have remarkable persistence in the body.

Although extensively metabolized in the liver, ultimately yielding water-soluble glucuronides which are excreted by the kidneys, the benzodiazepines do not induce liver enzymes, nor do they exert a major pharmacokinetic influence on other coincidentally administered drugs. However, pharmacodynamic potentiation of other CNS depressants, notably ethyl alcohol, can be important.

Tolerance and dependence

There are prescribing guidelines for oral benzodiazepines, and these include suggested maximum treatment periods and sensible upper dose limits. Adherence to these usually avoids serious abuse problems with these agents.

Tolerance and dependence (the former manifested by a patient-driven progressive increase in daily consumption of the drug, the latter by significant withdrawal symptoms when abruptly stopping or reducing medication) do occur but are usually predictable, and should therefore be avoidable. Problems are particularly likely to occur when insomnia has been treated every night for a prolonged period, especially in the elderly; and when daytime anxiety has been continuously treated with a relatively short-acting benzodiazepine. The use of higher doses of the longer acting benzodiazepines may also be associated with 'withdrawal symptoms', if the high dose is stopped or reduced abruptly. This is because at higher doses, e.g. 100 mg daily of diazepam, its pharmacokinetics may alter and the drug disappear more quickly from the body, thus delivering the same circumstances as one meets when discontinuing treatment with the short-acting drugs.

Pharmacodynamic tolerance appears to be a prerequisite of dependence, signalled by a need to increase the dose to maintain the pharmacological effect. This may be explained by a change in receptor sensitivity due to the drug's continuing presence in the tissues in excess of some threshold. This threshold almost certainly differs between patients. If the medication is stopped or its dose reduced abruptly (particularly if using a shorter acting benzodiazepine) the re-adaptation or return of the receptor to normal sensitivity may proceed more slowly than the drug's disappearance from the body. A sense of 'withdrawal' is then created, with accompanying drug craving by the patient. This clearly is an over-simplification of the clinical and biochemical events, but both tolerance and dependence can be minimized by adhering to published guidelines on dose and duration of treatment. The continuous daytime treatment of anxiety symptoms should be maintained using an agent with a prolonged duration of action from which eventual drug withdrawal should be carried out 'stepwise' over a period of several weeks. In patients with a previous history of alcohol or other substance abuse, benzodiazepines should be avoided. If anxiety must be treated pharmacologically in such cases, a modest dose of a sedative neuroleptic such as chlorpromazine or promazine should be substituted. The antidepressants amitriptyline and mianserin are also sedative and may be used at night to promote sleep.

Other adverse effects

At the time of maximal effect from a hypnotic dose of a benzodiazepine, lassitude, increased reaction time with motor incoordination, impairment of mental coordination, confusion and anterograde amnesia may all occur in varying degrees. These effects are potentiated, or may occur at lower doses, if another CNS depressant such as ethyl alcohol is co-administered. High doses (or overdose) are not accompanied by respiratory depression, unless other CNS depressants are present. They can, however, increase anoxia and hypercarbia in patients with existing obstructive sleep apnoea.

It follows that for any patient prescribed benzodiazepines, whether by oral or parenteral administration, driving a motor car or operating other hazardous machinery must be avoided for at least 24 h after stopping medication. Muscular weakness, blurred vision, headache, vertigo and gastro-intestinal symptoms are other, much less frequent, adverse effects, and again they will be enhanced by other CNS depressants.

There are a number of psychological effects that may accompany the use of short-acting benzodiazepines in insomnia. The normal pattern of sleep onset and the subsequent appearance and number of episodes of rapid eye movement (REM) sleep are frequently disturbed. Deficits in the overall proportion of REM sleep can lead to persistent tiredness or hangover effect upon waking the next day, features that may be made worse if sleep was promoted with a higher than normal dose, or with a longer acting drug. With repeated (every night) medication, some tolerance to these effects develops, to the extent that the proportion of REM returns to near normal. When medication is ceased, whether or not there is a return of the initial insomnia, sleep may be punctuated by nightmares and vivid dreams, and these can, in susceptible circumstances, lead to the appearance of symptoms of anxiety and tension during the working day. Adherence to the published guidelines on dose and duration of treatment of insomnia should keep these effects to a minimum.

Other anxiolytic sedatives: chemical variants

In recent years, several new and chemically different anxiolytic sedatives have been introduced. Of these zopiclone and zolpidem are important recent additions (see *Figure 3.1*).

Zopiclone and **zolpidem** produce qualitatively similar pharmacological effects to the benzodiazepines, and are believed to act by occupying the same, or similar, closely associated receptors and promoting the actions of the inhibitory neurotransmitter GABA at the $GABA_A$ receptors. At the time of their introduction, hopes were expressed that they would be devoid of the tolerance, dependence and other adverse effects that may accompany the use of benzodiazepines. Partly because both drugs are short acting, partly because they are only licensed for the treatment of insomnia, and partly because it is now possible to avoid tolerance and dependence even when giving benzodiazepines by careful selection of patients and treatment protocols, hard evidence of withdrawal effects or dependence upon these agents has not been demonstrated clinically. Both agents are effective in the treatment of insomnia: they act rapidly following oral administration, and their duration of action is suitably short. It is reported that they exert less interference on the stages of sleep (including the proportion of REM sleep) than do conventional benzodiazepines, and there is some evidence that their beneficial effects on insomnia may persist after stopping treatment.

Chloral hydrate has been used as a sedative or hypnotic agent for over a hundred years. It is rapidly absorbed after oral administration, being metabolized in the liver to trichloroethanol which is believed to be the active form. Its effects are less selective than the benzodiazepines, indeed it is more reminiscent of ethyl alcohol and the barbiturates, and is believed to interact with $GABA_A$ receptors in a similar manner. In overdose, its sedative and hypnotic effects are followed progressively by anaesthesia and coma, with death occurring following respiratory arrest. Although chloral hydrate syrup was once a popular 'over the counter' sleeping potion, chloral hydrate itself is irritant to mucous membranes, giving rise to an unpleasant taste and possible epigastric distress, nausea and occasional vomiting – effects usually avoided by administration after a light meal. Derivatives of chloral hydrate include cloral betaine and triclofos sodium. These formulations are intended to avoid the direct gastro-intestinal effects of chloral hydrate itself. There has been a recent revival of interest in these products for treatment of insomnia in the elderly, since the market withdrawal of triazolam in the United Kingdom.

Clomethiazole is another sedative drug useful for treating insomnia in the elderly. It has a rapid onset and short duration, and thus has minimal hangover effects. Like the benzodiazepines, it can interfere with sleep patterns, and its repeated use at night, followed by withdrawal, causes subsequent sleep disturbances characterized by bizarre dreams and nightmares. It is also useful as an anticonvulsant in status epilepticus, as a sedative in the restless elderly, and in assisting with the acute withdrawal from alcohol dependence in younger adults. The intravenous preparation is very dilute and has caused fluid overload and hypo-osmolarity of the plasma when given in large quantities.

Sleeplessness, or more correctly fear of sleeplessness, is a powerful psychological deterrent to recovery from physical and other causes of ill health. It is inevitable that assistance in achieving a prompt and predictable sleep is both requested by patients and given by physicians. There is no ideal anxiolytic or hypnotic, but prescribing guidelines help the benzodiazepines to meet most of the requirements.

Neuroleptics, major tranquillizers, anti-psychotics

The phenothiazine promethazine is profoundly sedative, yet increasing doses do not cause sleep, stupor or anaesthesia. The sedative or tranquillizing side effects of promethazine prompted further research for an agent of potential use in severe psychotic mental illness, resulting in the introduction in 1952 of the first phenothiazine neuroleptic, chlorpromazine. Such was the impact of this discovery that, within five years, it is estimated that more than 10 000 papers and publications appeared about new neuroleptic agents and their clinical potential in severe mental illness.

Today there is a substantial array of neuroleptics. Neuroleptics are used to treat psychotic patients with conditions such as schizophrenia and mania, while anaesthetists may use them in premedication, as an anti-emetic, in the technique of neuroleptanalgesia and in assisting with the cooling required for some forms of cardiovascular surgery

Table 3.1 Classification of neuroleptic agents into older or traditional neuroleptics* and atypical, newer neuroleptics†

Older, traditional neuroleptics
Phenothiazines:
 • with aliphatic side-chain (e.g. *chlorpromazine*)
 • with piperidine side-chain (*thioridazine*)
 • with piperazine side-chain (*fluphenazine*)
Thioxanthines:
 • with aliphatic side-chain (*chlorprothixine*)
 • with piperazine side-chain (*flupentixol*)
Butyrophenones
 (*haloperidol, droperidol*)
Atypical, newer neuroleptics
Various structures:
 (*clozapine, sulpiride, risperidone, olanzapine*)

* Where a non-specific dopamine-receptor antagonism is a major phenomenon in pharmacological properties.
† Where a combination of anti-serotonergic and selective antidopaminergic functions appear to contribute to drugs with fewer adverse effects, which improve 'negative' effects and are useful in resistant schizophrenia).

and neurosurgery. They may assist in providing analgesia in terminally ill patients when combined with an opioid drug; they may also be used in the treatment of phantom limb pain and some painful psychosomatic conditions of the back.

Neuroleptics structurally related to the three-ring structure of phenothiazine (for example, chlorpromazine, thioridazine, fluphenazine) or the later butyrophenone haloperidol, are looked upon as the traditional neuroleptics (see *Table 3.1* and *Figure 3.5*). Their anti-psychotic actions are generally attributed to a profound antagonism of dopamine function in the mesolimbic and related forebrain. They exert a more marked control of the 'positive' rather than 'negative' symptoms of schizophrenia and related psychotic conditions and they do not differentiate between different dopamine receptors, thus causing a wide range of adverse effects linked to the suppression of other dopaminergic activities in

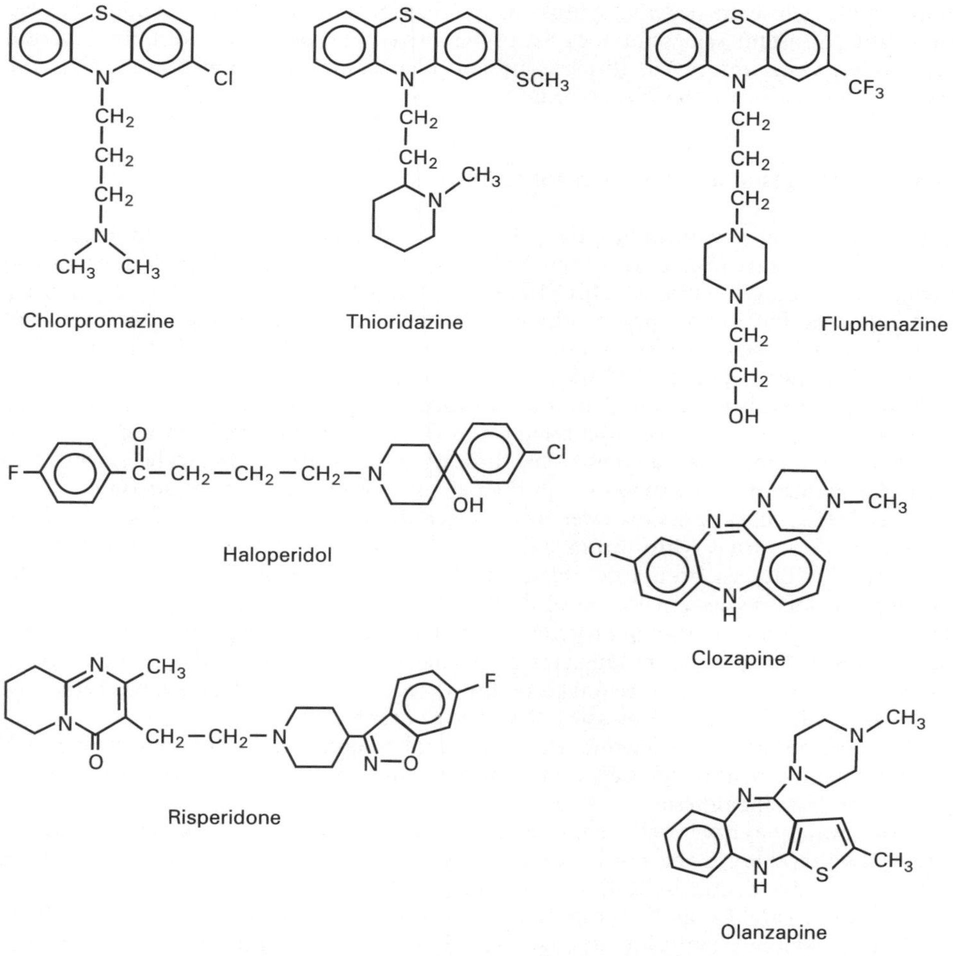

Figure 3.5 Structural formulae of old and new neuroleptics. Chlorpromazine, thioridazine and fluphenazine (phenothiazines) and haloperidol (butyrophenone) are traditional neuroleptics. Clozapine, risperidone and olanzapine are atypical structurally and pharmacologically

the brain. Many of them also possess an array of peripheral adverse effects although, for some agents such as chlorpromazine, these peripheral effects may be turned into useful clinical applications.

More recently, '*alternative*' or '*non-traditional*' neuroleptics have appeared. While the antagonism of dopaminergic function in the mesolimbic forebrain remains an important plank of their useful clinical anti-psychotic effects, an ability to modify other neuro-transmitter systems is a recognized desirable feature. Some agents possess antagonist properties at serotonin (notably 5-HT_2) receptors; others may affect α_2-adrenoceptors; while useful advances are also gained by sparing the (predominantly) D_1 dopaminergic receptors in the basal nuclei and in the tubero-infundibular pathway to the hypothala-mus. The former avoids the more severe extrapyramidal effects and the latter the endocrine disturbances. Some of the newer agents, perhaps because of their additional control of serotonergic and adrenergic transmission in the brain, are also claimed to be more active against the negative symptoms of schizophrenia. Certainly the opportunities for treating resistant schizophrenics with alternative neuroleptics or with combination therapy has vastly improved. Risperidone and olanzapine may soon become first-line drugs in the treatment of schizophrenia.

Neuroleptanalgesia and neuroleptanaesthesia

Neuroleptanalgesia was introduced in 1959 and has found a useful place in anaesthetic practice. It is a state produced by combining a potent neuroleptic drug with an opioid analgesic, commonly fentanyl. This mixture of drugs has been used in three basically different ways. For minor surgery where the stimulus is not too painful, an amount of analgesic can be given which is not enough to depress respiration dangerously. The technique is often supplemented with a local anaesthetic.

However, provided that ventilation is controlled, very large doses of analgesic can be given without producing loss of consciousness. This has, therefore, been used for adult patients undergoing artificial ventilation through a tracheal tube. It can be extended to the performance of major surgery with the patient in a mentally accessible state.

Nevertheless, most patients prefer to be unconscious, and it has been a short step to combining these drugs with nitrous oxide to produce what may be termed 'neurolept-anaesthesia'. This has been recommended for cardiopulmonary bypass in which the technique is less depressant to the cardiovascular system than other techniques and in which the analgesia and tranquillity can be extended into the postoperative period. It has also achieved wide popularity for neurosurgical anaesthesia. The technique produces no increase in CSF pressure or cerebral blood flow and, indeed, when fentanyl has been used as the analgesic, falls in CSF pressure have been observed.

The combination of neuroleptic drug, an opioid analgesic and a benzodiazepine such as midazolam can also be used to produce unconsciousness. This has been termed 'narconeurolept-anaesthesia'.

These techniques have been recommended for poor-risk and elderly patients. However, a long slow recovery is the norm. Additionally, many elderly patients have Parkinson's disease, a relative contra-indication to neuroleptic drugs.

In intensive care, haloperidol can be used to control the restlessness of so-called 'ICU psychosis', a state of confusion and agitation thought to be multifactorial in origin, and seen after a long episode of sedation and ventilation in intensive care. It is given intra-venously in doses of 5 mg, repeated at 10-minute intervals up to a maximum of 100 mg/day.

This is not the place to provide a full review of the newer neuroleptic drugs, but some outline is necessary for those agents most likely to assist the anaesthetist, and their important features are reviewed here rather than as individual monographs.

Chlorpromazine possesses a range of central and peripheral pharmacological actions. As a non-specific dopamine receptor antagonist, it blocks all dopaminergic pathways in the CNS: blockade of dopaminergic receptors in mesolimbic system and related forebrain areas probably underpins its clinically useful antipsychotic actions. On the other hand, blockade of dopaminergic receptors in the basal ganglia leads to extrapyramidal effects, although clinically these are less troublesome with chlorpromazine; blockade of dopaminergic function in the hypothalamus interferes with endocrine function.

Chlorpromazine's neurotransmitter blocking actions spread much wider than this, however, exerting antagonistic effects at serotonin (5-HT), adrenergic, cholinergic (muscarinic) and histaminergic receptors. So broad are chlorpromazine's pre- and post-synaptic actions that it has been described as a 'membrane stabilizing' agent. Furthermore, all of these properties are extended to the peripheral nervous system. The drug thus shows little fundamental difference from its immediate ancestor, promethazine, although there is a considerable shift of balance of pharmacological potency towards the CNS.

Chlorpromazine is profoundly sedative, perhaps as a consequence of its blocking actions on 5-HT and histamine function in the brain. This limits the drug's usefulness for long-term treatment of psychotic illness but makes it more useful in initial treatment or in crisis situations, in which a very wide dose range is available for safe treatment. Its anti-muscarinic actions limit the appearance of drug-induced Parkinson-like effects. It is also a useful anxiolytic when benzodiazepines are contra-indicated.

In the periphery, its membrane stabilizing properties make it useful in controlling nausea and vomiting, in acute anaphylactic or allergic and inflammatory conditions where sedation and anti-anxiety effects are useful companions; it suppresses itching and will control most instances of intractable hiccup. Combined with opioid analgesics, it makes it possible to reduce the dose or extend the duration of action of most opioids, particularly in terminal pain. It causes some vasodilatation and consequent minor fall in blood pressure.

Absorption of phenothiazines following oral administration is generally good. If in doubt, parenteral administration increases bioavailability. The drugs are highly lipophilic and substantially protein bound, and they accumulate predominantly in the CNS, the lungs and other well-perfused organs and tissues. They cross the placenta and enter the fetal circulation; they also pass into human milk. Plasma half-lives are long, and the pharmacological effects of single doses usually exceed 24 h. The exact duration of pharmacological effect is difficult to predict because of their complex and parallel (alternative) routes of hepatic oxidative metabolism which may proceed at different rates, producing metabolites of differing biological potency and, of course, with quantitative differences between patients. The eventual products are hydrophilic metabolites which are excreted by the kidneys, sometimes over several days or weeks. Chlorpromazine can also cause a long-lasting cholestatic jaundice.

Promazine and to a lesser extent **thioridazine** share a similar balance of central and peripheral actions, making them versatile drugs for short-term treatment of a wide variety of clinical needs, and the most likely agents to assist in the general management of patients pre- and post-surgically.

Fluphenazine is a phenothiazine with a piperazine side chain. The balance of central to peripheral effects is weighted heavily towards the CNS, and more specifically orientated toward antagonism at all dopamine receptors. It thus provides a potent, long-term, sedation-free treatment for schizophrenia and related psychoses, but does trigger extrapyramidal and endocrine adverse effects. It is also available as an intramuscular depot injection of the ester, fluphenazine decanoate, which provides long-term stable medication for 3–5 weeks' duration. Patients administered a depot injection of this type must first be shown to be responsive to the more conventional (oral) form of medication, before transfer to the depot.

Flupentixol is a thioxanthene neuroleptic which shows structural and pharmacological and clinical similarities to fluphenazine. It too is available as a depot injection, flupenthixol decanoate.

Haloperidol was the first of the butyrophenone neuroleptics, and remains the most widely used. Although structurally different from the three-ring structure of the phenothiazines (see *Figure 3.5*), a close chemical affinity can be seen by comparing three-dimensional models of the butyrophenone and phenothiazine drugs. Haloperidol does have some significant pharmacological differences from chlorpromazine: its peripheral effects are much reduced, while its central effects are more specific. It has no demonstrable antihistaminic or anticholinergic actions, and its antagonism at α-adrenoceptors is much reduced. In marked contrast, it does exert profound antagonistic activity at dopamine receptors, D_1 and D_2, rendering it simultaneously a potent anti-schizophrenic agent but one which also elicits marked extrapyramidal and endocrine adverse effects.

At equivalent anti-psychotic doses (5 mg haloperidol is roughly equivalent to 100 mg chlorpromazine), haloperidol causes minimal sedation and is the better agent for the long-term control of previously diagnosed psychotic conditions, including providing long-term prophylaxis against relapse. In addition to schizophrenia, haloperidol is used against other psychoses including mania and hypomania, paranoia, aggression, hyperactivity syndromes and self-mutilation disorders, and in certain organic conditions following upon brain damage. Other conditions in which it may be of value include intractable hiccup, Gilles de la Tourette syndrome, nausea and vomiting. It is also used in comparable conditions in children. In addition to oral preparations, haloperidol is available as an intramuscular depot injection, doses of 50 mg (initially) up to 300 mg providing about 4 weeks maintenance therapy.

Droperidol is a related butyrophenone neuroleptic which, as an injection, may be used in neurolept-analgesia (with an opioid analgesic such as fentanyl); in premedication; to control vomiting elicited by chemotherapy, and for the rapid calming of manic and/or agitated patients. It is also effective in small (<2.5 mg) doses given as premedication to reduce the incidence of postoperative nausea and vomiting.

Atypical, new neuroleptics

Although the non-sedative phenothiazines currently remain important agents in the control of schizophrenia and related psychotic conditions, they have always suffered two major disadavantages: they poorly control the negative symptoms of schizophrenia, if at all, and they induce serious and intrusive extrapyramidal effects. Consequently, compliance and cooperation with treatment strategies is at best unpredictable. These serious flaws have been addressed in various ways by the newer atypical or non-traditional neuroleptics described below.

Clozapine was introduced in the 1960s, and represented the first challenge to the well-established neuroleptics. From our knowledge today of the dopamine receptor subtypes, it is clear that clozapine has only a modest antagonistic action at D_1 receptors, which are believed to be the predominant post-synaptic receptors found in the basal ganglia and the hypothalamus; its adverse effects on the extrapyramidal and endocrine systems are thus markedly less. In contrast, clozapine is an effective D_2 receptor antagonist, receptors which are important in the mesolimbic forebrain, and it is thought that therein lies its major contribution to the control of the symptoms of schizophrenia. Clozapine also possesses central antimuscarinic and antiserotonergic properties at $5\text{-}HT_2$

receptors. Because of clozapine's propensity to cause agranulocytosis, there is a requirement for routine white blood cell counts and thus its use has been restricted. Nevertheless it has established itself in clinical use as an effective neuroleptic of modest potency, offering an alternative in patients with distressing and intrusive extrapyramidal effects induced by traditional agents, and also in patients where resistance is recognized and/or there is a need to alleviate negative symptoms.

Sulpiride shows a high degree of specificity for D_2 receptors, although extrapyramidal symptoms do occur in about 10 per cent of patients.

Several newer agents have become available in the early 1990s. It remains to be seen which, if any, of these become first-line medication.

Risperidone combines marked antagonism at 5-HT_2 and α-adrenoceptors with blockade at D_2 receptors, although the first may be the predominant effect. Risperidone has proved to be an anti-schizophrenic drug which is effective in previously treatment-resistant patients. Claims that it attenuates the negative symptoms as emphatically as the positive symptoms of schizophrenia require further confirmation, although quantifying the incidence and severity of negative symptoms is notoriously difficult. Risperidone also has some antihistaminic activity and modifies adrenergic function at α_1- and α_2-receptors. The contribution these additional properties make to clinical activity is unknown, but it is clear that risperidone is an antagonist at D_1 receptors only at the higher clinical doses. It is thus possible to prevent both extrapyramidal and endocrine effects even in long-term treatment.

Olanzapine blocks α-adrenoceptors, 5-HT_2, muscarinic-, and D_2 receptors, also sparing the D_1 receptors and avoiding the extrapyramidal adverse effects. Olanzapine has been shown to be a clinically effective anti-schizophrenic drug, and there is perhaps better evidence for this agent's ability to control both 'positive' and 'negative' symptoms.

From a review of the pharmacological actions and clinical effects of not only these, but still newer agents such as **quetiapine, amisulpride, seroquel** and **sertindole**, it appears that a combination of selective D_2, 5-HT_2 and α-adrenoceptor antagonism in the CNS produces agents which may be clinically effective in resistant schizophrenia, improve 'negative' as well as 'positive' symptoms and are relatively free from adverse effects on the extrapyramidal system and endocrine function. The importance of antagonism at other CNS neurotransmitter receptors, for example histamine and acetylcholine has yet to be determined.

Neuroleptics or anti-psychotic substances are important in anaesthesia for two reasons:

- Specific examples may be administered to assist in the management of the patient, for example in premedication, during anaesthesia and postoperatively.
- Patients for anaesthesia may present with ongoing neuroleptic medication. Most neuroleptics can profoundly affect the response of various physiological systems to anaesthetics and anaesthetic adjuvants. Whether to continue or discontinue such existing neuroleptic therapy requires planning. Where depot preparations have been recently given, such a choice may not be available in a surgical emergency.

Intravenous induction agents

Drugs with various chemical groupings are capable of inducing rapid loss of consciousness when given parenterally, and include thiopental, methohexital, ketamine, etomidate, propofol and midazolam.

The usefulness of such drugs for this purpose is determined by certain physical properties that they have in common and it is convenient to consider them together rather than scattered throughout the text under their various chemical groupings.

The thiobarbiturates were the first group of drugs to be widely employed as intravenous induction agents and thiopental, the most popular member of this group, was the only satisfactory agent for the induction of anaesthesia for nearly 30 years. Then came the methylated barbiturates, but only methohexital was sufficiently free of excitatory side effects to be of value. Yet another approach has been what has been termed 'dissociative' anaesthesia with ketamine, which has an unusual mode of action. There is a loss of consciousness and an intense analgesia associated with muscle relaxation and yet the pharyngeal and laryngeal reflexes remain brisk. The principal drawback to its use has been the intense dreaming and psychomotor activity which may occur, but it is still very popular in very deprived surroundings where there is no anaesthetist or no proper anaesthetic equipment.

A somewhat different approach has been the development of steroids with anaesthetic activity, but none is available at the moment for clinical use (see below).

γ-Hydroxybutyrate was used as an intravenous induction agent in the 1960s. An intravenous dose of 50–60 mg/kg induces general anaesthesia within 5 minutes, which lasts 1–2 h. This is usually accompanied by a slight rise in blood pressure and a bradycardia; respiration slows and may be irregular. Recovery is clear headed, as it is metabolized to CO_2 and water with no active metabolites. However, its use was associated with a high incidence of myoclonia and vomiting. The drug has no action at $GABA_A$ receptors, but has partial agonist activity at $GABA_B$ receptors.

Unfortunately, γ-hydroxybutyrate is being increasingly used for recreational purposes and has a high abuse potential. It is rapidly absorbed by mouth and produces a state of euphoria and relaxation. Overdose is associated with coma and seizure activity. It cannot be detected by toxicological tests and a high incidence of suspicion must be held in patients showing these features. It has been used in some centres in the treatment of narcolepsy.

The development which has done most to change practice has been the introduction of propofol in an acceptable formulation. In Britain it is now the most commonly used intravenous induction agent, being associated with a more clear-headed recovery and a lower incidence of laryngospasm, causes less nausea and vomiting and because it may be given more safely to asthmatic patients than thiopental. Its rapid metabolism makes it suitable for continuous intravenous anaesthesia, a technique for which barbiturates had proved unsuitable.

Pharmacokinetics of intravenous induction agents

If a drug is to be of value as an intravenous induction agent, then there are certain properties it must possess. Only the non-ionized fraction of the drug is able to penetrate the blood–brain barrier; a protein-bound drug is also unable to cross into the brain and all the intravenous anaesthetics are to some extent protein bound. The degree of ionization of a drug will depend on body pH and the pK_a of the drug. The pK_a is the negative logarithm of the dissociation constant of the drug and at 50 per cent ionization, the pK_a is the same as the pH. The stronger an acid, then the lower the pK_a; the stronger a base, the higher the pK_a. This becomes important when a drug has a pK_a that is close to body pH, when small changes in the latter cause a large change in the degree of ionization of a drug. Thus thiopental, which is a weak acid, has a pK_a of 7.6 and at the normal pH of blood is about 60 per cent un-ionized. In conditions of acidosis, more of the thiopental will be in the un-ionized form and a greater sensitivity to the drug can be expected.

Intravenous induction agents which readily cross the blood–brain barrier will produce sleep in one arm-brain circulation time, although ketamine is significantly slower in onset than the other agents when given intravenously. Midazolam has a much slower onset of action due to its lower lipid solubility. Ketamine is also unique in that effective narcosis can be produced by the intramuscular route, although this usually takes 2–4 minutes and occasionally longer.

The distribution of the intravenous induction agents will depend on their lipid solubility and the blood flow to the various tissues of the body. As these drugs are all highly fat soluble, and as the brain, together with the heart and viscera, belongs to the vessel-rich group, they will rapidly enter the brain and produce unconsciousness. These well-perfused viscera will subsequently be depleted of the drug by redistribution to lean tissues, such as muscle and bone. The blood supply of fat is so poor that it plays little part in the initial distribution of the drug which results in early awakening. However, by 2–4 h, 67–75 per cent of the dose of thiopental which is still in the body is deposited in fat.

The initial distribution from the vessel-rich group to the lean tissues is the principal mechanism leading to recovery of consciousness following a single induction dose of thiopental, although hepatic metabolism does play some role. The metabolic pathways for thiopental, however, are easily saturated so that on repeat administration, metabolism becomes a zero-order process. Recovery will then depend on redistribution: as more thiopental is given and the lean tissues become saturated with the drug, they lose the ability to assist in redistribution away from the brain. Prolonged coma and recovery can therefore be expected on repeated administration of thiopental and it is thus unsuitable for use by continuous infusion. Similar remarks also apply to methohexital, although the time course will be slightly different. With non-barbiturates, such as etomidate and propofol, redistribution plays a role in recovery after a single dose, but metabolism is of greater importance. The rapidity of metabolism of these drugs, which follows a first-order process, means that they can be given by continuous infusion and still allow rapid recovery.

A number of factors can alter the clinical effects of the intravenous anaesthetics, but one of the most important is the volume of the central pool into which the drug is injected. In conditions of hypovolaemia, the concentration of the drug will be increased and its distribution altered. Blood supply to the brain is maintained, but that to many of the other vessel-rich groups will be reduced by vasoconstriction. The brain will thus receive a greater proportion of any intravenously administered drug than usual and this explains the marked sensitivity of shocked patients to thiopental, for example.

Steroids

It has been known for many years that some steroids possess hypnotic properties. Their attraction has been their high therapeutic index and a number have been used clinically. Unfortunately, each has been associated with a number of adverse effects and none is available at the moment for clinical use.

Eltanolone (pregnanolone) is the most recent steroid shown to have anaesthetic properties in animals. It is not soluble in water and is presented as an emulsion. Initial studies in human volunteers have shown pregnanolone to be similar to Althesin, with rapid induction of, and recovery from, anaesthesia following a dose of 0.05 mg/kg. Haemodynamic changes were minor and there was slight depression of ventilation. Unfortunately, a number of patients developed severe myoclonic activity and further investigations have been abandoned.

Other sedatives and hypnotics

Barbiturates

Barbiturates were introduced near the beginning of the twentieth century but are of decreasing therapeutic importance. They are used as their soluble salts.

Classification

The barbiturates are structurally related to one another. Within the basic barbiturate skeleton (*Figure 3.6*), substitutions in three sites affect potency, duration of action and convulsant or anticonvulsant properties. They have traditionally been classified according to the duration of action of a single hypnotic dose into long, medium, short and ultra-short acting. Long- and medium-acting drugs are used as sedatives. In fact, it may be impossible to distinguish between the hypnotic effects of drugs in each category. The Medicines Control Agency has recommended the adoption of an international agreement in which barbiturates which have traditionally ended in -one in the United Kingdom, will in future terminate in -al (see Appendix).

In general, the duration of action reflects the speed of redistribution and mode of elimination by the body; the more brief the action, the greater the amount broken down in the liver prior to renal excretion.

There is little justification for the continued prescription of barbiturates as sedatives and hypnotics, mainly because of the dangers of overdose, their tendency to produce habituation, and the fact that safer alternatives are now available.

Pharmacology

Central nervous system   The barbiturates appear to act at all levels of the CNS, but the basis of their clinical usefulness is the greater sensitivity of the cerebral cortex and reticular activating system compared with that of the vital medullary centres.

Sleep induced by hypnotic doses of barbiturates closely resembles normal sleep, but the EEG shows characteristic changes. There is an initial diminution in the REM sleep. With continued usage this recovers, and after stopping the administration there is a rebound increase in REM sleep. Narcotic doses, however, produce other changes in the EEG which depend on dosage. Initial fast activity gives way progressively to slow-wave high-voltage activity with superimposed bursts of fast activity (the K-complex), and then to periods of electrical silence punctuated by bursts of activity (burst-suppression). With increasing doses, the intervals of electrical silence become progressively longer.

The barbiturates have no significant analgesic action, and in lower concentrations may actually have an antianalgesic effect. Their use in hypnotic doses in the presence of severe pain may produce restlessness and delirium. This propensity makes the use of barbiturates unsuitable for use as sole anaesthetic agents.

In adequate doses all barbiturates can prevent convulsions but barbiturates with a phenyl group show some specific anticonvulsant action, and phenobarbital and methylphenobarbital are used in the treatment of epilepsy, their prolonged action being an important factor in clinical management.

Barbiturate skeleton

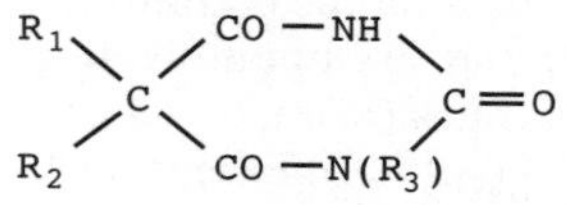

Thiopental

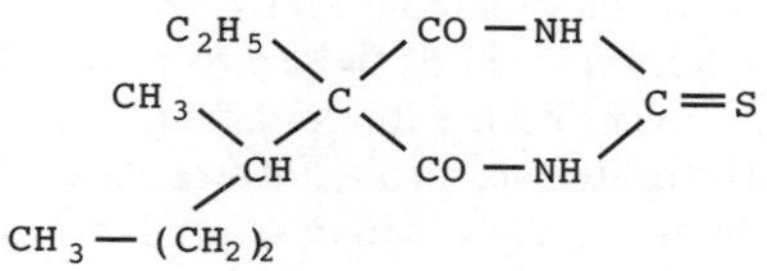

Methohexital

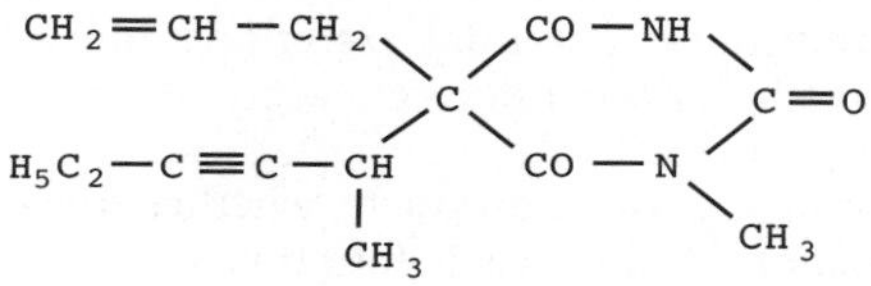

Phenobarbital

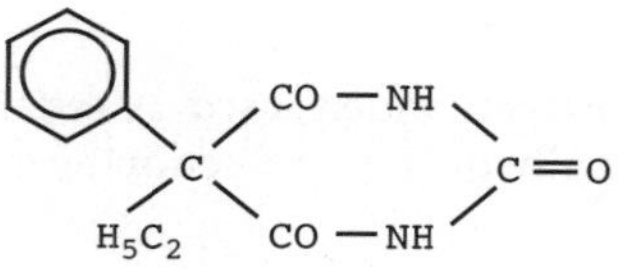

Figure 3.6 The barbiturate skeleton and some commonly used barbiturates

Autonomic nervous system   The barbiturates have only minor effects on the autonomic nervous system when given in the usual doses.

Cardiovascular system   Normal hypnotic doses of barbiturates have little effect upon the cardiovascular system, but a slight fall in blood pressure and pulse rate may occur. Larger doses cause a fall in blood pressure, due mainly to a direct depressant action on the vasomotor centres. The severe cardiovascular complications of overdose of barbiturates are mainly secondary to respiratory depression.

Respiratory system   The barbiturates are respiratory depressants, the chief action being a reduction in the sensitivity of the respiratory centre to carbon dioxide. They have no antitussive effect.

Placenta   All the barbiturates cross the placental barrier.

Metabolism   Oxygen uptake is reduced and metabolic rate diminished. Most barbiturates cause increased activity of liver microsomal enzymes. This is particularly the case with phenobarbital, for which purpose it is a commonly employed research tool. This property is utilized therapeutically in Gilbert's disease (inherited hyperbilirubinaemia).

Fate in the body   After absorption, the barbiturates are distributed in all tissues and fluids of the body. In the blood, they are bound to the plasma albumin fraction, the amount varying for different barbiturates (from 70–80 per cent in the case of thiopental to negligible amounts in the case of barbital). Except for barbital and phenobarbital, equilibrium between the brain and plasma is rapidly attained. With thiopental, the CSF concentration rapidly reaches the plasma concentration.

The barbiturates are eliminated both by hepatic metabolism and by renal excretion. Most are removed by a combination of these two routes. In general, the shorter acting drugs are metabolized by the liver and the longer acting ones are removed mainly by renal excretion.

The classic barbiturates are broken down solely by oxidation of their alkyl side chains and give rise to hypnotically inactive compounds. Thiobarbiturates also undergo desulphuration to yield barbiturates with a hypnotic activity similar to that of the original substances. After thiobarbiturate anaesthesia, hypnotically active substances can be detected in the plasma for 3–5 days, but for no longer than 24 h with pentobarbital and N-methylbarbiturates. The total excretion time of demonstrable metabolic products is 3–7 days with the thiobarbiturates, which is similar to that found with the long-acting barbiturate hypnotics.

Renal clearance of these products, whether free or conjugated with glucuronic acid, is by a combination of glomerular filtration and back-diffusion, similar to that of urea.

Indications

Barbiturates have been widely used as sedatives, hypnotics and basal narcotics, but are now used principally only as induction agents and anticonvulsants.

Routes of administration

Barbiturates are readily absorbed from the gastro-intestinal tract, especially the sodium salts. Rectal administration may be employed when oral administration is impracticable. Intravenous administration is now confined to thiopental and methohexital.

Precautions

Barbiturates induce increased synthesis of δ-aminolaevulinic acid synthetase, and are therefore contraindicated in porphyria. They should be used with caution in severe liver and kidney disease. They are best avoided in the presence of pain unless combined with a suitable analgesic. Contra-indications to the use of thiobarbiturates are discussed under thiopental.

Natural idiosyncrasy to the barbiturates is rare, but acquired idiosyncrasy or sensitization may occur, particularly in subjects with a tendency to allergy.

Chronic toxicity may occur due to cumulation, leading to drowsiness, slowness of thought, failing memory, incoherent speech, mental depression, confusion and disorientation.

Barbiturates are drugs of habituation and withdrawal symptoms occur when their administration is withheld. This complication occurs more frequently with the short-acting compounds given in high dosage.

Poisoning

Acute barbiturate poisoning due to overdose, usually taken with suicidal intent, still occurs. Accidental deaths can result from taking alcohol with barbiturates. Overdose gives rise to various degrees of central depression and their sequelae. In mild cases, respiratory exchange is usually adequate, and although the patient may be restless or in a deep sleep, bodily functions are within normal limits. Little or no treatment is necessary. In more severe cases coma is marked, respiration may be inadequate, the skin is cold and moist and often cyanotic, the pupils react sluggishly and may become dilated, cardiovascular depression may cause a fall in blood pressure, and reflexes are depressed or absent. Core temperature is often low. Hypostatic pneumonia may develop later. The hypophyseal–hypothalamic mechanism of release of antidiuretic hormone is stimulated and this, together with the lowered blood pressure, decreases the rate of renal excretion of barbiturates.

Treatment Conservative management is employed comparable to the management of the anaesthetized patient. Ventilatory support, if required, and maintenance of normal blood volume and fluid balance are essential. Myocardial depression, which may be seen in severe cases, is treated with infusions of inotropic drugs. The use of analeptics is avoided. Gastric lavage is only worth while if the drug has been taken orally within the previous 4 h.

Forced diuresis in the treatment of drug overdosage

If a drug is excreted by the kidneys, the fall in plasma concentration, once equilibrium has been attained, is exponential and the half-life of a drug in plasma is governed by its volume of distribution in body fluids and the rate at which it is cleared by renal excretion:

$$\text{Half-life} = \log_e 2 \times \frac{\text{Volume of distribution in ml}}{\text{Renal clearance in ml/minute}}$$

$$(\log_e 2 = 0.69)$$

The rate of its elimination from the body can be increased by inducing a high urine output and, in the case of some drugs, by altering urine pH.

Drugs that pass readily through lipid membranes may have their clearance reduced by back-diffusion from tubular fluid to peritubular blood. During diuresis the concentration of the drug in the distal part of the nephron is kept relatively low and there is, therefore, a relatively small concentration gradient for back-diffusion and a relatively high clearance.

The excretion of acidic or basic drugs may be considerably altered by urine pH. This is because the non-ionized moiety is much more diffusible than the ionized moiety. Raising the urine pH will increase the ionization, and hence the clearance, of acidic drugs; lowering it will do so for basic drugs. These increases of clearance with pH can be very large. For example, salicylate clearance can be increased approximately four-fold for each rise of one unit in urine pH.

Forced diuresis is only of value in certain well-defined instances of drug overdosage. It has little to offer in the management of overdosage with short- and medium-acting barbiturates or any of the tranquillizing drugs that have superseded them. It is most applicable to salicylate and phenobarbital overdosage, when it should be combined with measures designed to render the urine alkaline.

Methods of increasing urine output include intravenous infusion of large quantities of crystalloid fluid and administration of diuretics such as furosemide or mannitol. Both of these strategies are potentially dangerous in the presence of certain drugs or certain medical conditions. Alkalinization of the urine can be achieved by an intravenous infusion of sodium bicarbonate. It will not be successful if there is concomitant hypokalaemia. The use of acetazolamide to alkalinize the urine is not recommended because of the systemic metabolic acidosis that will occur.

In barbiturate overdose, the main dangers are related to depression of ventilatory drive, airway reflexes, fluid balance control and temperature regulation. Supportive treatment of these is routine in modern intensive care, and attempts to increase the rate of elimination of the barbiturate must balance the small risk of a somewhat prolonged stay in the intensive care unit with the very real dangers inherent in forced alkaline diuresis. The patients who are most likely to benefit from attempts to reduce plasma barbiturate levels are those with such severe poisoning that toxic effects are evident on the central nervous and cardiovascular systems. Unfortunately, these are the very patients who will tolerate forced alkaline diuresis least well. In practice, mild alkalinization with sodium bicarbonate (with no forced diuresis) is reasonably safe in moderate levels of poisoning, and severe cases will be treatable only with haemofiltration, haemodialysis or charcoal haemoperfusion. Of these, the first is the most commonly available and is also the least hazardous in the presence of cardiovascular depression.

Anticonvulsants

Since convulsions may be produced by a number of different metabolic and pathological conditions as well as by convulsant drugs or by electrical stimulation of the CNS, it is not surprising that anticonvulsants in general do not form a well-knit group. The correct antidotes for convulsions due to asphyxia or to hypoglycaemia are obvious and are aimed at their cause, but where convulsions are due to a cause that cannot be rapidly remedied, then recourse must be had to substances that prevent the CNS discharges, or sometimes only the peripheral motor function.

A large number of CNS depressants will control convulsions, but many of these do so only in doses that produce profound sedation or even anaesthesia. For example, this is true of many barbiturates and clomethiazole. Others produce a useful degree of motor depression in doses that have demonstrable but not incapacitating soporific effects, for example phenobarbital, methylphenobarbital and the benzodiazepines. A few drugs, such as carbamazepine and phenytoin, exert anticonvulsant actions at dose levels that do not cause overt drowsiness. Carbamazepine is additionally of interest in that it is effective in the control of the paroxysmal pain of trigeminal neuralgia in many patients.

A more recent development has been stimulation of inhibitory transmission. GABA (γ-aminobutyric acid) is a major CNS transmitter with inhibitory effects at interneuronal synapses and its concentration can be increased by inhibition of its catalytic enzyme. Vigabatrin is a synthetic derivative of GABA and an irreversible inhibitor of GABA transaminase which is now available as an anticonvulsant.

In the case of electroconvulsive therapy for the treatment of depression, it is thought to be disadvantageous to quell the electrical activity and only the peripheral motor manifestations are a hazard. These are controlled with muscle relaxants, the usual choice being suxamethonium, although rocuronium may offer advantages.

Convulsions encountered occasionally by the anaesthetist include those caused by drugs. The most common are local anaesthetics and some other anti-arrhythmic drugs, particularly those with anticholinergic actions, psychotropic drugs, particularly chlorpromazine, analeptics and radiographic contrast media. Convulsions are almost always

Table 3.2 Types of epilepsy and drugs of choice

Type of epilepsy	Drugs
Grand mal	Phenytoin, phenobarbital, primidone, vigabatrin
Petit mal (3 Hz spike and wave)	Sodium valproate, ethosuximide
Focal epilepsy (motor and sensory)	Phenytoin, phenobarbital, vigabatrin
Temporal lobe (psychomotor)	Carbamazepine, pheneturide, sultiame
Myoclonic and infantile spasms	Clonazepam, sodium valproate
Neonatal fits	Phenytoin, phenobarbital

associated with high brain concentrations. These are best treated with diazepam, midazolam or a small dose of thiopental.

Drug treatment of epilepsy

Not all the manifestations of epilepsy involve overt motor seizures; the most appropriate drug therapy is dependent on the type of epilepsy and a general guide is given in *Table 3.2*. Side effects are common with anti-epileptic drugs, particularly when starting treatment. Changes of dosage should be gradual and made under regular supervision. Estimation of plasma levels of some drugs, particularly of phenytoin, can help to avoid toxic effects.

Many of these compounds also interfere with folate production and cause megaloblastic anaemia. The incidence of congenital malformation is roughly three times higher than normal in children born to women being treated with anticonvulsants.

Phenobarbital is a barbiturate (for structural formula see *Figure 3.6*) whose duration of action may be as long as 8–16 h. Hangover effects can be marked when other than minimal doses are given. Besides having powerful sedative action on the CNS, it specifically depresses the motor cortex and so has an anticonvulsant action which makes it useful in epilepsy. Part is broken down by the liver and other tissues, but the majority is excreted unchanged in the urine, the rate of excretion being increased if the urine is alkaline.

Phenobarbital is given by mouth. The sodium salt has the same action as the acid, but being soluble in water can also be given parenterally. A dose of 15–30 mg 2–3 times a day is generally sufficient for the control of epileptic seizures, and may be combined with phenytoin. Larger doses up to 200 mg are sometimes necessary.

In status epilepticus and in the treatment of convulsions due to overdose of analeptics, such as amfetamine, 60–200 mg of the sodium salt may be given intravenously or intramuscularly and repeated if necessary. When given intravenously the solution should be diluted, 20 mg being made up to 10 ml. Solutions for injections should be freshly prepared in CO_2-free water or decomposition with precipitation of phenobarbital will occur. (Phenobarbital is also one of the most potent of those agents which induce proliferation of microsomal enzymes in the liver and thus influence the metabolism of other drugs.)

Phenytoin does not cause general depression of the CNS, but is powerfully anti-epileptic and experimentally is one of the most effective substances in opposing electrically induced convulsions. Phenytoin is the drug of choice for all forms of epilepsy except petit mal, where it may have an adverse effect. It exerts its effects by its ability to stabilize excitable cell membranes in the CNS. This effect is also seen in peripheral nerves and in the excitable tissues of the heart.

It is used alone rather than in combinations whenever possible, because its metabolism can be influenced by hepatic microsomal enzyme induction caused by other drugs (see above). It is also an enzyme inducer itself. The most effective combination clinically is with phenobarbital. It often has little effect on the EEG either in the normal person or in grand mal, and the latter condition may be well controlled without any corresponding improvement in the EEG pattern.

The pharmacokinetics of this drug are of importance for two reasons. First, because of slow absorption and distribution there is a considerable delay in the establishment of a steady-state concentration of the drug. Secondly, the breakdown of the drug does not increase with higher plasma levels, as is normally the case with first-order reactions which are usual in drug metabolism. Below plasma levels of 10 µg/ml elimination follows this pattern, but at higher concentrations the metabolic pathway becomes saturated and any further increase in concentration has no effect on breakdown rate. This stays constant, rather like the situation with the metabolism of alcohol. This critical level is close to the therapeutic level and, since the rate of metabolism is determined by multifactorial genetic influences, normal doses cause continued accumulation in some individuals until toxic blood levels are reached. For this reason, adjustment of dose by reference to plasma concentrations must be employed.

In adults, initial dosage is 100 mg 3 times a day by mouth, increasing if necessary up to 600 mg per 24 h. Infants and children need smaller doses: the aim is to achieve a plasma level of 10–20 µg/ml (40–80 mmol/litre), although seizure control can be achieved at lower plasma levels in some cases. Above 20 µg/ml toxic effects such as ataxia and nystagmus are evident; above 40 µg/ml lethargy becomes apparent.

A wide variety of hypersensitivity and haematological reactions have been reported and these necessitate stopping the drug. Megaloblastic anaemia is due to altered folate absorption and metabolism and responds to folic acid. After several months of treatment, young patients sometimes develop a hypertrophic condition of the gums, the cause of which is not known.

Administration during pregnancy leads to a typical abnormality, the fetal hydantoin syndrome, which typically includes wide-set eyes, a broad jaw and finger deformities. There is a three-fold higher incidence of fetal malformations than normal in children born to mothers taking this drug, but the cessation of effective therapy is potentially more dangerous to both mother and child.

Phenytoin is also useful in the treatment of arrhythmias due to digitalis. A dose of 50–100 mg of phenytoin may be given intravenously every 15 minutes until a satisfactory response is achieved, up to a maximum of 15 mg/kg. Digitalis-induced ventricular arrhythmias are suppressed at plasma concentrations of 8–16 µg/ml.

Sodium valproate is an effective anticonvulsant which has been used in the treatment of most forms of epilepsy. It is particularly effective in petit mal, for which it may be the drug of choice.

The mechanism of the antiepileptic effect of sodium valproate is not known, although it is probably associated with an increased concentration in the brain of the inhibitory transmitter GABA. The optimum therapeutic serum concentration has not yet been clearly established, but levels of 200 µg/ml should be exceeded only with extreme caution.

The serum concentration of other anticonvulsants may increase when sodium valproate is added. It displaces phenytoin from plasma protein binding sites but also increases phenytoin metabolism. Sodium valproate potentiates the actions of monoamine oxidase inhibitors and tricyclic antidepressants.

For adults the initial daily dose is 300 mg orally twice daily, increasing to a maximum of 2.6 g/day. In children and infants the dose must be scaled down appropriately. Perioperatively, administration may be continued by using slow intravenous boluses of the same dose as the patient is receiving chronically. For initiation of valproate therapy in neurosurgery or in the intensive care treatment of recurrent convulsions, 400–800 mg intravenously can be given 3 times daily. It is not used in the treatment of status epilepticus.

After several years of trouble-free usage, there have been reports of serious complications such as fulminant hepatic failure and pancreatitis. Raised transaminases occur in up to 44 per cent of patients, but are usually transient and often are present without clinical manifestations. The only other drug interactions of which anaesthetists should be particularly aware are reversible haemo-static defects, including decreased platelet adhesiveness, mild hypofibrinogenaemia and thrombo-cytopenia.

Carbamazepine is chemically and pharmacologically related to the tricyclic antidepressants. It may well prove to be the drug of choice for temporal lobe epilepsy but, despite clinical improvement, there may be a deterioration in the EEG. It is the drug of choice for the treatment of trigeminal and other neuralgias and has been said to be effective in the control of intractable hiccup. Initially, 100–200 mg may be given once or twice a day, increasing to 600–800 mg daily until an optimal response is obtained. A wide range of adverse reactions have been reported, ranging from thrombocytopenia to hepatocellular jaundice. It also exhibits toxic effects similar to those of other tricyclic antidepressants.

Ethosuximide is used for the control of petit mal, or absence seizures, which are associated with 3 Hz spike and wave discharges in the EEG. It should not be given without such evidence unless an 'absence' has been observed. An initial oral dose of 250 mg is given two to three times daily. This may be gradually increased up to 2 g daily as required. The most common side effects involve the gastro-intestinal tract (nausea, etc.) and the CNS (drowsiness). Its sole use may unmask tonic–clonic seizures and it is usually combined with phenytoin or primidone.

Primidone has a similar action to phenobarbital, although it is not a barbiturate. In fact, a considerable element of its anticonvulsant activity can be attributed to the formation of phenobarbital as an active metabolite by oxidation. It does, however, have some anticonvulsant action itself. The commonest side effects are sedation, vertigo, nausea, ataxia and nystagmus. At the start of treatment, 125 mg may be given daily in divided doses for 3 days. The dose can then be increased gradually up to 250 mg 4 times a day as required.

Benzodiazepines which are effective as anticonvulsants include chlordiazepoxide, diazepam, nitrazepam and clonazepam. Of these, diazepam and clonazepam are of particular value in the management of status epilepticus.

Acetazolamide, a carbonic anhydrase inhibitor, is a diuretic which is effective in many types of epilepsy in some patients, particularly when added to other therapy.

Sultiame is another carbonic anhydrase inhibitor, but it has few obvious advantages over acetazolamide.

Vigabatrin has been shown to reduce the frequency of seizures (although rarely abolish them) and has been found to be most effective in partial seizures with or without secondary generalization (the commonest form of chronic adult epilepsy). Because of the mode of action as a CNS enzyme inhibitor, there is no clear correlation between the plasma concentration of the drug and its effectiveness.

MONOGRAPHS

ALCOHOL

Ethanol (96 per cent) (rINN) and Alcohol (96 per cent) (USP) *Chemical name*: ethyl alcohol

Pharmacology

Ethanol (ethyl alcohol) is a depressant of the CNS. Inhibitory mechanisms and self-criticism are depressed first and this accounts for the apparent stimulation observed in some people early in its course of action. The subsequent order in which the CNS is depressed is the same as for general anaesthetics, but alcohol is too dangerous for use as such because the safety margin between full anaesthesia and full medullary depression is too narrow. It is also a gastric irritant. Central vasomotor and respiratory effects are important contributors to the cardiovascular depression caused by alcohol poisoning. Skin vasodilatation and increased sweating contribute to a loss of body heat, although the subject feels warmer, subjectively.

The body can metabolize alcohol only at a constant rate of about 10 ml/h, to carbon dioxide and water via acetaldehyde and acetate. This catabolic process can be speeded up by the injection of soluble insulin. Methyl alcohol, present with ethyl alcohol to the extent of about 4 per cent in methylated spirit, is much more toxic, being oxidized to formic acid which affects the optic nerves, causing blindness.

The oxidation of the intermediate metabolite, acetaldehyde, can be inhibited by disulfiram, and this has been utilized in the treatment of chronic alcoholism. This enzyme may be lacking in some people, notably those of Chinese extraction. The concentration of alcohol in urine or breath can be used to make a rough quantitative estimate of the content in the blood. The legal limit in the driver of a motor vehicle in Great Britain is 80 mg/100 ml, although there is no doubt that most people's faculties would be critically impaired by blood levels lower than this, especially when the level is rising. The legal limit is much lower in many other countries. Excretion by the kidney is hastened by a diuresis which is consequent upon a central depression of the release of antidiuretic hormone from the posterior pituitary.

Chronic alcoholics are frequently very resistant to anaesthesia. This resistance may be due to several factors. Repeated alcohol ingestion induces proliferation of enzyme systems in the liver which enhances the metabolic breakdown of other drugs. To some degree, however, the resistance may be an example of cross-tolerance, a pharmacodynamic adaptation in the CNS found with many other depressants given repeatedly over long periods.

Cirrhosis of the liver occurs from excessive continued intake of alcohol, and is mainly the result of a deficiency of essential metabolites consequent upon a diminished food intake.

The uses of alcohol as an anaesthetic are only of historic interest. Its only current therapeutic use is intravenously to control delirium tremens following alcohol withdrawal.

Chloral and triclofos. The action of these drugs is due to trichloroethanol, which is produced as a result of hepatic metabolism. Chloral is widely used as a sedative in hospital paediatric practice. In moderate doses, it has no effect on the cardiovascular system or on respiratory drive. It is used as an adjunct to sedation with opiates and/or benzodiazepines in paediatric intensive care, in an attempt to reduce the amounts of these which need to be given, because withdrawal problems are few with chloral and common with opiates and benzodiazepines. Triclofos is reputed to be associated with fewer unwanted gastro-intestinal effects than chloral. It has been suggested that these drugs are especially useful as hypnotics in the elderly, but there is no objective evidence to support this suggestion.

ALIMEMAZINE (TRIMEPRAZINE)

Alimemazine tartrate (rINN) and trimeprazine tartrate (BAN)

Alimemazine has pharmacological actions intermediate between promethazine and chlorpromazine. It has a greater antihistamine action than promethazine while its central actions, including anti-emetic activity, are similar to those of chlorpromazine. It has some anti-adrenergic activity, and blood pressure may be moderately depressed. It also possesses a powerful antispasmodic effect.

It is used as an antipruritic and sedative in dermatology and general medicine, and as a premedicant, especially for children. It is pleasantly formulated as a syrup containing 6 mg/ml.

It is given by mouth in a total daily dose of 10–40 mg in dermatological conditions, and 1–2 mg/kg 1–2 h before operation for full sedation and premedication.

Large doses cause a somewhat flushed appearance with circumoral pallor. On at least two occasions it has been incriminated as a possible trigger of the malignant hyperthermia syndrome.

CLOMETHIAZOLE

Clomethiazole and Clomethiazole edisilate (rINN)

Pharmacology

Clomethiazole is basically an anticonvulsant, but is also a powerful sedative and hypnotic with anti-emetic properties. Rapid intravenous infusion in healthy volunteers causes little change in cardiac output; blood pressure is little changed or rises, but a consistent effect is a marked rise in pulse rate. Respiratory depression and hypotension may follow large or rapidly administered doses.

Indications

It has been used intravenously to control delirium tremens and status epilepticus, to sedate patients in intensive care units, as a sedative to accompany regional analgesia and in the management of pre-eclamptic toxaemia.

Dosage and administration

Clomethiazole may be given intravenously as a 0.8 per cent solution in 5 per cent dextrose for status epilepticus or to severely agitated patients at a rate of 8–20 ml/minute, depending on the clinical state of the patient, 40–60 ml usually being adequate. Up to 1 litre may need to be administered in a 12-h period. Other fluid intake should be restricted if

2 litres need to be given in 24 h in pre-eclamptic or epileptic patients, to minimize dangers from overhydration.

It may be used orally for the treatment of alcohol withdrawal symptoms, commencing with up to 2 g initially followed by 1 g every 3–4 h, the dose being progressively reduced over a period of about 8 days. It can also be used as a hypnotic, particularly in the elderly where the lack of hangover is an advantage.

Precautions and side effects

Rapid intravenous injection should be avoided and the strength of the solution should not exceed 0.8 per cent or thrombophlebitis may occur. A tingling sensation in the nose or sneezing may occur after the first administration.

DIAZEPAM

Diazepam (rINN)

Physical characteristics

Diazepam is insoluble in water; the solution for injection (5 mg/ml) contains several organic solvents, mainly propylene glycol, ethanol, and sodium benzoate in benzoic acid. The solution is rather viscid and dilution with water or saline causes cloudiness and is not recommended. It should not be mixed with other drugs. These solvents can cause incoordination and depression of post-synaptic reflexes.

Diazemuls is a preparation of diazepam in soya bean oil, which has been emulsified in water by means of egg yolk phosphatides and acetylated monoglycerides.

Pharmacology

Central nervous system Diazepam is a benzodiazepine which is a potent tranquillizer, muscle relaxant and anticonvulsant. These properties are due to its effect on the ascending reticular activating system and spinal internuncial neurones, as well as the effect on the limbic system. Patients remain alert after small doses but high doses cause drowsiness, and amnesia and unconsciousness can be produced if it is given intravenously. It can be given in doses that cause a state of extreme drowsiness but in which the patient is still accessible and there is marked amnesia. When combined with other drugs as premedicant, the incidence of amnesia is increased. A dose of 0.2 mg/kg reduced the MAC (see pages 127–8) for halothane by 35 per cent from 0.73 to 0.48 per cent. Doubling the dose of diazepam brings no further reduction in anaesthetic requirements. The oil/water formulation has a considerably higher LD_{50} in animals. The pharmacokinetics of both formulations are identical.

Respiratory system Intravenous injection of 0.14 mg/kg depresses the sensitivity of the respiratory centre. The breathing frequency falls and there is a decrease in the slope of the carbon dioxide–ventilation curve.

Cardiovascular system Following intravenous injection of 0.2 mg/kg at the rate of 10 mg/minute, the only significant change is a tachycardia which may persist for some time. There is no effect on cardiac output or any marked effects on blood pressure.

Indications

The indications for this drug are numerous. It has been used as a premedicant, both intramuscularly and by mouth, and intravenously to induce anaesthesia. For the latter indication it has largely been superseded by midazolam. If it is used for this purpose, due allowance must be made for the prolonged drowsiness which it causes. It is employed intravenously in sub-anaesthetic doses as a sedative for patients with dental phobia, to cover unpleasant procedures in intensive care units, and to accustom patients to artificial ventilators. It has been employed as the sole agent for cardioversion, and has been recommended for cardiac catheterization in children. It is also employed as a sedative during carotid angiography. In fact, in almost every conceivable situation in which rapid sedation might be of benefit, diazepam has proved of value and exhibited a high degree of safety. It is also used orally in the treatment of psychosomatic illness, and has been used in the treatment of tetanus.

It is more effective than pentobarbital in treating and preventing lidocaine-induced convulsions, and can now be regarded as a drug of first choice in the treatment of convulsive states of all kinds, being associated with a much lower overall mortality.

Dosage and administration

Diazepam may be given by mouth in tablet form or as a syrup and by intravenous injection. Oral doses for anxiety states vary from 10 to 30 mg daily in divided doses. For premedication, 10–20 mg may be given 1–1.5 h before operation. When given orally the maximal effect is reached in 60 minutes and there is some suggestion that the oral route is more effective than the intramuscular one. For acute sedation, 0.2 mg/kg is usually adequate, but doses up to 0.6 mg/kg may be needed to induce unconsciousness. In the treatment of tetanus, doses of about 5 mg/kg/24 h are given by mouth or nasal tube in syrup form. Elderly and debilitated patients require about half the usual dosage, and when the drug is given intravenously it should be injected slowly at a rate not exceeding 10 mg/minute.

Precautions

The consumption of alcohol should be avoided by patients under treatment, or during the day on which an intravenous dose has been given. Diazepam injection cannot be diluted and precipitates when mixed with most other agents. It is painful when injected intramuscularly; there may also be complaints of pain on intravenous administration, particularly if injected into a peripheral vein. It has been reported that the incidence of thrombosis is about 6 per cent if injected into the antecubital vein and up to 23 per cent for a vein in the hand or wrist. Slow injection or dilution with the patient's own blood is said to reduce the incidence. Pain is virtually absent using Diazemuls.

Other benzodiazepines

The Committee on the Review of Medicines (CRM) divides these drugs into long-acting benzodiazepines whose plasma half-lives (of drug plus active metabolites) exceed 10 h, and short-acting ones. Long-acting drugs include nitrazepam, medazepam, flurazepam, diazepam, clorazepate and chlordiazepoxide. The CRM suggests that short-acting benzodiazepines are more suitable than long-acting ones for the treatment of insomnia. Lorazepam, temazepam and oxazepam are in this category.

Nitrazepam is frequently prescribed as a hypnotic, although it is in the long-acting category. It rapidly induces sleep which usually lasts from 6 to 8 h. Nitrazepam 5–10 mg before retiring is a common dose for adults, but should be reduced to 2.5–5 mg in elderly patients. It is associated with day-after sedation and accumulation occurs with regular nightly administration.

Like other long-acting benzodiazepines, it may affect patients' reaction time next morning, so driving performance and operation of machinery can be impaired. Summation with other centrally acting depressants such as alcohol is possible.

Medazepam has a pharmacological profile similar to nitrazepam. It is used in the treatment of anxiety. The initial recommended dose is 5 mg 3 times a day.

Temazepam is suitable for night sedation, being short acting, and is also used for premedication. Like diazepam, it depresses the ventilatory response to carbon dioxide. The dose is 10–60 mg.

DROPERIDOL

Droperidol (rINN)

Pharmacology

Droperidol is a substituted butyrophenone closely resembling haloperidol and certain phenothiazine derivatives. It is described as a neuroleptic and produces a state of mental calm and indifference with little hypnotic effect. Compared with haloperidol it acts faster, has a shorter duration of action and is less toxic. It is a powerful anti-emetic, whose action is localized to an area in the chemoreceptor trigger zone, but it does not antagonize motion sickness. It is frequently included in very small doses in PCA systems primed with an opioid, to control nausea and vomiting.

Large doses produce extrapyramidal side effects which may be delayed for some time after administration. Other actions are similar to haloperidol.

On rapid intravenous injection there is a moderate fall in systemic arterial pressure of short duration which is mediated by a direct action on the blood vessels. For a short period this hypotension cannot be reversed by α-adrenergic stimulating drugs, suggesting that the site of action of droperidol is at the α-adrenoceptors. With oral or intramuscular administration such an effect is not seen, presumably because a high concentration of drug at the receptor is avoided. In ordinary use the marked cardiovascular stability argues against any significant α-blockade. However, it can provide some protection against experimental shock.

Droperidol is metabolized in the liver.

Dosage and administration

For premedication, 5–10 mg is given intramuscularly 1 h before operation. Up to 10 mg may be given intravenously in conjunction with a potent analgesic to initiate neurolept-analgesia.

Precautions

Precautions and side effects are similar to those listed under haloperidol. It is of interest that dystonic reactions have been reported 24 h or more after administration. These are relieved by diphenhydramine, sedative drugs, and those usually given for the relief of Parkinsonism.

ETOMIDATE

Etomidate (rINN)

Physical characteristics

Although etomidate is soluble in water, for clinical use it is supplied in 35 per cent propylene glycol giving a solution of pH around 4.2; its pKa is 4.1. It differs from many drugs used in anaesthesia in that it is supplied only as the (+)-enantiomer.

Pharmacology

Pharmacokinetics   Etomidate is rapidly redistributed following intravenous injection with a distribution half-life ($t_{1/2}\alpha$) of 2–4 minutes. The elimination half-life ($t_{1/2}\beta$) is between 1–4 h. It has a volume of distribution of 2.0–4.5 litres/kg and is about 75 per cent protein bound. Etomidate is metabolized in the liver mainly by ester hydrolysis and also by N-dealkylation. All metabolic products are inactive. Only a very small amount of etomidate is excreted unchanged in the urine.

Nervous system   Etomidate causes a reduction in cerebral metabolic requirements for oxygen, together with a decrease in cerebral blood flow and intracranial pressure. The hypnotic properties of etomidate are associated with a lowering of the median frequency on the EEG and burst suppression at higher doses, similar changes to those seen with thiopental. Although myoclonic activity is frequently seen at induction of anaesthesia with etomidate, these are not reflected by EEG changes. It has been shown to have anticonvulsive properties and although no seizure activity has been observed on the EEG in patients with a history of convulsive disorders, it is best avoided in patients with a history of epilepsy.

Cardiovascular system   Etomidate is the most cardiovascularly stable of the currently available induction agents, being associated with only a slight fall in blood pressure and little change in heart rate. Cardiac output and myocardial contractility are little changed and this also is the case in patients with ischaemic heart disease.

Respiratory system   The degree of respiratory depression following etomidate is less than that following barbiturates and the incidence of apnoea after an induction dose is also less. Coughing, hiccups and laryngospasm are rarely seen.

Adrenocortical function   Etomidate is a potent inhibitor of 11β- and 17α-hydroxylase activity with a resultant marked depression in cortisol output. Although this is of little consequence following single bolus injections, infusions of etomidate to sedate severely injured patients in the intensive care unit have been associated with an increased mortality. As a result, etomidate has no product licence to be used by continuous infusion in the United Kingdom.

Indications

Because of the high incidence of side effects, etomidate is a rarely used induction agent in the United Kingdom. Probably its sole use is in induction of anaesthesia in patients with an unstable cardiovascular system, for example for myocardial revascularization procedures. Recovery following etomidate is faster than following thiopental, but is negated by the side effects and an increased frequency of nausea and vomiting during recovery. It is safe to use in patients with porphyria.

Dosage and administration

Etomidate in a dose of 0.2–0.3 mg/kg intravenously produces sleep in one arm–brain circulation time. Injection is associated with an incidence of local pain, which can be severe and is commoner the smaller the vein. It is reported to occur in 10–30 per cent of cases. This pain can be virtually eliminated by formulation as an emulsion, but this preparation is only available in a few European countries and not in the United Kingdom. Involuntary muscle movements are also a feature of induction of anaesthesia with etomidate and can be severe. The incidence is reduced, but not abolished, by sedative premedication. These movements can persist into the recovery period.

Precautions

Etomidate is best avoided in patients with epilepsy or a history of adrenocortical insufficiency.

FLUMAZENIL

Flumazenil (rINN)

Pharmacology

Flumazenil is a water-soluble benzodiazepine which acts as an antagonist specifically at benzodiazepine receptors. It acts by competitively displacing benzodiazepines from their receptors without changing their bioavailability or kinetics. As well as antagonizing the effects of pure benzodiazepine agonists, it also antagonizes the partial agonists, inverse agonists and partial inverse agonists (see *Figure 3.2*, page 74). Flumazenil itself is virtually without effect on the normal CNS, large doses being well tolerated in volunteers.

Flumazenil is a relatively short-acting drug with an elimination half-life in the order of 5 minutes. It has a plasma clearance of 0.92 litre/minute.

Indications

The main use of flumazenil is for reversal of benzodiazepine sedation following endoscopic procedures. It will produce rapid recovery and is short acting. This is rarely of concern if used to antagonize a short-acting drug such as midazolam. However, with longer acting benzodiazepines re-sedation is a distinct possibility after a single dose of flumazenil and great care must be taken when it is used under these circumstances. The possibility of re-sedation must also always be borne in mind even when midazolam has been used.

In patients who have been sedated in the intensive care unit with large doses of a benzodiazepine over a period of time, flumazenil may be used to completely reverse the effects, thus temporarily providing a 'window' during which neurological assessment can be carried out. Repeat administration or a continuous infusion may be necessary to maintain benzodiazepine reversal following long-acting drugs or after large doses.

Flumazenil may be used in the treatment of benzodiazepine overdose and can also be used as a diagnostic test when the nature of an apparent drug overdose is not known.

Dosage and administration

To reverse the effects of a benzodiazepine, the drug is given initially in a bolus of 0.2 mg intravenously and then in 0.1 mg increments until the desired end-point is reached. A total dose of 0.5 mg is usually sufficient. Following massive benzodiazepine overdose, or in the intensive care unit where a very large dose may have been used, 1 or 2 mg may have to be given to produce arousal. Flumazenil may be given by continuous intravenous infusion, the rate being adjusted to produce the desired effect. Rates up to 1 mg/h may be necessary to maintain a patient in a 'safe' condition.

FLUPHENAZINE

Fluphenazine hydrochloride (rINN)

Pharmacology

Fluphenazine is a piperazine phenothiazine. It is a more potent antiemetic than chlorpromazine and has a longer duration of action. It exhibits the pharmacological spectrum of the phenothiazines.

Indications

It is used for the control of postoperative nausea and vomiting and in schizophrenia. Fluphenazine enanthate or decanoate are long-acting preparations especially used in schizophrenia.

Dosage and administration

Fluphenazine hydrochloride 1 mg once or twice a day orally is the usual dose for control of postoperative nausea. It has been used to prevent postoperative vomiting, in a dose of 5 mg intramuscularly 30–45 minutes before the end of the operation. In schizophrenic patients an intramuscular dose of 0.5 ml of the decanoate or enanthate formulation (12.5–25 mg fluphenazine decanoate or enanthate) can provide adequate maintenance for 2–3 weeks. Some patients require larger doses, up to 4 ml every 2 weeks.

Precautions

These are similar to those for othger phenothiazines. Parkinsonian-like states and acute dystonic reactions can occur. With long-term therapy, tardive dyskinesia may develop.

Flupentixol has similar actions to fluphenazine. It is a thioxanthene. It is of interest that the stereoisomers differ in activity. The cis-isomer is the more potent in schizophrenia. Depot injections of the decanoate are used in schizophrenia. *Cis*-clopentixol decanoate is a related compound, also used in maintenance therapy in schizophrenia.

HALOPERIDOL

Haloperidol (rINN)

Pharmacology

Haloperidol is a substituted butyrophenone, its actions resembling those of droperidol. It is classified as a neuroleptic and produces a cataleptic state with little hypnotic action. Its duration of action is longer than that of droperidol, and lasts up to 24 h. It is a powerful anti-emetic, and in its ability to block apomorphine-induced vomiting is 50 times as potent as chlorpromazine.

Haloperidol potentiates both barbiturates and analgesics and blocks the CNS effects of amphetamine in animals. The EEG is not altered by normal doses.

It has virtually no anti-adrenergic activity. Blood pressure remains stable and hypotension does not occur, even after intravenous administration. There is no effect on respiration following recommended doses. Although extrapyramidal side effects may occur, toxic effects have not so far been reported.

Haloperidol, like other butyrophenones, is metabolized in the liver. Metabolites have been identified in both urine and faeces.

Indications

The drug is used in psychiatry for psychomotor manifestations such as delusions, hallucinations, paranoia and mania. It can also be used in ITU psychoses. It may be used for premedication and for the production of neuroleptanalgesia.

Dosage and administration

The drug is given orally for psychiatric indications in doses of 1.5–6 mg daily. For neuroleptanalgesia, 2.5–5 mg is given intravenously prior to the chosen analgesic, usually phenoperidine or fentanyl.

Precautions

Haloperidol should be avoided in patients with lesions in the basal ganglia, including spastic syndromes associated with arteriosclerosis. In such patients, and in normal subjects receiving high doses, extrapyramidal reactions may occur. These may be promptly alleviated by either soporific or anti-Parkinsonian drugs. High doses may be antisoporific. Solutions should be protected from light.

KETAMINE

Ketamine hydrochloride (rINN)

Ketamine is a white crystalline powder supplied as a colourless solution in concentrations of 1 per cent, 5 per cent and 10 per cent, the latter two containing 0.1 per cent benzethonium as a preservative. The pH varies from 3.5 to 5.5 and the pK_a is 7.5. The available preparation is a mixture of the S(+) and R(−) isomers in equal concentrations.

Pharmacology

Ketamine is a parenteral anaesthetic agent with an atypical profile of actions. It produces what has been described as dissociative anaesthesia in which the patient appears to be awake but does not respond to stimuli, even painful ones.

Pharmacokinetics

Ketamine is rapidly and extensively distributed throughout the body and the plasma concentration after intravenous injection best fits a two-compartmental model. The distribution half-life is 11–17 minutes and the terminal half-life 2½–3½ h. The initial volume of distribution is 20–100 litres and that at a steady state 100–400 litres. Total body clearance is about 1200 ml/minute. Ketamine undergoes extensive and complicated metabolism in the liver and only about 4 per cent appears unchanged in the urine.

Induction of anaesthesia   Unlike other agents, ketamine is effective both intravenously and intramuscularly. There is dissociation between the thalamic and limbic systems. Ketamine is devoid of hypnotic properties, but causes amnesia and intense analgesia. This state becomes apparent about 1 minute after intravenous injection and 5 minutes after intramuscular injection. Following a single intravenous injection, this 'state' usually persists for 15–20 minutes. Consciousness does not appear to be lost, but there is complete amnesia. Unlike with other general anaesthetic agents, muscle tone is not reduced, but usually increased and involuntary movements may occur which are unrelated to the surgical stimulus; the eyes tend to be open. Vocalization may also occur. Analgesia is intense and permits surgery with ketamine as the sole agent; it also persists longer than the dissociative state. The analgesia is thought to be related to the potent blocking properties of ketamine at N-methyl-D-aspartate (NMDA) receptors. Following intramuscular injection, the dissociative state takes about 5 minutes to develop and lasts correspondingly longer.

Analgesia may precede the onset of anaesthesia and persists after the return of consciousness. During this period, bizarre hallucinations may occur, associated with the loss of body image and if stimulated, the patient may react violently and irrationally. The occurrence of vivid and sometimes unpleasant dreams is frequently reported after ketamine anaesthesia, although the incidence is less in children. It is conventional to avoid any stimulation of patients recovering from ketamine anaesthesia in order to reduce the incidence of these emergence reactions, which can also be achieved with any sedative medication.

Nervous system   The EEG changes following ketamine differ from the other intravenous anaesthetics in that not all the CNS is depressed simultaneously. There is initially fast activity which then changes to slow theta activity. Also, unlike other agents, ketamine increases cerebral oxygen consumption, cerebral blood flow and intracranial pressure. Intra-ocular pressure is also increased following ketamine.

Cardiovascular system   Following intravenous injection of ketamine, 1.5–2.0 mg/kg, there is an increase in arterial blood pressure of around 15–25 per cent, with similar increases in heart rate, cardiac output and pulmonary artery pressure. These changes occur over 3–5 minutes and then gradually return to baseline over the next 10–20 minutes. Similar changes occur after subsequent doses. After intramuscular ketamine, the changes are more protracted and occur to a lesser degree. Although there is an increase in circulating norepinephrine (noradrenaline) after ketamine, these changes are caused by CNS stimulation with an increase in sympathetic outflow. Myocardial oxygen consumption is increased by ketamine and it is contraindicated in patients with ischaemic heart disease. These cardiovascular changes can be attenuated by prior administration of drugs with vasodilator properties and by α- and β-adrenoceptor blockers.

Respiratory system   Respiratory depression is rare after usual doses of ketamine given to unpremedicated patients, but may occasionally accompany rapid administration to very sick patients. Laryngeal and pharyngeal reflexes are depressed, but to a much lesser degree than with other agents and the absence of depression of muscle tone results in self-maintenance of the airway being a usual feature of ketamine anaesthesia. The latter is also accompanied by bronchodilatation. Increased salivation is a feature in the absence of anticholinergic administration.

Other systems   Adverse renal and hepatic effects have not been reported following ketamine. Nausea and vomiting are common after its sole use.

Indications

Ketamine may be used as an induction agent prior to general anaesthesia, although its routine use is limited by the associated side effects. It is an effective agent in poor risk patients and those with a tendency to hypotension, e.g. relative hypovolaemia. Its use should be considered in asthmatics. Its chief indication would appear to be in situations in which there might be difficulty in maintaining the airway, such as burns or trauma. It may be used by the operator/anaesthetist and for surgery under adverse circumstances, e.g. at major accident sites and in developing countries at sites which lack proper anaesthetic equipment or more appropriate drugs. It has been used successfully for neurodiagnostic procedures and as a sedative in children undergoing cardiac catheterization. It has received little success as a postoperative analgesic in low doses, e.g. 50 μg/kg/minute, but infusions have been successful in the avoidance of artificial ventilation in patients with status asthmaticus.

Dosage and administration

An intravenous injection of 2 mg/kg produces surgical anaesthesia within 30–60 s, lasting 5–10 minutes. Repeated doses may be given without significant cumulative effects. An intramuscular dose of 10 mg/kg produces surgical anaesthesia within 3–4 minutes, lasting 15–30 minutes. Repeated intramuscular injections result in a prolonged recovery time. In neonates, intramuscular doses need to be increased to 12.5 mg/kg. Epidural injection has been reported to produce satisfactory analgesia, but is little used.

Precautions

Ketamine should be avoided in patients with a history of cerebrovascular accidents, myocardial ischaemia and hypertension. A severe sustained increase in blood pressure has been reported in patients receiving thyroid replacement therapy. It is contraindicated in the presence of raised intracranial pressure and penetrating eye injuries. Stimulation of the patient during emergence from anaesthesia should be avoided.

Ketamine isomers

Ketamine is only available commercially as a racemic mixture. The S(+) isomer is 3–4 times more potent than the R(–) form. The former has been shown to produce more effective anaesthesia than the R(–) isomer or the racemic mixture. The S(+) form was associated with fewer adverse emergence reactions and less agitated behaviour than the R(–) form, while the latter was associated with more postoperative pain. It is possible that the S(+) isomer will be developed as a separate anaesthetic agent.

LORAZEPAM

Lorazepam (rINN)

Physical characteristics

Lorazepam is insoluble in water. For parenteral use it is dissolved in polyethylene glycol and propylene glycol.

Pharmacology

Central nervous system   Lorazepam is a benzodiazepine of short or intermediate duration of action with actions similar to those of diazepam. In the acute treatment of anxiety neurosis it causes fewer undesirable side effects. It produces anterograde amnesia; an intravenous dose of 5 mg invariably produces this effect for up to 24 h. Lorazepam has no analgesic properties.

Respiratory system   There is an enhanced ventilatory response to carbon dioxide challenge, suggesting that lorazepam may have a stimulant effect upon respiration.

Cardiovascular system   There are no marked changes in blood pressure, pulse rate or peripheral resistance.

Musculoskeletal system   Lorazepam, like diazepam, has muscle-relaxant properties, probably central in origin.

Fate in the body   Absorption of orally administered lorazepam is rapid, maximum blood concentrations occurring after 2–4 h and its actions persist for 12–18 h. Almost 80 per cent of the administered dose can be recovered in the urine over 5 days, mostly as the glucuronide which is the principal metabolite.

Indications

In anaesthetic practice, lorazepam is used in a similar manner to diazepam. However, the absence of depressant effect upon ventilation and its potent amnesic activity may be advantageous. Most investigations to date have described its value in pre-anaesthetic medication. Orally, doses from 1 to 5 mg have generally been found to have similar or superior actions to equipotent doses of diazepam. Sedation, relief of anxiety and amnesia are produced. Similar doses, given intravenously, have also been used. The relatively long duration of action limits its use when rapid and complete recovery is desired. Postoperatively it virtually abolishes emergence reactions when given intravenously after ketamine anaesthesia.

Dosage and administration

Lorazepam is approximately five times as potent as diazepam on a weight-for-weight comparison. Oral doses for the treatment of anxiety range from 1 to 3 mg, 2 or 3 times daily. Doses up to 5 mg orally or intravenously are used for pre-anaesthetic medication. Since it has an intermediate duration of action it may be given simultaneously to all patients on an operating list several hours before the start of the list.

Precautions

Lorazepam, like other benzodiazepines, may potentiate the effects of other CNS depressants and may have a prolonged action. It is not recommended for use in children. After intravenous injection of lorazepam, thrombosis or thrombophlebitis can be produced. The incidence of thrombophlebitis is less following lorazepam than diazepam. In general practice and psychiatry, the long-term use of lorazepam is associated with a relatively high incidence of dependence and withdrawal symptoms.

METHOHEXITAL

Methohexital and Methohexital sodium (rINN)

Methohexital is a methylated oxybarbiturate (for structural formula see *Figure 3.6*) which occurs as a white crystalline powder and is supplied mixed with anhydrous sodium carbonate, when it is readily soluble in water giving a solution of pH 10–11. Methohexital exists as as two pairs of stereoisomers. The α-pair causes much less skeletal muscle activity and only this pair is now included in the commercial formulation.

A dose of 1.0–1.5 mg/kg intravenously produces sleep in one-arm brain circulation time. Induction of anaesthesia is often accompanied by involuntary muscle movements, which are rarely severe, resembling convulsions; this is a feature of all methylated barbiturates. Clinical recovery is quicker than following equipotent doses of thiopental, but slower than following propofol. Respiratory depression occurs as with thiopental and is dose related. There is a tendency for a decrease in arterial blood pressure, but there is usually an accompanying tachycardia and, as a result, little change in cardiac output.

Pain on injection is a feature of methohexital and is commoner when given in small veins; the incidence can be reduced by giving a small dose of lidocaine just before. It does not cause venous thrombosis. Accidental intra-arterial injection causes little damage as it is used as a 1 per cent solution compared to 2.5 per cent for thiopental.

Methohexital used to be employed for similar indications to thiopental, but especially for minor surgery because of the more rapid recovery. It is now little used as it has been replaced by propofol. Probably the sole indication for methohexital is for electroconvulsive therapy as the duration of the convulsion is not reduced as with propofol.

MIDAZOLAM

Midazolam hydrochloride and maleate (rINN)

Midazolam is a water-soluble benzodiazepine whose solubility is pH dependent. Below 4.0 it is freely water soluble and forms a stable solution. At physiological pH, the ring structure closes and the drug becomes lipid soluble and rapidly penetrates the blood–brain barrier. It should not be mixed with acidic drugs. It is available for injection either in 2 ml ampoules at a concentration of 5 mg/ml or 5 ml ampoules containing 2 mg/ml.

Pharmacokinetics

At body pH, midazolam is highly lipophilic and is rapidly redistributed after intravenous injection, with a steady-state volume of distribution of 0.8–1.7 litres/kg. The kinetics fit a two-compartmental model with an elimination half-life of 2–3 h. This is much shorter compared to other benzodiazepines. The $t_{1/2}\beta$ is more prolonged in the elderly and half-lives of over 10 h have been described. It is virtually entirely metabolized by the liver and less than 1 per cent is excreted unchanged in the urine. Only one of the metabolites of midazolam (α-hydroxymidazolam) is biologically active, but as its half-life is less than that of the parent compound, it is not clinically important.

Pharmacology

Central nervous system

The actions of midazolam are qualitatively similar to those of other benzodiazepines and are exerted by its attachment to benzodiazepine receptors in the CNS. It blocks EEG arousal from stimulation of the brain stem and reticular system. Intravenously it provides dense anterograde amnesia which lasts up to 30 minutes following doses used for sedation.

The effect of midazolam given intravenously varies from mild sedation to full general anaesthesia, depending on the dosage used. The dose necessary to produce the latter varies considerably, up to 0.6 mg/kg being necessary in some young unpremedicated patients. The elderly, on the other hand, are particularly sensitive to the effects of midazolam. The drug is highly protein bound and slight variations in plasma protein concentrations can have a marked influence on the pharmacodynamically active free-drug levels in the plasma.

Cardiovascular system Midazolam is generally less depressant to the cardiovascular system than other intravenous anaesthetic agents and it has proved to be a safe induction agent in poor-risk patients. It causes a slight fall in systemic vascular resistance and arterial blood pressure with little change in cardiac output. The lesser effects on the cardiovascular system may be due to its slower onset of action than other induction agents.

Respiratory system In healthy subjects midazolam, in a dose of 0.075 mg/kg intravenously, produces only a transitory and non-significant depression of the CO_2 response curve. However, concomitant use of other CNS depressants may lead to a more significant degree of respiratory depression, and in patients with chronic obstructive airways disease the respiratory depressant effect of midazolam may be greater than in normal subjects.

Indications

Midazolam has largely replaced diazepam in anaesthetic practice. Intramuscularly it is an effective premedicant, but the main use of midazolam has been to produce sedation during relatively unpleasant procedures such as upper intestinal endoscopy, bronchoscopy, dental work carried out under local anaesthesia and major surgery performed with the aid of regional anaesthesia.

When used for sedation it is frequently combined with small doses of fentanyl or other opioid. Due to potentiation of the effects of the two drugs, respiratory depression is an ever present danger and these patients must be cared for by a dedicated, trained person.

It has been used for induction of anaesthesia, the main difference from thiopental being the delay in onset of anaesthesia. Although the α-hydroxy metabolite is biologically active, its half-life is shorter than that of the parent compound. Thus, because of its relatively short plasma half-life and high plasma clearance, midazolam has been used, both intermittently and by continuous infusion, to produce long-term sedation in patients in the intensive care unit.

Co-induction   Combinations of sedative drugs with intravenous anaesthetic agents have a synergistic action, although the exact mechanism is unknown. Several studies have shown that this also occurs between midazolam and propofol. Thus a dose of midazolam of 0.13 mg/kg reduces the ED_{50} for propofol anaesthesia by 52 per cent (Short *et al.*, 1992). Therefore, by using small doses of midazolam which themselves have no hypnotic properties, a significant reduction can be achieved in the induction dose of propofol. By using co-induction techniques, it is possible to reduce the incidence of side effects associated with the use of either drug alone.

Dosage and administration

Only injectable midazolam is currently available in the United Kingdom, and intramuscularly a dose of 0.07–0.08 mg/kg produces satisfactory anxiolysis and sedation when used for premedication. For 'conscious sedation' during endoscopy, doses of 0.07–0.1 mg/kg are generally satisfactory, whereas induction of anaesthesia requires from 0.3 to 0.6 mg/kg to produce unconsciousness. By continuous infusion it is usually administered in a strength of 1 mg/ml, the rate being adjusted to obtain the desired effect; there is a considerable inter-individual variation in dose requirements. Midazolam is available in tablet form (15 mg) in other countries, for night sedation.

Precautions

The elderly are particularly sensitive to the effects of midazolam and this, combined with its slow onset of action, can easily result in overdose. This is especially important when the person administering the midazolam is also performing the endoscopy; deaths have occurred from a combination of respiratory depression and obstruction. Despite the known pharmacokinetics of midazolam (data obtained in healthy volunteers), prolonged sedation has followed cessation of its use in the intensive care unit. Conjugates of its main metabolite, α-hydroxymidazolam, have been shown to accumulate in renal failure and because some of these conjugates have actions similar to the parent compound (particularly the glucuronide) they have been assumed to be responsible for this prolonged sedative effect which is commonly observed in critically ill patients (Bauer *et al.*, 1995).

Bauer, T.M., Rity, R. and Haberthur, C. *et al.* (1995) Prolonged sedation due to accumulation of conjugated metabolites of midazolam. *Lancet*, **346**, 145–7

Short, T.G., Plummer, J.L. and Chui, P.T. (1992) Hypnotic and anaesthetic interactions between midazolam, propofol and alfentanil. *British Journal of Anaesthesia*, **69**, 162–7

PROPOFOL

Propofol (rINN)

Physical characteristics

Propofol is a hindered phenol and is virtually insoluble in water. It is presented as a 1 per cent w/v aqueous emulsion containing 10 per cent w/v soya bean oil, 1.2 per cent w/v egg phosphatide and 2.25 per cent glycerol (this is very similar to Intralipid).

Pharmacokinetics

Propofol is highly lipid soluble and after a single injection is rapidly redistributed from the highly perfused organs such as the brain to less well perfused areas such as muscle and bone. It enters the highly lipophilic compartments such as fat much more slowly because of their poor blood supply. The initial fall in blood levels due to redistribution has a half-life ($t_{1/2\alpha}$) of 2–4 minutes, and elimination half-life ($t_{1/2\beta}$) representing metabolic clearance from blood, is of the order 30–50 minutes. The context sensitive half-time (half-life), context being the duration of a propofol infusion, is about 25 minutes for infusions up to 3 h duration and up to 50 minutes for prolonged infusions. Propofol only leaves the very lipophilic compartments when the blood level falls below the levels in the other compartments. The steady-state volume of distribution is 400–700 litres and transfer into the central compartment is very slow resulting in a long-half life ($t_{1/2}$ of 4–7 h or even longer). The plasma concentration during this time, however, is very low and well below levels that have a clinical effect. The plasma clearance of propofol is 23–29 ml/kg/minute compared to 3.4 ml/kg/minute for thiopental and 11.7 mg/kg/minute for etomidate.

Propofol is rapidly metabolized in the liver to produce water-soluble glucuronide and sulphate conjugates which are excreted in the urine. The metabolic clearance of propofol exceeds hepatic blood flow, indicating extrahepatic sites of metabolism. The occasional appearance of green urine in patients receiving propofol infusions is due to the presence of a quinol as a metabolite.

Pharmacology

Induction of anaesthesia Propofol is an intravenous anaesthetic agent that produces sleep in one arm–brain circulation time. Induction of anaesthesia is usually trouble free, but occasionally involuntary muscle movements occur; very rarely these movements are severe and resemble convulsions. Injection of propofol may be accompanied by pain along the vein; the reported incidence varies between 28 per cent and 90 per cent. Pain is commoner when the small veins on the dorsum of the hand are used. Numerous methods have been tried to reduce the incidence of pain, including injection into fast-running infusions, use of propofol at 4°C or body temperature and aspirating a small amount of blood into the syringe prior to injection. The simplest method of reducing the incidence is mixing 10–20 mg of lidocaine with 200 mg propofol, but this is not 100 per cent effective.

Nervous system In common with other intravenous anaesthetics (except ketamine), propofol causes an increase in cerebrovascular resistance with a resultant decrease in cerebral blood flow and also a reduction in the cerebral metabolic requirements for oxygen. This also occurs in patients with raised intracranial pressure due to head injury. Although most studies have found a reduction in intracranial pressure following propofol, this must be balanced against the fact that there is also a reduction in mean arterial pressure and thus possibly a reduction in cerebral perfusion pressure.

Induction of anaesthesia with propofol is accompanied by dose-dependent effects on the EEG. Initially there is a decrease in median frequency accompanied by an increase in amplitude. As anaesthesia deepens there is an increase in β and then δ waves. Despite the fact that involuntary movements can occur following induction of anaesthesia with propofol, there is no evidence that propofol produces epileptiform activity and it has been used successfully to terminate attacks of status epilepticus. Little information is available on its use in known epileptics, but it is probably best avoided in these patients.

Cardiovascular system   Propofol has a greater depressant effect on arterial blood pressure than equivalent doses of thiopental. The fall is due to a marked drop in systemic vascular resistance, cardiac output being little changed. The reduction in arterial pressure is accentuated in the elderly, in hypertensive patients and by rapid administration of the drug. Unlike thiopental and methohexital, there is little increase in heart rate following propofol. This is due to a resetting of the baroreflex mechanism which allows an unchanged heart rate at a lower arterial blood pressure.

Respiratory system   Following bolus doses, propofol is a potent respiratory depressant. The incidence and duration of apnoea is greater than with equivalent doses of thiopental and is accentuated by narcotic premedication. Propofol depresses the sensitivity of the respiratory centre to carbon dioxide and during infusions of the drug this depression is dose related.

Laryngeal and pharyngeal reflexes are depressed to a greater degree by propofol compared to thiopental. Oral airways are well tolerated and tracheal intubation has been achieved with propofol alone. The main advantage of this property is that it allows earlier and easier insertion of the laryngeal mask airway than following thiopental induction, the incidence of gagging being lower. Increasing the dose of thiopental does increase the ease of laryngeal mask insertion, but at the expense of a greater reduction in blood pressure and prolonged recovery. Using a target controlled infusion scheme, it has been shown that a laryngeal mask can be inserted successfully within 3 minutes in all patients at blood levels of propofol between 6 and 8 mg/ml, haemodynamic effects being acceptable.

Uterus and placenta   Propofol has little effect on the pregnant uterus. It rapidly crosses the placenta but is an acceptable induction agent for Caesarean section, having no greater effect on the fetus than thiopental.

Liver and kidney function   No evidence of any adverse function has been reported following intermittent injections of propofol.

Adrenocortical function   Single induction doses of propofol do not affect cortisol or aldosterone production in response to ACTH. No adverse effects have been found during infusions of propofol.

Recovery   Recovery from propofol anaesthesia is faster than that associated with other induction agents and is accompanied by a lower incidence of nausea and vomiting. Evidence suggests that propofol might have a direct anti-emetic effect and sub-hypnotic doses have been used successfully to control severe postoperative nausea and vomiting and that following cancer chemotherapy. Subhypnotic doses have also been used to treat severe pruritis associated with intrathecal opioids. The feasibility of using propofol for these two indications is such that it will only occasionally be used.

Indications

Induction of anaesthesia   A single dose of propofol results in acceptable induction of anaesthesia in the majority of patients. Falls in arterial blood pressure and the incidence of apnoea are related to the dose used and the rate of injection. Pain on injection can be controlled with lidocaine. Its pharmacokinetic properties render it the drug of choice for day-case anaesthesia, while the depression of laryngeal and pharyngeal reflexes yields optimum conditions for insertion of a laryngeal mask airway.

Total intravenous anaesthesia   Concerns about the possible toxic effects of inhalational anaesthetics and their metabolites, and of the adverse effects of environmental pollution, have led to a technique where the three components of general anaesthesia (hypnosis, analgesia and muscle relaxation) are provided solely by the intravenous route. The properties of propofol make it the ideal agent to provide the hypnotic component.

The aim of the technique is the same as for inhalational agents, namely to achieve the desired blood level of the drug as quickly as possible, to maintain it there for the duration of the operation and then to cease administration to allow reduction in blood levels, allowing recovery of consciousness to occur. It is possible to maintain anaesthesia by intermittent bolus injections, but this results in large fluctuations in blood level with the risk of cardiorespiratory depression immediately after an injection when blood levels are high and awareness just before injection when blood levels are much lower. The easiest way to achieve a constant blood level is to start the infusions at the desired rate, but under these circumstances it takes 4–5 half-lives before a steady-state concentration is reached. Propofol has three half-lives and it is a combination of these that determines the time to a steady-state plasma concentration. It takes 40–45 minutes to approach a steady–state level when given by a constant rate infusion (Gepts *et al.*, 1988) and is manifestly too long for its use in clinical practice. In order to achieve the desired plasma level rapidly, a loading dose must be given to fill the volume of distribution and then a decreasing infusion until the steady state is reached, when the infusion rate then equals the rate of elimination of the drug.

Although computer schemes have been derived to determine the infusion rate, many manual infusion schemes are available, which have been verified by measurement of propofol blood levels. One of the most popular is that described by Roberts *et al.* (1988) where following a bolus dose of 1 mg/kg, an infusion is commenced at 10 mg/kg/h for 10 minutes, 8 mg/kg/h for 10 minutes and 6 mg/kg/h thereafter. This scheme was designed to achieve a blood level of propofol of 4 μg/ml within 2 minutes and then to maintain it there. As the level of surgical stimulation is not constant during an operation, so the blood level of the anaesthetic will need to be altered to meet surgical demands, just as with inhalational anaesthesia. There are a number of factors which influence the blood level: rate of metabolism; age and physiological fitness of the patient; enzyme induction or inhibition. The blood level required will also depend on the type of surgery and the presence or absence of other drugs, e.g. premedication, nitrous oxide, dose of analgesic.

Target controlled infusions (TCI)   By incorporating a pharmacokinetic model into a computerized delivery system and entering into this pharmacokinetic parameters such as age, weight and desired plasma concentration of propofol, a system has been developed which will infuse the drug at the desired rate to achieve and maintain the chosen plasma level (White and Kenny, 1990). Such a system has been shown to succeed in producing predicted plasma levels which correlate satisfactorily with measured levels. To use such a system, it is necessary to have some knowledge of required blood levels of propofol to meet the differing demands of surgery and anaesthesia. Anaesthetists are used to working with blood levels of inhalational agents as these are indicated by the end-tidal concentrations, but there is no on-line system of measurement for intravenous anaesthetics. It has been shown that a chosen blood level of 5 µg/ml will induce anaesthesia in 90 per cent of patients premedicated with temazepam within 3 minutes. During maintenance of surgical anaesthesia, the blood levels required usually vary between 4 and 8 µg/ml, but this must be adjusted according to the patient's response. Choosing an increased blood level results in an increased infusion rate until the new level is reached, while choice of a reduced concentration results in the infusion stopping and then starting again at the appropriate time. TCI is much easier to use than manual infusion schemes.

Sedation   Propofol is an ideal agent to produce sedation for patients undergoing surgery under regional anaesthesia or for diagnostic procedures during radiology or MRI scanning. Following a bolus dose, an infusion rate of 1.5–4.5 mg/kg/h (representing a blood level in the region of 1–4 µg/ml) is usually necessary, depending on the chosen level of sedation. When used to produce sedation in the intensive care unit, rates of 0.3–4.0 mg/kg/h are normally satisfactory. Methods have now been described to allow patients to control the infusion in a way similar to patient controlled analgesia. Patient acceptance of such techniques is high. The method can also be used with target controlled infusion systems; an initial target of 1 µg/ml is chosen and optimum sedation is achieved at a level slightly less than this (Irwin *et al.*, 1997). There is considerable inter-individual variability in the amount of propofol used.

Dosage and administration

The induction dose of propofol will vary according to the rate of administration and the clinical condition of the patient. Elderly patients are more susceptible and a dose of 1.0 mg/kg may suffice, whereas fit healthy young adults may require 2.5 mg/kg or more. Premedication will reduce the dose. Slow administration will also minimize the cardiovascular and respiratory effects of the drug.

During total intravenous anaesthesia, the dose of propofol will vary according to the type of surgery and much more will be needed for upper abdominal surgery than body surface surgery. The dose will probably vary between 4 and 8 mg/kg/h. Target controlled infusions are much easier to use, but more propofol is consumed than with manual schemes. Less drug is needed to produce sedation. Use of a 1 per cent solution can on occasion result in a large fluid and lipid load and a 2 per cent solution of propofol is now available.

Precautions

These are as for all intravenous anaesthetic agents. Care must be taken in patients with cardiac disease or who are hypovolaemic. Propofol has no vagolytic properties and bradycardia is common. It is best avoided in epileptics and it has no product licence for use in obstetrics.

Propofol is not recommended for sedation in children. Serious adverse effects and even death have been reported in a small number of children with upper respiratory tract disease who have been given propofol in doses which were in excess of those used in adults. No causal relationship with propofol has been established when used in these patients. Use in children is, in fact, outwith its product licence.

When used as the anaesthetic agent for electroconvulsive therapy (ECT), the duration of seizure activity is much shorter than when methohexital or thiopental is used. As the efficacy of ECT is thought to be related to the duration of the seizure, propofol is not recommended for this treatment.

Gepts, E., Jonckheer, K., Maes, V., Sonck, W. and Camu, F. (1988) Disposition kinetics of propofol during alfentanil anaesthesia. *Anaesthesia*, **43** (Suppl.), 8–13

Irwin, M.G., Thompson, N. and Kenny, G.N.C. (1997) Patient-maintained propofol sedation. Assessment of a target-controlled infusion system. *Anaesthesia*, **52**, 525–30

Roberts, F.L., Dixon, J., Lewis, G.T.R., Tackley, R.M. and Prys-Roberts, C. (1988) Induction and maintenance of propofol anaesthesia. A manual infusion scheme. *Anaesthesia*, **43** (Suppl.), 14–17

White, M. and Kenny, M. (1990) Intravenous propofol anaesthesia using a computerised infusion system. *Anaesthesia*, **45**, 204–9

THIOPENTAL

Thiopental sodium (rINN)

Physical characteristics

Thiopental sodium occurs as a yellowish-white hygroscopic powder with a bitter taste and a faint smell of garlic. Its structural formula is given in *Figure 3.6* (page 89). It is always supplied mixed with anhydrous sodium carbonate, the mixture being readily soluble in water, giving a solution of pH 10–11. The sodium carbonate is added because thiopental is soluble only in strongly alkaline solutions. Thiopental sodium must be stored in a well-closed container and solutions should be freshly prepared.

Pharmacology

Thiopental is the sulphur analogue of pentobarbital. It was first used in the USA in 1934 by Lundy and Waters, and was introduced into Great Britain in the following year by Jarman and Abel. It has been described as an ultra-short-acting barbiturate, but the brevity of its effects is due to redistribution rather than to rapid elimination.

Nervous system When given by intravenous injection it rapidly diffuses into the brain and produces its effects within 30 s. While having strong hypnotic actions, its analgesic action is poor, and the respiratory centre is readily depressed. These characteristics make it difficult to assess the level of anaesthesia, especially as reactions to stimuli such as surgical incision can occur in the presence of apnoea and apparent deep depression of the CNS. In small doses thiopental has an anti-analgesic action, the pain threshold being actually lowered. The dose that will produce this effect is between 25 and 100 mg in healthy adults, but larger doses when they have become redistributed with the passage of time and reach a corresponding plasma level will have a similar action.

If a given dose is injected rapidly, consciousness returns at a higher plasma level than if the same dose is injected more slowly. This was at one time attributed to 'acute tolerance', a concept that is difficult to visualize in either pharmacological or physiological terms. It is more likely to be an artifact of the pharmacokinetics of 'slug' administration, a mode of administration that results in an exceedingly rapid entry into and exit from the CNS. This causes for some time a distortion of drug distribution between the brain and the peripheral circulation which does not occur with slower rates of administration.

Autonomic system   Vagal tone is not depressed with small doses of thiopental but because reflex vagal activity is often marked the impression may be gained that tone is actually increased.

Cardiovascular system   Thiopental depresses the myocardium and cardiac output decreases as the plasma concentration of the drug rises. Cardiac irritability is unaffected. There is usually a mild initial fall in blood pressure which returns to normal within a few minutes, but when the drug is injected rapidly or in large doses, severe hypotension may occur. This is mainly due to peripheral vasodilatation caused by depression of the vasomotor centre, but direct depression of myocardial contractility also plays a part. Such depression of blood pressure is more marked in the presence of cardiovascular disease, especially hypertension.

Respiratory system   Respiration is markedly depressed by thiopental. Following a few deep breaths a short period of apnoea is common, respiration being resumed with a diminished rate and depth. The degree of respiratory depression depends on the dose of thiopental administered and the speed of administration, and it is enhanced by the previous administration of other central depressants such as morphine and its derivatives. The sensitivity of the respiratory centre to carbon dioxide is considerably reduced. There is a mild degree of bronchial constriction, but secretions are not increased.
    Laryngeal reflexes are not depressed by thiopental and laryngeal spasm will therefore result in the presence of any stimulus e.g. presence of blood or mucus. Pharyngeal reflexes are depressed but not to the same extent as by equipotent doses of propofol and laryngeal mask insertion is easier following the latter drug.

Musculature   Skeletal muscle tone is markedly reduced when central depression is at its height. Smooth muscle is unaffected during light anaesthesia, but large doses cause depression of activity.

Uterus and placenta   Small doses of thiopental have little effect on the pregnant uterus, although contractions are depressed by large doses. It rapidly crosses the placental barrier; the fetal blood level is related to maternal blood level but is considerably lower. It is temporarily markedly raised shortly after a 'slug' of drug is administered to the mother.

Fate in the body   After injection, the level of thiopental in the plasma reaches its maximum rapidly. It is immediately taken up by nervous tissue and other tissues with a high blood flow. It then begins to diffuse more slowly from the plasma to other tissues, mainly liver, kidney and muscles. Most of the thiopental eventually ends up in fat, but the blood supply of this is so poor that it can play no part in the lowering of brain concentration leading to early awakening. As the plasma level falls, the concentration in the brain falls likewise and consciousness returns. At this time most of the original dose injected is still present unchanged in the body, having merely been redistributed from brain to other tissues.
    If a second dose of thiopental is given, then recovery from its effects will take longer. As there already is thiopental in the tissues responsible for its redistribution from the brain, then it will take longer for the drug to leave the brain (to take a simplistic view, the concentration gradient between the brain and these tissues is less, so it diffuses out

more slowly). As further repeat doses are given, so the concentration in these tissues increases and they lose their ability to 'remove' thiopental from the brain. Recovery thus gets longer and longer following repeated doses i.e. cumulation occurs. Thiopental is therefore unsuitable for repeat use and administration by continuous infusion.

In the blood, thiopental is bound to plasma proteins. Decreased binding occurs in malnutrition and other severe wasting illness and this accounts for a large increase in sensitivity to thiopental. The amount bound depends to a great extent upon the blood pH. Increasing the plasma pH by hyperventilation will increase the plasma concentration of free thiopental, and will therefore increase the effects of a given dose.

Thiopental is almost entirely metabolized in the liver. Breakdown products are excreted by the kidneys and alimentary tract. Traces are excreted unchanged in the urine. Destruction in the body is slow, 10–15 per cent per hour, and nearly 30 per cent of the original dose may remain after 24 h. Consequently, if further thiopental is given there will be a cumulative effect.

Liver and kidney function   No permanent effects have been recorded.

Metabolism   Oxygen consumption falls in proportion to the depth of anaesthesia. In the absence of surgical stimuli there are no effects on the endocrine system.

Indications

Practically all types of operation have at one time been attempted under thiopental, but respiratory depression and the slow recovery time associated with the use of large doses have led to its abandonment as a sole agent for anaesthesia in favour of more satisfactory methods. Thiopental is now only used for induction of anaesthesia and in the treatment of status epilepticus.

Dosage and administration

Thiopental is normally given intravenously in a 2.5 per cent solution. It can be given per rectum in a 5 per cent or 10 per cent solution.

The dose of thiopental required to produce a given depth of narcosis varies considerably according to the age and condition of the patient, and even healthy patients vary in their response. The rate of injection is also important; the faster the injection, the quicker and deeper is the response and the quicker is the recovery. Only the smallest dose necessary to produce the desired effect should be given.

For the induction of anaesthesia in fit adults, a dose of 3–5 mg/kg is usually required; half the dose may be injected over a period of 15 s, and after a pause long enough to note the effect the injection is continued until the desired level of narcosis is reached. Respiration must be assisted if unduly depressed.

For basal narcosis by the rectal route in children, the dose is calculated on the basis of 1 g of thiopental per 22 kg of body weight. It is given in 5 or 10 per cent solution. and is normally effective within about 15 minutes of administration.

Precautions

There are a considerable number of hazards associated with thiopental anaesthesia; its potency makes it a highly dangerous drug in inexperienced hands. It is very easy to give an overdose, especially to sick and elderly patients.

It should never be given to patients in the sitting position, as even a small overdose can cause severe hypotension. It should never be given rapidly to any but fit and robust patients. An apparatus capable of ventilating the lungs should always be readily available when thiopental is being used.

It is an unsuitable drug for use in outpatients, but if a more appropriate drug is not available, patients must be allowed to rest for as long as possible after recovering consciousness. They should be accompanied home by a responsible person and told not to take alcohol for 24 h, drive, or operate machinery.

Atropine or an atropine-like drug should always be given before or with thiopental to depress vagal reflexes and mucous secretions. Central depressants such as morphine or pethidine are often given before thiopental to reduce the dose of thiopental required.

It is probably true to say that, apart from patients with porphyria, there is a safe dose of thiopental for everyone. Apart from absence of suitable veins for its administration it is generally considered to be contraindicated in the following situations:

- porphyria;
- if the airway is obstructed in conditions such as Ludwig's angina, and where an adequate airway cannot be guaranteed;
- in severe shock;
- in uncompensated heart disease, and constrictive pericarditis;
- in status asthmaticus.

In some of these conditions, general anaesthesia would, of course, be a hazard in any case.

Relative contraindications, where special care should be exercised both as regards size of dose and the rate of administration, are as follows:

- decreased circulating blood volume – severe haemorrhage, burns, dehydration;.
- severe anaemia;
- cardiovascular disease – conditions affecting the myocardium, severe hypertension;
- severe liver disease;
- dystrophia myotonica;
- myasthenia gravis;
- adrenocortical insufficiency, even when controlled by cortisol;
- cachexia and severe toxaemia;
- raised blood urea;
- raised plasma potassium;
- reduced metabolic rate, as in myxoedema.

Smaller doses than normal will be required in the elderly, and in subjects who have been heavily premedicated with narcotics and other central depressants. The dose in obstetric cases should be restricted to the minimum necessary for induction.

Complications

Laryngeal spasm   This is uncommon unless the patient is stimulated and even then is likely to be seen only when painful procedures are undertaken under thiopental alone. Its occurrence in other circumstances suggests the proximity of blood, saliva or stomach contents to the laryngeal inlet.

Bronchospasm   This may occur in asthmatics whose vagal reflexes are particularly sensitive.

Extravascular injection This causes pain and swelling which is less severe with the 2.5 per cent than with the 5 per cent solution. Treatment consists of infiltrating the area with lidocaine and hyaluronidase. The arm should be kept at rest.

Intra-arterial injection This usually results in intense pain shooting down the arm, blanching of the skin and disappearance or weakness of the radial pulse. Delayed and permanent sequelae include gangrene of parts of the arm, hand and fingers which may require amputation. Intra-arterial thiopental results in precipitation of crystals of the drug, due to the discrepancy in pH between the drug and the blood, which block the small vessels of the hand, with possible retrograde thrombosis, and release of norepinephrine (noradrenaline) from the vessel wall. As a 5 per cent solution of thiopental contains twice as much drug as a 2.5 per cent, then the incidence of serious sequelae is greater.

Thrombophlebitis This complication sometimes occurs after injection of thiopental, but is less likely to occur if the 2.5 per cent solution is used. Treatment is symptomatic and may require rest and warmth.

Overdose An overdose of thiopental will produce apnoea or serious respiratory depression. Cardiovascular collapse may also occur. Respiratory insufficiency requires controlled respiration with oxygen until normal respiration is resumed. Analeptics should not be given. Thiopental may cause an anaphylactoid reaction but it is very rare – about 1 in 15 000 administrations.

References and further reading

ABPI's Compendium of Data Sheets (1998–99 edn) *Datapharm Publications Ltd, London (Refer for individual products)*

Baldessarini, R.I. (1996) Drugs and the treatment of psychiatric disorders: psychosis and anxiety. In *Goodman and Gilman's 'The Pharmacological Basis of Therapeutic'*, 9th edn, Chapter 18, pp. 399–430 (Eds: Hardman, J.G., Limbird, L.E. and Gilman, A.G.). New York: McGraw-Hill

Hobbs, W.R., Rall, T.W. and Verdoorn, T.A. (1996) Hypnotics and sedatives; ethanol. In *Goodman and Gilman's 'The Pharmacological Basis of Therapeutic'*, 9th edn, Chapter 17, pp. 361–396 (Eds: Hardman, J.G., Limbird, L.E. and Gilman, A.G.). New York: McGraw-Hill

Iqbal, N. and Van Praag, H.M. (1995) The role of serotonin in schizophrenia. *Eur. J. Neuropsychopharmacology,* **5**(suppl), 11–23

Liddow, M.S., Williams, G.V. and Goldman-Rakic, P.S. (1998) The cerebral cortex: a case for a common site of action of antipsychotics. *Trends in Pharmacological Sciences,* **19**, 136–140

Siegel, E. and Buhr, A. (1997) The benzodiazepine binding site of GABA$_A$ receptors. *Trends in Pharmacological Sciences,* **18**, 425–429

Whitwam, J.G. (1987) Benzodiazepines. *Anaesthesia,* **42**, 1255

4

General anaesthetics

The word 'anaesthesia' means absence of sensation, and general anaesthesia therefore implies unconsciousness. General anaesthetics include any agents capable of producing total insensibility in a reversible manner. In fact, the term 'general anaesthetic' has come to mean an agent whose actions are qualified in far more detail than this, especially with regard to good relaxation of skeletal muscles, lack of toxicity to tissues, minimal after-effects and a recovery that is complete and predictable.

Stages of anaesthesia

Certain stages are recognized to describe the depth of anaesthesia. These stages were first described for anaesthesia induced with ether given by the semi-open method in unpremedicated patients, and are modified when agents other than ether are used or when premedication is employed. Four stages are described which can be recognized both during induction of, and recovery from, anaesthesia.

Stage I: stage of analgesia   This stage lasts from the commencement of induction until loss of consciousness. Respiration is quiet, but often irregular. Reflexes are still present. This stage is utilized during obstetric analgesia, when sub-anaesthetic concentrations of nitrous oxide or a volatile agent are administered.

Stage II: stage of excitement or delirium   This stage lasts from the loss of consciousness to the onset of surgical anaesthesia. The patient is unconscious and uncooperative, but may talk, move the limbs, or even become violent. Respiration is irregular and breath-holding may occur: the irregular respiration may result in an irregular rate of absorption of anaesthetic vapour. Reflexes in response to stimuli are active. Retching may occur and, if the stomach is not empty, vomiting may result. Premature surgical stimulation may cause excessive release of epinephrine (adrenaline), with a danger of ventricular fibrillation. The more quickly and smoothly the patient can be brought through this stage, the less likely are these reactions.

Stage III: stage of surgical anaesthesia   This stage extends from the onset of regular respiration, commonly termed 'automatic', until respiratory failure occurs from a toxic concentration of anaesthetic agent in the CNS. This stage is divided into the following four planes:

Plane 1. Movements cease and respiration becomes regular and automatic; the eyelid reflex is lost. Eyeball movements are marked. The pharyngeal reflex disappears late in this plane, but the laryngeal and peritoneal reflexes are still present, and so is muscle tone.

Plane 2. The eyes become fixed centrally; muscle tone is decreasing but all muscles of respiration are still functioning. The laryngeal and peritoneal reflexes disappear during this stage.

Plane 3. Onset of paralysis of intercostal muscles, with respiration becoming purely diaphragmatic. Good muscle relaxation.

Plane 4. Respiration becoming gradually depressed with paralysis of diaphragm. A tracheal tug may be present. Muscle relaxation is full.

Stage IV: stage of medullary paralysis, with respiratory arrest and vasomotor collapse.
The pupils are widely dilated and the skin is cold and ashen. The blood pressure is very low and the pulse feeble. Respiration is gasping and finally ceases.

These stages are usually well defined with ether or chloroform, but are much less clearly marked when more modern agents are used. If anaesthesia is induced with an intravenous barbiturate, the stages become telescoped, the patient passing rapidly into Stage III, Plane 2, and the intermediate stages are not recognized. With the introduction of muscle relaxants and powerful analgesics. there is no indication for 'deeper' levels of anaesthesia.

Surgical anaesthesia

Surgical anaesthesia should be a state of harmless and reversible insensibility which allows operations of considerable magnitude to be carried out without hindrance to the surgeon or detriment to the patient. It is convenient to consider this anaesthetic state as consisting of a triad of sleep, analgesia and muscular relaxation. 'Sleep' in this context differs from natural sleep, where subjects can be awakened by simple and not necessarily painful stimuli, such as touch and noise. By definition, the anaesthetized patient cannot be roused by stimuli of any intensity. Different patients undergoing different surgical procedures will require different degrees of analgesia and muscular relaxation.

It has so far not proved possible to find any single drug that will produce all these effects without causing unpleasant or undesirable side actions. Single anaesthetic agents are rarely used today except for very short and minor operations. The aim now is to use several agents, each for its specific pharmacological actions and in minimal doses so as to produce a state of 'balanced anaesthesia'. A common practice is to use thiopental or propofol to produce initial brief but deep sleep; to maintain sleep and provide analgesia with nitrous oxide supplemented either with low concentrations of a volatile anaesthetic and incremental doses of a systemic analgesic; and to use neuromuscular blocking agents to produce the required degree of muscular relaxation. In this way patients will be enabled to regain protective reflexes and recover consciousness within a few minutes of the end of an operation and suffer minimal postoperative side effects and complications.

Mode of action of anaesthetics

A large number of chemical substances are capable of producing general anaesthesia, and many attempts have been made to produce a single theory of action that would embrace them all. These compounds have no common chemical structure, thus no structure– activity relationships can be defined. Many are also chemically unreactive and unlikely to occupy specific receptors. In most theories, attempts have been made to correlate anaesthetic potency with some physical property of the anaesthetic agents. The majority of these theories imply a major site of action at the neuronal cell membrane. More recent research has indicated that these theories are largely incorrect and may actually have been misleading.

The lipid solubility theory followed the observation by Meyer and Overton that the narcotic potency of members of a chemical series is proportional to their oil/water partition coefficients. This led people to believe that the fat layers of the neuronal cell membrane were the site of action of anaesthetic agents. While the observations of Meyer and Overton were undoubtedly true, it does not mean that the anaesthetic state results from the effects of substances dissolving in the fatty neuronal membranes.

Other theories suggested that anaesthetic agents could form hydrates (also known as clathrates) which would form microcrystals in the cell membranes and affect their function. At body temperature, however, very high pressures are necessary for clathrate formation. Anaesthetic agents have been shown to affect Na^+ and K^+ movement in neuronal membranes, but these changes are very small at concentrations relevant to general anaesthesia. Similarly Ca^{2+} channels are little affected by anaesthetics in clinical concentrations. The suggestion that anaesthetics act by causing reversible dispersal of microtubules has also been disproved. The discovery that the anaesthetic state could be reversed by pressures of 50 atmospheres or more led to suggestions that anaesthesia was due to expansions of molecular sites, but again, whereas pressure reversal is a fact, it does not explain anaesthesia.

More recent work, particularly by Franks and Lieb (1994), has concentrated on the molecular and cellular aspects of general anaesthesia. Basically it is suggested that at clinical concentrations the main effects of anaesthetics are on ligand-gated ion channels rather than voltage-gated ion channels.

GABA$_A$ receptors   General anaesthetics might act by potentiating inhibitory transmission. Most anaesthetics are very effective, at clinical concentrations, at potentiating responses to GABA. This has been shown for the barbiturates, propofol, alfaxalone and the inhalational agents halothane, enflurane and isoflurane, and most evidence now suggests that GABA$_A$ channels are a major site of action for most general anaesthetics, with the exception of ketamine. The effects are probably largely mediated at post-synaptic membranes. There is little evidence that anaesthetics affect second messenger systems.

Glutamate receptors   Glutamate is the major excitatory transmitter in the CNS. One of the selective agonists at this receptor is *N*-methyl-D-aspartate (NMDA). Good evidence now exists that ketamine exerts its effect by inhibiting the NMDA receptor.

Molecular sites   Many drugs act by binding to proteins and there is now evidence, following work with a lipid-free enzyme, firefly luciferase, that general anaesthetics do the same. This is supported from observations on stereoselectivity. Although protein binding appears to be the mechanism of action of anaesthetics, there is no information so far as to the site of binding on the membrane proteins.

Franks, N.P. and Lieb, W.R. (1994) Molecular and cellular mechanism of anaesthesia. *Nature*, **367**, 607–14

Uptake and distribution of inhalational agents

After administration via the lungs, the rate of entry of general anaesthetics into any tissue depends upon:

- the rate of entry into the circulation;
- the steepness of the concentration gradient between blood and the tissue concerned;
- the blood supply of the tissue;
- the affinity of that tissue for the anaesthetic.

All anaesthetics readily diffuse into the CNS. The attainment of adequate brain tension of an anaesthetic depends upon the balance between the rate of entry of anaesthetic into the blood and its removal into other tissues.

The progress of an anaesthetic can in theory be divided into three phases. During induction, the anaesthetic agent is being taken up into body tissues across the concentration gradients that exist. Eventually, tissues come into equilibrium with the inspired tension, and in the maintenance phase there is no net uptake of anaesthetic. During recovery, inspired tension is reduced to zero and elimination of anaesthetic occurs across the reversed tension gradient. In practice, because of the long time constants of some body tissues, equilibrium is rarely achieved during clinical anaesthesia. Uptake of most anaesthetic agents continues for many hours, albeit at a lower rate.

The rate of uptake of an anaesthetic agent, and thus the duration of induction, is determined by the rate at which the alveolar anaesthetic tension approaches the inspired anaesthetic tension. Small and negligible differences exist between the tension of an anaesthetic in alveolar gas, arterial blood and brain but, because of dilution, large differences can exist between inspired and alveolar tensions. The important factors that determine alveolar anaesthetic tension are the solubility of the agent in blood, the inspired tension, alveolar ventilation, cardiac output and venous anaesthetic levels.

Blood solubility

This is best expressed in terms of the partition coefficient of the agent between blood and gas at body temperature (*Table 4.1*). Agents with a high blood/gas partition coefficient are removed in large quantities from alveoli by pulmonary capillary blood, reducing the mass and therefore the tension of agent left in the alveoli. As arterial blood is in near tension equilibrium with the alveoli, blood and brain tensions thus rise slowly. In

Table 4.1 Chemical structure and properties of the inhalational anaesthetics

Drug	Chemical formula	Molecular weight	Boiling point (°C)	Saturated vapour pressure at 20°C	Partition coefficients at 37°C Blood/gas	Oil/gas	MAC% (v/v)
Nitrous oxide	N_2O	44.0	−88.5	38760	0.47	1.4	110.0
Cyclopropane	C_3H_6	42.1	−32.9	4800	0.46	11.8	9.2
Halothane	$CF_3CHClBr$	197.4	50.2	243.3	2.3	224	0.75
Trichloroethylene	C_2HCl_3	131.4	86.7	64.5	9.15	970	—
Diethyl ether	$(C_2H_5)_2O$	74.1	34.6	44.2	12.1	65	1.92
Enflurane	$CHFClCF_2-O-CF_2H$	184.5	56.5	171.8	1.9	96	1.68
Isoflurane	$CF_3CHCl-O-CF_2H$	184.5	48.5	235.9	1.4	91	1.15
Sevoflurane	$CF_3CF_3CH-O-CH_2F$	192.0	58.5	160	0.6	42	2.0
Desflurane	$CF_3CFH-O-CF_2H$	168.0	24.0	700 (22°C)	0.42	18.7	6.0

contrast, insoluble agents such as nitrous oxide and sevoflurane are removed in only small quantities from the alveoli. Alveolar tension thus rapidly approaches inspired tension and induction of anaesthesia is rapid.

Inspired tension

The prolonged induction phase seen with soluble agents may be shortened to some extent by initially increasing the inspired anaesthetic tension. In this way an adequate blood tension can be attained long before equilibrium between inspired and alveolar tensions has occurred. Because of the complexities of pulmonary gas exchange, the rate of uptake of an anaesthetic is not a simple function of its inspired tension. This is discussed in the concentration effect below (*Figure 4.1*).

Alveolar ventilation

An increase in alveolar ventilation, by increasing the mass of anaesthetic presented to the alveolar membrane, will increase the rate of uptake. This factor is of greater importance with soluble agents. Blood is so readily saturated with insoluble agents that the availability of an increased mass of anaesthetic has little effect on the rate of uptake, whereas with soluble agents blood leaving the lungs generally has a largely unsatisfied anaesthetic capacity. Doubling alveolar ventilation during diethyl ether anaesthesia will nearly halve the duration of the induction phase.

Cardiac output

An increase in cardiac output allows more agent to be removed from the alveoli by blood and thus increases the inspired–alveolar tension gradient. When cardiac output is

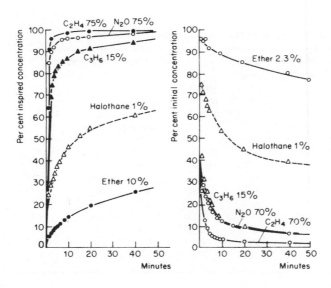

Figure 4.1 Differences between anaesthetics in the rate at which alveolar concentration approaches that inspired. The curves on the left represent induction, and those on the right, recovery. The actual inspired concentration during induction is noted on the respective curves. Alveolar concentrations at the start of recovery are noted on the respective curves. The curves for recovery assume complete tissue equilibrium (From Papper and Kitz, 1963)

reduced, less anaesthetic is removed from the lungs and alveolar tension approaches inspired tension more rapidly. However, these effects of changes in cardiac output are seen only in the early stages of induction. When cardiac output rises, a greater mass of agent is extracted from the alveoli and presented to the tissues, which become saturated more rapidly. The concomitant rise in venous anaesthetic level limits further anaesthetic uptake in the alveoli. During clinical anaesthesia, changes in cardiac output are often accompanied by widespread alterations in the distribution of blood, which can have complex and often unforeseeable effects on anaesthetic uptake.

Venous anaesthetic levels

The amount of anaesthetic that is removed from the alveoli is also a function of the arteriovenous anaesthetic tension difference. At equilibrium, arterial and mixed venous tensions are equal and uptake is zero. Arteriovenous difference is due to tissue uptake and depends upon the solubility of an agent in tissues and upon tissue blood flow. Tissue/blood coefficients of anaesthetics vary throughout the body, being highest in lipid tissues. Body tissues can be divided into three compartments. Initially, tissues of the vessel-rich group play a dominant part in uptake. These tissues comprise the brain, heart, kidney, hepatoportal system and endocrine glands. Uptake by muscle and skin proceeds at a slower rate. The vessel-poor tissues consist predominantly of fat which, because of its poor blood supply and its affinity for anaesthetic agents, often continues to take up anaesthetic for many hours after all other body tissues have reached equilibrium.

Papper, E.M. and Kitz, R.J. (1963) *Uptake and distribution of Anaesthetic Agents*. New York: McGraw-Hill

Concentration and second gas effects

A relationship exists between the rate at which the alveolar tension of any agent approaches the inspired tension and the actual inspired concentration. In theory, the rate of uptake of all agents is equally rapid when they are administered in 100 per cent concentration; under these circumstances anaesthetic uptake will still leave a 100 per cent anaesthetic mixture within the lung and will not reduce the alveolar tension. With lower inspired tensions, the duration of the uptake phase is progressively increased. When uptake of an agent occurs from the lung, alveolar volume is potentially reduced and additional gaseous inflow occurs in order to maintain intrapulmonary pressure. The effect on the rate of uptake of this additional inspiratory flow is greatest with high inspired anaesthetic concentrations. This 'concentration effect' is most marked with agents that can be given over a wide range of inspired concentrations and which can be taken up in large volumes, such as diethyl ether and nitrous oxide.

Closely related to the concentration effect is the 'second gas' effect. Removal of anaesthetic from the alveoli by the uptake process increases the fractional concentration and therefore the tension of other components of alveolar gas. Uptake of one agent can therefore increase the rate of uptake of a second agent.

A mathematical treatment of many of the factors concerned in anaesthetic uptake can be obtained from the general equation describing the determinants of the alveolar concentration of an inhaled gas. This states that

$$F_{Ax} = F_{Ix} \frac{-V_x}{V_A}$$

where F_{Ix} and F_{Ax} are the fractional concentrations of gas x inhaled and in alveolar gas, respectively: V_x is the uptake of gas x per unit time; and V_A alveolar ventilation per unit time. When x represents any anaesthetic, this equation shows that the alveolar concentration will be reduced if uptake increases or if alveolar ventilation falls. Uptake in this equation is a function of blood solubility, cardiac output and venous anaesthetic levels. This equation does not describe the concentration effect or the second gas effect.

Rubber solubility

Some anaesthetic agents have quite high solubility in rubber and uptake into rubber of breathing systems could produce large initial differences between the anaesthetic concentration entering the breathing system and that leaving and entering the patient. Nowadays, with the advent of single-use plastic breathing systems, such problems do not normally arise.

Excretion of volatile anaesthetics

During elimination of volatile anaesthetics by the lung, the factors concerned in uptake operate in a reverse fashion. Alveolar tension is the resultant of the amount of agent released to the alveoli from blood and the amount removed by alveolar ventilation. Insoluble agents are readily released from blood and removed by alveolar ventilation, leading to rapid recovery. Soluble agents, because of their affinity for blood, are removed from the body more slowly.

The duration of the recovery phase is also related to the mass of anaesthetic present in body tissues, and will thus be affected by the duration of anaesthesia and the tissue solubility of the agent. High fat solubility of an agent may lead to the presence during recovery of a large reservoir of anaesthetic which, because it is contained in poorly perfused tissues, is released only slowly to the blood. For example, nitrous oxide and cyclopropane have nearly identical blood/gas partition coefficients and recovery after a brief administration takes a similar time with both agents. If administration is prolonged, the higher lipid solubility of cyclopropane becomes a more dominant factor, and recovery from this agent is then much slower than after nitrous oxide given for a similar period of time.

Metabolism of volatile anaesthetics

General anaesthetics were traditionally considered to be inert substances, undergoing no chemical reaction in the body and being excreted in an unchanged form. The lungs are the major route of elimination, small amounts of unchanged agent appearing in the urine, sweat and other secretions. Strong evidence has now accumulated to show that all volatile agents undergo biotransformation to a varying extent, and both volatile and non-volatile metabolic products of inhaled anaesthetics have been demonstrated in experimental animals and man.

Biotransformation of drugs in general is a process aimed at reducing the lipid solubility and increasing the water solubility of administered substances. It is not surprising that the inhalational anaesthetics, which have a high lipid affinity and in the main are hydrophobic, should undergo some transformation in the body. As with all drugs, biotransformation of anaesthetics occurs in the liver and is effected by microsomal enzymes, especially cytochrome P-450. The commonest transformation is an oxidation resulting in ether cleavage or dehalogenation. Halothane appears to be an exception in undergoing reduction as well as oxidation. Initial transformation is followed by conjugation to form glucuronides. The fraction of anaesthetic transformed varies greatly between agents, ranging from nearly 50 per cent for methoxyflurane to 0.2 per cent for isoflurane, and probably less than 0.01 per cent for nitrous oxide.

Enzyme induction by phenobarbital increases the rate of breakdown. Metabolic transformation of anaesthetics is reduced by treatment with non-specific enzyme inhibitors such as SKF S25A. There is some evidence to show that high concentrations of anaesthetics inhibit their own biotransformation.

Biotransformation of inhalational anaesthetics may have important clinical implications. The nephrotoxicity of methoxyflurane was related to the liberation of inorganic fluoride during metabolism of this compound. The lethal results of prolonged exposure of a variety of experimental animals to fluroxene was due to the production of trifluoroethanol. One type of hepatitis following halothane is due to production of a genetically determined metabolite.

Evaluation of anaesthetic potency

The term 'potency' can be used to refer to different attributes of anaesthetic agents. A potent agent may be considered as one that produces its effects in low concentrations. By this definition, methoxyflurane and trichloroethylene are the most potent and nitrous oxide the least potent inhalational agents. This use of the term ignores the lengthy period for which these 'potent' agents may have to be administered in order to attain their low effective blood concentrations. In a different sense, potency may refer to the rapidity with which anaesthesia can be produced. Here, nitrous oxide and sevoflurane would be considered as agents of high potency, while methoxyflurane and trichloroethylene would be classed as agents of low potency. A third method of comparison is to class as potent those anaesthetics capable of producing deep anaesthesia down to Stage IV of the Guedel classification. By this definition, nitrous oxide becomes the least potent of all agents.

Because of the obvious confusion which can arise when the term is used in different ways, any statement of anaesthetic potency should define the criteria by which potency is being evaluated.

Further confusion is possible when attempting to define the concentrations of inhalational agents required to induce and maintain anaesthesia. The inspired concentration, which is easy to measure, often bears a complex and unknown relationship to alveolar and arterial concentrations. The concentration required for induction often depends upon how much time it is considered desirable to spend in going through this phase: induction of anaesthesia with diethyl ether can be achieved with equally effective end-results using inspired concentrations varying from 5 to 50 per cent. Surgical anaesthesia has no sharp end-points, and difficulties arise in determining the concentrations necessary to produce this stage of anaesthesia.

These potential confusions have been eliminated by the use of the concept of 'minimum alveolar (anaesthetic) concentration' (MAC). This is defined as the alveolar concentration of an agent which will prevent response to specified stimuli in 50 per cent of subjects. MAC can be converted into a partial pressure (as a percentage of 1 atm) and then represents the tension of anaesthetic at its site of action in the brain. Average MAC values for most of the commonly used agents are given in *Table 4.1.*

The MAC is unaffected by duration of anaesthesia and changes in $Paco_2$, or Pao_2 over a wide range. It is affected by age; halothane has a MAC of 1.08 per cent in infants and 0.64 per cent at age 81 years. MAC is affected by drugs that alter CNS catecholamine levels: D-amfetamine raises MAC, whereas catecholamine depleters such as reserpine reduce it. MAC is also affected by temperature. Other inhalational anaesthetics reduce the MAC of any agent in a simple subtractive manner. The addition of 70 per cent nitrous oxide reduces the MAC of halothane by about 60 per cent. Narcotic analgesics lower MAC in a non-additive fashion. Premedication with 10 mg of morphine lowers the MAC of halothane by about 7 per cent.

Pharmacology

While the various anaesthetics each have their own pharmacological actions, certain generalizations may be made concerning the physiological changes produced by anaesthesia, whatever the causative agent.

Central nervous system

The paralysis of function of the CNS begins at the cortical level and descends, but fortunately irregularly. The order is cortex, basal ganglia, cerebellum, spinal cord (sensory then motor), medulla. In the medulla the respiratory centre is completely depressed before the vasomotor centre, but only just before with some anaesthetics. It must not be thought that any given level of the CNS is fully depressed before any depression of the next begins; all levels suffer some effect right from the start of anaesthesia, although in some circumstances there may be a phase of reflex stimulation of some areas associated with the depression of other controlling influences. At a neurophysiological level, anaesthetics appear to exert most of their influence at the thalamic level, inhibiting transmission from the periphery to the brain.

A point with important practical consequences is the implication of a 'safety margin'. Usually this is stated to be wide if the concentration of anaesthetic required to cause medullary paralysis and cardiac arrest is great compared with the concentration required for surgical anaesthesia, but such a fascination with figures does not take into consideration the relative ease and rapidity with which concentrations may be increased for some anaesthetics without the signs of severely deepening anaesthesia being very obvious.

Autonomic system

Autonomic balance At first there may be stimulation, later there is normally depression of this system, but the action on the sympathetic and parasympathetic is often unequal; thus the tone of one or the other may predominate and there may appear to be either a parasympathomimetic or sympathomimetic effect.

Gastro-intestinal tract Nausea and vomiting, much more frequent during recovery than during induction, are mainly of central origin. Anaesthetic agents also depress gastro-intestinal motility and secretion.

Cardiovascular effects

In general, the deeper the anaesthesia the more obvious is the depression of the vasomotor centre, but the precise cardiovascular effects of general anaesthetics vary very much from substance to substance. All anaesthetics cause progressive myocardial depression with increasing dose, but in the intact animal this may be completely masked by sympathetic over-activity, for example, as a response to hypercapnia.

Some of the halogenated hydrocarbons, particularly halothane, increase cardiac irritability. Cardiac irregularities are not uncommon during their use, especially in the presence of an increased carbon dioxide tension, hypoxia, or an increase in circulating epinephrine.

Heart rate   In the first two stages of anaesthesia the rate is increased, but the better the pre-anaesthetic sedation and the shorter the duration of these early stages, the less marked is the over-activity of the sympathetic nervous system. Even in surgical anaesthesia ether usually causes an increased heart rate by sympathetic stimulation, while halothane generally causes a slow rate, by increasing vagal tone.

Cardiac output and the distribution of blood flow   Cardiac output is decreased during anaesthesia, apart from a temporary rise during induction if accompanied by excitement. Total cardiac output may fall to 3 litres/minute or less. Local autoregulatory mechanisms ensure that cerebral and coronary blood flows are well maintained. In early and light anaesthesia, in the absence of oligaemia or dehydration, there is a marked increase in skin blood flow and, with most anaesthetics, in muscle flow also. This is probably due to a central depression of vasomotor tone, although certain anaesthetics, notably chloroform and halothane, have a direct vasodilator action as well as a central effect. Both liver and kidney suffer considerable reductions in blood flow in deep anaesthesia, and oliguria or even suppression of urine formation can occur. However, during 'balanced' anaesthesia, urine flow can easily be maintained by adequate parenteral fluid therapy. Since the total peripheral resistance is not markedly reduced, the splanchnic vessels, by inference, are believed to be constricted, and the flow reduced. A major determinant of this is the degree of sympathetic over-activity induced by the anaesthetic agent.

Blood pressure   Light surgical anaesthesia may usually be achieved with blood pressure relatively unaltered or slightly reduced. Occasional increases may be due to carbon dioxide retention or stimulation of the too lightly anaesthetized patient. Falls in pressure during light anaesthesia may be due to unrecognized hypovolaemia. Progressive hypotension during prolonged light anaesthesia is often due to unreplaced fluid loss. Deepening the level of anaesthesia tends to cause a fall in blood pressure, often proportionate to depth, and due to progressive vasomotor paralysis and direct myocardial depression.

Respiration

All anaesthetics depress the medullary respiratory centre when present in sufficient concentration and reduce its sensitivity to carbon dioxide, but there are variations within the pattern of steadily increasing depression, and with some anaesthetics there are even phases of respiratory stimulation.

The tendency for respiration to be shallower and more rapid in anaesthesia is often ascribed to effects upon the lung stretch receptors which inhibit inspiration, and upon intrathoracic receptors which initiate inspiration when expiration occurs (deflation reflex). These reflexes are much less effective in man than in other species.

Some hypoxaemia exists for hours or days after anaesthesia and surgery; the causes are many, and include the site of operation, the degree of pain and changes in ventilation/perfusion relationships. It is related to pre-existing lung disease, age and the nature of the operation, and probably reflects a continuation after operation of impairment of gas exchange in the lungs.

Metabolism

Metabolism is depressed during anaesthesia, oxygen uptake and carbon dioxide output by tissues falling to basal levels.

Temperature

The hypothalamic regulation of heat loss is depressed and body temperature varies with the environment: hypothermia or hyperthermia can result. Serious loss of heat may occur in newborn infants. Hyperthermia is particularly dangerous in older children who are already febrile.

Electrolyte and water balance

Pituitary and adrenocortical systems appear to be affected in such a way that there is retention of water and sodium in the body and a loss of potassium following surgery, due to the stress of surgical trauma. There are no specific effects with well-conducted anaesthesia.

Kidney function

All potent inhalational agents cause a reduction in renal blood flow and glomerular filtration rate in proportion to the dose. The association between the metabolic production of inorganic fluoride ions and high-output renal failure has been known for years. Enflurane is metabolized to a small extent and occasional cases of renal failure have been reported following its use. It should not be used in patients with renal impairment. Sevoflurane is metabolized to a slightly greater extent than enflurane and fluoride levels greater than 50 μmol/litre have occasionally been measured after sevoflurane, but there has been no evidence of postoperative clinical renal dysfunction. This is almost certainly due to the fact that sevoflurane, like enflurane (but unlike methoxyflurane), undergoes minimal intrarenal defluorination. Although fluoride is also the major metabolite of isoflurane, the extent of its metabolism is so small (0.2 per cent) that the amount of fluoride produced is believed to be unlikely to cause renal damage.

Liver function

Disturbances of liver function are known to occur postoperatively and in the majority of cases can be traced to events that occurred during surgery. Hypoxia and hypotension are factors that will aggravate any tendency to liver dysfunction. Occasionally liver damage occurs when there has been no obvious precipitating cause and suspicion falls on the anaesthetic agent used, particularly if this has been a halogenated hydrocarbon.

Voluntary muscle

With most anaesthetics the degree of relaxation of voluntary muscle depends on depression of the CNS, but with all modern potent agents there is also a potentiation of the effects of non-depolarizing relaxants.

Uterus

In labour, concentrations of anaesthetics that are merely analgesic do not affect uterine action. Halothane may be given in concentrations up to 0.5 per cent for Caesarean section, but in concentrations greater than this it causes relaxation of uterine muscle and is unsuitable when uterine contraction is desirable. Enflurane and isoflurane also do not relax the uterus in light planes of surgical anaesthesia.

Transplacental passage

All of the general anaesthetics cross the placental barrier and reach the fetus, giving degrees of depression proportional to their concentration. The tensions in the fetus lag behind those in the mother so that duration of administration also has an effect. With low concentrations there is no clinical problem and certainly any effect is minor when set against the danger of unintended awareness of the mother.

Anaesthetic hazards

The dangers to the patient of drugs used to produce anaesthesia are obvious. While the introduction of agents with fewer side effects and the better understanding of the use of these agents have greatly reduced the hazards of general anaesthesia, constant care must be exercised in the use of these potent and potentially lethal drugs. In recent years, increasing interest has been paid to the potential relationships between the metabolism of anaesthetic agents and their toxicity. A low level of metabolic transformation is a desirable attribute of any new inhalational anaesthetic.

Anaesthetic drugs are potentially hazardous, not to the patient alone but to all who may be exposed to them. Addiction to inhalational anaesthetics is rare but well recognized, and virtually all agents have been implicated in such addiction. Trichloroethylene addiction is commoner among workers in industries where this agent is used as a solvent than in personnel with access to this drug through medical practice.

Trace concentrations of inhalational anaesthetics

Despite the fact that there is no evidence of any deleterious effects of trace amounts of volatile and gaseous anaesthetics in humans, in the United Kingdom the Health and Safety at Work Act and the Control of Substances Hazardous to Health regulations have laid down Occupational Exposure Standards for inhalational anaesthetic agents. It is important to realize that the exposure limits are an average in terms of an 8 h reference period (8 h time-weighted average). The acceptable levels in parts per million (ppm) are:

- nitrous oxide 100 ppm;
- enflurane 50 ppm;
- isoflurane 50 ppm;
- halothane 10 ppm.

No levels have been published for sevoflurane and desflurane. It is unlikely that levels as high as these will be reached in a modern, air-conditioned operating theatre with scavenging of waste gases. The permitted levels differ in different countries.

Inhalational anaesthetics in small doses might be expected to have deleterious effects on mental performance, but the evidence is contradictory and on balance the effect, if any, is not clinically significant.

Halogenated hydrocarbon anaesthetics

Many halogenated hydrocarbons with useful anaesthetic properties have been described. Chief among these are halothane and trichloroethylene.

The substitution of halogen atoms for the alkyl hydrogen atoms in hydrocarbons usually leads to the production of compounds with enhanced narcotic activity. Increasing halogen substitution leads to increasing narcotic action, but when halogen substitution is continued to the total exclusion of hydrogen, narcotic activity declines. Thus, in the methane series, methyl chloride is a more potent narcotic than methane and activity increases with increasing chlorine substitution to reach a maximum with chloroform. Carbon tetrachloride, however, is less potent than chloroform.

Increasing narcotic potency due to halogenation is accompanied by increased side effects, especially cardiac irritant and hepatotoxic effects. This again is well exemplified by the methane series, protoplasmic toxic effects increasing with increasing chlorine substitution to reach a maximum with carbon tetrachloride.

The pure bromo- and iodo-derivatives of hydrocarbons tend to be rapidly hydrolysed into the corresponding alcohol or re-converted into the parent hydrocarbon and are therefore of little clinical use. In the past, halogenation has been largely confined to the insertion of chlorine into hydrocarbon molecules. Most modern anaesthetic agents have been produced by fluorine substitution, either alone or together with other halogens.

Anaesthetic gases

The most widely used anaesthetic gas is nitrous oxide. Cyclopropane is still used for the induction of children in a few centres; ethylene and acetylene have been used in the past. Xenon has anaesthetic properties very similar to those of nitrous oxide, but its prohibitive cost has precluded its clinical use.

By definition, the anaesthetic gases have a vapour pressure above ambient pressure at room temperature and there are no limitations upon the concentrations that may be administered. These gases are stored in cylinders, usually compressed to a liquid form at moderate pressure.

Nitrous oxide and cyclopropane differ in many of their anaesthetic properties. They have in common the property of low blood solubility. Because of this, induction with these agents is more rapid than with any of the volatile anaesthetic liquids, with the possible exception of sevoflurane.

MONOGRAPHS

DESFLURANE

The chemical structure and physical properties are shown in *Table 4.1*. It differs from isoflurane in that the sole chlorine atom is replaced by fluorine.

Physical characteristics

Desflurane is a halogenated methyl-ethyl ether. It boils at 23.5°C which is very close to room temperature. It therefore requires a sophisticated vaporizer which is heated and pressurized and an electrical supply is essential. This makes it much larger and heavier than other vaporizers, but more accurate than those produced for other agents. The blood/gas solubility is the lowest of all inhalational anaesthetics at 0.42. Rapid changes in blood level therefore occur when the inspired concentration is altered. Very rapid inhalational induction is theoretically possible, but limited by its irritant properties. Recovery is faster than following any other volatile anaesthetic.

Pharmacology

Central nervous system   The CNS effects are similar to those of other agents and there is no evidence of excitatory activity. It causes cerebral vasodilatation and an increase in cerebral blood flow. There is a dose-dependent decrease in cerebral metabolic rate and oxygen consumption.

Respiratory system   Desflurane is a respiratory depressant, causing a dose-dependent decrease in tidal volume and an increase in respiratory rate, with a resultant increase in arterial carbon dioxide tension.

Cardiovascular system   The effects are very similar to isoflurane in that there is an increase in heart rate, decreases in systemic vascular resistance and mean arterial pressure, while cardiac output is maintained. There is no evidence of a coronary steal phenomenon. Cardiac rhythm is not affected. Rapid increases in inspired desflurane concentration are often associated with transient cardiovascular stimulation, as evidenced by increases in heart rate and blood pressure. This has been ascribed to the irritant effect of desflurane on the respiratory mucosa. To avoid this in relevant patients, the inspired desflurane concentration should only be increased slowly, thus negating one of the benefits of its low blood/gas solubility coefficient, namely rapid changes in depth of anaesthesia.

Muscular effects   Desflurane produces muscular relaxation in relation to the depth of anaesthesia. Like other ethers, it potentiates the action of non-depolarizing neuromuscular relaxants. There have been no reports of malignant hyperthermia developing in susceptible patients, but it is probably wiser to avoid the agent in such patients.

Liver and Kidneys   Desflurane has no direct effect on these organs.

Metabolism   Desflurane strongly resists metabolism which only occurs to a very small amount in humans. There is no significant increase in serum fluoride concentration even after prolonged use. Small, but statistically significant, increases in serum trifluoroacetic acid levels occur, but these are much lower than following isoflurane anaesthesia.

Indications

The low blood/gas solubility of desflurane would indicate its use for rapid induction of inhalational anaesthesia and also rapid recovery; the former would be particularly useful in children. Unfortunately, its irritant properties preclude its use for the latter purpose. Only a few centres use the drug for day-case anaesthesia. Overall, desflurane seems to have attained little favour among anaesthetists in the United Kingdom and its future is uncertain.

ENFLURANE

Enflurane (rINN)

Physical characteristics

Enflurane is a halogenated ethyl-methyl ether and an isomer of isoflurane. It is a colourless liquid of specific gravity 1.5 which is stable and not affected by ultraviolet light, and may safely be stored in clear glass bottles. The vapour has an ethereal odour, and vapour concentrations above 6 per cent are flammable. Because of its low blood/gas partition coefficient (1.9), induction of anaesthesia is rapid, depth of anaesthesia may readily be controlled and prompt recovery follows withdrawal.

Pharmacology

Central nervous system   Although it is a potent anaesthetic, enflurane can also produce marked central stimulant actions, and therein differs from other inhalational anaesthetics. During enflurane administration the EEG commonly shows episodes of paroxysmal activity and periods of burst suppression. Such abnormal EEG activity is seen more commonly in children than in adults. These EEG responses are a function of anaesthetic depth and are exacerbated by a reduction in $P\text{CO}_2$. They may persist for up to 30 days after its administration. Seizures have been reported up to 1 week after enflurane anaesthesia. However, under conditions of normocapnia, enflurane does not exacerbate preexisting epileptic activity. These EEG abnormalities should be regarded as signs of overdosage, possibly associated with hypocapnia.

Cardiovascular system   Light enflurane anaesthesia is usually accompanied by a slight decrease in arterial pressure and increase in heart rate. Cardiac output, stroke volume. peripheral resistance and myocardial contractility are reduced during light (1.0 MAC) enflurane anaesthesia in man. While the cardiovascular effects of this level of enflurane anaesthesia are similar to those of halothane, deepening anaesthesia often produces profound cardiovascular depression with little evidence of adaptation with time. The spontaneous appearance of cardiac arrhythmias is uncommon during enflurane anaesthesia and the amount of epinephrine (adrenaline) needed to produce ectopic ventricular contractions during enflurane anaesthesia is some five times that needed during halothane anaesthesia.

Respiratory system   Enflurane commonly causes respiratory depression. This is usually the result of a reduced tidal volume associated with a slight increase in rate. During enflurane anaesthesia respiratory rate is slower and tidal volume greater than during halothane administration. Enflurane is a more powerful respiratory depressant than either halothane or isoflurane. Respiratory depression is dose related and some recovery occurs over a period of time. The respiratory depressant effects of enflurane are partly antagonized by the stimulus of surgery.

Neuromuscular transmission Enflurane can produce a marked degree of muscular relaxation and can be used alone to provide adequate operating conditions for abdominal surgery. The concentration of enflurane needed for this may, however, produce severe cardiovascular depression. Neuromuscular blocking agents are potentiated more by enflurane than by halothane anaesthesia.

Liver and kidneys It is now known that metabolic adducts of enflurane may act as immunogens and provoke hepatic necrosis, but instances of unexplained hepatitis after enflurane have been reported very much less frequently than after halothane.

Renal blood flow and glomerular filtration rate are reduced by enflurane, the changes being of the same order as with other volatile anaesthetics. Inorganic fluoride is produced during enflurane metabolism, although the concentrations are far less than with methoxyflurane. A few cases of renal failure have been reported after enflurane anaesthesia and it may be wise to avoid using this agent in patients with pre-existing renal disease.

Metabolism Enflurane undergoes much less metabolic degradation than halothane. As with methoxyflurane, inorganic fluoride is the most important product of its metabolism, fluoride levels being related to the inspired enflurane level and the duration of exposure. Maximal serum fluoride levels are in the order of 25 μmol/litre and they decline more rapidly than after methoxyflurane. Serum fluoride levels of 50 μmol/litre are needed to produce nephrotoxicity but significant reductions in the maximum urine-concentrating ability can occur when serum fluoride levels are in the order of 20 μmol/litre. These effects of enflurane are not of great clinical importance in well-hydrated patients with normal renal function.

Indications

Inspired enflurane concentrations of 3–4 per cent are required for induction of anaesthesia and of 1–3 per cent for maintenance, lesser concentrations being needed in the presence of nitrous oxide. Both induction and recovery from anaesthesia are more rapid than with halothane. The central stimulant effects of enflurane have not caused major problems. The relative lack of myocardial sensitization to catecholamines and the rarity of cardiac arrhythmias during enflurane anaesthesia make this agent suitable for use when catecholamines are being used for haemostatic purposes or when high catecholamine levels are anticipated, as in patients with phaeochromocytomas. Although in unstimulated subjects severe cardiovascular and respiratory depression are seen at only moderate levels of enflurane anaesthesia, surgical stimulation usually counters these effects. Because of potential nephrotoxicity, enflurane should be avoided in subjects with pre-existing renal disease or during procedures in which renal function may be compromised.

ETHER

Diethyl ether (rINN)

Diethyl ether is a colourless, highly volatile liquid with a pungent odour. It has a specific gravity of 0.714 and a vapour density of 2.6. Diethyl ether is highly flammable and its vapour forms flammable mixtures with air, oxygen and nitrous oxide. With the exception of nitrous oxide, ether is the oldest inhalational anaesthetic still in use. It was first used by Crawford Long in 1842 and by Morton in 1846, since when it has enjoyed considerable popularity, and for many years was the anaesthetic of choice for major surgery.

Pharmacology

During induction of anaesthesia there is depression of the cortex and the medulla and spinal cord. Paralysis of the respiratory centre precedes that of the vasomotor centre by a considerable margin. There is stimulation of the sympathetic system, with an increase in circulating catecholamines.

During light planes of diethyl ether anaesthesia there are usually only minor changes in blood pressure, cardiac output and peripheral resistance. During deeper anaesthesia, myocardial depression and paralysis of the vasomotor and other vital centres may lead to circulatory failure. Thus this agent does not afford the patient in shock or with haemorrhage a wide margin of safety. The innocuous effects of light diethyl ether anaesthesia are due to the sympathetic stimulation produced by this agent.

Unlike other inhalational agents, diethyl ether produces respiratory stimulation until the deepest planes of surgical anaesthesia are reached. The cause of this stimulation is unknown. Arterial $P{CO_2}$ levels of 30 mmHg (4 kPa) are commonly met during clinical diethyl ether anaesthesia. When the alveolar concentration of diethyl ether rises above 6 per cent, respiratory depression usually ensues.

The vapour of diethyl ether is irritant to the respiratory tract. Laryngeal spasm is not uncommon during induction. Bronchial secretions are increased but are prevented by the previous administration of adequate doses of atropine. Diethyl ether may be useful in some cases of asthma and bronchitis because of its property of producing bronchial muscle relaxation.

Salivary and gastric secretions are increased at first, but are decreased during deep anaesthesia. Bowel movement is decreased, due in part to stimulation of dilator fibres and also to depression of plain muscle. Nausea and vomiting are common with diethyl ether, their incidence varying with the length of operation and the depth of anaesthesia.

Skeletal muscle tone is markedly reduced, especially during the deeper levels of anaesthesia. This is due mainly to depression of transmission at the neuromuscular junction by an action similar to that of non-depolarizing muscle relaxants.

Liver function is depressed, and some impairment may persist for several days. Irreversible damage does not occur.

Renal vasoconstriction causes a reduction in renal plasma flow and therefore of glomerular filtration rate. A further tendency to oliguria is due to tubular reabsorption of water caused by raised levels of antidiuretic hormone.

Glycogen is mobilized by the liver, and hyperglycaemia follows. This effect is mediated by increased sympathetic activity. Some degree of metabolic acidosis may occur due to decreased tissue perfusion produced by increased sympathetic activity. Many of the changes in blood chemistry observed after diethyl ether, such as decreased serum bicarbonate, increased lactate, rise in lactate/pyruvate ratio, and decreased serum potassium, are qualitatively similar to those produced by physiological amounts of epinephrine (adrenaline).

The pregnant uterus is not affected during light anaesthesia, but is relaxed during deep anaesthesia. Diethyl ether passes rapidly from mother to child and may cause depression of respiration in the infant.

About 15 per cent of an inhaled dose of diethyl ether is metabolized in the liver, via acetaldehyde and ethanol, to carbon dioxide and water.

Anaesthetic properties

Diethyl ether is a potent inhalational anaesthetic. Because of the high solubility of this agent in blood, induction is slow and may be further prolonged by breath-holding and coughing due to the irritant effect of the vapour. Muscular relaxation is good during deep anaesthesia. When light anaesthesia is used in association with muscle relaxants, smaller doses of non-depolarizing agents than usual are required because of the curare-like action of diethyl ether. Respiration is often of a blowing or tugging nature during deep anaesthesia and is sometimes an embarrassment to the surgeon during upper abdominal surgery. In the inadequately atropinized patient, bronchial and salivary secretions are troublesome.

Capillary bleeding is more prominent during diethyl ether anaesthesia than in more modern forms of balanced anaesthesia. Coagulation time may be shortened but the bleeding time is unchanged; the prothrombin time is somewhat prolonged. As with other general anaesthetic agents, there is a polymorphonuclear leucocytosis. Recovery is slow after prolonged administration.

Indications

Since the introduction of the muscle relaxants, the popularity of ether has waned. It is, however, a very safe and reliable anaesthetic and may be used for operations in all branches of surgery and obstetrics, especially where good muscle relaxation is required. It is a particularly useful agent for those working in remote parts of the world where elaborate apparatus is not available, provided that attention is given to the risk of fires.

Dosage and administration

Diethyl ether may be given on an open mask or by means of a vaporizer. Vapour strengths of up to 20 per cent are required for induction; light anaesthesia can be maintained on strengths in the region of 3–5 per cent, but deep anaesthesia may require concentrations up to 10 per cent or more in resistant subjects. There is a tendency to cross-tolerance with alcohol.

Accurate administration of known vapour concentrations is not possible with the Boyle type of vaporizer. The EMO inhaler, however, will deliver known concentrations between 0 and 25 per cent under all normal conditions, and when relaxants are used it has been found that 3 per cent diethyl ether vapour in air will maintain unconsciousness. Patients anaesthetized with 3 per cent diethyl ether vapour regain consciousness very quickly and the incidence of nausea and vomiting is no greater than with the conventional nitrous oxide–oxygen–relaxant technique.

Precautions

Diethyl ether should not be used in cases of diabetes mellitus and severe liver disease, and its use is inadvisable in patients with fever under hot and humid operating conditions. This particularly applies to children and those who have been atropinized: such patients are liable to have convulsions. If these occur the anaesthetic should be withdrawn, the patient should be cooled by sponging with cold water if hyperthermia is present, and small doses of thiopental or diazepam should be given intravenously until convulsions cease. Small doses of a muscle relaxant may also be employed in resistant cases.

When used on an open mask or with air, the large mass of diethyl ether in the inspired atmosphere inevitably leads to hypoxaemia. To prevent this, a small flow of oxygen should be added under an open mask or to air draw-over vaporizers.

The flammability of diethyl ether contraindicates its use in the presence of diathermy, and care to avoid static discharge must be taken in hot dry climates.

HALOTHANE

Halothane (rINN)

Physical characteristics

Halothane is a colourless liquid with a sweet, non-irritant odour. It has a specific gravity of 1.87 and a vapour density of 6.8. Halothane is non-flammable and non-explosive. Some decomposition occurs on exposure to light, but it is more stable in the presence of thymol 0.01 per cent w/w and when stored in amber glass bottles. It is unaffected by soda lime and can be used in a closed circuit. It is absorbed by rubber.

Pharmacology

Central nervous system   CNS depression follows the pattern of all general anaesthetics, but the stage of excitement is minimal and often absent. Paralysis of the vasomotor centre follows that of the respiratory centre much less rapidly than with chloroform, but more readily than with ether. Halothane is much less soluble in the phospholipids of brain cells than in the neutral fats of adipose tissue: this, together with its low blood/gas partition coefficient, accounts for the relatively rapid recovery of consciousness. A characteristic feature of the use of halothane in neurosurgical anaesthesia is an increase in cerebral blood flow and in intracranial pressure. This is more marked in the presence of an intracranial space-occupying lesion, and in association with hypoventilation.

Autonomic system   The sympathetic system is depressed more than the parasympathetic system; the tone of the latter therefore preponderates. Sympathetic ganglia are mildly blocked, and the block produced by hexamethonium and trimetaphan is potentiated. Mild β-adrenergic stimulant effects of halothane have been demonstrated on the cardiovascular system.

Cardiovascular system   The outstanding effect of halothane on the cardiovascular system is a reduction in blood pressure proportional to the depth of anaesthesia. This hypotension reflects the myocardial depressant action of halothane. Eger *et al.* (1970) showed that during controlled ventilation halothane caused a reduction in cardiac output, with reductions in both stroke volume and myocardial contractility, while right atrial pressure rose. Prolonged anaesthesia was associated with a recovery of cardiovascular function, due to a sympathetic stimulant action of halothane. During spontaneous ventilation there is much less cardiovascular depression than during controlled ventilation. This difference reflects the rise in carbon dioxide levels associated with spontaneous ventilation during halothane anaesthesia and a consequent β-adrenergic stimulation. During spontaneous ventilation, recovery of cardiovascular function with prolonged anaesthesia still occurred.

Bradycardia is not uncommon during induction and may be associated with hypotension; both may be reversed with small doses of atropine or glycopyrolate. The most common arrhythmias seen during halothane anaesthesia are nodal rhythm and ventricular extrasystoles. These often occur under deep anaesthesia with spontaneous ventilation and are related to the concomitant hypercapnia. Like other hydrocarbon anaesthetics, halothane sensitizes the myocardium to the dysrhythmic effects of catecholamines.

Respiratory system   The usual respiratory response is a reduced tidal volume associated with an increased respiratory rate, resulting in a diminished alveolar ventilation. During light anaesthesia there may be no change or even a fall in the rate of breathing and the response is variable from patient to patient. Halothane does not provoke salivary or bronchial secretions, and coughing is not easily provoked.

Muscular system   The effect of many competitve muscle relaxants is potentiated, but that of suxamethonium is diminished. The potentiation of non-depolarizing relaxants by halothane is less than that produced by isoflurane, enflurane and sevoflurane.

Renal function   Halothane has no particular effect on renal function as distinct from that of other anaesthetic agents.

Liver function   All forms of surgery are probably followed by some detrimental effects on liver function, but these are minor and may not even be detectable. The extent of surgery has an influence: surface surgery has little effect, whereas vascular or cardiac surgery are commonly followed by a rise in serum bilirubin and transaminases. Patients with existing liver damage may deteriorate further. Furthermore, surgical or anaesthetic complications, such as hypoxaemia, hypotension, sepsis and blood transfusion may also be associated with hepatic dysfunction. However, the introduction of halothane into clinical practice was soon followed by anecdotal reports linking it with much more severe liver damage in the postoperative period. This stimulated a number of studies of liver function after surgery, mainly retrospective, in order to identify the existence of a problem, but because of their non-prospective, non-randomized nature and the very rarity of the condition, they failed to throw any light on the matter.

A controversy about the nature, or indeed the reality, of 'halothane hepatitis' raged for many years. The introduction of other inhalational anaesthetics has made this of less practical importance and contributed to a great decline in the use of halothane in developed countries. Summarizing the many reports concerning patients who have become jaundiced after surgery, unexplained hepatitis with clear evidence of cellular damage was present in the great majority of those who had received halothane. Certain associated features were apparent: the majority had been exposed to halothane previously and most within the previous four weeks. Some had had unexplained hepatitis following a previous halothane anaesthetic, the latent period becoming shorter after each administration. The condition appears to be commoner in older patients, particularly if they are obese and female.

Thus hepatic necrosis following halothane is a rare, but often fatal, definite entity. This led the Committee on Safety of Medicines to make the following recommendations on the use of halothane:

- a careful anaesthetic history must be taken to determine any previous exposure and reactions to halothane;
- repeated exposure to halothane within a period of at least three months should be avoided unless there is a clear-cut case for its use;

• a history of unexplained jaundice or pyrexia following exposure to halothane is an absolute contraindication to its further use in that patient.

Where newer inhalational agents are available, few anaesthetists would now choose halothane except, possibly, in children. In countries in which newer alternatives to halothane are not an option, however, some guidance on its safe use is necessary. With an incidence of severe hepatic failure believed to be between 1:10,000 and 1:35,000, the risk of repeating the use of this agent has to be set against the undoubted risks associated with surgery in any situation where no alternative exists. The absence of any reaction such as mild pyrexia or mild jaundice on a previous occasion, and an interval between exposures of at least six months should reduce the risk even further.

Mechanism of 'halothane hepatitis' There appear to be two mechanisms by which halothane can exert its hepatotoxic effect and each gives rise to a syndrome which is commoner in adults than children. The first is characterized by a raised serum level of liver transaminases of which glutathione-*S*-transferase is by far the most sensitive in this situation. It has a short half-life of under 90 minutes and two peaks have been described, one within 3–6 h of exposure and one after 24 h. It has been suggested that these are related to two different processes, the first being related to necrosis of centrilobular hepatocytes and the second caused by metabolites of halothane or an immunological response. The first rise in transaminases is a relatively common reaction of low morbidity and may not be solely a direct toxic action of halothane but related to reductions in portal and hepatic blood flow associated with its use. The second rise is uncommon and associated with a repeat exposure, usually after a short interval, and may progress to fulminant liver failure with high mortality. This is most likely to be an immunologically mediated reaction in which, following a previous exposure, a metabolite of halothane has acted as a hapten which has combined with a liver cell protein to which the body has created an antibody. If indeed it is an immune response, then no totally safe interval can be relied on, and the safest course of action is never to repeat halothane.

Uterus and placenta The contractility of the uterus is inhibited rapidly by inspired concentrations of 2–3 per cent; the myometrium regains its normal tone soon after withdrawal of halothane.

Fate in the body Compared with previously used liquid anaesthetic agents, halothane had a relatively low blood/gas solubility coefficient. Even so, the arterial tension took a considerable time to approach the inspired tension; it is only due to the fact that a sufficiently high vapour pressure exists at room temperature, relative to its potency, that induction can be made rapid by giving much higher concentrations during induction than are necessary for maintenance (over-pressure technique). The concentration in organs with a very rich blood supply, such as the heart and brain, closely follows arterial tensions. However, areas with a poor blood supply and high solubility, such as adipose tissue, take up the anaesthetic for a considerable time and it has been estimated that it would take 20–30 h at a constant inspired tension for the whole body to come to equilibrium.

Halothane is metabolized in the body by hepatic microsomal enzymes. Both oxidative and reductive metabolic pathways exist. Dechlorination and debromination appear to be the initial steps in its breakdown. Trifluoracetic acid, *N*-trifluoroacetyl-2-aminoethanol and *N*-acetyl-L-cysteine can be isolated from the urine of patients given halothane. Bromide has also been shown to be released, but negligible amounts of inorganic fluoride are formed. Enzyme induction and a consequent greater breakdown of halothane has been shown to occur after pretreatment with phenobarbital, and followed repeated exposure to halothane. Metabolic pathways for halothane are rapidly saturated and its metabolism is depressed by high concentrations.

Anaesthetic properties

Halothane is a potent inhalational anaesthetic. The deeper the level of anaesthesia, the greater the degree of respiratory depression and hypotension. Induction is smooth and not unpleasant for the patient, as the vapour is non-irritant, consciousness is quickly lost and surgical anaesthesia can be produced in 2–5 minutes with little excitement; intubation is normally possible at this stage. Induction with a small dose of thiopental, however, is a more common practice, and is more pleasant for the patient.

Maintenance of anaesthesia with vapour strengths of the order of 0.5–2 per cent provides good operative conditions. Respiration is usually quiet; a rapid respiratory rate is often a sign of overdose. Muscle relaxation is usually good, but the deep anaesthesia required to produce adequate relaxation for upper abdominal surgery is often accompanied by marked cardiovascular depression. The hypotension associated with halothane anaesthesia reduces capillary bleeding and gives a relatively bloodless field. The degree of hypotension will be dependent on the depth of anaesthesia and will also be affected by the patient's posture.

Other advantages of halothane anaesthesia are suppression of salivary and bronchial secretions, suppression of sympathetic activity, and rapid recovery when the anaesthetic is withdrawn. The speed of recovery, however, is dependent on the concentration of the vapour employed and the length of administration, and can be considerably delayed if deep anaesthesia is maintained for long periods. Shivering often occurs during recovery, and restlessness is not uncommon in the immediate postoperative period due to the poor analgesic action of the drug.

Indications

Since its introduction, halothane has been widely used for every type of operation. Until recently it was the most widely used volatile anaesthetic. Its use has now started to decline, due mainly to medicolegal fears concerning the risk of hepatitis but also because newer agents are perceived to have advantages. However, there is no evidence that the overall risk to the patient is any less with alternative agents. It is most useful in operations where considerable but not full muscular relaxation is required. Uraemia resulting from intrinsic renal disease is not a contraindication to its use.

Dosage and administration

Inspired concentrations of 2–3.5 per cent are necessary for induction, and anaesthesia can be maintained with inspired concentrations of 0.5–2.5 per cent. The concentrations required will depend to a considerable extent on the degree of previous sedation, and whether nitrous oxide is used in the vaporizing gases. It may be given by the open drop method, by the OMV inhaler (with air), and by calibrated vaporizers. The latter are recommended as they give accurate vapour concentrations under normal working conditions irrespective of temperature, flow rate and the amount of fluid in the vaporizer. Halothane can be used in a closed circuit, the vaporizer being either outside or inside the circuit. If the vaporizer is outside the circuit it must be capable of putting out 40–80 ml/minute of halothane vapour, with a fresh gas flow of 500 ml/minute or less. For this purpose a vaporizer calibrated to give 10 per cent halothane vapour has been used in the past. If the vaporizer is inside the circuit it will only be safe if it is relatively inefficient and has a small capacity; halothane concentration in the circuit is a function of the patient's minute volume. Dangerously high concentrations will be attained if ventilation is assisted or controlled.

Precautions

Although, on rare occasions, halothane may cause liver damage, its use should not be prejudiced solely on this account. There is no evidence that liver damage is more likely in the presence of existing liver disease. In the present climate of opinion, however, an unexplained pyrexial illness, unexpected liver damage after halothane anaesthesia or exposure within the last 3 months contraindicates a second exposure.

It is recommended that the patient should be atropinized before induction with halothane to decrease vagal tone; this will prevent bradycardia and a serious fall in blood pressure. Atropine 0.6 mg may be given in the normal way 30 minutes before operation, or intravenously during induction. Hyoscine is not effective in depressing the cardiac vagus in normal doses. Heavy sedation with morphine or its derivatives is inadvisable as they tend to cause an increase in respiratory depression and hypotension. If hypotension associated with bradycardia occurs during anaesthesia, atropine should be given intravenously. If the pulse rate is within normal limits and blood pressure falls unduly, the inspired concentration of halothane should be reduced.

Should controlled ventilation be necessary, care must be taken that high concentrations of vapour are not forced into the patient's lungs. If the vaporizer is within the circuit it must be turned off before controlled ventilation is started.

Ganglion blocking agents such as trimetaphan have been used with halothane, but it must be remembered that halothane potentiates their action and they must therefore be given cautiously. Epinephrine should not be given to patients during halothane anaesthesia, unless special precautions are taken (see page 356).

Eger, E.I., Smith, N.T., Stoelting, R.K., Cullen, D.I., Kadis, L.B. and Whitcher, C.E. (1970) Cardiovascular effects of halothane in man. *Anesthesiology*, **32**, 396

ISOFLURANE

Isoflurane (rINN)

Physical characteristics

Although isoflurane was first synthesized in 1965, only two years after its isomer enflurane, problems in its purification delayed its introduction. A suggestion that this agent might be carcinogenic further delayed clinical use of isoflurane. The physical properties of isoflurane resemble those of enflurane, but it has a lower boiling point and a higher vapour pressure, and is less soluble in blood (partition coefficient 1.4). Like enflurane, isoflurane is stable in the presence of ultraviolet light.

Pharmacology

Central nervous system The CNS effects of isoflurane are similar to those of most other volatile anaesthetic agents. Unlike enflurane it does not have any convulsant actions, even at deep levels of anaesthesia with hypocapnia. Cerebral blood flow is increased during moderate to deep isoflurane anaesthesia. While the rise in cerebral blood flow is less with isoflurane than with halothane or enflurane, large rises of intracranial pressure can occur with all three agents in the presence of a space-occupying lesion.

Respiratory system   Isoflurane is capable of producing profound respiratory depression in the spontaneously breathing subject. This is evidenced by a dose-related increase in $P\text{CO}_2$ and a reduced ability to respond to an imposed carbon dioxide load. The degree of respiratory depression is more than that seen with halothane but less than that produced by enflurane. This respiratory depression is countered by surgical stimulation, and during routine clinical use only moderate rises in $P\text{CO}_2$ occur when isoflurane is given to spontaneously breathing subjects.

Circulatory system   Isoflurane has little effect on cardiac contractility, as evidenced by no change in right atrial pressure, the ballistocardiogram IJ wave and dP/dt. Cardiac output is little changed but there is a dose-dependent fall in arterial blood pressure due to a reduction in systemic vascular resistance. Heart rate increases and occasionally tachycardia is troublesome. Heart rhythm is stable and isoflurane does not increase the sensitivity of the myocardium to epinephrine (adrenaline).

Isoflurane has been implicated in a 'coronary steal' phenomenon, where, because of its coronary vasodilator properties, blood is diverted away from ischaemic areas when there is a stenosis in a coronary artery supplying that area. However, controlled trials have now indicated that isoflurane does not appear to have any deleterious effects under these circumstances and that the drug can be used in patients with myocardial ischaemia.

Muscular effects   Isoflurane alone can produce a good degree of muscular relaxation, and has been used without muscle relaxants during upper abdominal surgery. Isoflurane also potentiates the effects of muscle relaxants rather more than either enflurane or halothane, but less than sevoflurane.

Liver and kidneys   Isoflurane produces negligible changes in liver function, as evidenced by studies of changes in liver function tests and enzymes during and following administration of this agent. There have been no documented cases of antibodies to isoflurane metabolites associated with liver damage, even though TFA is an oxidative product of its metabolism.

Similarly, the effects of isoflurane on the kidney resemble those of other inhalational agents and include a reduction in renal blood flow and glomerular filtration, with a full recovery of renal function after anaesthesia.

Metabolism   Less than 1 per cent of administered isoflurane is metabolized. However, serum fluoride levels rise slightly after administration. The minimal biodegradation seen with isoflurane can be related both to the stability of its molecule and to its rapid elimination from the body after stopping administration.

Indications

Isoflurane has been used to anaesthetize without incident a wide range of patients for a large variety of procedures. and perhaps approaches the ideal inhalational agent more closely than any other agent. The marked muscular relaxation and stable cardiovascular system are particular advantages of isoflurane. Because of its lower blood solubility, induction with isoflurane can be more rapid than with halothane, although the pungent odour of isoflurane leads to a greater incidence of breath-holding and coughing and may limit the rate of induction.

A further advantage of isoflurane over halothane and enflurane is its lack of deleterious side effects, especially those relating to hepatic and renal function. The lack of toxicity of isoflurane is related to the low level of metabolic breakdown of this agent.

Dosage and administration

Isoflurane has a MAC of 1.15 per cent. Concentrations of 1.5 per cent – that is, 1.3 times the MAC – can be used to maintain light anaesthesia. Higher concentrations are needed if any significant level of relaxation is desired. The inspired concentration of isoflurane can be greatly reduced if the agent is given together with 60–70 per cent nitrous oxide. Under these circumstances isoflurane MAC falls to about 0.5 per cent. Isoflurane should be administered from a calibrated vaporizer. Halothane and isoflurane have nearly identical vapour pressures and a calibrated halothane vaporizer can be used to deliver almost accurate concentrations of isoflurane. However, hazards can arise if a vaporizer specifically designed for one agent is filled with a different agent and this practice is not recommended.

NITROUS OXIDE

Nitrous oxide (rINN)

Nitrous oxide is a colourless gas with a slightly sweetish odour. It has a density compared to air of 1.5 and a critical temperature of 36.5°C. It is neither flammable nor explosive, but will support combustion. It is supplied in blue cylinders, compressed to a liquid at a pressure of 650 lbf/in^2 (4485 kPa).

Nitrous oxide, or laughing gas, was first used as an anaesthetic agent at the beginning of the nineteenth century, and is still in widespread use. It was prepared by Priestley in 1772. Humphry Davy tried it on himself in 1799, noticed the anaesthetic properties and suggested it be used to allay pain. It was not until 1844 that it was first used in clinical practice by Colton and Wells in the USA.

Pharmacology

Many of the effects that have been ascribed to nitrous oxide alone were the direct result of hypoxia rather than those due to the agent itself. In the presence of adequate oxygen the effect on the body systems is not great.

Nervous system   CNS depression is similar to that caused by all general anaesthetics, but paralysis of the respiratory and vasomotor centres does not occur if normal oxygen requirements are satisfied.

Cardiovascular system   Animal evidence would suggest that nitrous oxide is a myocardial depressant, but human evidence of any such effect is sparse. If 70 per cent nitrous oxide is substituted for 70 per cent nitrogen in patients undergoing coronary artery surgery no significant changes in haemodynamic performance or myocardial wall motion are seen.

Respiratory system Although psychic factors operate during induction of nitrous oxide anaesthesia, ventilation usually increases. Hypoxia, painful stimuli or relief of pain may mask the slight respiratory effects of nitrous oxide. There is a mild depressant effect of nitrous oxide on alveolar ventilation and the ventilatory response to added carbon dioxide.

Muscular system Depression of skeletal muscle tone is minimal and plain muscle is unaffected.

Uterus and placenta There is no detectable effect with clinical concentrations.

Haemopoietic system Prolonged administration of nitrous oxide depresses bone marrow function. It is known that nitrous oxide converts the cobalt in vitamin B_{12} from the monovalent to the bivalent form, thus rendering it inactive. Megaloblastic changes in bone marrow have followed inhalation of 60 per cent nitrous oxide for as little as 6 h. It is possible to prevent these megaloblastic changes by administration of folinic acid.

Agranulocytosis consistently follows exposure to nitrous oxide for 4 days or longer. Nitrous oxide also interferes with the synthesis of DNA. This property is probably responsible for the fetotoxicity attributed to nitrous oxide.

Other effects There is no effect on kidney or liver function. Nausea and vomiting are likely to occur if anaesthesia is associated with hypoxia. Nitrous oxide crosses the placental barrier but does not cause respiratory depression in the fetus.

Fate in the body Nitrous oxide is rapidly excreted by the lungs. A small amount diffuses through the skin. Intestinal bacteria can break nitrous oxide down, eventually to nitrogen: some 0.004 per cent of administered nitrous oxide is metabolized in man.

Anaesthetic properties

Nitrous oxide is a weak anaesthetic, as can be deduced from its indirectly determined MAC of 110 per cent. When used with air it is impossible to produce anaesthesia without some degree of hypoxia. With oxygen at near atmospheric concentration, the first plane of surgical anaesthesia can be reached in average subjects, although difficulties can occur with alcoholics, habitual takers of narcotics, and fit, powerfully built adults. Induction is rapid and not unpleasant, but hallucinations and some violence in the second stage are not uncommon. Arterial blood reaches approximately 90 per cent saturation in 10 minutes, there being a net gas uptake of about 1 litre/min during induction. Full equilibrium does not occur for several hours, and uptake continues at a greatly diminished rate for the entire course of most clinical administrations. Recovery is rapid (1–4 minutes) even after prolonged administration.

Because of the limited depth of anaesthesia attainable with nitrous oxide, relaxation is poor and insufficient for major surgery. Limb movements are apt to occur following painful stimuli.

Indications

Nitrous oxide is still occasionally used with oxygen as a sole agent for short minor procedures, such as dental extractions, although there is an increasing tendency to supplement its actions with low concentrations of more powerful volatile agents. With supplementary agents it is widely used for all branches of major surgery. Two advantages accrue from using potent agents with nitrous oxide: 60–70 per cent nitrous oxide will reduce to approximately two-thirds the alveolar concentration of other agents needed to maintain light anaesthesia: and because of the marked initial net uptake of nitrous oxide, there is a noticeable second gas effect which initially hastens the uptake of other agents.

Sub-anaesthetic concentrations of nitrous oxide are widely used to produce analgesia. Employed mainly in obstetrics, this practice is applicable in other situations that require controllable and easily administered pain relief, such as trauma, and for the relief of pain associated with chest physiotherapy postoperatively. It is also effective as a sedative in dentistry.

Dosage and administration

Nitrous oxide can be given as a 1:1 nitrous oxide/oxygen mixture, delivered either from pre-set intermittent-flow machines, such as the Lucy Baldwin, or from pre-mixed cylinders attached to an Entonox demand flow head. Nitrous oxide and oxygen in other ratios can be given by many different types of apparatus.

Although anaesthesia for major surgery may be maintained with nitrous oxide, oxygen and muscle relaxants alone, this technique is prone to allow unintended awareness and supplementation with a low concentration of a volatile agent or a narcotic analgesic is strongly advised.

Precautions

The most obvious problem arising with nitrous oxide administration is hypoxia. An inspired oxygen concentration of 20 per cent or even slightly less is usually safe for induction, especially if 3–5 minutes of pre-oxygenation is performed. The 'second gas effect' due to nitrous oxide uptake effectively increases arterial oxygen tension during the first few minutes of administration. Such oxygen concentrations are inadequate during prolonged administration; because of the inevitable ventilation/perfusion abnormality during general anaesthesia, inspired oxygen concentrations of at least 30 per cent should be given. During upper abdominal and thoracic surgery, especially in patients with pre-existing cardiac or respiratory disease, an inspired oxygen concentration of at least 50 per cent may be needed to ensure adequate arterial oxygenation. These considerations of necessity limit the concentration of nitrous oxide that can be administered.

Hypoxia can occur during recovery from nitrous oxide administration if patients breathe air. 'Diffusion anoxia' is due to the rapid elimination into the alveoli of large volumes of nitrous oxide and a consequent diminution in alveolar oxygen concentration. Although usually mild, diffusion hypoxia may present a risk to the patient with depressed or impaired cardiac or respiratory function. Diffusion hypoxia is only important when an appreciable volume of nitrous oxide has been taken up. It can easily be prevented by administration of low concentrations of added oxygen during the initial phase of nitrous oxide elimination.

During nitrous oxide anaesthesia, any closed gas-filled cavity in the body will expand, due to the exchange of small volumes of nitrogen from the cavity for larger volumes of nitrous oxide from blood. Expansion of a pneumothorax, pneumopericardium or pneumoperitoneum may have serious consequences. Gas-filled obstructed intestine will also expand, although a poor blood supply will limit the rate, and therefore the significance, of nitrous oxide passage into the intestine. Air accidentally entering the circulation during nitrous oxide anaesthesia will greatly increase in volume. Air injected during pneumoencephalography will also expand and may raise the CSF pressure. Nitrous oxide diffusing into the middle ear may interfere with middle ear mechanics.

Prolonged nitrous oxide administration depresses bone marrow function.

Pre-mixed cylinders Although nitrous oxide readily liquefies under pressure, mixtures of nitrous oxide and oxygen can be prepared that will remain gaseous when pressurized. Under these circumstances nitrous oxide may be considered as being dissolved in oxygen. A constant composition mixture is released from such pre-mixed cylinders as long as they are above their critical temperature. The stability of these mixtures decreases as the nitrous oxide fraction is increased and only re-mixed cylinders containing 50 per cent nitrous oxide (Entonox) are in use. If cooled below –8°C (the critical temperature), the contents separate into liquid nitrous oxide and gaseous oxygen. The cylinders will then initially deliver a high oxygen-containing mixture, but eventually nearly pure nitrous oxide will emerge. Ideally, these cylinders should not be stored in situations in which such temperatures are possible. If accidentally exposed to low temperatures, they should be brought indoors to warm up, and inverted several times to re-establish the stable mixture.

SEVOFLURANE

Physical characteristics

Sevoflurane is a methyl-propyl ether and unlike other volatile agents is not a chiral compound and thus does not exist as optical isomers. Its boiling point is 58.6°C and saturated vapour pressure at 20°C is 160 mmHg. It has a blood-gas partition coefficient of 0.69 and as a result, coupled with the fact that it is non-irritant and virtually odourless, induction of anaesthesia is rapid. The low blood-gas solubility also means that change in the level of anaesthesia is also rapid. It has a MAC value of 1.71–2.05, being higher in children and reduced in the presence of nitrous oxide.

Pharmacology

Central nervous system Like other volatile anaesthetics, sevoflurane causes a dose-dependent depression of the CNS. It preserves cerebral blood flow and reduces the cerebral metabolic requirements for oxygen. The effects on the EEG are similar to most other agents and there is no evidence of convulsive or epileptiform activity.

Respiratory effects Sevoflurane is not irritant to the upper airway and bronchi. Tidal volume is progressively decreased by increasing concentrations. Respiratory rate increases, but not enough to compensate for the reduction in tidal volume and hence minute volume decreases. It inhibits the pulmonary vasoconstrictor response to hypoxia.

Cardiovascular system There is a dose-dependent depression of the cardiovascular system, with a decrease in arterial blood pressure, systemic vascular resistance and negative inotropic effects. Unlike isoflurane and desflurane, sevoflurane is not associated with an increase in heart rate. It has less coronary vasodilator properties than isoflurane and does not cause a steal phenomenon in experimental animals with appropriate coronary artery anatomy. It does not potentiate epinephrine (adrenaline)-induced arrhythmias.

Muscular effects   Like other inhalational agents, sevoflurane produces some degree of muscular relaxation in relation to the depth of anaesthesia. It potentiates the action of non-depolarizing neuromuscular blocking drugs in a manner similar to other ethers. There have been, to date, four instances of malignant hyperthermia associated with the use of sevoflurane and although no definitive cause–effect has yet been established, it would be wiser to avoid the drug in patients susceptible to the condition.

Liver and kidneys   Liver and kidney blood flow are well preserved under sevoflurane anaesthesia. It has no detrimental effect on overall hepatic function and has a low potential for hepatotoxicity. There is no effect on blood urea and serum creatinine, although there is some evidence of minor tubular damage when more sophisticated tests of renal function, e.g. urinary γ-glutathione-*S*-transferase, are used. These changes, however, are transient and no cases of serious renal or hepatic damage have been reported after sevoflurane anaesthesia.

Metabolism   Approximately 3 per cent of inhaled sevoflurane is metabolized by the cytochrome P-450 system in the liver. It is defluorinated to free fluoride (F^-) and hexafluoro-isopropanol, the latter being rapidly conjugated to its glucuronide.

There has been concern over the metabolism of fluorinated anaesthetics to inorganic fluoride since the demonstration that renal toxicity, in the form of a high-output renal failure, could follow methoxyflurane anaesthesia. Toxicity occurred when free F^- levels exceeded 50 μmol/litre and this was therefore accepted as the toxic level of fluoride. Sevoflurane is metabolized to a slightly greater extent than enflurane and F^- levels of 15–25 μmol/litre can be expected after exposure of one MAC hour. Levels greater than 50 μmol/litre have occasionally been measured after sevoflurane, but there has been no evidence of postoperative clinical renal dysfunction. This is almost certainly due to the fact that sevoflurane, like enflurane but unlike methoxyflurane, undergoes minimal intra-renal defluorination.

Sevoflurane and CO_2 absorbents   Carbon dioxide absorbents (soda lime and Baralyme®) degrade sevoflurane and five breakdown products can be produced experimentally, named compounds A, B, C, D and E. Clinically, the only important one is compound A, which is fluoromethyl-2,2-difluoro-1-(trifluoromethyl)vinyl ether. This substance can cause proximal tubular injury in rats, but this has not been reported in man.

Formation of compound A is particularly likely to occur at low fresh gas flows and the amount produced is related to the dose of sevoflurane, time of exposure and temperature of the absorbent material. There is some evidence that production is increased when the absorbent is dry and also that more is produced when Baralyme is used rather than soda lime. The amount of compound A produced in clinical practice is well below that which causes toxicity in animals. Compound B is less toxic and only formed after prolonged anaesthesia at very low flows. In the USA, the minimum recommended fresh gas flow during sevoflurane anaesthesia with CO_2 absorption is 2 litres/minute; no such restriction is imposed in the United Kingdom.

Several million closed circuit anaesthetics with sevoflurane have now been given, but there have been no reports of toxicity related to compound A.

Indications

Because of its physical properties, sevoflurane has many of the features of an ideal volatile anaesthetic agent. The fact that it is non-irritant and has a low blood-gas solubility means that induction of anaesthesia can be achieved rapidly by inhalation, which makes it particularly useful in children, where it now competes with halothane. It is also suitable for 'vital capacity' induction by inhalation of a single large breath of a high concentration, e.g. 8 per cent in oxygen. It is beginning to replace halothane as the induction agent of choice in patients with upper airway obstruction. Little information is available as yet on its effects in patients with pre-existing renal disease and therefore, at the moment, it is probably wiser to avoid the drug under these circumstances. The biggest drawback to its use is probably its expense and it should only be used in low flow systems with CO_2 absorption.

XENON

All anaesthetic agents in routine use have undesirable side effects. An ideal agent would be completely inert. Such a substance is xenon, which is one of the inert gases. It has been known for many years that xenon possesses anaesthetic properties, ones which cannot be explained in terms of actions on receptors (see Chapter 1). Induction and recovery from anaesthesia is rapid and it has a MAC value of around 70 per cent, which is a considerable advantage over nitrous oxide in that hypoxia is not a problem. It is not explosive, is non-toxic and does not undergo biotransformation. When compared with equiconcentrations of nitrous oxide (70 per cent in oxygen), xenon proved to be a more potent analgesic, reducing fentanyl requirements, and was associated with greater cardiovascular stability. Recovery following anaesthesia for over 1 h averaged 4 minutes in the xenon group and 7 minutes in those who received nitrous oxide. The concentrations used, however, were not equipotent. (Lachmann et al., 1990).

Xenon has none of the drawbacks of nitrous oxide and the main reason why it has not been used is expense. Furthermore, no anaesthetic machines are equipped for administration of the gas. However, xenon is coming down in price and with the increased use and efficiency of closed circuit techniques, xenon may eventually find a place in anaesthetic practice. Its mode of action has not been elucidated.

Lachmann, B., Armbruster, S., Schairer, W., Landstra, M., Trouwborst, A., van Daal, G.-J., Kurama, A. and Erdmann, W. (1990) Safety and efficiency of xenon in routine use as an inhalational anaesthetic. *Lancet*, **335**, 1413–5

Agents mainly of historical interest

With the development of new drugs, many of the agents which for many years had been the 'backbone' of anaesthetic practice have ceased to be available. Some were regarded as too toxic and their use could not be justified in the presence of the more modern, albeit considerably more expensive, alternatives, for example chloroform, fluroxene, methoxyflurane. Some were explosive, for example ether, cyclopropane, and their use can no longer be justified in the presence of modern operating theatre equipment. However, diethyl ether is still widely used in the developing world. Others, like trichloroethylene, ceased to be used because the alternatives were much more useful and easier to administer.

Chloroform

This was first used clinically by Simpson in 1947. It was highly potent, but had the propensity to cause death from vagal effects or ventricular fibrillation. It was very easy to use and much of its bad reputation was due to its administration in an uncontrolled fashion. One of its major disadvantages was its effect on the liver, usually appearing 24–48 h after administration. Centrilobular necrosis occurred, which could be massive and was more likely in starved, dehydrated and toxic patients.

Cyclopropane

Cyclopropane is a highly explosive, colourless gas with a vapour density of 1.45. During anaesthesia, always administered via a closed system, blood pressure and cardiac output tend to be maintained. It is a potent respiratory depressant and the $P\text{CO}_2$ is increased. Arrhythmias are common.

Ethyl chloride

This is a gas at room temperature, but is usually stored under pressure in glass containers. The effects are similar to chloroform, but control of the inspired concentration is difficult; arrhythmias frequently occurred and deep anaesthesia could rapidly and uncontrollably be obtained. It is also flammable. When sprayed on the skin it evaporates and can cause refrigeration anaesthesia.

Fluroxene

This is a colourless liquid with a not unpleasant smell. Its vapour is heavier than air and is both flammable and explosive. Introduced clinically in 1954 under the name of Fluoromar, it enjoyed wide popularity in North America.

Significant metabolic transformation of fluroxene occurs. Repeated exposures of experimental animals to fluroxene invariably led to death following one to three exposures. A further disadvantage of fluroxene is its potential mutagenic action.

Methoxyflurane

This is a fluorinated methyl ethyl ether. However, its very low saturated vapour pressure and a boiling point of 104°C did not make for easy use. The major problem was significant (50 per cent) metabolic breakdown, especially to inorganic fluoride. As a result, high-output renal failure was a feature of prolonged methoxyflurane anaesthesia when the serum inorganic fluoride levels exceeded 50 µmol/litre. Unlike the other fluorinated ethers, methoxyflurane was also defluorinated in the kidneys and this is now thought to be the reason for its high local toxicity.

Trichloroethylene

Trichloroethylene is a colourless liquid with a specific gravity of 1.47 and a vapour density of 4.35. Its vapour is not flammable in the presence of air, but under certain conditions will ignite in the presence of oxygen in concentrations of 10–65 per cent. It is decomposed by alkalis and heat and therefore cannot be used with soda lime in closed circuits.

Its action on the CNS is the same as that of all general anaesthetics. Apart from its anaesthetic properties it is a powerful analgesic, formerly used in midwifery.

Depression of cardiac muscle is minimal and blood pressure is usually unchanged. The pulse rate is usually slower but cardiac irritability is increased. The sensitivity of the heart to epinephrine (adrenaline) is increased. Arrhythmias are rare during controlled ventilation but not uncommon during spontaneous ventilation.

Respiratory effects of trichloroethylene become prominent at any but the lightest planes of surgical anaesthesia. Tidal volume is decreased and respiratory rate usually increased. This is probably central in origin, and represents in an exaggerated form the respiratory response evoked by the majority of inhalational anaesthetics.

Skeletal muscle tone is slightly depressed but there is little effect on plain muscle and little effect on the uterus. It rapidly passes from the mother into the fetal circulation.

Trichloroethylene undergoes a significant degree of metabolic transformation, being first oxidized to chloral hydrate and then either further oxidized to trichloroacetic acid or reduced to trichloroethanol. Both chloral hydrate and trichloroethanol have hypnotic properties.

Although a powerful analgesic, trichloroethylene is a relatively weak anaesthetic and suitable only for the production of light anaesthesia. The vapour is non-irritant and induction with this agent is not unpleasant. Vapour strengths of 0.2–1.5 per cent are required to produce light anaesthesia. Normal doses of muscle relaxants may be used.

Even though trichloroethylene is not commercially available as an anaesthetic agent, anaesthetists working in underdeveloped surroundings find that some industrial sources of it are effective and not toxic.

Vinyl ether

This is a highly volatile liquid, lighter than water. The vapour is highly flammable and explosive when mixed with air (1.7–27 per cent) or oxygen (1.8–85 per cent). Vinyl ether is highly unstable.

Many of the actions of vinyl ether resemble those of diethyl ether. Induction, as would be expected with a low blood-gas partition coefficient, is more rapid, respiration is not stimulated, and the vapour is less irritant. Many cases of centrilobular hepatic necrosis have been reported following prolonged administration of vinyl ether.

5

Systemic analgesics

Pain

Pain is an important protective phenomenon. Although an oversimplification, it is widely accepted that pain comprises two major components: a nociceptive stimulus (the physical component) which allows us to determine when and where the pain arises, and its underlying features such as sharp or nagging, acute or prolonged; and a second reactive component (the psychological component) which is generated at cortical and sub-cortical levels in the brain. This component is usually secondary to (and consequent upon) the perception of a nociceptive stimulus. The contribution to pain made by the psychological component is dependent upon our past experiences, and the interpretation we place on the pain. It is thus important in determining the level of suffering aroused by the painful stimulus, and is substantially dependent upon levels of fear and apprehension. The level of clinical suffering is thought to be a product of the nociceptive and psychological components and attenuation of either component can lead to clinical relief. The perception of pain and the degree of suffering can vary considerably between individuals, and the contribution of fear (and ignorance) to an individual patient's suffering cannot be exaggerated.

Doses of analgesics required to suppress experimental pain in volunteers are usually significantly greater than those required to alleviate suffering in patients with most forms of cancer pain. It thus seems that the psychological component (which is usually dominant in cancer or terminal pain) is more sensitive to analgesic intervention. This is consistent with lower doses being required to prevent or delay the recurrence of clinical pain than are required to reverse established pain.

Not only does the perception of pain vary significantly between patients, but the level of pain or suffering in individual patients may also vary from day to day, according to the environment, their social expectations and their mood generally. While there are some objective, external markers of a patient's suffering (verbal, behavioural, motor, autonomic), the approach to treatment and dose must be based primarily upon what the patient tells us. If the patient says the pain is bad, then it is bad. A different approach is required when the patient makes it clear that their pain is tolerable, implying that the suffering is minimal.

Nomenclature

There is currently no consistency in the usage of the terms 'opiate' and 'opioid'. Originally, only drugs which were derived from opium itself were regarded as opiates. Drugs with similar actions were therefore classed as opioids. This had little logic, as heroin (diamorphine) is not found in opium, but everyone would regard it as an opiate since its actions follow from its conversion to metabolites which are found in opium.

Throughout this text we have attempted to conform to more modern usage, namely to use opiate as a noun and opioid as an adjective. Thus heroin is an *opiate* mainly active at *opioid* receptors.

Pain pathways

Following the nociceptive stimulation of sensory and pain nerve endings, impulses are conveyed into the spinal cord by two parallel routes. The first is a fast-conducting myelinated 'A-delta' fibre which is probably responsible for our determining where the pain is, and the nature or type of sensation. The second pathway is a slower conducting unmyelinated 'C' fibre. Both pathways synapse in the dorsal horn of the cord, before discharging their information into ipsilateral ('A' fibre) and contralateral ('A' and 'C' fibres) ascending spinothalamic pathways. The contralateral spinal pathways are important in ascribing the sensation of 'pain' to the initial stimulus. Critically, the tranmission of the original 'A' fibre sensory stimulus through to the contralateral 'pain pathway' is normally blocked, unless the level of stimulation of the parallel sensory 'C' fibres exceeds a predetermined level – the 'gate control' theory of Melzack and Wall. Thus, at low or sub-threshold levels of stimulus intensity, cells in the substantia gelatinosa are recruited by collateral 'A' fibres and these in turn appear to release endorphins which prevent both the main 'A' fibre neurones and the slower 'C' fibre neurones stimulating 'T' or transmission cells in the cord, from which the contralateral spinal pathway is normally stimulated and a pain stimulus is finally implemented. However, at higher stimulus intensities, the 'C' fibre neurones overcome the impediment raised by the substantia gelatinosa cells, at which point the stimulus assumes 'painful' characteristics on reaching the brain.

Nociceptive stimulus intensity is markedly increased in sub-acute or chronic pain, when inflammatory mediators substantially increase the 'C' fibre sensory input, causing supersensitivity. Increased sensitivity to chronic pain is also created by changes in the *s. gelatinosa* cells. In neuropathic pain (chronic pain of long standing, with significant pathological changes occurring at the site of sensory or nociceptive input), a range of new transmitter substances also become involved, and there is a dramatic 'wind up' in sensitivity to all modalities of sensory stimuli originating at or close to the sites of pathology.

There are also important descending largely inhibitory bulbospinal tracts which synapse with the 'T' cells to reduce the sensory stimuli. These descending pathways appear to arise in the median Raphe nuclei from serotonergic and GABA-ergic neurones, and may play an important part in determining inter-patient differences in pain sensitivity, or even differences in pain awareness in the same individual under altered circumstances. Regarding the role of serotonin in pain, it should be noted that procedures which attenuate serotonin function in the CNS, such as serotonin depletion or blockade, may induce hyperalgesia or attenuate the analgesic effects of morphine. Conversely, procedures which increase serotonin function will reduce inherent pain sensitivity and enhance the analgesic effects of opiates at opioid receptors. The instillation of small amounts of serotonin into the peri-aqueductal grey matter of experimental animals exerts a powerful analgesic effect which can be blocked by the opioid antagonist naloxone, suggesting that opioid and serotonergic functions are interdependent in this area of the CNS.

Analgesics

A wide range of drugs can alleviate pain: an anti-infective agent which relieves the pain associated with a localized infection, or an agent that reverses anginal pain through an increase in coronary flow in the heart may be described as relieving pain *aetiotropically*; other agents may alleviate or prevent pain by inducing general anaesthesia, *symptomatically*. In both types of attenuation, the agent is relieving pain as a consequence of some other non-analgesic primary pharmacological action. In contrast, an *analgesic* is an agent which prevents or alleviates pain as its principal therapeutic indication.

There are a number of potential sites at which to block the pain pathways. An agent may reduce the inflammation and other localized physiological reactions associated with local trauma, thus lowering the sensitivity of 'C' fibres to stimulation. Examples would be the non-steroidal anti-inflammatory drugs such as aspirin or ibuprofen. Drugs may also inhibit transmission in the dorsal horn, by enhancing the properties of the substantia gelatinosa cells that block pain transmission through the release of endorphins onto local opioid receptors. Both of these examples would result in a reduction of the physical component or nociceptive stimulus gaining access to the brain. Subsequently, each synapse in the upwards pain transmission pathway is theoretically open to pharmacological intervention, but the suppression of the psychological reaction to pain by opioid analgesics seems likely to occur by a combination of actions at opioid receptors in both the limbic system and sensory cortex.

Despite almost a century's research to find better analgesics, it remains convenient to classify them primarily according to their main site of action, namely 'central' and 'peripheral', notwithstanding that the peripheral effects of some opioids and the central effects of some non-steroidal anti-inflammatory drugs contribute to their overall clinical analgesic effects.

Centrally acting analgesics

The dried exudate or latex from the opium poppy, *Papaver somniferum*, has been used for several thousand years as a sedative, anxiolytic and analgesic. It also has a range of actions on the peripheral nervous system, including a profound reduction in gastro-intestinal motility – a boon or bane, according to a patient's circumstances. *Tincture of laudanum* (alcoholic tincture of opium) has been used alone or added to other medicines for several hundred years, its popularity diminishing only with the isolation of morphine (the most abundant and most active alkaloid in opium) and the introduction of the hypodermic syringe in the mid-19th century.

While the introduction into medicine of morphine was a landmark in the development of pain control, the many additional pharmacological properties and their adverse effects quickly led to a realization that it was not a panacea. A constant supply of new synthetic alternatives has ensued. The main purpose has been, variously, to increase analgesic potency (or reduce intrusive adverse effects, in particular to reduce physical dependence or 'addiction' liability); increase the extent and predictability of absorption following oral administration; and to increase duration of action. During this work, exceedingly potent analgesics were discovered (e.g. etorphine (Imobilon) and carfentanil) with a clinical dose measured in micrograms rather than milligrams. It was also recognized that the body showed stereoselectivity for different isomers of morphine and its analogues. These twin observations led to the proposition that the body contains discrete opioid receptors to which morphine-like drugs (opiates) bind to exert their principal pharmacological actions.

Endorphins

It was quickly established that the body also produced natural ligands for these receptors, subsequently collectively named endorphins, of which two penta-peptides leu-enkephalin and met-enkephalin were the first discovered.

At the present time, three principal families of endorphins are recognized – the enkephalins, the dynorphins and β-endorphins. Each family is derived from a distinct precursor polypeptide and each family has a characteristic anatomical distribution. Pro-enkephalin and pro-opiomelanocortins (POMC), precursors respectively of the enkephalins and β-endorphins, are found in CNS sites associated with pain transmission and suppression, and more than one family may be expressed in a given pathway. Endorphins and their precursors are also found at peripheral sites, including the adrenal medulla, gastro-intestinal tract, nerve plexuses and in certain exocrine glands. In addition to these families of peptides, there are also claims that morphine and codeine themselves also occur naturally in mammalian species including man. However, the veracity and significance of these claims remain to be demonstrated. The discovery and identification of the endorphins has not led to a range of new and improved analgesics, but there have been significant advances in our understanding of the role and location of different opioid receptors and greater insight into the probable mechanisms underlying tolerance and physical dependence and the roles of conventional neurotransmitters such as serotonin (5-HT) in pain and its suppression.

Opioid receptors

Currently three, possibly four, main classes of opioid receptor are recognized – mu (μ) (and subclasses μ_1 and μ_2), kappa (κ), delta (δ) and possibly sigma (σ) (The receptor terms mu, kappa and delta may be replaced by OP3, OP2 and OP1, respectively, following a review of opioid receptors by the *International Union of Pharmacology* (IUPHAR) in 1996.)

Opioid receptors are found at high densities in five areas of the CNS, namely the brain stem (where they mediate respiratory control, cough reflexes, nausea and vomiting and some autonomic effects); the medial thalamus (poorly localized deep pain); spinal cord (substantia gelatinosa cells and the arrest of nociceptive input); hypothalamus (temperature and neuroendocrine function) and the limbic system (influencing mood and emotional behaviour). Agonist actions in these CNS areas on all three main opioid receptors bring about the full range of observed desirable and adverse pharmacological actions, but the control of serious pain associated with fear and emotional reaction appears to follow upon activity at μ_1-receptors in the medial thalamus and limbic system. Drugs classified as 'full agonists' in *Table 5.1* thus possess a high efficacy at μ_1-receptors.

The different roles of the subclasses of opioid receptors are now emerging. Thus, μ_1-receptors are found predominantly at supraspinal sites, whereas μ_2-receptors are found in the spinal cord and at peripheral sites. This is consistent with μ_1- and spinal μ_2-receptors contributing to pain relief, while respiratory inhibition and constipation follow upon agonist actions at μ_2-receptors in the respiratory centre and gastro-intestinal tract, respectively. Three subclasses of κ-receptors, κ_1 κ_2 and κ_3 have been identified by a combination of *in vivo* animal studies and *in vitro* receptor binding techniques. κ_1-receptors appear to be important in spinal analgesia (and make some contribution to the analgesic actions of morphine and diamorphine), whereas κ_3-receptors are important in supraspinal analgesia, information that may become more relevant as new analgesics with agonist activity specific to κ-receptors are identified. Evidence for the roles of subclasses

Table 5.1 Principal opioid receptors, their subtypes and physiological roles*

Common name	IUPHAR† designation	Subtypes	Functional consequences of agonist action	Typical agonist
μ (mu)	OP_3	μ_1, μ_2	Supraspinal analgesia (μ_1) Spinal analgesia (μ_2) Sedation (μ_1) Respiratory inhibition (μ_2) Slowed GI transit, constipation (μ_2) Increased feeding (μ_1, μ_2) Increased prolactin secretion (μ_1) Increased growth hormone secretion (μ_2) Inhibits acetylcholine release (μ_1) Inhibits dopamine release (μ_2)	β-endorphin (μ_1, μ_2) Enkephalins (μ_1, μ_2) Morphine (μ_1, μ_2) Pethidine (μ_1, μ_2) Fentanyl (μ_1, μ_2) Diamorphine (μ_1, μ_2) Etorphine
κ (kappa)	OP_2	κ_1, κ_3	Supraspinal analgesia (κ_3) Spinal analgesia (κ_1) Slowed GI transit, constipation (κ_1, κ_3) Increased feeding (κ_1, κ_3) Sedation (κ_1, κ_3) Increased diuresis (κ_1) Psychotomimetic effects (κ_1, κ_3)	Dynorphins A and B Ethylketocyclazocine
δ (delta)	OP_1	δ_1, δ_2, δ_3,	Supraspinal analgesia (δ_1, δ_2) Spinal analgesia (δ_2) Increased growth hormone release (δ_1, δ_3) Inhibition of dopamine release (δ_1, δ_3)	Enkephalins Etorphine

* Information continues to emerge on the specific physiological roles of the opioid receptors and their subtypes. Analgesics (agonists) show specificity between μ-, κ- and δ-receptors, but not between subtypes. An analgesic with agonist effects at μ_1- but not μ_2-receptors might show some clinical advantages, but no such agent is available for clinical use. Naloxone and naltrexone are effective antagonists at all main opioid receptors (From Pasternak, 1993.

of δ-receptors is so far less conclusive, although both δ_1 and δ_2 have been identified. A report that a specific receptor exists for morphine-6-glucuronide has yet to be confirmed. *Table 5.1* summarizes our present knowledge of the physiological roles of different opioid receptors (and their subtypes), and provides some examples of known endogenous and exogenous agonists at these receptors.

Centrally acting analgesics can be classified in several ways, but that in *Table 5.2* is based upon both chemical structure and pharmacology. The accompanying *Figure 5.1* illustrates the structures of principal natural and synthetic centrally-acting analgesics.

Table 5.2 lists analgesics as 'agonists', 'partial agonists', 'antagonists' and 'non-opioid analgesics'. These terms require some explanation.

Opioid agonists

Although several separate opioid receptors exist (and specific agonists have been identified at each of these), it is widely accepted that the control of clinical pain, especially the suffering associated with terminal illness, may be effected by drugs with a strong agonist action at μ-receptors. Thus, morphine and diamorphine are full agonists at μ-receptors,

Table 5.2 Classification of some principal opiate analgesics based on their actions at μ opioid (OP3) receptors*

Agonists
Naturally occurring	Codeine
	Morphine
Semi-synthetic	Diamorphine
Wholly synthetic	Alfentanil
	Dextropropoxyphene
	Dihydrocodeine
	Fentanyl
	Methadone
	Pethidine
	Phenoperidine
	Remifentanil
Partial agonists	Buprenorphine
	Cyclazocine
	Nalorphine
	Pentazocine
Opioid antagonists	Naloxone
	Naltrexone
Non-opioid analgesics	Meptazinol
	Nefopam
	Tramadol

* Since agonist activity at μ opioid (OP3) receptors is of major importance in the relief of clinical pain, the above classification is based upon agonist or antagonist actions at these receptors. Agonist actions at δ (OP1) and κ (OP2) receptors contribute variously to spinal analgesia and certain adverse effects.

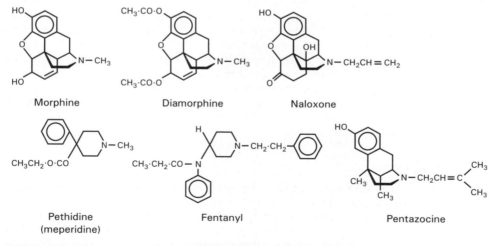

Figure 5.1 Chemical structures of some principal natural and synthetic centrally-acting analgesics. Morphine (naturally occurring) and diamorphine (semi-synthetic) exert analgesic activity and most of their main adverse effects through agonist actions at μ opioid receptors. Naloxone is an opioid antagonist at all known opioid receptors. Pethidine (meperidine) and fentanyl are wholly synthetic agonist analgesics, whereas pentazocine has mixed agonist/antagonist (partial agonist) properties

although their actions at other receptors (e.g. κ-receptors) do contribute to opiates' other desirable properties. However, activity at κ- and δ-receptors appears to be more important in determining some of their adverse effects. As doses are increased, for example following pharmacodynamic tolerance during opiate abuse, agonist activity at κ- and δ-receptors may become more intrusive.

The subcellular mechanism of opiate agonist actions at opioid receptors is still far from fully understood. The recent cloning of opioid receptors has confirmed that they belong to the G-protein coupled receptor superfamily, and thus transduce their signals through interactions with guanine nucleotide-binding proteins. All three opioid receptors appear to couple to various Ca^{2+} channels, and they are also known to regulate inwardly-rectifying K^+ channels and interact with Na^+/H^+ ion exchanges. The outcome of these subcellular effects may be largely pre-synaptic: inhibition of neurotransmitter release in the CNS through an enhancement of K^+ ion-induced membrane hyperpolarization and an inhibition of Ca^{2+} ion neuronal entry, both of which are preparatory events to the release of neurotransmitters from pre-synaptic sites.

Partial agonist analgesics

With the synthesis of N-allyl norcodeine in 1919 and later N-allyl normorphine (nalorphine) in 1943 came the realisation that morphine's and diamorphine's actions could be antagonized. Paradoxically, nalorphine on its own exerted some analgesic activity, although this quickly reached a ceiling and was associated with dysphoric mood and other adverse effects. Nevertheless it prompted the search for new derivatives which would maximize a modest analgesic action devoid of addiction liability, and the first benzomorphan derivative, pentazocine, was introduced in 1969.

Today, several synthetic morphine derivatives have been introduced, with a mix of low agonistic (low intrinsic) and antagonistic properties at the different opioid receptors. At the μ-receptor, they exert a partial agonist action, with efficacies ranging from 'low' (e.g. nalorphine) to 'moderate' (pentazocine) and 'high' (buprenorphine).

A significant advantage of the partial agonists is their relatively low abuse potential, a property assisted by their mildly unpleasant (dysphoric) effects in some patients. On the other hand, switching clinical pain relief from a partial agonist (e.g. pentazocine or buprenorphine) to relief with a full agonist such as morphine requires care, since larger initial doses of the agonist may be required to displace remaining molecules of the partial agonist. This is particularly true with buprenorphine whose long duration of action is at least partly due to continuing occupation of the opioid receptors. There is no pharmacological rationale therefore to attempting basic clinical pain relief with a partial agonist occasionally 'topped up' with a pure agonist. Indeed failure to relieve pain at all may be a consequence of such combinations.

Opioid antagonists

Naloxone (and a more recent, longer acting drug naltrexone) are pure opioid antagonists; that is, despite high affinity for opioid receptors, these agents possess no intrinsic activity. This means that, although occupying the opioid receptors, they do not bring about the receptor perturbations that develop into intracellular biological responses; their efficacy or intrinsic activity as agonists is thus described as 'zero', a property they possess at all three (μ-, κ- and δ-) opioid receptors. Opioid antagonists reverse the effects of agonists such as morphine, diamorphine and pethidine, by competing for the receptors and, once in occupation, the antagonist prevents the actions of any agonist. Naloxone is relatively short acting, so that having reversed the effects of an agonist, the agonist's effects may reappear once the naloxone has been eliminated and this explains why opioid inhibition of respiration in the newborn rapidly responds to the first administration of naloxone but the respiratory difficulties may reappear later, depending on the dose and timing of agonist administration earlier in labour.

While opiate overdose or intoxication should never be the consequence of rational medication, emergencies do arise from accidental or deliberate overdose, or through opiate abuse. The use of naloxone in a procedure called 'rapid anaesthetic antagonist opiate detoxification' is decribed in the Monograph on naloxone.

Absorption and fate of opiates in the body

In small to modest doses, morphine is rapidly demethylated in the liver. Following oral administration, there is a classical 'first-pass' effect, effectively reducing oral bioavailability to about 30 per cent. Larger doses, given orally in sustained or delayed release forms, to some extent overwhelm the hepatic demethylating process, thus enhancing the oral bioavailability beyond that of morphine in simple tablet, capsule or solution form. Oral delayed release preparations do provide effective analgesia. They also permit a reduced frequency of administration to two or three times a day during terminal or other unremitting pain, and are thus an effective alternative for domiciliary use. Predictably, morphine is more potent rectally or by any parenteral route. It can also be given extradurally or intrathecally, when its analgesic actions may be limited to spinal μ_2- and certain κ-receptors producing a prolonged analgesia.

The major metabolic pathway of morphine is hepatic conjugation to the glucuronide, morphine-6-glucuronide, which is pharmacologically active; the desmethylated drug, desmethyl-morphine-6-glucuronide, is not. The metabolite morphine-6-glucuronide makes a considerable contribution to morphine's actions, particularly during chronic treatment. While the plasma half-life of morphine is about 3 h in young adults, that of the active glucuronide metabolite is nearer 8–10 h. Thus, during chronic administration its plasma levels comfortably exceed those of the parent drug. This situation is exacerbated in patients with renal failure, when the glucuronide's persistence is even more marked. Because renal function diminishes with age, lower doses of morphine are usually indicated. Morphine is eliminated by the kidneys as a glucuronide after some enterohepatic circulation of both morphine and its glucuronide metabolites. This is another factor contributing to a prolonged 'tail' to the duration of morphine's effects.

The morphine analogue codeine has much lower affinity at opioid receptors but better oral bioavailability which, coupled with the fact that a proportion is demethoxylated to form morphine (and in turn morphine-6-glucuronide), means that codeine is an effective pro-drug. The enzyme responsible for the codeine-to-morphine conversion, CPY2D6, is missing from about 8 per cent of the Western European population. Thus, about 1 in 12 patients might find codeine useless, or be tempted to use rather higher than normal doses to achieve analgesic effects. There is also some speculation that codeine's activity as an anti-tussive agent may relate to better affinity of codeine itself at modified receptors.

Diacetylmorphine (diamorphine, heroin) is rapidly deacetylated to first mono-acetylmorphine (MAM) and thence morphine itself. Both diamorphine and MAM are more lipid soluble than morphine, and thus more easily enter the CNS. Since MAM is pharmacologically active, the greater potency of diamorphine and its more rapid onset of action are attributable to the combined effects of MAM and morphine.

In addition to oral, buccal, rectal, parenteral and spinal routes of administration, there is a growing interest in the transdermal administration of analgesics. The advantages are prolonged and continuing availability of the analgesic throughout the day, no first-pass metabolism, and a stable plasma (and tissue) level of the drug. Replenishment of the dose of drug can be carried out in the ambulant patient or in the domiciliary situation. The prerequisites are a drug potent enough to achieve clinical effects at 5 mg or less, per day, and high lipid solubility (although studies with assisted penetration may soon dispose of the need for high lipid solubility). Fentanyl is just such a potent, highly lipid soluble synthetic opiate which is available in self-adhesive skin patches. The rate of administration of drug is controlled by the skin patch area of contact, and over a 72 h period can deliver up to 100 µg of fentanyl per hour. This approximates to a 24 h dose of 2.4 mg, which is equivalent to about 400 mg of morphine given orally. After 72 h the patch should be replaced. Peak plasma levels of fentanyl usually occur between 24 and 72 h after applying the first patch, after which they remain very stable with successive patches.

The pursuit of new synthetic opioid derivatives has several objectives which include greater potency, longer duration of action, better bioavailability by mouth and fewer acute and chronic adverse effects. Since these objectives have only been met in part, the introduction of new opioid derivates is likely to continue. Monographs of individual analgesics of importance to anaesthetists follow at the end of the chapter.

Tolerance, physical dependence and addiction

These phenomena relate to chronic or extended use, rather than that associated with the normal postoperative situation.

Tolerance

In the clinical situation, morphine, diamorphine and other full agonist opiates may occasionally be prone to tolerance, that is, a clinical situation in which a constantly repeated dose of analgesic achieves progressively less relief of suffering; or the dose needs to be continuously increased with successive administrations to maintain the same level of relief.

First, morphine and its close congeners may suffer a pharmacokinetic tolerance during the first 10–14 days' administration in some patients, the extent of this tolerance varying markedly between patients. This tolerance is attributed to some (limited) induction of hepatic metabolizing enzymes which reaches a plateau. Its effects are limited and usually call for only minor changes in dose or frequency of dosing with opioid analgesic.

Secondly, morphine may be subject to a pharmacodynamic tolerance in which the pharmacological action of morphine at its receptors is reduced because of compensatory or adaptive changes. It is far more difficult to predict the speed of onset or intensity of this form of tolerance and it can occur more quickly with certain opiates (generally the fast-acting, short-duration ones) and to some drug effects (for example, euphoria following injected diamorphine) than to actual pain relief. Some steps may be taken to minimize the risks of pharmacodynamic tolerance developing. For example, it is easier to prevent pain or the recurrence of pain than it is to reverse pain by waiting for its return. Further, if a patient is allowed to suffer the progressive return of pain (for example, by using a fixed 3- or 4-hourly regimen on the ward for administering analgesics), this can induce a drug-seeking or anticipatory behaviour which maximizes the possibility of tolerance developing. Pharmacodynamic tolerance can be minimized by making sure the patient stays free from pain through the use of adequate doses of analgesic given as often as is necessary. It should also be remembered that developing pathology may generate a need for greater pain relief, and this should not be confused with the development of tolerance to the drug. Finally, the appearance of pharmacodynamic tolerance may occur more easily or more quickly in a small proportion of the population: it is not a common problem unless the patient has had a history of drug abuse involving alcohol and/or opiate substances.

Patients and relatives should be reassured that serious tolerance to the effects of opioid analgesics is uncommon, and will not interfere with providing proper pain relief.

Physical dependence or addiction

Physical dependence is manifest more in the withdrawal from drug effects than in their use and follows upon the development of pharmacodynamic tolerance. In pre- or postoperative circumstances it is difficult to create clinical conditions from which opioid dependence can occur, but where opiates are being used chronically for unremitting pain, those procedures which minimize the development of pharmacodynamic tolerance will also minimize the appearance of physical dependence. This includes the use of procedures which prevent the reappearance or recurrence of pain, whether by using adequate doses, or long-acting analgesics, or continuous medication with other agents (e.g. via skin patches, or using patient controlled analgesia, PCA). Prevention of suffering takes a higher priority than concerns about inducing drug dependence. Terminally ill patients in pain are dependent on drugs for relief.

Whether in acute or chronic pain relief, patients' and relatives' natural concerns about 'addiction' should be anticipated, and efforts made to reassure them of the rarity of this event. In a widely quoted study reported from the Boston Collaborative Surveillance Program, only four cases of addiction occurred in almost 12,000 hospitalized patients receiving opioid analgesics. Clinical tolerance to, and dependence upon, opioid analgesics has recently been reviewed by Collett (1998).

Collet, B.J. (1998) Opioid tolerance: the clinical perspective. *British Journal of Anaesthesia*, **81**, 58–68

Intrathecal and extradural opiates

The discovery of opioid receptors in the dorsal horn of grey matter in the spinal cord in the mid-1970s was soon followed by the demonstration in animals of prolonged analgesia resulting from local application of opiate drugs to the cord. Since 1979, intrathecal and extradural opiates have been used extensively in man in the management of chronic and acute pain. The site of action of the drugs is probably on presynaptic opioid receptors in the substantia gelatinosa, where they inhibit release of nociceptive transmitters such as substance P from the small nerve endings.

Use of opiates in this way has several distinct advantages over spinally administered local anaesthetics. There is no autonomic blockade and hence no hypotension, no loss of any other modality of sensation and no motor block. Tachyphylaxis is not a problem and the results of accidental intravenous administration are easier to treat. Analgesia is effective and prolonged and achieved with much smaller doses than when used systemically. A specific antagonist is also available in the form of naloxone.

There is no difference in the quality of analgesia between the drugs used, but merely in the speed of onset, duration of action and incidence of complications, which are all explicable by the different pharmacokinetic properties of the agents. On injection into the extradural space, some of the drug will escape through the intervertebral foramina, some will dissolve in epidural fat and some will be absorbed into the systemic circulation. Most of the drug is lost to dural transfer and the extent to which this occurs depends largely on the fat solubility of the agent used. Thus a poorly fat-soluble drug like morphine will cross the dura only slowly and this will result in a slow onset of analgesia. It will only slowly be leached into the spinal cord and will tend to linger in the cerebrospinal fluid (CSF) and be available for rostral spread. With such an agent, long-duration, diffuse analgesia can be expected with a high incidence of side effects. This is borne out by clinical experience. On the other hand, much more of a fat-soluble drug such as fentanyl would be lost to dural transfer and as it would rapidly cross the dura and be leached into the spinal cord, it would be expected to produce rapid onset, segmental analgesia of shorter duration than morphine, with a lower incidence of side effects; again, this is borne out by clinical experience.

It would therefore seem much more logical to inject the drug directly into the CSF. Typical doses are 0.1 mg morphine, 0.2 mg diamorphine or 0.5 μg fentanyl.

There is little convincing evidence that spinally applied opiates produce better quality analgesia than by more conventional routes of administration, although analgesia is achieved with smaller doses of drug. However, the incidence of complications is high. Pruritus, nausea and vomiting occur in up to 50 per cent of patients. Particularly troublesome is the 30–40 per cent incidence of urinary retention that occurs in patients who are not catheterized. But the most disturbing complication is respiratory depression, especially as its appearance may be delayed for several hours after drug administration. It is commoner after morphine than the other drugs, the reported incidence in large series varying from about 0.1 per cent to over 3 per cent. It may be delayed as long as 16 h: it is readily reversed by naloxone. As would be expected, it is much rarer following fat-soluble drugs and can come on within 30 minutes, indicating an effect due to systemic absorption. Although the incidence after these drugs is not known, because of the absence of large reported series, it must be remembered that delayed respiratory depression has been reported following diamorphine, methadone, hydromorphone and fentanyl. The nature of the complications after intrathecal and extradural opiates has important implications for the management of these patients after surgery.

Non-opioid, non-NSAID centrally-acting analgesics

A number of synthetic agents have been introduced which appear not to rely wholly upon opioid receptor mechanisms. Drugs with agonist activity at opioid receptors mimic the effects of endogenous endorphins: these in turn may enhance or reduce neuronal traffic involving neurotransmitters such as acetylcholine, norepinephrine (noradrenaline), dopamine and serotonin. It follows that drugs which interfere with cholinergic or aminergic transmission in the CNS may *inter alia* reduce pain. It may also be that analgesics produce pain relief by a similar mechanism.

Tricyclic antidepressants such as imipramine and amitriptyline have been used, particularly in Europe, in some chronic pain conditions, including post-herpetic pain and some arthritic and back pain, either alone or in combination with an opiate or non-steroidal anti-inflammatory drug (NSAID). Curiously, the onset of their 'analgesic' effects may occur significantly more quickly (2–3 days) than their antidepressant actions. An enhancement of central serotonergic function has been offered as one explanation for these effects, but there is also some evidence from animal studies to suggest an opioid mechanism. Rather less experience is available, so far, with the more selective serotonin re-uptake inhibiting (SSRI) antidepressants such as fluoxetine. Carbamazepine is an agent structurally related to the phenothiazines and tricyclic antidepressants, which is used in chronic back conditions and post-herpetic pain associated with the face.

Of the agents specifically introduced as analgesics, meptazinol is a drug with some passing structural resemblance to pethidine, but has mixed pharmacological properties: at μ opioid receptors it exerts a modest partial agonist activity assisted by some central muscarinic actions and is useful in moderate pain associated with the postoperative period. It has not demonstrated any advantages over other partial agonists. Nefopam (once known as fenazoxine) is used in mild to moderate pain, and compares with codeine and propoxyphene. Its mechanism of analgesic action is largely unknown: it is not an opioid agonist, but does promote central serotonin function by inhibiting 5-HT re-uptake, which is consistent with our knowledge of the role of serotonin in pain suppression.

Peripherally-acting analgesics

The analgesic, antipyretic and anti-inflammatory properties of certain salicylates particularly acetylsalicylic acid (aspirin) were discovered in the late nineteenth century, since when they have proved to be relatively safe and predictable medicines. Their irritant effects upon the gastro-intestinal tract, coupled with their relative lack of potency in some chronic progressive painful conditions such as arthritis, prompted a major search for newer agents, and the range of agents available was considerably widened by the new drugs introduced in the 1960s and 1970s. Chemically, they are a heterogeneous group, although many of them are derivatives of organic acids. Their prototype is aspirin: although originally referred to as aspirin-like drugs, the acronym NSAIDs is now widely used, internationally, to define the class.

Although it was known that NSAIDs inhibit a wide range of enzyme catalysed reactions *in vitro*, it was not until Vane and associates in 1971 showed that aspirin and certain other NSAIDs inhibited the synthesis of prostaglandins, that any fundamental inhibitory effect upon the inflammatory process could be demonstrated.

Inflammation is a normal, protective response to tissue injury, whether caused by mechanical, thermal or chemical insults, infectious agents, antigen/antibody reactions or ischaemia. Inflammation is the body's reaction to local injury: it is designed to remove the irritants and prepare for tissue repair, and involves both cellular and vascular events. Mediators of inflammation are derived from injured tissues and migrating cells, and include the prostaglandins and other eicosanoids, cytokines, histamine, bradykinin and other neuropeptides, complement components and components of the kinin cascade. Although erythema, oedema, hyperalgesia and actual pain are common to the inflammatory process, three phases are recognized: an acute transient phase, a delayed sub-acute phase and a chronic proliferative phase. The time scales of these successive phenomena differ according to the initiating agent, the inflammatory agents recruited and the location.

Prostanoids (prostaglandins and other 20-carbon eicosanoid derivatives) are the products of the cyclo-oxygenase metabolism of arachidonic acid, the latter being one of the first 'products' of cell wall injury. Following its release from the injured cell wall, arachidonic acid may be chemically transformed along one of several different pathways. Two of these are important in the development of inflammation:

- The **lipoxygenase pathway**. Leukotrienes and the hydroperoxy-eicosa-tetranoic acids (HPETEs) are the products of this pathway and this leads also to phagocyte mobilization; inhibitors of 5-lipoxygenase, such as docebenone, piripost and zileuton, are undergoing clinical trials against asthma and related inflammatory conditions.

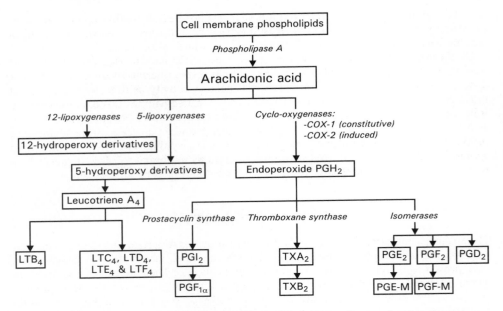

Figure 5.2 Arachidonic acid metabolism to show major products of lipoxygenase and cyclo-oxygenase pathways.

Principal enzymes are shown in italics. Arachidonic acid is formed as a result of cell injury. Leucotrienes appear as a result of 5-lipoxygenase activity, and it is now accepted that a mixture of LTC_4 and LTD_4 makes up a material earlier known as 'slow reacting substance of anaphylaxis' (SRS-A) – their principal actions include vasconstriction in, and plasma exudation from, small vessels. Thromboxane A_2 is also a potent vasoconstrictor, and (when sourced by platelets) prevents platelet aggregation. In contrast, prostaglandins exert a variety of effects: PGE derivatives are vasodilators, PGFs are vasoconstrictors, while PGDs have mixed effects. PGI_2 is a powerful vasodilator and by controlling platelet aggregation also contributes to the anti-thrombogenic properties of the intact vascular wall. The PGs' individual roles become clearer and more coherent when their effects on the cardiovascular system, blood elements, kidney and other organs are interpreted in relation to the tissues and organs in which they are released and subsequent local actions.

Glucocorticoids exert some anti-inflammatory effect indirectly by reducing the activity of phospholipase A and the appearance of arachidonic acid following cell injury, but their principal effects are to prevent the expression of new COX-2 enzyme during the inflammatory reaction to injury. Most NSAIDs in current clinical use are non-selective inhibitors of both COX-1 and COX-2 enzymes

- The **cyclo-oxygenase pathway**. The various prostaglandins and thromboxanes are produced by this pathway which is a target for NSAID inhibitory activity.

The relative importance in acute and chronic inflammatory conditions of these two metabolic pathways of arachidonic acid, and the identity of the products formed, vary from tissue to tissue as a result of different types of cell insult. (Cytochrome P-450 also transforms arachidonic acid to a series of metabolites with vascular, renal, endocrine and other effects, but the overall significance of this third metabolic pathway remains obscure.)

Within the cyclo-oxygenase pathway a number of prostaglandins have been identified in the development of the inflammatory response, and are of particular importance in the early stages; for example, in the appearance of erythema and increased local blood flow. Prostaglandins are released whenever cells are damaged, and local bradykinin (from plasma kininogen) and various cytokines assist in this release by promoting arachidonic acid metabolism. Prostaglandins sensitize pain receptors to mechanical and chemical stimulation, thus lowering the threshold at which sensory 'C' fibres are recruited into the initiation and transmission of painful stimuli. The prostaglandins PGE_2 and $PG1_2$ are two of the most active as mediators of hyperalgesia (enhanced nociceptive sensitivity), and sensory neurones (and some central neurones, see below) express receptors sensitive to both of these. *Figure 5.2* summarizes the main pathways of metabolism of arachidonic acid following its appearance as a consequence of cell injury, and the main products of the enzymes 5-lipoxygenase and cyclo-oxygenase.

The principal therapeutic effect of NSAIDs derives from their ability to suppress the formation and appearance of prostaglandins and related prostanoids such as thromboxane in the inflammatory process. This they achieve by selectively inhibiting the cyclo-oxygenase pathway. They exert no similar effect upon the lipoxygenase pathway, so that leucotrienes and the appearance of other inflammatory mediators are not affected by NSAIDs. Two main cycloxygenase isoenzymes have been identified, COX-1 (a mainly constitutive, preformed enzyme) and COX-2 (largely induced in inflammatory conditions by cytokines). Aspirin and other existing NSAIDs prevent prostaglandin, prostacyclin and thromboxane production, as a result of their inhibition of both COX-1 and COX-2, although there is an increasing likelihood that COX-2 selective inhibitors may soon become available. It must be noted, however, that assigning wholly constitutive functions to COX-1 and pathology-induced functions to COX-2 is an oversimplification.

COX-1 isoenzyme is physiologically present in blood platelets, where it is essential for the synthesis of thromboxane A_2 (TxA_2). Pharmacological inhibition of TxA_2 synthesis leads to a loss of normal platelet aggregation induced by certain stimuli. COX-1 is also responsible for the production of prostacyclin, which when released by the endothelium is anti-thrombogenic and when released by the gastric mucosa is cytoprotective. This cytoprotection extends to both exogenous and endogenous agents. In the kidney, prostaglandins are produced mainly in the renal medulla, the ascending loop of Henle and the cortex, and influence total renal blood flow, renal distribution of blood, sodium and water reabsorption and renin release.

In contrast, COX-2 is a predominantly 'inducible' enzyme. It is found as a tissue constituent only in small amounts, for example in normal lung, kidney and fetal membranes. Most of its activity follows upon a 20-fold 'induction' following the detection of cell injury, involving agents such as endotoxins, interferons and tumour necrosis factor. The anti-inflammatory cytokine IL-10 down-regulates COX-2 expression.

There is therefore an important rationale behind the search for COX-2 selective inhibitors, because these would target the isoenzyme mainly responsible for the appearance of inflammatory prostaglandins, and in parallel lead to a substantial reduction in adverse effects. Thus, COX-1 enzyme, if unaffected, would continue to synthesize prostaglandins important in gastro-intestinal protection, platelet function, regulation of blood flow and kidney function, while the inhibition of the COX-2 isoenzyme would prevent the emergence of prostaglandins which induce inflammation, fever and pain. Sodium salicylate and meloxicam are partially COX-2 selective, and clinical evidence is emerging to quantify the extent to which such drugs possess an improved adverse effects profile. There are some early worries that, although COX-2 specific inhibitors may indeed exert less upper GI tract irritation, conversely they may increase irritation of the epithelium of the colon.

Aspirin's inhibition of cyclo-oxygenase activity (unlike the inhibition exerted by most of its NSAID-derivatives) is the result of a covalent binding to the enzyme. Consequently, there is an irreversible, long-lasting suppression of prostaglandin synthesis until fresh cyclo-oxygenase enzymes are synthesized. An interesting consequence of this irreversibility is a prolonged suppression of thromboxane synthesis by platelets: because of their inability to synthesize new protein (new enzyme), they remain incapable of further thromboxane synthesis throughout their 8–11-day life span. This is important in preventing platelet adhesion and the initiation of clot formation. A dose as little as 40 mg per day is sufficient to indefinitely impede this process. Other NSAIDs combine with COX-1 and COX-2 in a less permanent manner, being reversible or competitive inhibitors.

Aspirin and other NSAIDS, being organic acids, are well absorbed orally. They are highly bound to plasma proteins which delays their metabolism or elimination by the kidneys. Aspirin may be described as a *hit-and-run* drug because its pharmacological effects (cyclo-oxygenase inhibition) persist, particularly with larger doses, after its elimination from the body. For the newer (reversible) agents, their duration of action is determined by their pharmacokinetics and they can be subdivided into short-acting (less than 6 h) and long-acting (greater than 10 h) subgroups. This has implications for their frequency of administration and, importantly, the ability to maintain relatively constant concentrations at effective sites.

As organic acids (or their derivatives), aspirin and the other NSAIDs accumulate at sites of inflammation, a useful if unplanned pharmacological feature. Less useful is their non-selective inhibition of both COX-1 and COX-2 enzymes. COX-1 is a constitutive enzyme and thus plays a role in other non-inflammatory processes whose inhibition may be deleterious to human physiology. An important example is in the gastro-intestinal tract where prostaglandins and prostacyclins play important protective roles against the irritating actions of gastric acid. Heartburn, dyspepsia and indigestion are common and overt consequences of chronic NSAID treatment. More insidious and serious is the associated ulceration and bleeding that follow upon the loss of gastro-intestinal protection by COX-1 derived prostacyclins (which suppress gastric acid secretion) and the cytoprotective effects of the prostglandins, leading to anaemia or worse.

Central effects of NSAIDs

The NSAIDs are thought to be primarily peripherally acting drugs, firstly, because entry into the CNS is limited for most NSAID compounds because of their protein binding, their polar nature and consequent low lipophilicity, although the presence of fever may enhance penetration of some of these agents into the brain. Secondly, the painful and inflammatory conditions against which they are most frequently used are usually very localized, for example, pain associated with headache, myalgia and arthralgia. However, both isoforms of cyclo-oxygenase (as well as prostaglandin receptors) are found in a number of regions of the CNS, including the mid-brain peri-aqueductal grey matter. A recent study has shown that opioid potentiation of descending inhibitory GABA-ergic influences on nociceptive pathways in the mid-brain peri-aqueductal grey matter may itself be enhanced further by NSAIDs. NSAIDs are known to potentiate clinical opioid analgesia, and this synergism in the CNS appears to be linked mainly to the former's inhibition of COX-1.

Therapeutic use of NSAIDs and related drugs

These agents are commonly used to allay or reduce 'mild pain', when they are most frequently (but not only) used for a few hours or just one or two days. Such pains are commonly musculoskeletal in origin. The drugs are commonly used for clinical conditions in which fever and inflammation are important accompaniments of pain. Such conditions are often acute, but when they have become chronic they are often seriously disabling conditions in which chronic inflammation and perpetual pain are prominent features.

Numerous clinical trials have compared new NSAIDs with aspirin or with each other, often with conflicting results. Newer NSAIDs are usually more potent, may be less irritant to the gastro-intestinal tract in some patients, and may be longer acting. However, despite considerable effort, an adverse effect-free 'once daily' drug has yet to emerge, although some agents do have extended half-lives.

NSAIDs are the drugs of first choice in the active stages of rheumatoid arthritis and arthritides such as ankylosing spondylitis. They are also more effective than simple analgesics in relieving the symptoms of osteoarthritis when there is secondary inflammation. NSAIDS reduce the pain and stiffness, perhaps also the early swelling, associated with both acute and chronic inflammatory conditions. They do nothing to treat or reverse the underlying disease process. NSAIDs act upon the inflammatory process within 18–24 h, and peak effects are usually achieved within 1–2 weeks of starting treatment. Changing or alternating between different NSAIDs is unlikely to increase effectiveness, unless it permits a higher dose through a reduction in attendant adverse effects.

Their principal adverse effect, common to all NSAIDs to a greater or lesser extent, is gastro-intestinal erosion, bleeding and ulceration, caused by their non-selective blockade of the synthesis of protective prostaglandins in the gastro-intestinal tract. Gastro-intestinal effects are perhaps most noticeable with aspirin, indomethacin and phenylbutazone but they remain a significant hazard with all NSAIDs depending on the individual patient, their dietary habits, the dose regimen used and duration of treatment.

A procedure recommended for all oral NSAIDs is to administer them after a significant meal, when immediate gastro-intestinal effects may be minimized. A consequence of this, however, will be a modest but significant delay in absorption, and time to peak plasma (and tissue) levels. In the acute clinical situation, the conflict between obtaining a prompt beneficial effect and the need to minimize gastro-intestinal symptoms must be weighed carefully.

Less common adverse effects include tinnitus (particularly in the elderly and following high doses for a prolonged period), onycholysis, photosensitivity and the displacement of certain other drugs from protein binding, thus enhancing their effects. The most notorious example is warfarin. Aspirin inhibits thromboxane synthesis by platelets, which can delay or prevent their aggregation and, in small doses, is used prophylactically to prevent microthromboemboli. Aspirin can conversely cause renal damage and, occasionally, an asthma-like airways hypersensitivity. Bone marrow suppression, hepatic toxicity and the Stevens–Johnson syndrome are uncommon and unpredictable consequences of NSAID medication. Renal toxicity may ultimately be a problem with all NSAIDs administered for prolonged periods or in high doses.

NSAIDs in infants and children

For most of the twentieth century, aspirin has been a simple and widely used domicilary antidote to childhood musculoskeletal pains and fevers, but its possible association with Reye's syndrome has seen its formal withdrawal as an analgesic, antipyretic, anti-inflammatory agent in children below the age of 8 years. This is unfortunate because it is otherwise safer than paracetamol or alternative NSAIDs, and the evidence for aspirin precipitating Reye's syndrome is at best weak.

The niche left by aspirin's withdrawal has largely been filled by paracetamol. It has recently been suggested that it is often used at sub-optimal doses, and that one should give a loading dose (up to 30 mg/kg, orally or rectally) followed by regular oral or rectal doses up to a total of 90 mg/kg daily, depending upon the general health of the child. Liver toxicity is a possibility at doses above 150 mg/kg/day. Paracetamol and codeine combined is more effective than paracetamol alone, while other NSAIDs such as ketorolac, ibuprofen and diclofenac have been found useful in combating postoperative pain in children.

The Monographs in the second part of this chapter cover only a small proportion of all the drugs available, but an attempt is made to provide information about drugs that are commonly used, are used for specific indications or which possess unique or uncommon properties.

The Royal College of Anaesthetists has published *Guidelines for the Use of Non-Steroidal Anti-inflammatory Drugs in the Perioperative Period* (1998).

Therapeutic uses of prostaglandins

Where an NSAID causes unacceptable gastro-intestinal irritation, it may be possible to offer protection through the administration of a second agent. Recently, the co-administration of the synthetic PGE_2 analogue misoprostol has proved advantagous in preventing or delaying the gastro-intestinal side effects of chronic treatment with high doses of NSAID for long-term conditions such as arthritis. Misoprostol protects the gastro-intestinal mucosa by inhibiting basal, stimulated and nocturnal acid secretions; it reduces the volume of gastric secretions, it reduces the proteolytic activity of gastric fluid, and increases bicarbonate and mucous secretion. At the recommended doses (up to 800 µg daily), misoprostol achieves this gastro-intestinal protection without increasing inflammatory conditions or hyperalgesia, or attenuating the effect of NSAIDs elsewhere. More recently, the new anti-H_2 antagonist ebrotidine has been introduced in Europe, with licensed indications which include the prevention of gastropathies induced by NSAIDs. Other therapeutic uses of prostaglandins are discussed in Chapter 16.

Analgesic nephropathy

There is a clear lack of correlation on this subject between experimental work in animals and clinical experience. In acute experiments in rats, a large number of aspirin and phenacetin derivatives cause renal damage which, however, is confined to the proximal convoluted tubule. Phenacetin alone in animals has only rarely induced papillary necrosis, but aspirin does so readily. In man, the evidence is the reverse. Numerous cases of analgesic nephropathy have been reported in patients taking mixtures containing phenacetin; by contrast, considering the enormous consumption, relatively few cases have been reported in patients taking aspirin alone.

Anaesthestists should be alert for possible analgesic nephropathy in patients undergoing major surgery, particularly gastric surgery for ulceration. Dehydration and renal ischaemia are both capable of exacerbating experimental nephropathy and they may occur in surgical patients for a variety of reasons. There have been clinical reports of a high mortality in surgical patients with known analgesic nephropathy, and agents that are less likely to cause renal vasoconstriction are therefore indicated, combined with adequate fluid therapy.

Treatment of migraine

Migraine is a relatively common illness, with an incidence of about 1 in 16 for men and 1 in 6 for women. Because many of those suffering from mild and or infrequent attacks never seek professional advice, the true incidence of migraine is difficult to calculate. Many patients recognize 'trigger' factors which may be dietary or stress related, but in women may also be associated with decreasing oestrogen levels late in the menstrual cycle. The disease usually has its onset in early adulthood, becoming less frequent again with advancing age, and up to 80 per cent of cases are thought to be familial.

In its classical form, migraine consists of a severe throbbing unilateral headache that is preceded by a quite characteristic 'aura' which may involve visual disturbances, photophobia, hyperacusis, polyuria or diarrhoea. Other symptoms include nausea and occasionally vomiting. Although the symptoms of a mild attack may be of limited duration and severity (typically less than an hour, in which the aura is quickly replaced by a headache), severe migraine attacks may last for 1 or 2 days, and may include repeated episodes occurring within the space of a few hours. Symptom patterns, severity and frequency of attack differ greatly between patients. Medication may be used to prevent a threatened attack or reverse an established attack or a combination of these in severe, frequent attacks.

The pathophysiology of migraine remains obscure, but is thought to involve one or more vasomotor mechanisms, whether causal or consequential to an as yet unidentified underlying phenomenon is not clear. One theory suggests that the attack begins in serotonergic (5-HT) and adrenergic neurones, causing vasoconstriction in the associated cerebral and extracerebral vasculature, which in turn initiates the prodromal phase or the initial aura. As a consequence, a perivascular inflammation develops, characterized by the release of autocoids such as histamine, prostaglandins (for example PGE_2) and substance P, with the consequential vasodilatation associated with the severe localized headache and the other, later symptoms of migraine. The traditional use of ergotamine, which *inter alia* has mixed serotonin agonist/antagonist actions, and the more recent introduction of synthetic serotonin agonists such as sumatriptan, suggest that the underlying phenomenon may be related to abnormalities in the response of cerebral and extracerebral vessels to serotonin. Most theories of the causes of migraine also invoke adrenergic and dopaminergic mechanisms.

Very substantial advances have recently been made in the characterization of serotonin (5-HT) receptors, a recent review concluding that up to fourteen separate receptors, assigned to seven separate subclasses, can now be identified on the basis of their structural, recognitory and transductional properties. Of these, $5-HT_1$ and $5-HT_2$ receptors (more particularly the $5-HT_{2C}$ and most recently the $5-HT_{2B}$ receptors) appear to be most important in eliciting the initial vasoconstrictor and subsequent vasodilator vasomotor effects associated with migraine. The precise subclasses of 5-HT receptors involved in vasoconstriction and the subsequent vasodilatation of migraine are currently under review, as some $5-HT_1$ receptors have been reassigned to the $5-HT_2$ class.

Mild to modest attacks of migraine, in which there may be no aura, or the aura is rapidly replaced by a severe localized headache and minimal other symptoms lasting no more than 1–2 h, are effectively treated with an NSAID such as aspirin or ibuprofen, or with paracetamol, and patients frequently obtain these by over-the-counter purchase. Occasionally, more stubborn attacks may require the addition of an anti-nauseant such as metoclopromide or domperidone (agents which can also accelerate the absorption of the NSAID) and perhaps a benzodiazepine anxiolytic. Tolfenamic acid (200–400 mg orally) is a recent new NSAID licensed for the acute treatment of migraine, but it has no proven advantages over standard, cheaper, NSAIDs.

More severe, classical migraine is best treated with a serotonin agonist at 5-HT$_1$ receptors, of which sumatriptan, introduced in the late 1980s, was the first of several now available. Traditionally, ergotamine has been used to treat acute migraine. It possesses a range of pharmacological actions, of which its mixed agonist/antagonist effects at α-adrenergic and 5-HT receptors are thought to contribute to its anti-migraine effects. Even modest overdoses, however, are associated with significant adverse effects, in which these same receptors and additional agonist actions at dopaminergic receptors occur in both the central and peripheral nervous systems.

Sumatriptan is a synthetic 5-HT$_1$ agonist and an effective anti-migraine treatment. The effective dose is 50–100 mg orally or 6 mg subcutaneously in the majority of patients. It is also available as a nasal spray (10–20 mg) and suppository. Sumatriptan should be reserved for patients who do not respond to NSAIDs (alone or with an anti-emetic). Adverse effects include dizziness, muscle weakness and neck pain: in about 5 per cent of patients there is some chest discomfort which resembles angina. Sumatriptan and other serotonin agonists are contraindicated in patients with known coronary ischaemia or Prinzmetal's angina. Sumatriptan has revolutionized the treatment of classical severe migraine, although its relatively short duration of action may permit the reappearance of symptoms. A maximum daily dose of 300 mg orally should not be exceeded.

Zolmitriptan (2.5 mg orally initially, repeating after 2 h if necessary up to a maximum of 15 mg per day) may have a slightly longer duration of action which could be useful in persistent migraine.

Naratriptan is a more recently introduced serotonin agonist (2.5 mg orally at onset, repeat once after 4 h if symptoms persist), while the properties of enzatriptan and eletriptan have still to be fully evaluated. From all that is currently known of their pharmacodynamic and pharmacokinetic properties, sumatriptan, zolmitriptan, naratriptan, rizatriptan and eletriptan produce qualitatively similar clinical effects. They should not be used in combination with ergotamine, although modest doses of NSAIDs are permissible. Sumatriptan and the other agents should not be used where a patient is currently receiving medication with a serotonin-selective re-uptake inhibitor (SSRI) or MAOI antidepressant, or with lithium salts. They should not be used where coronary ischaemia exists, where hypertension is uncontrolled, and caution should be exercised where there is concomitant renal or hepatic impairment.

Structures and classification of commonly used NSAIDs:

Table 5.3 provides a list of the more commonly used NSAIDs, whilst *Figure 5.3* contains the structures of aspirin and newer NSAIDs, illustrating the basic 'organic acid' commonality of structure.

Table 5.3 Classification of NSAIDs (based on differences in the chemical stem – after Goodman and Gilman, 1996)

(a) Salicylic acid derivatives, e.g. aspirin, sodium salicylate, diflunisal
(b) *para*-Aminophenol derivatives, e.g. paracetamol (acetaminophen)
(c) Arylpropionic acids, e.g. ibuprofen, flurbiprofen, ketoprofen, naproxen
(d) Indole and indene acetic acids, e.g. indomethacin
(e) Heteroaryl acetic acids, e.g. diclofenac, ketorolac
(f) Anthranilic acids (fenamates), e.g. mefenamic acid
(g) Enolic acids, e.g. piroxicam (oxicams), phenylbutazone (pyrazolidinediones)
(h) Alkanones, e.g. nabumetone

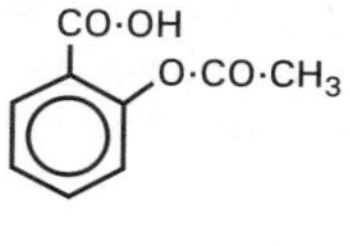

Aspirin

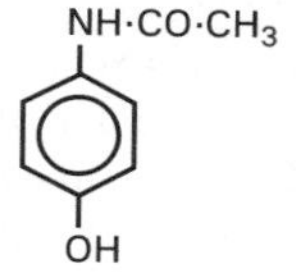

Paracetamol (acetaminophen)

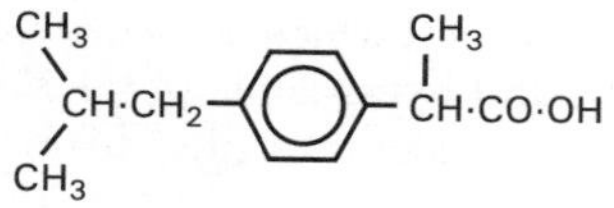

Ibuprofen

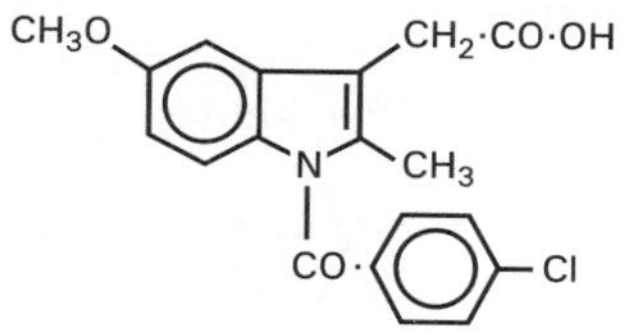

Indomethacin

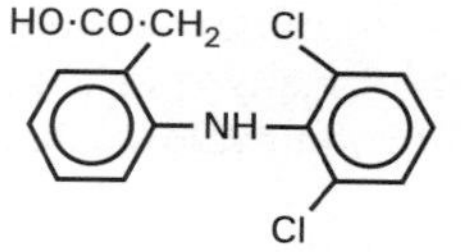

Diclofenac

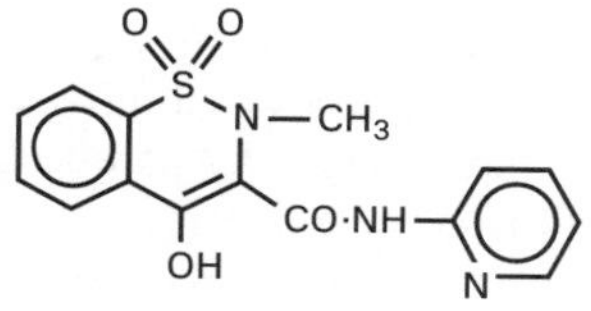

Piroxicam

Figure 5.3 Chemical structures of some principal non-steroidal anti-inflammatory drugs (NSAIDs)

Included in the monograph section below are descriptions of NSAIDs from each group and short notes on the principal differences claimed for other members of the group.

MONOGRAPHS

ACETYLSALICYLIC ACID

Aspirin (rINN)

Pharmacology

Aspirin exerts analgesic, anti-inflammatory and anti-pyretic effects, primarily by inhibiting the production of prostglandin derivatives, through an irreversible blockade of COX-1 and COX-2 enzymes in the arachidonic acid cascade. While the anti-inflammatory effects are almost entirely exercised at peripheral sites, the anti-pyretic effects are mediated via the hypothalamus, and the analgesic effects are mediated at both peripheral and central sites.

Acetylsalicylic acid is one of the most potent of the salicylate drugs as an analgesic. It is about 50 per cent more effective and toxic than sodium salicylate in doses containing equal amounts of salicylate. Analgesia is usually adequate for pain from integumental structures, for example bones, joints, muscles and teeth, but poor for visceral pain.

The analgesic action is confined to a small dose range below which there is little effect, and above which an increase in dose produces toxic effects with little increase in analgesia. There is no graded response as with the morphine group. Analgesia is mainly due to its peripheral anti-inflammatory effect, but there are some additional central effects at dorsal horns and peri-aqueductal grey areas.

Acetylsalicylic acid, like the other salicylates, has an anti-pyretic action which occurs only in pyrexia and which is mediated via the hypothalamus, invoking increased heat loss by sweating and hyperaemia of the skin. It is also a primary metabolic stimulant, but the rapid fall in temperature due to profuse sweating normally overcomes the stimulant effect. If sweating fails to occur, as in the presence of electrolyte depletion, hyperpyrexia will result.

In addition to these effects, the drug has an anti-inflammatory action. The possible mechanisms by which drugs such as acetylsalicylic acid exert this action are discussed on page 163–5.

Salicylates have important effects on carbohydrate metabolism. Large doses may reduce glycosuria in diabetic patients; in normal subjects hyperglycaemia and glycosuria occur. They also inhibit the action of many enzymes including succinate dehydrogenase, α-ketoglutaric dehydrogenase and hyaluronidase, and uncouple oxidative phosphorylation.

Acetylsalicylic acid has a paradoxical dose-dependent action on the excretion of uric acid. At daily doses of 1–2 g, net excretion is diminished because the drug depresses active tubular excretion more than reabsorption. Above 4–5 g per day, however, the effect on tubular reabsorption dominates, and the net effect is enhanced excretion. The side effects of such doses make it an unsuitable drug for this purpose. Salicylates inhibit the uricosuric action of probenecid (but not its capacity to inhibit tubular excretion of penicillin) and the activity of other uricosuric drugs such as sulfinpyrazone. No entirely satisfactory explanation for this has been advanced.

Acetylsalicylic acid is a common cause of bleeding from gastric erosions. Patients in whom there is strong circumstantial evidence that the drug precipitated the bleeding may subsequently show a normal susceptibility. It also inhibits platelet aggregation and there is now some evidence that the rare severe gastric bleeding episodes that are associated with this drug are a manifestation of an abnormally increased susceptibility of the platelets to this inhibiting action. Chronic bleeding occurs in about 50 per cent of all patients who take 4 g or more of acetylsalicylic acid per day. The loss is usually between 3 and 10 ml/day, although in some there is sufficient bleeding to cause an iron-deficiency anaemia. Most of the available preparations, including the soluble ones, are equally responsible, but effervescent aspirin and aloxiprin cause significantly less bleeding. In large and repeated doses salicylates tend to cause haemorrhages by prolonging the prothrombin time, an effect antagonized by vitamin K. Doses of 3–4 g/day also shorten erythrocyte survival time.

Absorption, distribution and fate   Absorption is mainly from the upper part of the small intestine, although some is absorbed from the stomach when the contents are particularly acid. Sodium bicarbonate has often been given with salicylates to prevent the tendency for free salicylic acid to cause gastric irritation, but although it may help in this respect it increases urinary excretion, and therefore to obtain the same blood level with bicarbonate a larger dose is necessary.

After absorption, salicylate is rapidly distributed throughout all the body tissues; it is secreted in saliva, milk and bile and crosses the placental barrier. Acetylsalicylic acid is detectable for only a short time in the plasma after absorption, as the ester is rapidly hydrolysed to salicylic acid. Salicylate is found in the urine; between 60 and 90 per cent is in the free form when the urine is alkaline and it is almost entirely conjugated with glycine as salicyluric acid and with glycuronic acid when the urine is acidic. Ferric chloride will give a reddish-violet colour in a urine containing excreted salicylate, even after boiling, which distinguishes it from the colour obtained in ketonuria.

Indications

Acetylsalicylic acid may be used for the relief of minor degrees of pain such as that of rheumatism, fibrositis, headache and toothache. It is the drug of choice in the treatment of acute rheumatic fever.

It may be employed alone, but is often combined with codeine to produce a slightly greater analgesic effect.

Dosage and administration

The dose of acetylsalicylic acid is 0.3–1 g. In adults 0.6 g is usually given in tablet form when required and repeated at 4-hourly intervals if necessary. A plasma level of 30 mg/100 ml is necessary for an adequate therapeutic effect.

In acute rheumatic fever, as much as 12 g may be given in the first 24 h, after which the dose is reduced to about 5 g/day.

Precautions

Acetylsalicylic acid, especially when given in large or repeated doses, may cause tinnitus and dizziness, gastric irritation and bleeding. The latter complication can be minimized by use of the aluminium preparation aloxiprin; acetylsalicylic acid is best avoided altogether in the presence of known gastric or duodenal ulceration. The drug should be avoided in infants in whom it has been implicated in inducing malignant raised intracranial pressure – Reye's syndrome.

Aspirin sensitivity, so-called, is manifest as wheezing, sometimes accompanied by urticaria and rhinorrhoea. It occurs in up to 2 per cent of all asthmatics. It seems likely that this is in fact a consequence of prostaglandin synthetase inhibition: antibodies to aspirin are not involved and cross-reaction to all other prostaglandin synthetase inhibitors occurs. PGE_2 is a bronchodilator and PGF_2 is a bronchoconstrictor; the synthesis of the former is preferentially blocked by these drugs, thus allowing bronchoconstriction to preponderate. Because of this effect, caution should be exercised in prescribing acetylsalicylic acid to known asthmatics, particularly children.

Aspirin poisoning

This is the commonest cause of death by poisoning in children under the age of 4 years. Two clinical phases can be described which depend on the speed of development of three different toxic mechanisms.

In the first phase there is an initial direct stimulation of the respiratory centre, with the development of a respiratory alkalosis. This induces renal compensation in which hydrogen ion is conserved, and bicarbonate, sodium and potassium are excreted. As a consequence, serum bicarbonate levels fall and the pH is shifted back towards normal at the expense of buffering capacity. At the same time, tissue metabolism is stimulated directly and the increase in carbon dioxide production maintains the hyperpnoea. Oxygen consumption can go up by 100 per cent. Hyperthermia will develop if sweating is limited by dehydration, and tetany may also be induced.

The second clinical phase is dominated by effects on carbohydrate and lipid metabolism. The general stimulation of metabolism increases the demand for glucose. However, at least two essential enzymes of the Krebs cycle – succinic dehydrogenase and α-ketoglutaric dehydrogenase are inhibited by salicylates. This blocks normal glucose metabolism and metabolic requirements become increasingly dependent on fatty-acid catabolism, with consequent overproduction of ketoacids. This metabolic acidosis now comes to dominate the clinical picture and, as a result of the previous cation loss and dehydration, can be neither buffered nor effectively compensated for by the kidney.

In young children, and in cases of severe poisoning, the first phase of alkalaemia may have passed before the patient reaches hospital, but in adults and older children this phase lasts 12–24 h.

Acute renal failure, possibly due to tubular necrosis, has been reported, and a review of the literature suggests that renal damage in aspirin poisoning may be commoner than is generally appreciated.

Treatment   Treatment should include gastric aspiration, lavage and full supportive therapy. Repeated blood-gas measurements are needed to guide therapy. Rapid alkalinization of the urine, accompanied by a forced diuresis with osmotic diuretics increases the rate of excretion of salicylates to values comparable to exchange transfusion or dialysis. The regimen of forced diuresis combined with alkalinization of the urine, as described for barbiturate poisoning on page 91, is suitable for older children and adults. Small children aged 1–4 years (the commonest age group in which salicylate poisoning occurs accidentally) are usually in a state of metabolic acidosis on admission. Their relatively high rate of water loss, often exaggerated by hyperpyrexia, makes osmotic diuretics unsuitable. Initial rehydration may be with 80–100 ml/kg of 5 per cent dextrose plus 3 mmol/kg of sodium bicarbonate (6 ml/kg of 4.2 per cent solution) in the first 2–3 h, followed by a similar volume of fluid containing a further 1 mmol/kg of bicarbonate during the rest of the 24 h; 2–4 g of potassium chloride should also be given during this period.

Adults characteristically exhibit respiratory alkalosis and virtually never develop metabolic acidosis regardless of the severity of the poisoning. Although the danger of tetany if sodium bicarbonate is given in such cases has probably been overemphasized, little may be gained by doing so if the urine is already alkaline. Tubular excretion of bicarbonate is the normal renal response to overbreathing and sodium bicarbonate should not be given unless arterial blood pH is less than 7.5 and urinary pH less than 7.6. Paper indicator strips of the appropriate range are sufficiently accurate for monitoring urinary pH. In adults, the arterial pH tends to rise with increasing blood salicylate levels. In severely alkalotic patients (arterial pH >7.6), intravenous calcium may be given to reduce the risk of tetany.

Curarization and mechanical ventilation are extremely valuable in severe aspirin intoxication in children. This should be considered if coma, hyperthermia (>40°C) and tetany occur. In severe cases in which a diuresis cannot be obtained because of renal failure, dialysis will be necessary.

Benorilate

Benorilate is a paracetamol–aspirin combination, the two agents linked chemically to form an ester. Given by mouth, benorilate is absorbed largely unchanged, to be broken down in the plasma by non-specific esterases to give both paracetamol and salicylate. This 'pro-drug' is considerably more lipid soluble than aspirin, it avoids direct gastro-intestinal irritation, and there is some evidence of unchanged benorilate gaining access to inflamed sites such as arthritic synovial and other inflamed joints where it exerts anti-inflammatory and analgesic effects.

Benorilate is available as a tasteless white liquid suspension, as granules for suspension in water or as tablets: it is readily absorbed from the gastro-intestinal tract, although large volumes of the liquid suspension can be nauseating. The drug has a prolonged half-life, and is normally administered only twice a day, 8 g of benorilate yielding the equivalent of 4–5 g of aspirin and about 3 g of paracetamol. Toxic effects are likely to be those associated with high doses of aspirin and paracetamol.

The drug was developed primarily to reduce the incidence and seriousness of gastro-intestinal tract effects in patients requiring long-term anti-arthritic or anti-inflammatory medication. Benorilate should not be used for the alleviation of acute or short-term pain, when the more rapid onset of aspirin or other NSAIDs is more desirable. The recent introduction of the PGE_2 derivative misoprostol, the anti-H_2 receptor blockers such as cimetidine or ranitidine, or the anticipated specific COX-2 inhibitors, have largely removed benorilate's main clinical indications of permitting the administration of high doses of aspirin while minimizing the attendant gastro-intestinal irritation.

ALFENTANIL

Alfentanil hydrochloride (rINN)

Pharmacology

Alfentanil is a synthetic derivative of fentanyl which was first synthesized in 1976. It is about 5–10 times less potent than fentanyl when compared as a single intravenous dose. It has all the pharmacodynamic properties of opioid drugs, but differs from them in several pharmacokinetic respects.

Pharmacokinetics   Alfentanil has a low lipid solubility with a partition coefficient (N-octanol) of 130 at pH 7.4. This, combined with its high degree of protein binding (90 per cent at pH 7.4), results in a low volume of distribution (approximately 30 litres). Because of the latter, a greater proportion of the drug remains in the plasma, from which it can be rapidly eliminated by hepatic metabolism. The elimination half-life is therefore short (75–95 minutes).

It is also a much weaker base than other opiates, with a pK_a of 6.8. Thus 89 per cent of the unbound drug in plasma at pH 7.4 is un-ionized and can rapidly cross the blood–brain barrier. Onset of action is therefore rapid after intravenous injection, while recovery is also rapid. The cardiovascular system remains stable even after high doses, although bradycardia may be seen.

Indications

Because of its rapid onset and short duration of action, alfentanil is the opiate of choice for short surgical procedures, doses of 5–10 µg/kg usually being satisfactory. For longer procedures lasting more than 30 minutes, it is best given by continuous intravenous infusion following a loading dose of 150 µg/kg. The infusion rate usually varies from 0.5 to 1.5 µg/kg/min; the rapid onset and clearance allows for rapid adjustment in analgesic levels to meet clinical requirements. To avoid respiratory depression postoperatively, the infusion should be stopped 15–20 minutes before the end of the procedure. High doses of alfentanil have been used in cardiac surgery in a similar way to fentanyl, with satisfactory results. Infusions of alfentanil into the epidural space provide good postoperative analgesia. It can also be given as a bolus of 500 µg just prior to intubation or insertion of a laryngeal mask airway, to block a hypertensive response.

Alfentanil has also been used by continuous intravenous infusion to provide long-term sedation in critically ill patients in the intensive care unit. Good-quality sedation can be obtained, but establishment of spontaneous ventilation can be time consuming.

Precautions

Side effects are as for other opioid drugs; it is a powerful dose-related respiratory depressant. There is a high incidence of muscle rigidity when it is given to conscious subjects. Facilities for treatment of respiratory depression must be immediately available.

BUPRENORPHINE

Buprenorphine hydrochloride (rINN)

Pharmacology

Buprenorphine is a semi-synthetic highly lipid soluble opiate derived from the naturally-occurring opium alkaloid thebaine; it has partial agonist analgesic properties at µ opioid receptors where its intrinsic activity or efficacy is high (if falling short of being a full agonist such as morphine). Because of its high lipid solubility, high receptor affinity and persistence at receptors, buprenorphine is active at low doses, whether given by intra-muscular or slow intravenous injection, or sublingually.

Because of its relatively high intrinsic activity, buprenorphine is not so obviously an antagonist of morphine analgesia, unless high doses of morphine are being used. Consequently, it is easier to progress from buprenorphine to full agonist analgesia (with morphine or diamorphine) than it is with pentazocine or other partial agonists. Buprenorphine ably substitutes for morphine and other µ-agonist analgesics in most clinical applications, providing a strong analgesia lasting somewhat longer than that of morphine, diamorphine or pethidine – sublingually, 0.2–0.8 mg in adults provides analgesia for 5–8 h (chewing and swallowing the tablet reduces its potency because of hepatic first-pass metabolism). By slow intravenous injection, buprenorphine is suitable for use in patient controlled analgesia (PCA), when peak analgesia can be achieved in about 30 minutes; drowsiness and some respiratory inhibition have appeared following intravenous administration of higher doses. These can be reversed with naloxone although several successive doses may be required because of the drug's persistence. The plasma half-life of buprenorphine is only some 5–6 h, but its persistence at receptors provides lasting analgesia beyond the half-life predictions.

Unlike morphine, buprenorphine produces no constipation and its inhibitory effects on respiration are associated with large doses. Its chief adverse effect is drowsiness, while nausea and vomiting are less common or intrusive. Interactions with the heart and cardiovascular system are slight. Buprenorphine ably substitutes for morphine and the other strong agonist analgesics except perhaps in severe or prolonged unremitting pain associated with terminal illness. If large doses of buprenorphine have been used, switching to a full agonist (e.g. diamorphine) under these conditions may require relatively high doses of the new agent until the buprenorphine has been fully displaced from the receptors.

Some care may be required when discontinuing prolonged treatment with buprenorphine, although serious withdrawal effects are unlikely except if discontinuing high doses, when progressive withdrawal may be advisable.

Fate in the body Burprenorphine is metabolized in the liver by *N*-demethylation and glucuronidation, the metabolites being excreted in the urine and mainly the bile and faeces.

Indications

It has been found to give satisfactory analgesia after surgery and was virtually indistinguishable from morphine when given either intravenously or intramuscularly by PCA. It is a useful analgesic when given sublingually to patients with cancer pain.

Dosage and administration

Buprenorphine is given by intramuscular or slow intravenous injection 0.3–0.6 mg 3–4 times per day. The duration of action of a single dose is 6–8 h. It may also be given sublingually 0.4–0.8 mg every 6–8 h.

Precautions

As with other opiate-like compounds, liver dysfunction can prolong its duration of action. Buprenorphine can cause drowsiness which may be potentiated by other central depressants, including alcohol. It may cause vomiting, and an interaction with monoamine oxidase inhibitors (MAOIs) is possible. Overdosage leading to respiratory depression is not easily reversed by naloxone, and doxapram may need to be administered as well. General supportive measures to maintain adequate oxygenation and ventilation may also be necessary.

Butorphanol (tartrate) is similar to buprenorphine in being a potent partial agonist analgesic. It also exhibits a ceiling effect. Butorphanol's actions are reversed by large doses of naloxone.
   The drug is well absorbed when given orally, but there is a marked first-pass effect. Peak levels in man occur 1.5 h after oral administration and 30 minutes after intramuscular administration. The elimination half-life in healthy subjects is about 3 h. The drug can be used for the relief of moderate or severe pain. A dose of 1–2 mg butorphanol is equivalent to 40–50 mg pethidine or 10 mg morphine.

CODEINE

Codeine phosphate (rINN)

Pharmacology

Codeine is a naturally-occurring alkaloid of opium, and possesses qualitatively similar properties to morphine but requires doses some 3–5 times higher to achieve comparable analgesia. Codeine produces less sedation, less nausea and vomiting and, in its usual applications, little respiratory depression. By mouth, it does cause constipation, which may be its most intrusive adverse effect in ambulatory patients.

Most of codeine's pharmacological actions depend upon its conversion to morphine. Its onset of action is thus slower. Its actions to suppress coughing are thought not to depend upon its metabolic conversion to morphine, and one of codeine's main clinical uses is as an anti-tussive. Since about 1 in 12 of people in Europe do not possess the hepatic enzyme CPY2D6, codeine will not be converted to morphine by them and will lack many of its predicted properties. Its anti-tussive effects, however, are less likely to be affected, since codeine itself is believed to exercise this property. However, where exceptionally high doses of self-administered codeine are encountered in a patient, one possible explanation is the absence of CPY2D6.

Codeine is also widely used to combat minor pain, for example that associated with toothache, sinus pain and other facial pain. In these circumstances, it may be usefully combined with aspirin (e.g. *Cocodaprin*) and paracetamol (*Co-codamol*) where there is some synergism between the peripherally-acting and centrally-acting analgesic actions.

Fate in the body Codeine has about 60 per cent bioavailability by mouth: about 10 per cent is converted to morphine (and, subsequently, the active morphine-6-glucuronide), which is thought to be mainly but not wholly responsible for codeine's morphine-like effects. The plasma half-life of codeine itself is no more than 2–3 h, although on prolonged use morphine-6-glucuronide is more persistent. Codeine metabolites and morphine metabolites are excreted in the urine.

Indications

Codeine phosphate is used in the treatment of minor degrees of pain, often in combination with other analgesics such as acetylsalicylic acid and paracetamol. Its main use, however, is as an anti-tussive and in the treatment of diarrhoea.

Dosage and administration

Codeine phosphate is given by mouth in a dose of 10–60 mg, but doses up to 100 mg are sometimes employed. Higher doses do not achieve a greater degree of analgesia. A common formulation is 250 mg each of aspirin and paracetamol and 8 mg of codeine phosphate.

Precautions

Precautions are basically the same as for morphine; side effects in the doses normally employed are rare and addiction is uncommon.

DIAMORPHINE

Diamorphine hydrochloride (rINN) – synonym: heroin hydrochloride

Pharmacology

Diamorphine is produced from morphine by acetylation, and may be described as a 'semi-synthetic opiate'. It is more lipophilic than morphine and a greater proportion of a dose gains access to the brain, and does so more quickly. Consequently, diamorphine is more potent and more rapidly acting than morphine. Linked with its rapidity of action, particularly by intravenous administration, diamorphine is also 'more rewarding' as a drug of abuse, and its manufacture, possession and use are banned in the USA and certain other countries. In the United Kingdom its availability as a therapeutic agent (albeit as a Controlled Drug) has been maintained and justified on the basis of its value in the control of severe terminal pain.

Diamorphine itself is believed *not* to bind to μ opioid receptors, but to be rapidly metabolized to 6-monoacetyl-morphine (MAM) and subsequently, more slowly, to morphine and morphine-6-glucuronide. MAM is pharmacologically active, however, rapidly enters the brain and contributes to the greater potency and the more rapid onset of action of diamorphine.

Pharmacologically, diamorphine's actions are identical to those of morphine, although there are subtle differences: optimal doses are about half those of morphine, when it is less of a respiratory depressant, and produces nausea, vomiting and constipation less frequently. Like morphine, it reduces anxiety and fear and frequently induces a sense of euphoria. It is also more susceptible to pharmacodynamic tolerance. Since its duration of action is shorter than that of morphine, patients will be maintained pain free only by more frequent administration.

Indications

As our understanding of the circumstances that can precipitate opioid tolerance and physical dependence increases, and as we become more adept at preventing the appearance or reappearance of pain, there is evidence that diamorphine is more frequently and confidently used in postoperative pain. This includes administration by mouth, parenterally, epidurally and by patient controlled analgesia (PCA) systems. It is normally given subcutaneously in doses of 5–10 mg, but is also included in Brompton Hospital mixtures because it is better absorbed by mouth than morphine. Precautions and treatment of overdose are as for morphine.

DICLOFENAC

Diclofenac sodium (rINN)

Pharmacology

Diclofenac is a cyclo-oxygenase inhibitor which has a useful enhancement of potency, combining analgesia with good anti-inflammatory activity. It is rapidly absorbed by mouth, although a substantial amount is removed by hepatic first-pass metabolism. Peak plasma levels are reached after about 2–3 h and the plasma half-life is about 2 h. Extensive plasma protein binding (>99 per cent) and the drug's ability to enter synovial spaces give it a duration of effective action which exceeds expectations. In suppository form, absorption from the rectal mucosa is rapid, giving peak plasma concentration after about 1 h. Peak plasma concentrations tend to be lower than those following the enteric-coated tablets.

Hepatic hydroxylation with subsequent glucuronidation and sulphation are followed by elimination via the kidneys and bile.

Indications

Diclofenac is effective for moderate pain of musculoskeletal origin, including tendonitic and bursitic conditions, and rheumatoid and osteorarthritis. The drug has achieved particular popularity for postoperative use to treat moderate pain following laparoscopy when the suppository may be inserted before or during the operation.

Dosage and administration

Diclofenac is available as conventional, dispersible and retard-release (enteric-coated) tablets in amounts up to 100 mg; it is also available as a solution containing 25 mg/ml for deep intramuscular injection or as suppositories (up to 100 mg).

A combined preparation of diclofenac (50 mg) with the PGE_1 analogue *misoprostol* (200 µg) as an enteric-coated tablet is available in the United Kingdom and Europe, and this combination provides substantial protection from gastro-intestinal side effects associated with long-term treatment.

Precautions and side effects

As well as the usual gastro-intestinal effects, it should be noted that long-term diclofenac treatment can raise plasma aminotransferase levels in about 15 per cent of patients. In consequence, plasma aminotransferase levels should be monitored during the first two months' of treatment. Other adverse effects can include skin rashes, allergic reactions, fluid retention and oedema, and CNS effects. These are occasionally marked, albeit qualitatively similar to the adverse effects of other NSAIDs. Intramuscular injections need to be given deeply to avoid skin ulceration with repeat injections given in different sites.

FENTANYL

Fentanyl citrate (rINN)

Pharmacology

Fentanyl is chemically related to pethidine, but is not a pethidine derivative. It is a potent narcotic analgesic and shares the same properties as other opiates, namely analgesia, sedation, respiratory depression, vagal stimulation, nausea and vomiting, constipation and physical dependence. When first introduced it was usually used with droperidol in the technique of neuroleptanalgesia. It is now used mainly on its own as the analgesic component of balanced anaesthesia and is probably the commonest drug used for this purpose.

Pharmacokinetics   Fentanyl is an extremely fat-soluble drug with a partition coefficient (*N*-octane) at pH 7.4 of 950 as compared to 21 for pethidine and 1 for morphine. It thus rapidly leaves the bloodstream and is widely distributed throughout the body. Its kinetics are best described by a three-compartmental model. When first introduced it was claimed to be a short-acting analgesic, but later work showed that this was not so. Several workers have remarked on the inconsistency of the reported pharmacokinetic constants for fentanyl. Clearance has been reported at values which vary from 160 to 1530 ml/minute, volume of distribution from 77 to 390 litres and elimination half-life from 2 to 7 h, the latter being longer than for morphine. Indeed one doubts whether the currently available pharmacokinetic data for fentanyl have any clinical applicability.

Metabolism Fentanyl is metabolized mainly in the liver, initially by dealkylation, to norfentanil, which has virtually no analgesic properties. This and the parent compound are then hydroxylated and excreted in the urine. The half-life is prolonged in the presence of liver disease and also in the elderly when drug metabolism is reduced.

Cardiovascular effects The haemodynamic effects of fentanyl are minimal, even in high doses. Small doses (up to 5 µg/kg) tend to cause a slight decrease in heart rate with little effect on arterial blood pressure. Even doses up to 100 µg/kg given to patients with valvular or ischaemic heart disease cause few circulatory changes. However, significant haemodynamic effects will occur following concomitant administration of other drugs such as nitrous oxide or benzodiazepines.

Respiratory effects In common with other opiates, fentanyl produces profound dose-related respiratory depression. Several workers have reported a biphasic respiratory depression following use of fentanyl during anaesthesia. Adams and Pybus (1978) described severe respiratory depression in three patients 2–4 h after low to moderate doses of fentanyl during anaesthesia; secondary peaks in plasma fentanyl concentrations have been demonstrated. The exact mechanism of this phenomenon is unknown, but a postulated entero-systemic recirculation is an unlikely explanation because of the high hepatic clearance of fentanyl.

Metabolic response to trauma In doses in excess of 50 µg/kg, fentanyl will completely abolish the endocrine and metabolic response to trauma, even after upper abdominal surgery. However, the profound and prolonged respiratory depressant effects after such doses necessitate artificial ventilation in the postoperative period and thus the method is not feasible after routine upper abdominal or thoracic surgery.

Muscle rigidity Intravenous fentanyl can cause rigidity of skeletal muscle, usually of the chest and abdomen, but it can affect the limbs and jaw. Truncal rigidity will impair ventilation. The complication is associated with larger doses of the drug, most patients becoming rigid after 15–20 µg/kg, which is usually coincident with loss of consciousness. The rigidity is abolished by neuromuscular blocking drugs.

Indications

Fentanyl is now one of the most widely used drugs as the analgesic component of a balanced anaesthetic technique. Doses of 50–200 µg can be used to supplement nitrous oxide in spontaneously breathing patients. During artificial ventilation, usual doses are 100–200 µg boluses, given when signs of inadequate analgesia appear. High-dose fentanyl anaesthesia requires doses in excess of 50 µg/kg and is associated with remarkable cardiovascular stability when used for cardiac anaesthesia. Although infusions of fentanyl are used, the prolonged half-life makes cumulation of the drug a distinct possibility.

Fentanyl is also a popular drug given by the epidural route for postoperative analgesia. Single bolus doses of 100–200 µg have been used, but delayed respiratory depression has been reported. More frequently an infusion at a rate of 1 µg/kg/h, adjusted if necessary, is used after a loading dose.

Precautions

Analgesic doses of fentanyl will always cause respiratory depression and facilities for its treatment must be immediately available.

Adams, A.P. and Pybus, D.A. (1978) Delayed respiratory depression after use of fentanyl during anaesthesia. *British Medical Journal*, **1**, 278

IBUPROFEN

Ibuprofen (rINN)

Ibuprofen is a proprionic acid derived NSAID of modest potency, combining anti-inflammatory, antipyretic and analgesic activity. Although somewhat better tolerated than aspirin or indometacin, ibuprofen in common with other presently available NSAIDs inhibits both COX-1 and COX-2 activity and, consequently, is associated with qualitatively similar adverse effects to this group of drugs. Gastro-intestinal sensitivity to ibuprofen is not significant at low to modest doses, but above a dose of 2 g/day, gastro-intestinal tract irritation rises sharply.

Ibuprofen is rapidly and almost completely absorbed following oral administration, reaching a peak plasma level after 60–90 minutes, with a plasma half-life extending to no more than 2 h, despite its almost complete plasma protein binding. The parent drug is hydroxylated and carboxylated, the glucuronides of which are almost totally eliminated by the kidneys. There is evidence of the parent drug crossing into synovial fluid where its stay can be prolonged despite falling plasma levels.

Dosage and administration

Ibuprofen is used in the treatment of rheumatoid arthritis and other similar conditions, and is useful in the treatment of patients intolerant to acetylsalicylic acid. At the start of treatment, 1.2 g may be given daily in divided doses. This is then followed by a maintenance dose of 200 mg 3–4 times a day.

Precautions

Ibuprofen has been available for about 40 years. Its adverse effects profile is good at single doses up to 400 mg, so much so that in both the United Kingdom and USA preparations containing up to 200 mg of ibuprofen per dose are available over-the-counter (OTC). In assessing the impact of toxicity following a suspected overdose of a prescribed NSAID, the concomitant administration of OTC-obtained ibuprofen (and aspirin and paracetamol) must also be considered.

Flurbiprofen is a second-generation more potent proprionic acid derivative of ibuprofen, used at lower clinical doses but possessing effectively similar pharmacological properties. It is well absorbed by mouth, is extensively protein bound, with a half-life of about 6 h, making it more useful for the treatment of chronic conditions. Like ibuprofen, hydroxylation precedes glucuronidation and excretion by the kidneys.

Naproxen also is a proprionic acid derivative. It too is rapidly absorbed following oral administration, reaching a plasma peak at 2–4 h after administration. Unusually, naproxen has a much longer plasma half-life (12–15 h), so that in chronic use its administration should be limited to twice daily. In the elderly the half-life is longer still, and the dose and/or frequency of administration will need adjustment. While its range of adverse effects mimic those of other NSAIDs (and particularly other proprionic acid derivatives), clinical experience suggests that gastro-intestinal effects are better tolerated, perhaps because of the reduced frequency of administration.

INDOMETACIN

Indometacin (rINN)

Pharmacology

Indometacin was introduced in the early 1960s and is a potent analgesic, antipyretic and anti-inflammatory agent, perhaps the archetypal representative of the NSAID family. It thus has clinical value in both acute and chronic conditions. The drug is well absorbed following oral administration (plasma peak at 2 h, unless administered after food), extensively plasma protein bound, and has a relatively short plasma half life of 3 h. There is some evidence of greater lipophilicity than with aspirin, with synovial levels matching plasma levels at about 5 h after administration.

The drug also exerts central effects which may contribute to both its beneficial (analgesic, antipyretic) and adverse effects (frontal headaches, dizziness, mental confusion, vertigo and somnolence). While indometacin's main pharmacological action is to inhibit both COX-1 and COX-2 sources of prostaglandin synthesis, there is also evidence of interference with neutrophil and leucocyte mobilization.

In chronic administration, up to 50 per cent of patients receiving recommended doses may suffer adverse effects, perhaps 20 per cent of patients become non-compliant or discontinue use. Gastro-intestinal tract effects are the most intrusive. Indometacin remains an effective analgesic, anti-inflammatory and antipyretic agent, but it warrants continuing vigilance and a careful evaluation of the balance between beneficial and adverse effects.

Indications

Indometacin is used in the treatment of rheumatoid arthritis and osteoarthritis, gout and other musculoskeletal disorders.

Dosage and administration

The initial dose is 25 mg 3 times a day, which is then gradually increased up to about 100 mg per day. It should be given with meals. Smaller doses may be combined with a corticosteroid. Alternatively the drug may be given as a suppository containing 100 mg.

Precautions

Prolonged use may be associated with haematopoietic consequences, which include neutropenia, thrombocytopenia and (rarely) aplastic anaemia. Indometacin may also impair renal function. Frontal headaches, dizziness, mental confusion, vertigo and somnolence have all been reported fairly frequently.

Indometacin should not be given to patients with active peptic ulceration, and should be used with caution if there is a history of peptic ulcer. Multiple ulceration, haemorrhage and even perforation of the upper gastro-intestinal tract have been reported. In the absence of such acute adverse effects, substantial occult blood loss can occur, leading to anaemia on continued use of the drug. If diarrhoea occurs, this too may be associated with bowel ulceration and bleeding.

The extended clinical experience with indometacin, almost 40 years, and the accumulated reporting, is partly responsible for the very detailed lists of adverse effects induced by indometacin. These may be quantitatively rather than qualitatively more important with indometacin than with other NSAIDs

MORPHINE SALTS

Morphine hydrochloride or sulfate (rINN)

Pharmacology

Morphine is the oldest analgesic known to man. It occurs naturally in commercial *opium*, which is the dried latex exudate of the fruit capsule of the poppy, *Papaver somniferum*. It is the most active and most abundant (8–15 percent by weight) of opium's active constituents, although the actual amount of morphine varies by geographical origin, with the altitude at which it is grown and according to its subsequent storage conditions. The first undisputed reference to the use of poppy juice is found in the writings of Theophrastus (300–200 BC). A phenanthrene alkaloid, morphine was first isolated by Serturner in 1803, but its full therapeutic impact awaited the introduction of the hypodermic syringe in the mid-19th century. Alcoholic tincture of opium, *laudanum*, has been used in the Western world since the middle ages when its use strayed far outside those of pain relief: the alcohol/morphine combination significantly enhanced the opium's sedative/hypnotic and anxiolytic properties. The wholly synthetic production of morphine was only achieved in the latter part of this century: organic synthesis is not a commercially feasible source of morphine, which remains one of the few powerful drugs currently in use which is obtained from a natural source. Its name derives from the Greek, *Morpheus*, the God of Dreams, while opium is the Greek word for *juice*.

Actions on the CNS Morphine exerts a range of stimulant and depressant actions at all levels of the CNS. Although depressant actions predominate, morphine is not anticonvulsant but is more likely to potentiate convulsant agents. Morphine's depressant actions on the cerebral cortex may produce calm, reducing fear and anxiety, but this may also be attended by a loss of mental concentration and ability to deal with complex reasoning or other thought processes. Mental and physical performances are impaired, especially for newly acquired skills, yet motor function is usually unimpaired. Morphine and its metabolite morphine-6-glucuronide exert a full agonist action at μ opioid receptors at several levels of the CNS, including the spinal cord, the peri-aqueductal grey, thalamic and cortical regions. Morphine's agonist actions at κ- and δ-receptors are much less important in its therapeutic effects, although spinal k-receptors may contribute to the spinal component of analgesia. On the other hand, the dysphoric and sometimes hallucinatory effects of higher doses of morphine may be attributable to effects at κ and δ opioid receptors at higher levels.

Analgesia and the relief from anxiety are the most powerful (and sought after) effects of morphine, whilet the suppression of cough is also therapeutically useful. A reduction in hunger, the depression of respiration, the induction of nausea and vomiting, possible disturbances to endocrine, temperature and cardiovascular controls, are all important adverse effects of central origin. Common adverse effects also include a feeling of body warmth, heaviness of the extremities, dryness of mouth, sweating and itching, especially of the nose.

The effect on the cerebellum is mainly depressant, causing an ataxic gait by inhibiting motor coordination. All morphine alkaloids have a strychnine-like action and spinal reflexes are stimulated. Thus it depresses the CNS from above downwards, and stimulates from below upwards. In clinical doses this mixture of excitement and depression is of no significance, except in rare cases when morphine given postoperatively, for example, may excite rather than sedate a patient.

Various medullary areas are affected. The respiratory centre is depressed and becomes less sensitive to the stimulant effects of carbon dioxide. This effect is detectable even after the smallest effective analgesic doses of morphine and after overdosage it is the cause of death. The cough centre is also depressed, but various morphine derivatives (e.g. codeine and diamorphine) do this relatively more in proportion to their other actions.

In contrast, the chemoreceptor emetic trigger zone and the parasympathetic portion of the oculomotor nucleus are stimulated. Nausea therefore occurs, and nearly 50 per cent of ambulant patients may be affected and 16 per cent may vomit. Nausea and vomiting are less common in patients who are at rest and receive morphine when pain is already present. In either case any preliminary stimulation of vomiting may be followed by depression, so that morphine can also have an anti-emetic action; other emetics are usually ineffective after morphine. Nausea and vomiting are therefore commoner with the first dose, or when doses are spaced at too great intervals.

The pupils are constricted by the effect on the oculomotor nucleus, which is probably due to the removal of an inhibitor tone to this nucleus from a higher level, and in morphine poisoning the pupils may be pin-point in size. This stimulant effect is not followed by depression, and such pin-point pupils dilate again only when the effect of the morphine wears off or is antagonized or when asphyxia supervenes. Mydriatics such as atropine or hyoscine or others with the same mode of action can counteract morphine miosis. Morphine has no local effect in causing pupillary constriction.

The vagal and vasomotor centres are not significantly affected by morphine in man. The effect on heart rate and blood pressure is discussed below.

Analgesia The analgesic effect reaches its peak about 20 minutes after intravenous injection and about 90 minutes after intramuscular or subcutaneous injection. The duration of action is about 4 h. The best effects are obtained when dosage precedes the onset of painful stimuli, in which case the pain threshold is demonstrably raised. When the drug is given after pain is established, relief is mainly due to alteration in the pattern of reaction to pain, which is still recognized by the subject but appears distant and does not give rise to anxiety. Under favourable circumstances sleep may ensue and dreams may be prominent. On the other hand, in the absence of pain small doses of morphine (5–10 mg), in contrast to the larger doses normally given, may actually increase anxiety and general discomfort. Continuous dull pain is relieved more effectively than sharp intermittent pain. The lightning pain of tabes dorsalis is one of the few types that resists morphine analgesia. In sharp contrast to the salicylates and related analgesics, morphine is effective against pain arising from viscera as well as from muscles, joints and integumental structures.

Morphine appears to relieve pain in at least four ways: by raising the threshold for pain; by altering the pattern of reaction to pain; by inducing sleep, which in itself raises the pain threshold to an appreciable extent; and by inducing hypercapnia, which produces a similar effect. Reduction in body temperature may also be a contributory factor.

Cardiovascular system Therapeutic doses have negligible effects upon heart rate and blood pressure, but larger doses slow the heart by depressing conduction; a stimulant action on the vagal nucleus may contribute to this effect. With anoxia and central vasomotor depression added, a fall in blood pressure will occur. In man the peripheral blood vessels are dilated by therapeutic doses, producing a feeling of warmth in the skin. Peripheral vasodilatation becomes more marked when morphine is injected rapidly intravenously and will cause a fall in blood pressure. All the alkaloids of opium produce a histamine-like weal when injected intradermally, and histamine release may well be a factor in producing vasodilatation and hypotension, as can be shown in the cat.

Respiratory system All phases of respiratory activity are depressed by therapeutic doses of morphine. The rate, minute volume and tidal exchange are decreased. The diminished minute volume is primarily due to the slower rate of breathing. After intravenous injection, morphine produces a reduction in amplitude of respiration in nearly all subjects; when given by other routes, the depth of breathing may be increased or decreased, but is usually unaltered. With overdose, Cheyne–Stokes type of periodic breathing may be seen. From work in dogs it is thought that morphine causes 'pharmacological decerebration' by inactivating cortical and subcortical suppression mechanisms which modify the activity of more caudally located respiratory centres.

Although minute ventilation is decreased by morphine, it is important to note that its analgesic effect vastly improves its efficiency where it has been fast, shallow and inefficient, due to pleuritic pain. Similarly, where the lungs are oedematous, as in left ventricular failure, central depression by morphine prevents the Hering–Breuer reflex from initiating expiration before a useful inspiratory volume is reached. Bronchial constriction by a central vagal action is normally too slight to matter, but it can be dangerous in bronchial asthma.

Gastro-intestinal tract and biliary tract Morphine is constipating yet stimulant to the gastro-intestinal muscle. The tone of the visceral muscle is raised, especially that of the pyloric, ileocolic and anal sphincters. Segmenting contractions increase and truly propulsive activity diminishes. The delay of intestinal transit in the colon allows an increased absorption of water to take place and, finally, the normal defaecation reflex is inhibited more easily than usual because the distended rectum no longer produces the usual discomfort. In addition to the alleviation of pain, hunger and thirst are relieved or abolished, and vomiting if it occurs is not necessarily associated with the usual unpleasant emotional reactions even when it is violent and repeated.

The tone of the biliary musculature is raised and spasm may result, including that of the sphincter of Oddi. This extra spasm may increase pain originating in biliary colic already present and is unrelieved by the belladonna alkaloids.

Urinary tract Ureteric tone is increased as markedly as is that of the biliary tract, but it can be completely relaxed by the belladonna alkaloids. The detrusor musculature of the bladder is stimulated, but so is the sphincter, so that urgency may be created and difficulty also, but the central analgesic effect prevails. Catheterization may become necessary. Morphine, experimentally in dogs, can be shown to cause antidiuresis due to release of antidiuretic hormone and a reduction in the number of nephrons functioning, but whether this effect occurs in patients receiving therapeutic doses is uncertain.

Uterus The natural contractions during labour are not affected by analgesic doses, although the stimulant effect of oxytocic agents may be slightly diminished.

Placenta and fetus The placenta is permeable to morphine which can thus reach the fetus and depress the respiratory centre, making the initiation of respiration after birth difficult. Intra-uterine addiction can occur when the mother is addicted.

Metabolism Any fall in body temperature is usually the result of large doses and is due to lowered muscular activity, increased heat loss through cutaneous vasodilatation and sweating, and decreased metabolic rate. The last named is of the order of 10–20 per cent and is due to a decrease in oxygen consumption, which is of considerable benefit in cardiac disease. Hyperglycaemia and even glycosuria may be seen from epinephrine (adrenaline) release and, when there is respiratory depression, acidosis occurs with increased bicarbonate and lactic acid levels.

Fate in the body Although the most profound actions of morphine are on the CNS, only small amounts of morphine are believed to cross the blood–brain barrier. Ninety per cent of the drug is excreted by the kidneys in conjugated form within 24 h of administration. A small amount is excreted into the stomach and bile, and appears in the faeces. Traces can be detected in sweat and milk. Unlike codeine and the synthetic pethidine, *N*-demethylation is an unimportant route of metabolism, instead glucuronide conjugation occurs at both the 3- and 6-hydroxyl positions of morphine. Morphine-3-glucuronide is pharmacologically inactive, but morphine-6-glucuronide (M6G) retains its affinity for opioid receptors, readily crosses the blood–brain barrier and has a plasma half-life of about 6 h, so that it contributes very substantially to morphine's effects, particularly on repeated administration when M6G blood levels frequently exceed those of the parent drug. M6G is claimed to possess about four times the potency of the parent drug, unless compared following intraventricular injection in experimental animals when the increase is fortyfold. In patients with renal failure, M6G excretion is delayed, contributing to morphine's prolonged effects – and explains the need to use lower doses of morphine in older patients.

Tolerance An early pharmacokinetic-related tolerance to morphine (first 14–21 days) may occur in a few patients and is manifested by the need to increase the dose to maintain the same effect. The frequency and importance of this have been much exaggerated in the past. It should not be confused with the need to obtain an adequate dose to give full pain relief, nor with increasing pathology, and tolerance is a phenomenon more likely to occur in patients with a history of alcohol and/or opiate abuse. In the majority of patients given an adequate dose of morphine, tolerance should not be a problem in patients receiving postoperative pain relief.

Pharmacokinetic tolerance can give way to a pharmacodynamic tolerance, in which modifications to central and peripheral neurotransmitter and receptor functions are suspected. Again the incidence and importance of this have been much exaggerated. Patients do require increased doses if their pathology deteriorates, particularly in association with greater fear or anxiety about outcomes. Giving adequate doses of morphine to prevent recurrence of pain, to prevent drug-seeking, drug-craving or drug-waiting emotions, is important. It should be possible to reduce as well as increase morphine doses, to match pathological changes. Where patients have received morphine regularly for 7 days or more, it is prudent, when discontinuing opiate medication, to do so gradually over 48 h.

Addiction Pharmacodynamic tolerance to morphine is a prerequisite to the development of addiction, where similar and interacting neurotransmitter mechanisms are involved. Recent observations in patients receiving substantial doses of morphine for pain relief have shown that, as the pathological situation improves, so the doses of morphine can be gradually reduced. In a well-publicized surveillance of almost 12 000 postoperative, hospital patients, only four were shown to have developed physical dependence upon morphine.

Patients with a previous or existing alcohol or opiate abuse problem are at special risk, and there is a case for withholding opiate medication for as long as possible, provided that non-opioid drugs are providing adequate relief. There is no excuse for withholding such drugs in life-threatening or terminal conditions, or where pain relief cannot be obtained without the administration of an opiate.

In the small proportion of patients at risk of addiction, it can become established in as short a period as 10 days; if established, abrupt withdrawal can precipitate an abstinence syndrome within 10–12 h of the last dose of morphine. The injection of the antagonist naloxone can precipitate withdrawal effects within 30 minutes. Signs and symptoms include mydriasis, gooseflesh and cramps, insomnia, nausea, vomiting and diarrohea. Many of the effects are reminiscent of massive peripheral sympathetic stimulation, and the phenomenon has been referred to as the 'sympathetic storm'.

A patient with an existing or recent opiate abuse problem will lie about the history and exaggerate the pain in order to secure opiate administration. Drug histories must therefore be suitably authenticated if morphine medication is indicated. For the vast majority of patients, however, the incidence of tolerance and addiction to morphine is so low that it should not be a factor when considering the use of morphine for pain relief.

Abstinence syndrome When the addict is suddenly deprived of his supply of morphine, the well-known withdrawal symptoms occur. They usually commence about 10–12 h after the last dose, with yawning, sweating, and running of the eyes and nose. Then follows a restless irregular sleep for 18–24 h. The previous signs and symptoms then return, accompanied by mydriasis, gooseflesh and cramps and later by insomnia, nausea, vomiting and diarrhoea. Signs and symptoms reach their peak in 72 h and they decline over the next 7–11 days.

During the withdrawal period, tolerance to morphine is rapidly lost, and the syndrome may be terminated at any time by a suitable dose of morphine or related drug. The longer the period of abstinence, the smaller will be the dose required.

Indications

Morphine is used in the treatment of acute pain which may follow trauma, cardiac ischaemia, acute abdominal conditions and operations, and in severe chronic pain such as that which may occur in the terminal stages of cancer. It is also useful in the treatment of severe pleuritic pain and left ventricular failure. It was the first drug to be used as a sedative before anaesthesia and is still used in premedication.

Dosage and administration

Morphine may be given by mouth, but since absorption is slow and the effect variable, it is normally given by subcutaneous or intramuscular injection. The intravenous route can also be employed and it is a popular choice for patient controlled analgesia (PCA).

Acute pain   In the treatment of acute pain the official dose is 8–20 mg, but larger doses up to 30 mg may sometimes be required. In acute pain associated with shock, it should be given intravenously, as when given by the other routes its action is delayed owing to the poor circulation in peripheral tissues.

Chronic pain   In chronic pain, such as that associated with cancer, an initial dose of 15 mg may be given subcutaneously and repeated at 3 to 4-hourly intervals as required, but its tolerance develops the dose and frequency of administration should be increased and doses of 20–30 mg may become necessary.

In premedication   A dose of 10–15 mg according to the condition of the patient is usually given by subcutaneous or intramuscular injection 1–1.5 h before operation. It is normally better to avoid the use of morphine in the elderly.

Precautions

As morphine causes marked respiratory depression, it should not be given when there is increased intracranial pressure, and in conditions where respiration is already depressed or ineffective as in bronchial asthma and emphysema. It is also contra-indicated in adrenocortical insufficiency, severe liver disease, hypothyroidism, diverticulitis and other spastic conditions of the colon, biliary colic, in patients who are being treated with MAOIs, in cachectic or elderly patients, and during labour.

As morphine can be a drug of addiction, it should be used with due circumspection when repeated doses are likely to be required. This, of course, does not apply to the terminal stages of painful disease such as cancer, when duration of life can be only a matter of days or weeks.

Apart from respiratory depression, other side effects of morphine include drowsiness, confusion, nausea, vomiting and constipation. They are more marked when the patient is ambulant. Overdose causes respiratory failure, cardiovascular collapse and coma. Treatment consists of supportive therapy and the administration of naloxone 0.2–0.4 mg intravenously.

Artificial ventilation may be necessary and hypotension requires the administration of a pressor drug and fluids to increase the circulating blood volume.

Dihydrocodeine is closely related chemically to codeine and its analgesic potency lies between that of codeine and pethidine. A dose of 30 mg gives similar analgesia to 10 mg of morphine. Compared with morphine, its sedative effect is less, and its duration of action is slightly shorter. Dihydrocodeine may be used as a substitute for morphine or its derivatives in the treatment of postoperative and chronic pain in a dose of 30–60 mg. Side effects are less troublesome than with morphine but similar precautions should be taken regarding its use.

Other morphine derivatives include dihydromorphinone hydrochloride and oxymorphone hydrochloride. Their actions are similar to those of morphine and they have no particular advantages.

Opium in the raw state varies in consistency from being firm and plastic to brittle. It occurs as irregular masses of a chocolate or dark brown colour, having a strong characteristic odour and bitter taste. Powdered opium is a fine, or moderately fine, light brown powder.

The official preparation of powdered opium contains 10 per cent anhydrous morphine; the tincture and Dover's powder contain 1 per cent. Papaveretum contains 50 per cent anhydrous morphine. Nepenthe contains 0.84 per cent of anhydrous morphine.

Papaveretum is a preparation containing the water-soluble alkaloids of opium, standardized to contain 50 per cent anhydrous morphine. The other 50 per cent consists of the hydrochlorides of the remaining opium alkaloids (mainly papaverine, codeine, narcotine and thebaine). Morphine is normally prescribed as a salt and contains water of crystallization: 20 mg of papaveretum is, therefore, equivalent to 13 mg of a morphine salt. The other alkaloids do not exert much sedative or analgesic effect. It has been reformulated so that it now contains no noscapine, following evidence that this substance is genotoxic.

Historically, papaveretum has been presented in combination in a single ampoule with hyoscine (scopolamine) for premedication. This combination may cause severe depression in the elderly. A dose range of 10–20 mg is employed.

Nalbuphine is a partial opioid agonist whose effects are similar to those of pentazocine. It has typical central opioid effects, but can also act as an opioid antagonist. It is an agonist at κ-receptors, an antagonist at μ-receptors and has no effects on δ-receptors. It is equipotent with morphine and three to four times as potent as pentozacine. It is subjected to extensive first-pass metabolism and no oral preparation is available. It is used in doses of 10–20 mg for moderate to severe pain by subcutaneous, intramuscular or intravenous injection.

Nalbuphine has a low abuse potential, but symptoms of opioid withdrawal have occurred following cessation of use after prolonged administration. At therapeutic doses, nalbuphine causes respiratory depression which is equivalent to morphine. At higher doses (20–30 mg), there appears to be a ceiling effect on both its respiratory and its analgesic actions. Nalbuphine also causes miosis, sedation, nausea and vomiting and constipation. Haemodynamic effects are minimal. It can produce an abstinence syndrome in morphine addicts and will also reverse the respiratory depression produced by opioids.

NALOXONE

Naloxone hydrochloride (rINN)

Pharmacology

Naloxone is an opioid antagonist, displacing opiate agonist drugs and exerting antagonist effects at μ, κ and δ opioid receptors. In both animals and man, no agonist effects can be detected at non-toxic doses, and the drug is used to reverse the existing effects of morphine, diamorphine or other opiate overdose.

Administered alone, it elicits no detectable effects or symptoms unless a gross overdose is administered (e.g. 200 times the therapeutic dose). In usual therapeutic doses, it rapidly reverses opiate-induced analgesia, euphoria, respiratory depression, pupillary constriction, delayed gastric emptying, coma and convulsions. It has no antagonistic action against respiratory depression induced by other groups of drugs such as barbiturates.

Naloxone also antagonizes the analgesic, dysphoric and depressant effects of partial agonist drugs such as nalbuphine and pentazocine, as well as the weaker agonists such as codeine, dihydrocodeine, pethidine and dextropropoxyphene. However, the potency (affinity) and persistence of the partial agonist buprenorphine at opioid receptors makes it a difficult agent to reverse with naloxone, particularly because of naloxone's short duration of action. Indeed, in reversing the effects of any full, or partial, agonist opiate, clinical observations must continue beyond the initial reversal of symptoms, since these may reappear as the concentration of naloxone in the body falls.

Following intravenous injection, the effects of naloxone are apparent within 1–2 minutes. With a plasma half-life of about 60–90 minutes the agonist's effects may reappear after 45–60 minutes, depending on the nature and dose of agonist being reversed. Naloxone may also be given by intramuscular injection when the onset of effects are slower but also slightly prolonged. This may be of advantage.

Pharmacokinetics   The blocking effect is apparent 1–2 minutes after intravenous injection. The plasma half-life is between 1 and 1.5 h, so that the effect is apparent for about 45–60 minutes.

Indications

Naloxone is used to antagonize the respiratory depression and other effects of morphine-like full opiate and partial agonist opioid drugs. In parallel, naloxone will reverse the opiate-induced analgesia, euphoria, pupillary constriction, delayed gastric emptying, coma and convulsions. It will also antagonize the effects of partial agonists such as pentazocine, including the associated dysphoria and depressant effects. Other clinical uses of naloxone include the emergency reversal of accidental or deliberate opiate overdose, respiratory depression in the newborn following obstetric analgesia with an opiate, and terminating the effects of neuroleptanalgesia induced by agents such as phenoperidine or fentanyl. Naloxone may also be used as an investigative tool where narcotic overdose is suspected in unconscious patients, and in demonstrating narcotic addiction (when a prompt withdrawal reaction can be elicited).

Dosage and administration

Naloxone may be given subcutaneously, intramuscularly or intravenously; it is normally given intravenously in doses of 0.2–0.4 mg when a rapid action is required. In children the initial dose is 10–20 µg/kg. It can be given intramuscularly in a dose of 20–70 µg/kg for a more prolonged effect. In the neonate, doses of 0.2–0.4 µg/kg body weight are given: the prolonged effects of intramuscular administration may be particularly useful in the neonate depressed by pethidine placentally transferred from the mother.

Precautions

The duration of action after intravenous administration may be shorter than that of some of the agents whose effects it is required to antagonize. It will rapidly induce withdrawal symptoms if given to patients addicted to one of the narcotics.

Rapid anaesthetic antagonist opiate detoxification

Attempts can be made to accelerate the process of opiate detoxification by the administration of naloxone (or naltrexone). If naloxone is given to an opiate dependent patient, for example 0.4–0.8 mg i.m., symptoms of withdrawal will appear in 10–20 minutes, disappearing in about 1 h. After 4–6 h of total opioid receptor blockade, the precipitated withdrawal symptoms will have largely abated. These symptoms can be extremely severe, and are accompanied by intense sympathetic activity (the sympathetic storm) causing considerable distress to the subject and attendants.

At first, benzodiazepines were given prior to the administration of naloxone in order to suppress the withdrawal symptoms. More recently, inhalational anaesthesia or a propofol infusion have been used to completely suppress the opioid antagonist-precipitated symptoms. Thus, anaesthesia is first induced and naloxone given as a challenge. If no adverse reactions occur, the longer acting naltrexone (see below) is given; presynaptic α_2-adrenoceptor agonists such as clonidine may also be used to attenuate some of the withdrawal symptoms. Anaesthesia is maintained up to 24 h or more. Full supervision is required throughout, as for any anaesthetic procedure. Unfortunately, at least one death has been reported associated with this accelerated withdrawal procedure.

The Advisory Council on the Misuse of Drugs has reported that the efficacy of this treatment has not been established, and there is no evidence that the procedure is effective in the long term.

Naltrexone is a relatively pure opioid antagonist. It has a similar spectrum of properties and uses as naloxone, and is slightly longer acting. The predicted progressive replacement of naloxone as the 'standard' opioid antagonist has not been observed in clinical practice. It is, however, used for the long-term therapy of opioid addiction because, unlike naloxone, naltrexone has high oral bioavailability and a half-life of about 4 h.

It displaces all agonists and blocks the effects of subsequent opiate administration. It is given to addicts in a dose of 50 mg daily, but the dose is often increased at weekends!

NEFOPAM HYDROCHLORIDE

Nefopam hydrochloride (rINN)

Nefopam is an analgesic which is neither an opiate nor an NSAID. It has been reported to be approximately eight times as potent as aspirin and about half as potent as morphine. After parenteral intramuscular injection, the peak effect is reached after 1 hour.

The oral dose is 30 mg 3 times a day which can be increased up to 90 mg 3 times a day. By intramuscular or slow intravenous injection the dose is 20 mg, followed by further similar doses at 6-hourly intervals if necessary.

The drug can produce atropine-like effects – blurred vision, dry mouth, tachycardia. It should probably be avoided in patients with glaucoma or urinary retention. Convulsive disorders and myocardial infarctions are other contra-indications. After injection it can produce fainting and it is best administered to patients who are lying down and who remain so for about 20 minutes after injection. It can produce profuse sweating, insomnia and nausea.

PARACETAMOL

Paracetamol (rINN) and Acetaminophen (USP)

Pharmacology and metabolism

Paracetamol was first used as an analgesic and antipyretic in 1893, but its widespread use did not occur until the 1950s. Following its recognition as phenacetin's active metabolite, and the subsequent withdrawal of the nephrotoxic phenacetin from the United Kingdom, European and USA markets, paracetamol's clinical popularity rose substantially. Paracetamol is not an NSAID, since it lacks significant anti-inflammatory activity at non-toxic doses, but its antecedents can be traced back to the original 'coal tar analgesics' of the late nineteenth/early twentieth centuries.

Unlike phenacetin, prolonged use of paracetamol has not reliably demonstrated 'analgesic-abuse nephropathy', hence its steady rise in popularity as an over-the-counter (OTC) analgesic and antipyretic. Note, however, that paracetamol has little or no anti-inflammatory activity. It is rapidly absorbed, providing relief from minor pain in about 30–40 minutes; elimination by the kidneys is also rapid; 85 per cent of an oral dose can be accounted for as soluble glucuronic and sulphate hepatic conjugates. While its lack of anti-inflammatory activity is a clear deficiency, this must be balanced against its lack of irritation on the gastro-intestinal tract.

The exact subcellular mechanism of action of paracetamol remains obscure. Its failure to exert anti-inflammatory activity is probably related to its inability to block either of the cyclo-oxygenase enzymes (COX-1 and 2), nor does it interfere with neutrophil activation at the site of injury or inflammation. Its effects on fever appear to be mediated at the hypothalamic level, and it is possible that its analgesic effects are also mediated centrally.

Indications, dosage and administration

A dose of 0.5–1.0 g paracetamol by mouth provides about the same analgesia and antipyresis as 250–500 mg of aspirin, and it is usually administered at 4 h intervals. It may be used for the relief of minor degrees of pain as a substitute for acetylsalicylic acid. As will be seen from the larger dose, it is a weaker analgesic than aspirin but is less irritant to the stomach in those who cannot tolerate aspirin, and is generally less toxic in normal doses than any other drug in this group.

Paracetamol toxicity and overdose

This takes the form of a dose-dependent hepatic necrosis and may follow the ingestion of as little as 10–15 g. A single intake of over 25 g is potentially fatal. It is caused by a toxic metabolite (N-hydroxyparacetamol) which is slow to appear and belies the potential seriousness of the problem. It is inactivated by glutathione; toxicity results when the amount of this metabolite exceeds the stores of glutathione available for its inactivation. Regular consumers of alcohol or other drugs that induce liver microsomal enzymes produce metabolites at a greater rate and have an increased risk of developing hepatic damage.

Nausea, vomiting, anorexia and abdominal pain are the first symptoms to appear (in the first 24 h), with a 2–4-day latency occurring in overt signs of liver damage. Plasma aminotransferases may be very substantially raised, bilirubin levels also rise and the prothrombin time is lengthened.

Successful treatment means early treatment, usually in anticipation of the overt toxicity. Evidence or suspicion of overdose should be followed immediately by gastric lavage and the determination of plasma levels of paracetamol. Such estimations are of value within the first 10 h after ingestion as a guide to therapy. Hepatic damage is likely if the blood level is over 200 µg/ml at 2 h after ingestion or 120 µg/ml at 10 h after ingestion, and active therapy is indicated. Any compound rich in sulphydryl groups able to replenish hepatic stores of glutathione can be given, such as methionine, cysteamine and *N*-acetylcysteine: the last named has the advantage of being available for intravenous use. The initial dose should be 150 mg/kg in 200 ml of 5 per cent dextrose over 15 minutes followed by 50 mg/kg over 4 h and 100 mg/kg over the next 6 h. To be effective, treatment must be started within 10 h of ingestion of the overdose of paracetamol.

Although uncommon, prolonged use of paracetamol may cause nephropathy, and anaesthetists should be alert to patients undergoing major surgery, particularly gastric surgery for ulceration. Although at first covert, analgesic nephropathy may be revealed by agents causing dehydration or renal ischaemia. The avoidance of agents causing renal vasoconstriction and the provision of adequate fluid therapy are important precautionary steps.

PENTAZOCINE

Pentazocine hydrochloride (rINN)

Pharmacology

Pentazocine is a benzomorphan derivative, introduced in the late 1960s following attempts to mimic the potentially useful and avoid the adverse properties of the non-addicting 'antagonist' analgesic nalorphine. These objectives were largely achieved: pentazocine is a useful analgesic when used in appropriate clinical circumstances.

Pentazocine is described as a partial-agonist analgesic at µ opioid receptors. As such, 20–30 mg of pentazocine exert roughly comparable analgesic effects to 10 mg of morphine, although there is a 'ceiling' to these effects which higher doses will not overcome. Pentazocine is thus effective in combating postoperative pain, but not that associated with terminal illness. Pentazocine is only mildly sedative, does not constrict the pupil, and it has only modest opiate-like effects on respiration and the cardiovascular system. Constipation, nausea and vomiting are relatively uncommon. In higher doses, dysphoria is more likely to appear than euphoria, and in 30 years' experience, addiction has not been encountered in normal clinical circumstances. In the absence of respiratory depression and any rise in Pa_{CO_2}, pentazocine causes a small fall in intracranial pressure.

About 50–75 per cent of an oral dose is absorbed: an oral dose of 25–100 mg gives a peak plasma level in 1–3 h, and a subsequent plasma half-life of 4–6 h. A similar dose may be given intramuscularly. Pentazocine is sufficiently lipophilic to cross the blood–brain barrier and the placenta. Little of the drug is excreted unchanged, appearing in the urine as metabolites.

Indications

Pentazocine can be used for a range of painful conditions in which modest doses of narcotic (agonist) analgesics would normally suffice. It is suitable for postoperative pain and in chronic pain conditions where clinical circumstances suggest that the potentially addictive properties of morphine or diamorphine should be avoided.

Although itself an antagonist of full agonist analgesics, the analgesic and other effects of pentazocine may be in turn antagonized by naloxone. A pentazocine overdose is thus responsive to naloxone.

Precautions

Similar precautions should be observed as for morphine; overdosage can be reversed with naloxone. It is important to remember that levallorphan and nalorphine are ineffective.

Fortagesic is an oral proprietary combination of pentazocine (15 mg) and paracetamol (500 mg), for use in modest to severe pain associated with musculoskeletal disorders or injuries, and rheumatoid patients intolerant to the gastro-intestinal effects associated with aspirin and other NSAIDs.

Phenazocine is a benzmorphan derivative and has powerful analgesic properties. It has little sedative action. Although it is claimed that it causes less respiratory depression than morphine, reports are conflicting and there is probably little difference between the two drugs. Other side effects such as nausea, vomiting and constipation are possibly less prominent.

It may be used for the same purposes as morphine and is given intramuscularly in a dose of 1–3 mg.

PETHIDINE

Pethidine hydrochloride (rINN) and Meperidine hydrochloride (USP)

Pharmacology

Although structurally dissimilar to natural and semisynthetic opiates when represented in two-dimensional diagrams, computer-assisted three-dimensional imaging shows many spatial and dimensional similarities between pethidine and the phenanthrene structure of morphine.

Pethidine is a full agonist at opioid μ-receptors, and consequently shares many of the desirable and undesirable properties of morphine, albeit that some properties may be more or less expressed quantitatively. It may also inhibit norepinephrine (noradrenaline) and epinephrine (adrenaline) re-uptake into pre-synaptic neurones, which is responsible for some of its additional effects. It also has some atropinic (anti-muscarinic) properties.

Pethidine is well absorbed following oral administration, and therein lies its major therapeutic advantage: good analgesia can be achieved following oral administration with minimal sedative or depressant effects, 50–100 mg producing an analgesia lasting 3–4 h. Its potency thus lies between that of codeine and morphine.

Medullary and respiratory depression are likely to occur only at high doses, when they may also be accompanied by cerebral irritation and convulsions. Tachycardia and hypertension may also occur. Pupillary size is usually unaffected, while nausea and vomiting are uncommon. Euphoria and elevation of mood commonly accompany modest doses, while dysphoria is likely only when administered in the absence of pain.

For clinical purposes, equi-analgesia requires a dose 8–10 times that of morphine, but the duration of analgesia is only about three-quarters of that of morphine. All types of pain are relieved, but the drug is more effective in pain of visceral origin, probably because of its atropine-like action.

The drug is of value in the relief of intractable pruritus which may be aggravated by giving morphine. Morphine addicts will substitute with pethidine. Tolerance is not as complete as with morphine; the withdrawal symptoms are less severe and appear more rapidly. They resemble those of morphine (see page 185), twitching of skeletal muscle and extreme restlessness being particularly prominent.

Autonomic system There is a mild anticholinergic action, which produces an atropine-like effect.

Cardiovascular system Pethidine has a quinidine-like action which reduces cardiac irritability, and ventricular arrhythmias may often be prevented or controlled if already present. Blood pressure is normally unaffected, but sometimes falls; this may be due to relaxation of the muscle of vessel walls, histamine release or, in the case of overdose, vasomotor depression. The heart rate may be slightly increased.

Respiratory system Respiration is depressed in proportion to the dose given. The main effect is on the rate which may be markedly slowed; apnoea will follow large intravenous doses. The cough reflex is unaffected, but laryngeal reflexes are depressed. Bronchi are not affected, but will relax if in spasm. Secretions are moderately reduced.

Smooth muscle Minor effects are exerted on smooth muscles which cause spasm in some – for example, the sphincter of Oddi – and relaxation in others. Spasm, with the exception of biliary colic, is usually relieved. The atropine-like effect of the drug probably plays some part in this process.

Alimentary system There is little action on the bowel, but when in spasm it is relaxed. Unlike morphine, it has little constipating effect, but nausea and vomiting are not uncommon. In analgesic doses in labour, pethidine virtually suppresses gastric emptying.

Liver and kidney function Pethidine has no adverse action on the liver. Urinary output and peristaltic movements of the ureter are decreased.

Uterus and placenta Uterine contractions are unaffected. Pethidine crosses the placental barrier and can cause depression of respiration in the infant at birth.

Histamine release The action of liberation of histamine is a local one, a weal often being noticed along the course of the vein used for injection. Systemic effects are rare.

Fate in the body Pethidine is absorbed in 20–60 minutes when given by mouth, 15 minutes by intramuscular injection, and its effects are noticeable within 2–4 minutes when given intravenously. It is mainly detoxicated by hepatic metabolism, either by demethylation to norpethidine or by hydrolysis to meperidinic acid. Only about 5 per cent is excreted unchanged in the urine. Pregnant women, neonates and women on oral contraceptives excrete a higher proportion of unchanged drug. In severe liver disease (and in patients under treatment with MAOIs), the degradation of the drug is inhibited.

The urinary excretion of pethidine is pH dependent; if the pH is reduced below 5.0, as much as 25 per cent is excreted unchanged. Whereas only 1 per cent/h is excreted in urine at normal pH, the rate is increased to 4 per cent/h if it is highly acidic.

Indications

Pethidine is used for the treatment of acute pain in the preoperative and postoperative periods, the intractable pain associated with carcinoma, premedication before operation, as a supplement to nitrous oxide and oxygen anaesthesia, in the early stages of labour, and for minor procedures, such as painful dressings, which do not require full anaesthesia. Pethidine is also used to control the tachypnoea which may occur during halothane (and trichlorethylene) anaesthesia in patients who have not received an opiate premedication.

Dosage and administration

Pethidine may be given by mouth, intramuscularly, or intravenously. For analgesia, a dose of 50–100 mg is given orally or intramuscularly and repeated every 3–4 h as necessary. For premedication, an intramuscular injection of 50–100 mg is given 1 h before operation.

As a supplement to nitrous oxide and oxygen anaesthesia, the initial intravenous dose after induction is 10–15 mg, according to the age and condition of the patient. Supplementary doses are normally necessary every 20–30 minutes. In the treatment of tachypnoea, up to 25 mg may be given intravenously.

In obstetrics, an initial dose of 100 mg (or up to 150 mg in obese subjects) is given intramuscularly when labour pains have become regular. These doses may be repeated every 2–3 h as required. If delivery occurs while the drug could still be affecting the fetus, respiratory depression can be reversed by naloxone. There is some evidence that the intramuscular administration of a relatively large dose of naloxone to the baby is more beneficial than administration of the usual dose by intravenous injection. Behavioural improvements extend over several days and may be related to the earlier establishment of feeding and quicker urinary clearance of pethidine.

Precautions

Pethidine is contra-indicated in severe liver disease and in patients who are under treatment with MAOIs. Pethidine can partially inhibit the re-uptake of norepinephrine (noradrenaline) into nerve terminals: in the presence of MAOIs this can result in hypertension and coma.

Pethidine is a drug capable of causing addiction, and should be used in repeated doses for the relief of chronic non-malignant pain only in exceptional circumstances.

Side effects such as nausea and vomiting, excitement or depression, and confusion, are not uncommon, and ambulant patients must be warned to adjust their activities accordingly. Apart from respiratory depression, overdose of pethidine may cause convulsions, cardiovascular collapse and coma.

Naloxone (0.2–0.4 mg) should be given as an antagonist. Hypotension can occur without other symptoms following even relatively small doses, due to histamine release. If severe, a small dose of a pressor agent should be given.

If coma and other signs of overdose are associated with liver disease or the administration of MAOIs, the urine should be acidified as soon as possible. This may be accomplished by the intravenous infusion of 10 g of L-arginine hydrochloride dissolved in 500 ml of 5 per cent dextrose and given over 30 minutes.

Anileridine and **alphaprodine** are closely related to pethidine and have similar actions. The dose range of both these compounds is 30–60 mg, given by mouth or intramuscular injection.

Methadone is a wholly synthetic μ opioid agonist: the commercial form is a racemate of D and L forms, the L isomer being some 10-40 times more potent. This applies to both its useful and adverse effects. Methadone has pharmacological properties qualitatively similar to morphine. Like pethidine, methadone is well absorbed but relatively slowly by mouth: peak plasma levels are reached in about 4 h, more quickly after intramuscular or subcutaneous injection. About 90 per cent of the drug in the plasma is protein bound, so that the drug has an extended duration of action and a plasma half-life variously estimated at 15–40 h. This is useful in prolonged pain treatment and for overnight control of pain and cough.

Pharmacological effects can be demonstrated fully 24 h after a single dose, and prolonged relief of pain is still further enhanced by repeated administration with the subsequent drug accumulation in tissues. Methadone is useful in morphine substitution programmes, when only a low frequency of administration is required in support of opiate addicts. In the USA, the methadone derivative lα-acetylmethadol (levomethadyl acetate) has been introduced for morphine-substitution in addicts. Onset of action is delayed but duration of action is sufficiently prolonged that only one administration per day will sustain most addicts.

Phenoperidine is chemically related to pethidine and on a weight-for-weight basis is considerably more potent as an analgesic. It acts within 2–3 minutes when given intravenously and its effect lasts for 0.5–1 h. Some degree of analgesia persists for 4–6 h. In recommended doses the cardiovascular system remains stable but respiration is readily depressed; 2–5 mg given intravenously will cause apnoea. Other actions are similar to those of pethidine.

It is used as an analgesic supplement to nitrous oxide and oxygen anaesthesia, in neurolept-analgesia, and as a respiratory depressant to assist conscious patients to acclimatize to mechanical ventilation. It can also be used in place of other analgesics in the relief of severe pain.

Piritramide is a tertiary amine of the diphenylpropylamine series. It is a powerful narcotic analgesic but has little structural similarity to other drugs of this class. Its duration of action is about 6 h. Equi-analgesic doses depress ventilation to a lesser extent than morphine. Compared with morphine, vomiting is comparatively rare. A dose of 15 mg is approximately equivalent to 10 mg of morphine. The chief side effect appears to be drowsiness which may be an advantage in the postoperative period.

PIROXICAM

Piroxicam (rINN)

Piroxicam was one of the first 'oxicam' NSAIDs, which are derived from a group of enolic acids.

Pharmacology

Like aspirin, indometacin and naproxen, piroxicam exerts substantial anti-inflammatory, antipyretic and analgesic activity, yet may be somewhat better tolerated (at least initially) than aspirin or indometacin, making it more suitable for long-term treatment. In addition to cyclo-oxygenase enzyme (and prostaglandin synthesis) inhibition, there is some evidence that it at least partially suppresses the lipoxygenase pathway, since inflammation-induced neutrophil activation is also delayed in the presence of piroxicam. Evidence of interference with proteoglycanase and collagenase activities in cartilage has also emerged.

Piroxicam is rapidly and completely absorbed following oral administration. Peak plasma levels are reached in 3–4 h, and the drug is about 99 per cent plasma protein bound, which enhances its relatively long plasma half-life (about 12 h). Little unchanged piroxicam appears in the urine, renal elimination being achieved following the glucuronidation of its hydroxylated (inactive) metabolite.

Indications

Piroxicam is used in the treatment of rheumatoid arthritis and osteoarthritis. Its persistence in the body means that infrequent dosing (once daily) promotes optimum suppression of pain and inflammation in association with relatively constant tissue levels.

Piroxicam is a potent NSAID, comparable with indometacin but rather better tolerated by patients. While the gastro-intestinal irritation with piroxicam may be minimal at low to modest doses, gastro-intestinal-related adverse effects can become severe at sustained high dosage, emphasizing that it is a powerful suppressant of prostaglandin synthesis.

Dosage and administration

An oral dose of 20 mg/day, usually divided, is recommended for chronic conditions, allowing 10–14 days to elapse for maximum tissue levels to develop. At this time, concentrations in the plasma and synovial fluid are about the same.

Precautions

These are the same as for all NSAIDs

Meloxicam has recently been introduced to Europe and there are claims that it may be a partially selective COX-2 inhibitor, with a consequently lower incidence of COX-1-associated adverse effects, thus permitting some protection of the gastro-intestinal tract from irritation and erosion. Clinical evidence of this is awaited. Meloxicam is well absorbed following oral administration, is substantially plasma protein bound and peak plasma levels are reached after 3–4 h, with a plasma half-life of about 20 h. The drug can thus be administered just once daily (7.5 mg) or twice daily (7.5 mg twice), steady-state tissue levels being reached in 5–7 days. Little of the drug is eliminated unchanged, its metabolites appearing in roughly equal amounts in urine and faeces.

Tenoxicam is a similar, related new drug in the oxicam series. It is rapidly and completely absorbed following oral administration, extensively protein bound and has a very extended plasma half-life of about 70 h (3 days). Once-daily administration (20 mg) is thus sufficient to promote progressive accumulation of tenoxicam in plasma, synovial and other tissues. There is no evidence yet of selectivity or lack of selectivity of inhibition of either of the COX enzymes. The drug is promoted for sub-acute and chronic musculoskeletal and arthritic conditions. It should be noted that an injectable preparation is available when a 20 mg dose can be used to initiate early pain relief.

Ketorolac (as *ketorolac trometamol*) is another NSAID, acting through cyclo-oxygenase inhibition, but exerts minimal anti-inflammatory activity at analgesic doses. Available as 10 or 30 mg ampoules for i.m. or bolus i.v. injection, ketorolac has a licensed indication for the short-term management of moderate to severe postoperative pain, when it also has a useful opiate-sparing effect. Peak plasma effects following i.m. administration are achieved in less than 1 h (at about 5 minutes following an i.v. bolus), and the terminal half-life is about 5 h (prolonged where there is renal impairment). Analgesia is effective for about 4–6 h.

Ketorolac can prolong postoperative bleeding and is contra-indicated where haemorrhage may be significant, or in patients wlth a history of bleeding disorders (including those caused by previous or concomitant use of other NSAIDs).

Daily doses should not exceed 90 mg and this maximum should be reduced where there is renal impairment and/or in the elderly. Initial doses in postoperative pain relief should not exceed 10 mg (whether by i.m. or i.v. injection), although this dose may be repeated at 2-hourly intervals early in the postoperative period.

REMIFENTANIL

Remifentanil (rINN)

Remifentanil has a molecular weight of 412.9 Da and as it does not contain an asymmetric carbon atom it exists only in a single form.

Pharmacology

Metabolism Remifentanil is unique among opioids in having a methyl ester in the *N*-acyl moiety. As a result it undergoes rapid and widespread extrahepatic metabolism by blood and tissue esterases that are non-saturable. The primary metabolic pathway is by de-esterification to a carboxylic acid metabolite which has only a fraction of the opioid potency of the parent compound. It is a poor substrate for plasma cholinesterase and is not affected by anticholinesterases such as neostigmine. Its action will not therefore be potentiated by reversal of non-depolarizing relaxants.

Pharmacokinetics Remifentanil is very fat soluble, with a volume of distribution of around 22 litres (Egan *et al.*, 1966). This small volume of distribution, combined with the fact that it's action is terminated by metabolism rather than redistribution, results in an extremely rapid clearance of around 3 litres/minute. The context sensitive half-time of remifentanil is around 3 minutes irrespective of the duration of the infusion. Kapila *et al.* (1995) found that the context-sensitive half-time of remifentanil after a 3 h infusion was 3 minutes and the pharmacodynamic offset time was 5.4 minutes. The corresponding figures for alfentanil were 47.3 minutes and 54.0 minutes, respectively. The terminal half-life in these volunteers was an average of 11.8 minutes for remifentanil and 76.5 minutes for alfentanil. The pharmacokinetics appear to be little altered in patients with severe liver disease. These pharmacokinetic parameters indicate that remifentanil is an ideal drug for use by continuous infusion.

Pharmacodynamics Remifentanil is a potent, rapidly acting μ opioid agonist, nineteen times more potent that alfentanil, with all the features of such a compound. After intravenous injection there is rapid onset of intense analgesia and sedation. It also has all the complications of opioids and can cause profound respiratory depression, nausea, vomiting, bradycardia, hypotension, muscle rigidity and pruritus. Schüttler *et al.* (1997) found that infusions of remifentanil during abdominal anaesthesia were comparable to those of alfentanil in providing satisfactory analgesia. Its use during the recovery period, however, was accompanied by serious morbidity in terms of respiratory depression and muscle rigidity, with the advice that, certainly at the moment, the drug should not be used for this purpose.

All studies have confirmed the predictable and very short duration of action of remifentanil, which results in early severe postoperative pain. New and possibly sophisticated techniques will be required to solve these problems in the immediate postoperative period. As remifentanil contains glycine, which is a neurotransmitter, it has no licence for use by epidural or spinal routes.

Egan, T.D., Minto, C.F., Hermann, D.J., Barr, J., Muir, K.T. and Shafer, S.L. (1996) Remifentanil versus alfentanil: comparative pharmocokinetics and pharmacodynamics in healthy adult male volunteers. *Anesthesiology*, **84**, 821–33

Kapila, A., Glass, P.S.A. and Jacobs, J.R. et al. (1995) Measured context sensitive half-times of remifentanil and alfentanil. *Anesthesiology*, **83**, 968–75

Schüttler, A., Albrecht, S. and Breivik, H. *et al.* (1997) A comparison of remifentanil and alfentanil in patients undergoing major abdominal surgery. *Anaesthesia*, **52**, 307–17

Sufentanil is the thienyl analogue of fentanyl. It is the most potent of the newer opioids currently available for use in man. In animals it is approximately 2000 times as potent as morphine and 5–15 times as potent as fentanyl. It is extremely lipophilic (partition coefficient 1730 at pH 7.4) and is extensively taken up by tissues with a resultant large volume of distribution (1.74–5.17 litres/kg). Its elimination half-life of 120–165 minutes is between that of alfentanil and fentanyl.

It has all the features of opioid drugs and may be used as the analgesic component of a balanced anaesthetic technique. In minor surgery, doses of 2 µg/kg or less are usually used, while doses up to 8 µg/kg are used to supplement nitrous oxide during major surgery. High doses (15–50 µg/kg) have been used in cardiac surgery, where it provides excellent haemodynamic stability apart from occasionally causing a bradycardia. Recovery is more rapid than following fentanyl.

Sufentanil has been used epidurally for postoperative pain relief, the optimum dose being a bolus of 50 µg. This produces satisfactory analgesia within 7–8 minutes, with a duration varying from 140 to 410 minutes. Its epidural use is associated with all the usual complications, and profound respiratory depression has occurred within 10 minutes of injection. Precautions are as for all potent opioid drugs.

TRAMADOL

Tramadol hydrochloride (rINN)

Pharmacology

Tramadol is a racemic mixture of the two *cis* isomers. It was introduced in Germany in 1971 as a mild analgesic with activity at the µ opioid receptor (as assessed in animal experiments) and steadily established itself as market leader as an oral analgesic for moderate pain which, however, lacked dependence and addiction liability. In the preparation of submissions to the FDA and the CSM in the late 1980s, it became clear that further work was needed to explain several anomalies.

In summary, this work has shown that the R(+)-isomer has some activity at the µ-receptor and the S(−) isomer inhibits norepinephrine (noradrenaline) and 5-HT uptake. The significance of this is that these are the transmitters at the terminals of descending inhibitory neurones which act on the relay cells in the substantia gelatinosa, at which µ opioids are also inhibitory. The main metabolite of the R(+) isomer (+M1) has greater µ opioid receptor activity than the parent compound, but the amount produced in man is much less than in rats. This pathway depends on the enzyme CPY2D6 and approximately 8 per cent of Caucasians lack this enzyme. (This enzyme also transforms codeine into morphine and codeine is therefore ineffective as an analgesic in these subjects. These individuals also seem to experience fewer opioid side effects to tramadol but not less analgesia, suggesting that M1 is not a significant contributor to the analgesia in man).

More recent work has shown that parenteral tramadol given by patient controlled analgesia (PCA) can produce analgesia comparable to that produced by morphine in the immediate postoperative situation after abdominal surgery.

The mechanism of analgesia has been the subject of ingenious volunteer experiments using electrical stimulation of the sural nerve and recording the spinal reflex and the conscious assessment of changes in the pain threshold. Using naloxone to antagonize the opioid effect and yohimbine to antagonize the aminergic component, it has been shown that the opioid component contributes about 30–35 per cent of the analgesia and the aminergic component a similar amount. There is thus true potentiation, approximately one-third of the analgesia arising from the combination. The consequence is that, in proportion to the analgesic effect, the opioid side effects, particularly depression of ventilation, are extremely weak. Furthermore, the central aminergic action seems to counteract the 'liking' of the opioid component, as attested by trials in cured morphine addicts. As a consequence the drug is not a Controlled Drug in any market.

Tramadol has slightly stimulating central effects and small changes can be observed in the processed EEG after intravenous administration. However, these are not sufficient to cause awareness during general anaesthesia.

Pharmacokinetics

Single oral doses have 70 per cent bioavailability but the metabolic pathway is saturable and regular doses achieve 100 per cent bioavailability. Effective blood levels are reached in 30–60 minutes and last for 4–6 h: sustained-release formulations extend this to 8 h. Intravenous administration shortens the onset time to about 10 minutes.

Indications

In the United Kingdom tramadol is licensed for the treatment of moderate to severe pain. The indications are therefore potentially very wide. Its principal uses seem likely to be the treatment of chronic pain, both non-malignant, such as exacerbation of the pain of chronic arthritis, and for cancer, for which it is classed as a Step 2 drug in the WHO ladder. It can be given during anaesthesia with little effect upon respiration and would seem to be ideal for administration just before recovery from anaesthesia. It would also seem likely to find a useful niche as a safe 'second day' postoperative analgesic and as an analgesic to take home by patients following day-stay surgery.

Dosage and administration

For acute pain   Intravenous increments of 50–100 mg, until adequate relief is obtained, up to 400 mg. Doses of 3 mg/kg i.v. have been given without ill effect during the late stage of general anaesthesia in order to provide analgesia on awakening for the early postoperative period.

For chronic pain   50 mg orally initially, increasing up to 400 mg daily, in divided doses.

Precautions

Side effects are mostly on the CNS, with nausea and dizziness predominating. Side effects are minimized by increasing the dose gradually and tend to reduce with time. No specific anti-emetic has been identified as uniquely effective.

References and further reading

ABPI's Compendium of Data Sheets (1998–99 edn) London: Datapharm Publications Ltd. (Refer for individual products)

Dhawan, B.N. *et al.* (1996) International Union of Pharmacology, XII. Classification of opioid receptors. *Pharmacological Reviews,* **48**, 567–592

Grubb, B.D. (1998) Peripheral and central mechanisms of pain. *British Journal of Anaesthesia,* **81**, 8–11

MeReC Bulletin (1997) Acute treatment of migraine: new products, vol. **8**, number 10, Liverpool: NHS National Prescribing Centre Publication

Pasternak, G.W. (1993) Pharmacological mechanisms of opioid analgesics. *Clinical Neuropharmacology,* **16**, 1–18

Reisine, T. and Pasternak, G.W. (1996) Opioid analgesics and antagonists. In *Goodman and Gilman's 'The Pharmacological Basis of Therapeutics,* 9th edn, Chapter 23, pp. 521–555 (Eds: Hardman, J.G., Limbird, L.E. and Gilman, A.G.). New York: McGraw-Hill

6

Local anaesthetics

Local anaesthetics used in anaesthetic practice are one of the very few classes of drug that are injected into their site of action. Unlike the other drugs used in anaesthesia, for example volatile and intravenous agents, neuromuscular relaxants and opiates, they do not require the blood stream to carry them to their target site and under normal circumstances their blood levels are low. They therefore do not exert profound effects on other organs of the body.

Any substance which, when applied to nervous tissue, prevents conduction of a nerve impulse is strictly speaking a local anaesthetic, but the effect of those used in anaesthesia is reversible. Thus many antihistamines and especially some of the phenothiazines, have local anaesthetic properties, but are unsuitable for use because of tissue irritation. Prolonged or permanent interruption of nerve conduction can be achieved with protoplasmic poisons such as quinidine, alcohol, phenol or chlorocresol. Such substances are only used in the management of severe chronic pain states.

Mode of action

Experimentally, if an electrode is inserted through an axonal membrane, a potential difference is recorded between the inside and outside of the membrane such that the inside is negatively charged in the region of -70 mV. This is the resting membrane potential and is due to the differential distribution of ions across the membrane, there being a high concentration of sodium on the outside and this is actively prevented from entering the axon by the energy-dependent sodium pump. When the nerve is stimulated, the potential difference alters so that the inside becomes positive and the outside negative for a very brief period. In this state the nerve is said to be depolarized and this is due to the rapid influx of sodium ions followed by an efflux of potassium. This action potential lasts for milliseconds and the resting potential is rapidly restored by ion flux.

If a local anaesthetic solution is applied to the nerve, then the action potential becomes smaller and if the concentration is sufficiently high, is completely abolished. If the transmembrane potential is measured in this state it shows the normal resting potential, indicating that the local anaesthetic has exerted its effect by preventing the inward passage of sodium ions. These substances are believed to block the sodium channels from the inside of the axon. Local anaesthetics therefore act by stabilizing the axonal membrane and will stabilize all excitable membranes, such as those of the myocardium, skeletal muscle, smooth muscle, and not just the nerves. The reason for complete cessation of conduction in nerves is due to the high concentration of local anaesthetic that is injected

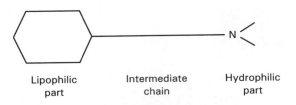

Figure 6.1 Basic chemical structure of local anaesthetics

Lipophilic part | Intermediate chain | Hydrophilic part

in their vicinity. The myocardium, central neurones, etc., are exposed to only very low concentrations carried there by the blood stream.

Nerve fibres also differ in their susceptibility to local anaesthetics. Thus it is the fine C fibres that are blocked first, followed by the Aδ fibres, both these groups subserving pain and temperature. Increasing the concentration results in loss of touch and vibration sense, while the highest concentrations used clinically are needed to block motor function and proprioception.

Chemistry

Local anaesthetics have a remarkably uniform chemical structure (*Figure 6.1*). They consist of a bulky, fat-soluble aromatic part joined by an intermediate chain to a terminal water-soluble part, which is usually an amine group.

It is by adjusting various parts of this structure that drugs of different potency are produced. Unfortunately, increases in potency are limited by increases in toxicity. Branching the intermediate chain tends to increase fat solubility e.g. etidocaine, whereas the bulkier the moiety in the terminal amino group, the greater the potency of the drug e.g. bupivacaine. The presence of the terminal amino group is necessary for solubility; absence results in a drug such as benzocaine which can only be used for surface analgesia.

Local anaesthetics are tertiary amine basic drugs which are poorly soluble in water. They therefore have to be prepared as the water-soluble salt of an acid, usually the hydrochloride, which is stable in solution. In solution, therefore, the local anaesthetic base will be in equilibrium with the water-soluble, positively charged cation, the amount of each present being determined by the prevailing hydrogen ion concentration, as shown in *Figure 6.2*.

The higher the hydrogen ion concentration, the more the equation will move from right to left and more of the drug will be in the water-soluble, cationic form; conversely, a decrease in acidity results in the equilibrium moving from left to right with a consequent increase in the amount of base present.

On injection into tissues, the amount of base and cation present depends on the pH of the tissues and the pK_a of the drug. The higher the pK_a of the local anaesthetic, the greater the amount of cation that is present at body pH. It is the cation component that is actually responsible for blocking nerve conduction, but being water soluble and

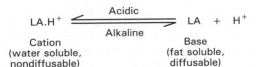

Figure 6.2 Dissociation of local anaesthetic salt in solution

positively charged, it diffuses poorly through the tissues. It is thought that local anaesthetics act inside the axonal membranes. The base will readily diffuse into the axon and
as intracellular pH is lower than extracellular, the base will dissociate into the cationic
form that will block sodium channels. Both forms of the local anaesthetic are therefore
necessary, the base to diffuse through tissues and the cation to block nerve conduction.

Attempts have been made to improve the onset and efficacy of local anaesthetics by
re-formulating them as a carbonated solution at a P_{CO_2} of 93.3 kPa. These solutions have
a higher pH than the hydrochlorides (6.5 compared to 6.0 or lower). The proportion of
free base is thus greater and the enhanced diffusion leads to a shorter latency and greater
intensity of block. Despite this, carbonated solutions have found little favour in clinical
practice.

Classification

Local anaesthetics are classified into esters or amides according to the nature of the
chemical linkage between the aromatic portion and the intermediate chain.

Local anaesthetics which are esters

Apart from cocaine, which is a naturally occurring compound, the ester drugs result from
the combination of para-aminobenzoic acid and an amino-alcohol (*Figure 6.3*).

The currently available drugs are shown in *Table 6.1*.

Local anaesthetics of the ester type are hydrolysed in the blood stream and the liver,
probably by plasma cholinesterase. They have short half-lives and consequently any toxic
reactions are of short duration. Metabolism is prolonged in the presence of severe liver
disease.

The esters tend to be unstable in solution and clinically they only diffuse poorly
through tissues. The pK_a values of the ester drugs (*Table 6.1*) are higher than those of
the amides. As a result, at body pH significantly more drug is in the ionized, poorly
diffusable form. True allergic reactions have been reported to their use, which are
extremely rare with the amide drugs.

Local anaesthetics which are amides

These drugs are formed from the combination of an aromatic amine such as aniline and
an amino acid (*Figure 6.4*). The currently available drugs are shown in *Table 6.1*.

The amides represented a significant advance in local anaesthetic pharmacology. They
are stable in solution and diffuse through tissues more readily than the esters; their pKa

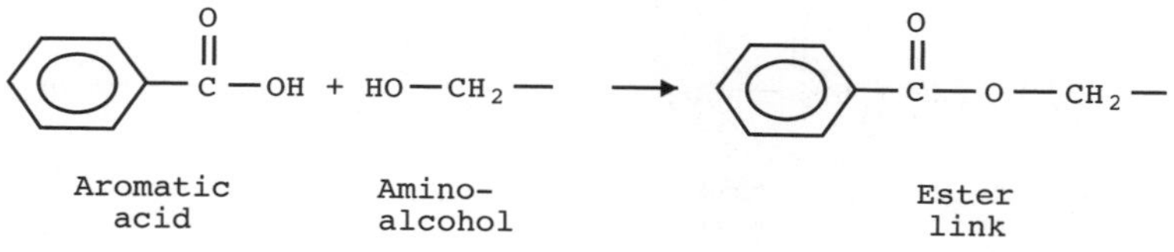

Figure 6.3 Ester link, resulting from the combination of an aromatic acid (usually *p*-aminobenzoic acid)
and an amino-alcohol with the elimination of water

Table 6.1 Local anaesthetic drugs

	Toxicity	pKa
Esters		
Cocaine	Very high	8.7
Benzocaine	Low	2.9
Procaine	Low	8.9
Chloroprocaine	Low	9.1
Tetracaine (amethocaine)	High	8.5
Amides		
Lidocaine	Medium	7.7
Mepivacaine	Medium	7.6
Prilocaine	Low	7.7
Cinchocaine	High	7.9
Etidocaine	Medium	7.7
Bupivacaine	Medium/High	8.1
Levobupivacaine	Low	8.1
Ropivacaine	Low	8.1

values are lower, as shown in *Table 6.1*. These drugs are metabolized in the liver and the appearance of metabolites of lidocaine after a bolus dose has been used as a test of liver function.

Eutectic mixture of local anaesthetics (EMLA)

A eutectic mixture is one in which the mixing of two substances of the same consistency produces a mixture of quite a different consistency. This is related to an alteration in the melting point of the mixture. A familiar example of this phenomenon is the mixing of common salt and ice, both of which are solids. However, on mixing, the ice melts and the salt dissolves in the water and thus the two solids change into a liquid. This is due to a lowering of the melting point of the ice.

It has been found that if the uncharged bases of prilocaine and lidocaine are mixed, a eutectic mixture is formed, the two powders becoming a paste. Substances are then added to make the mixture into a cream that is suitable for application to the skin. The cream therefore contains a very high concentration of the uncharged base which can diffuse through the skin.

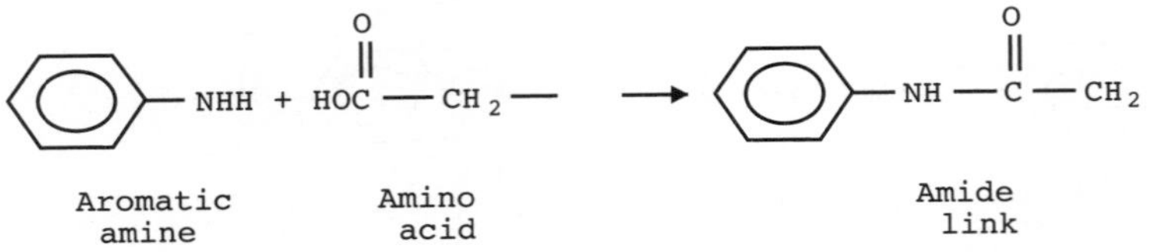

Figure 6.4 Amide link, resulting from the combination of an aromatic amine, e.g. aniline, and an amino acid with the elimination of water

Application for at least 45 minutes is required for adequate analgesia. EMLA cream can be used to permit pain-free venepuncture, particularly in children, and split-skin grafts can also be taken. The cream contains 2.5 per cent of each constituent and tends to produce some blanching of the skin.

Tetracaine (amethocaine) is also available in a formulation for producing surface analgesia of intact skin (see below).

Other pharmacological actions

Apart from the actions in producing local analgesia, these drugs have important actions on other systems in the body. These are only manifest if absorption is too rapid for destruction and excretion to maintain a safe equilibrium. The side effects most usually encountered are like those of atropine and quinidine.

Central nervous system Local anaesthetics can penetrate the blood–brain barrier and exert a similar stabilizing effect on central neurones. They will thus control status epilepticus if given intravenously in suitable doses. Under normal conditions, however, inhibitory neurones are more sensitive to the actions of these drugs than are the excitatory neurones and excitatory phenomena predominate. Overdose leads to tremors and restlessness, proceeding to clonic convulsions. Larger doses depress consciousness and ventilation. Cocaine has a special stimulant action on the cortex, a fact that renders it a dangerous drug of addiction.

Some local anaesthetics, especially procaine and lidocaine, have marked general analgesic properties. Even small doses of procaine used in local infiltration produce measurable, although transitory, degrees of general analgesia. Although procaine and lidocaine have been used in continuous intravenous infusions to produce controllable analgesia during surgical operations and the changing of painful dressings, their use in this way is limited by the small margin between the effective dose and that which produces convulsions and severe depression of the cardiovascular system.

Autonomic ganglia and myoneural junction Local anaesthetics can produce some degree of blockade of transmission at autonomic ganglia and at myoneural junctions. At both of these sites the block is probably in part an 'anti-release' phenomenon, due to depression of acetylcholine release, and partly a true non-depolarizing competitive block.

Cardiovascular system Local anaesthetics are also able to stabilize membrane permeability of excitatory tissue in the heart. They consequently increase the refractory period, prolong conduction time and depress myocardial excitability. They have thus found a useful role in the control and treatment of ventricular arrhythmias. Procainamide was originally introduced as a drug with greater stability for this purpose, but lidocaine is now widely employed.

All local anaesthetics except cocaine tend to cause peripheral vasodilatation by a direct action on arterioles; racemic bupivacaine has little effect although the S isomer has a greater vasodilator effect than the R isomer. By contrast, cocaine potentiates norepinephrine (noradrenaline) and causes vasoconstriction in skin and mucosa. Vasodilator effects, together with the cardiac action and the tendency to cause blockade of autonomic ganglia, tend to result in a fall in blood pressure if large doses or continuous infusions are given.

Local anaesthetics when given by spinal and epidural routes block preganglionic fibres as they leave the spinal cord in the anterior rami; this too will cause a fall in blood pressure, proportional to the number of nerves affected.

Respiratory system   Central stimulation causes some increase in the rate of respiration, but as the medulla becomes depressed, breathing becomes rapid and shallow. Bronchial musculature is relaxed.

Local anaesthetics also have an atropine-like spasmolytic effect on smooth muscle and a mild antihistamine action.

Fate in the body   All of the local anaesthetics are destroyed in the liver. Thus the toxicity of the various agents will vary in inverse proportion to liver function. Procaine and tetracaine are also inactivated by plasma cholinesterase. Those agents which are most slowly broken down will, to a small extent, appear unchanged in the urine.

A large number of local anaesthetics have been synthesized, but few have stood the test of time. Lidocaine and bupivacaine are the most commonly used agents in Great Britain at present. It is too early to evaluate the usage of ropivacaine. Prilocaine has a place as a relatively non-toxic agent for intravenous analgesia. Maximum doses and strength of solution are discussed under the appropriate headings of the drugs concerned.

The relative toxicity and potency of these agents to one another are difficult to determine with any accuracy, as they vary with the concentrations employed and with the routes of administration. Much of the experimental work has been done on different animal species and it is not surprising that figures quoted by different workers vary considerably.

Blood levels of local anaesthetics

Systemic toxic reactions are directly related to the blood level of the drug and this is influenced by a number of factors. Following injection into tissues, the resultant blood level is a balance between absorption of the drug and distribution and metabolism, both of the latter acting to reduce its blood levels. Initially, the amount of local anaesthetic in the tissues is sufficiently high that the blood level rises, overcoming the effects of redistribution and metabolism. As the local concentration decreases, the rise in blood level slows and eventually reaches a plateau. The combined effect of redistribution and metabolism then result in a gradual decrease in concentration. Once the drug has been evenly distributed throughout the body, the decline in blood level is then solely due to metabolism.

The factors that determine the blood level are:

- Dose of drug.
- Rate of administration.
- Site of injection. Absorption occurs rapidly and is more complete from vascular areas. Thus, head and neck blocks are associated with high blood levels, as are intercostal blocks.
- Presence or absence of a vasoconstrictor. The latter, by reducing local blood flow, will reduce absorption from the site of injection. Some drugs have an inherent vasoconstrictor action.

The individual drugs possess properties that will have some effect on their absorption. These include:

- the degree of protein binding in the tissues, as only the free drug is absorbed;
- the fat solubility, as the proportion dissolved in fat is unavailable for absorption;
- vasoactivity, in that vasoconstriction will delay absorption;
- pKa of the drug, which will determine the degree of ionization at the prevailing tissue pH.

Toxic effects

Toxic reactions to local anaesthetics are the result of excessively high blood levels of the drug. This may occur when a large dose has been injected into a very vascular area or when a normal dose is inadvertently injected intravenously; it may also result from premature release of the tourniquet during intravenous regional anaesthesia. The toxic threshold is considerably reduced in sick, frail and undernourished patients. Toxic levels are also more likely to be seen when there is reduced metabolism of the drugs in severe liver disease.

A variety of signs and symptoms occur, depending on the blood level and its rate of rise. For convenience these are divided into central nervous and cardiovascular effects, although both occur simultaneously.

Central nervous system

As the blood level increases a number of symptoms appear.

Cerebral cortex

- Sedation with the patient becoming drowsy. Lidocaine has been used in the treatment of status epilepticus.
- A variety of symptoms including circumoral paraesthesiae and pallor, fear, dizziness, excitement, tinnitus, anxiety. Some of these symptoms are similar to those of an overdose of epinephrine. In mild cases, these symptoms may pass off.
- Convulsions.

These signs and symptoms appear in this order only if the blood level increases gradually. If the blood level rises rapidly, as when an overdose is given into a very vascular area or following inadvertent intravenous injection, then the appearance of convulsions may be the first signs of toxicity.

Pons and medulla At the same time as the above symptoms are appearing there is increasing depression of the vital centres in the pons and medulla.

Cardiovascular system

With increasing blood concentrations there are a number of myocardial effects: increased refractory period, reduced excitability, prolonged conduction and decreased contractile force. Eventually ventricular fibrillation occurs. One of the serious consequences of bupivacaine overdose is the sudden appearance of ventricular fibrillation without warning.

Treatment

Convulsions should be treated with small divided doses of a benzodiazepine or short-acting barbiturate such as thiopental. If they are not controlled by small doses, a short-acting muscle relaxant should be given. Respiratory failure will require the administration of oxygen and controlled respiration, if prolonged, by the tracheal route. Circulatory failure should be treated by the administration of a pressor agent, or if this is ineffective, norepinephrine (noradrenaline) should be given by intravenous infusion.

MONOGRAPHS

BENZOCAINE

Benzocaine (rINN)

Pharmacology, indications and dosage

Benzocaine is the ethyl ester of *p*-aminobenzoic acid. The absence of a terminal amino group renders it insoluble; it is used as a local analgesic on mucous surfaces, and in various forms for surface analgesia of the mouth and throat, ear, and skin.

BUPIVACAINE

Bupivacaine (rINN)

Bupivacaine is the hydrochloride salt of (*dl*)-1-butyl-2'6'-pipecoloxylidide and is presented as the racemic mixture. It is four times as potent as lidocaine, is slower in onset, but has a significantly longer duration of action. It has a pKa of 8.1.

Pharmacology

Pharmacokinetics Bupivacaine is rapidly absorbed from the site of injection, but the rate of absorption is dependent on the vascularity of the site and the presence or absence of a vasoconstrictor in the solution. It has a long elimination half-life for a local anaesthetic (2.7 h) accompanied by a low plasma clearance (0.58 litres/minute); these tend to increase the risk of systemic toxicity. It is about 95 per cent protein bound, mainly to α_1-acid glycoprotein. Most of the drug is metabolized in the liver and only about 4–10 per cent appears unchanged in the urine. One of the metabolites is pipecoloxylidide (PPX) and others are the result of hydroxylation.

Pharmacodynamics The drug is slower in onset than other local anaesthetics, but has the longest duration of action of the existing drugs. The degree of motor block increases with increasing concentration, and at the highest available concentration (0.75 per cent) may outlast the sensory block.

Indications

Bupivacaine may be used for any nerve block with the exception of intravenous regional anaesthesia. It is particularly suitable for continuous epidural analgesia in labour. It is also of value for single-dose epidural injections for surgery.

Dosage and administration

Plain solutions of 0.75, 0.5 and 0.25 per cent are available, and also 0.5 per cent with epinephrine 1:200 000, and 0.25 per cent with epinephrine 1:400 000. Appropriate solutions may be used for all types of nerve blocks. Not more than 150 mg (30 ml of 0.5 per cent solution) should be given at one time or in any 4-hour period.

Toxicity

As with other local anaesthetics, toxicity is related to the plasma level of unbound drug and is most likely to be seen after inadvertent intravenous injection. The appearance of convulsions may be the first sign of toxicity under such circumstances. With local anaesthetics, CNS toxicity occurs at a lower dose than adverse cardiovascular effects, but under some circumstances this may not apply with bupivacaine. Cardiovascular toxicity is usually preceded by evidence of hypoxia associated with apnoea due to central depression, but on occasion bupivacaine causes primary ventricular arrhythmias, usually tachycardia but sometimes fibrillation. Because of its high degree of protein binding, cardiac resuscitation is difficult following bupivacaine toxicity.

Despite a considerable amount of research having been published on the topic, and despite various suggestions and recommendations, including bretylium, amiodarone and 1.8 per cent saline, no specific treatment has been shown to be more effective than general supportive measures alone.

Precautions

Because of its relatively greater toxicity on the heart in overdose it is not recommended for use intravenously for the technique of Bier's block in which accidental leakage into the circulation may occur.

Levobupivacaine (L-bupivacaine, S-bupivacaine). Concern over the toxicity of racemic bupivacaine led to investigations into the effects of the leavo enantiomer of bupivacaine, as studies have shown that most of the toxic properties of bupivacaine rest with the R-enantiomer.

Studies in laboratory animals have confirmed that levobupivacaine causes significantly less cardiotoxocity and fewer cardiac arrhythmias than the racemic mixture and at subconvulsant doses was significantly less stimulating to the CNS. These findings have been confirmed in a large number of animal studies. This higher level of safety of levobupivacaine over the racemic mixture has led to its clinical development. There appears to be no difference between the pharmacokinetics of the single enantiomer and those of the racemic mixture, and the onset, duration and degree of motor block also seem to be identical; levobupivacaine has identical potency to bupivacaine.

Many more studies are needed to see whether the margin of safety of levobupivacaine in regional anaesthesia is confirmed and to determine its eventual place in anaesthetic practice.

COCAINE

Cocaine or cocaine hydrochloride (rINN)

Pharmacology

Cocaine methyl benzoylecgonine, an ester of benzoic acid, is an alkaloid obtained from the leaves of *Erythroxylum coca*, a tree found in Peru, Brazil and other South American countries. The leaves have been chewed by the natives of these countries for centuries to produce euphoria and to increase their capacity for muscular work. Its local analgesic properties were discovered towards the end of the last century; its toxicity, however, was soon found to be too great for general use and an intensive search began for safer substitutes.

Cocaine has many actions in common with other local anaesthetics; it differs, however, in some respects.

Nervous system   There is marked central stimulation at first, which results in excitement, restlessness, euphoria and an increase in mental alertness. There is an increased capacity for muscular effort which is due to the loss of feelings of fatigue. Respiratory, vasomotor and vomiting centres are stimulated, and with increasing dosage convulsions will occur. Later, central stimulation gives place to depression, paralysis of vital centres, and death.

Cocaine blocks the re-uptake of norepinephrine (noradrenaline) into the pre-synaptic nerve terminal, the mechanism which is normally responsible for the termination of the action of the transmitter. It is therefore an indirectly acting sympathomimetic agent. Many of the signs of toxicity of cocaine can be explained in terms of excessive sympathetic activity. Centrally it also has marked dopaminergic effects.

Cardiovascular system   Slowing of the heart rate due to central vagal stimulation may occur after small doses. Larger doses induce all the signs of sympathetic stimulation, with tachycardia, peripheral vasoconstriction and hypertension; these persist until medullary depression or cardiac failure supervene. Ventricular fibrillation may occur quite early.

Respiratory system   Respiratory rate is increased, but depth is unaffected. As the dose is increased, the respiratory centre becomes depressed and respiration becomes rapid and shallow.

Musculature   There is no evidence of direct action on skeletal muscle, but smooth muscle is relaxed. Motor activity is well coordinated with small doses of cocaine, but as the dose is increased this activity increases and tremors and convulsive movements appear.

Mucous surfaces   When applied topically, cocaine produces excellent surface analgesia, with intense vasoconstriction. When applied to the eye, mydriasis occurs (sympathomimetic action) and the intra-ocular pressure is increased, but the effect is less than is seen with atropine. Cocaine has a deleterious action on the cornea, which may become clouded and pitted. This toxic effect is increased by the abolition of the normal protective eyelid reflexes. Because of this damage, and the tendency to produce mydriasis, cocaine has been replaced by other local analgesics in ophthalmology.

Fate in the body Cocaine is absorbed slowly on account of the vasoconstriction which it produces; in spite of this, toxic symptoms readily occur, as it is eliminated relatively slowly. It is mostly detoxicated in the liver, but a small quantity is excreted unchanged by the kidneys.

Indications

Cocaine can only be used with any degree of safety as a surface analgesic. It is still occasionally used for this purpose in nose and throat surgery and in ophthalmology.

Dosage and administration

Owing to its vasoconstrictor action, the use of epinephrine with it is not only unnecessary but increases the likelihood of cardiac dysrhythmias and ventricular fibrillation.

For surface analgesia, a 4 per cent solution is used for operations on the eye; 10 and 20 per cent solutions are employed for procedures on the nose and throat. It is stated that the 20 per cent solution is only slightly more toxic than the 10 per cent as absorption is slower. A dose of 100 mg (1.5 mg/kg) of the 10 per cent solution should not be exceeded in fit adults.

Precautions

Cocaine is rapidly absorbed from the nose and it is very easy to exceed the recommended dose when administered on gauze or wool plugs. It is advisable to administer a barbiturate before using cocaine, as it not only protects against the toxic effects of the drug but also acts as a sedative.

Cocaine is a drug of addiction; it differs from morphine and similar drugs in that it is taken for the euphoria and pleasing sensations it produces, rather than from the necessity to be free from withdrawal symptoms or pain. Present-day therapeutic uses of cocaine are unlikely to cause addiction.

An overdose of cocaine gives rise to excitement, restlessness and confusion. Headache, nausea and vomiting and abdominal pain are common. The pulse rate is increased and respiration is rapid and shallow. The temperature may rise and convulsions, coma and death may follow. Most, but not all, of these effects can be attributable to sympathetic over-activity, and the logical treatment is to diminish this both by central sedation and by competitive antagonism with adrenergic blocking agents. Both α- and β-receptor blocking agents may be needed. Propranolol 2–5 mg diminishes the tachycardia and protects against the onset of ventricular fibrillation, but has little effect on the hypertension. Phentolamine 5 mg should be given intravenously, and may need to be repeated every 15–20 minutes. Convulsions should be controlled with a small dose of thiopental; if this is ineffective, muscle relaxants and artificial ventilation will be required. Ventricular fibrillation, probably the most usual cause of sudden death in such cases, should be treated by cardiac massage and electrical defibrillation.

LIDOCAINE (LIGNOCAINE)

Lidocaine hydrochloride (rINN)

Pharmacology

Lidocaine is an aminoacyl amide and a derivative of acetanilide. It is an effective local anaesthetic with a rapid onset of action which is intense and lasts some 60–90 minutes.

It has a tendency to cause vasodilatation and this is normally counteracted by the addition of a vasoconstrictor. It has a potent action on mucous surfaces when applied topically and produces sedation with some lessening of reaction to pain when given intravenously. Less than 10 per cent is excreted in the urine and less than 7 per cent is excreted into the bile. The majority is broken down in the liver to monoethylglycine xylidide, and thence hydrolysed by liver amidases to 2,6-xylidine and 4-hydroxy-2,6-xylidine. Glycine xylidide is also formed. The rate of metabolism is doubled by pretreatment with phenobarbital.

Pharmacokinetics   Following a single rapid intravenous injection, the plasma level declines in two distinct phases. The first phase lasts approximately 30 minutes and exhibits a half-life of approximately 10 minutes. This decline primarily reflects a redistribution of the drug into various body tissues, including the heart. The rapid uptake into the heart is responsible for the immediate onset of anti-arrhythmic effect, and the rapid fall in blood levels is probably responsible for the short duration of action following a single intravenous bolus injection. The second phase manifests a half-life of approximately 90–120 minutes and is more representative of the clearance of the drug from the body.

Indications

Lidocaine is used for the production of local anaesthesia by infiltration, nerve, epidural and caudal block and topical application. It has been employed for spinal analgesia, but is not used extensively for this purpose in Great Britain. It is employed for the control of myocardial irritability and ventricular arrhythmias, particularly in the acute treatment following myocardial infarction. The anti-arrhythmic properties of this drug differ distinctly from those of other drugs in that the depressant action on ectopic foci is not accompanied by a significant slowing of the conduction of normal impulses. Furthermore, in normal therapeutic dosage there is no change in myocardial contractility, systemic arterial blood pressure or peripheral vascular tone.

Dosage and administration

Epinephrine, unless otherwise contra-indicated, is normally used with lidocaine to delay absorption and prolong the action.

Infiltration analgesia   A 0.5 per cent solution is commonly employed. The maximum dose is 100 ml (500 mg) with epinephrine and 40 ml (200 mg) without. If the operative field is such that larger amounts are necessary, a 0.25 per cent solution with epinephrine should be used, when 300 ml (750 mg) may safely be given.

Nerve block   A 1 per cent solution is used with epinephrine, up to 10 ml for single nerves and 15–30 ml for brachial plexus block.

Epidural and caudal block   A solution of 2 per cent lidocaine with 1:200 000 epinephrine produces a block similar in distribution and density to that produced by plain 0.5 per cent bupivacaine. However, its onset is more rapid and the duration of the block is less.

Spinal block   There is extensive experience outside the United Kingdom of using lidocaine for spinal anaesthesia. A 2 per cent isobaric solution produces an effect which is similar to that produced by isobaric 0.5 per cent bupivacaine with regard to distribution and intensity, but with a more rapid onset and shorter duration of action. There have been several reports (Hampl *et al.*, 1996; Corbey and Bach, 1998) of both transient and permanent radicular pain postoperatively which may be more common with continuous spinal anaesthesia and the use of 5 per cent hyperbaric solutions. One must bear in mind that this complication has also been reported after the use of spinal bupivacaine, although less commonly.

Surface analgesia   For the cornea, a 2 per cent solution is used. For the pharynx, larynx and trachea, a 2 per cent solution, maximum 8 ml, or a 4 per cent solution, maximum 4 ml, may be used. Analgesia of the mouth and pharynx may also be effected by the sucking of a lozenge (250 mg). A 2 per cent jelly is used for the urethra.

A 5 per cent preparation containing hyaluronidase, a 5 per cent ointment and a 2 per cent jelly are also available for surface application and for the lubrication of instruments used for endoscopy.

Intravenous local analgesia   25-40 ml of 0.5 per cent lidocaine is used for the arm. The average dose required is 30 ml. Up to 50 ml may be needed in the leg.

Toxic symptoms involving the CNS are not uncommon shortly after deflation of the tourniquet, particularly if the interval since administration is short. They are less likely in the sedated patient and are very rarely serious. In spite of this possible danger, this technique is often employed for the production of anaesthesia of the upper limb, especially for outpatients. Prilocaine is the preferred drug.

Treatment of arrhythmias

Because of the pharmacokinetic characteristics referred to above, lidocaine takes 6–8 h to reach a steady plasma level when given by continuous infusion. To obtain and maintain adequate blood levels it is necessary, therefore, to precede the infusion with a loading dose of 50–100 mg given by slow bolus injection. A further two such doses may be given at intervals of 15–20 minutes. The continuous infusion should run at a rate of 2.4 mg/min. A 0.2 per cent solution in 5 per cent dextrose is commonly employed.

Precautions

Precautions are as for other local anaesthetics.

Hampl, K.F., Schneider, M.C., Bont, A. and Pargger, H. (1996) Transient radicular irritation after single subarachnoid injection of isobaric 2% lidocaine for spinal anaesthesia. *Anaesthesia*, **51**, 178–81

Corbey, M.P. and Bach, A.B. (1998) Transient radicular irritation (TRI) after spinal anaesthesia in day-care surgery. *Acta Anaesthesiologica Scandinavica*, **42**, 425–9

PRILOCAINE

Prilocaine hydrochloride (rINN)

Prilocaine is a local analgesic closely related chemically to lidocaine. It is equally effective as an analgesic, its duration of action is longer, and it is less toxic. It is equally active on mucous surfaces by topical application, and systemic effects also are similar. It is broken down by amidases in the liver.

Prilocaine is an effective local analgesic but is less potent dose for dose than lidocaine. It is less toxic, but in large doses cyanosis due to the formation of methaemoglobin may occur, due to the action of the metabolite *o*-toluidine. This complication occurs only when doses of the order of 0.6 g are employed. Cyanosis usually disappears within 24 h. If treatment is urgent, methylene blue 1 mg/kg may be given intravenously.

Indications

Prilocaine is used for the production of local anaesthesia by infiltration, nerve, epidural and spinal block, by topical application, and intravenously for limb anaesthesia, for which purpose it has advantages over lidocaine as it is less toxic.

Dosage and administration

Prilocaine is available in 0.5–2 per cent solutions, with and without epinephrine, and also with felypressin, an analogue of vasopressin. This powerful vasoconstrictor is without effect on the myocardium and is much to be preferred as a local vasoconstrictor. Doses and volumes employed are similar to those of lidocaine; slightly larger maximum doses may be given – 400 mg of the 0.5 and 1 per cent solutions without epinephrine, 600 mg with epinephrine.

For intravenous analgesia a 0.5 per cent solution is used. For spinal use a 5 per cent solution in 6 per cent dextrose is used in a dose of 0.6–2 ml.

ROPIVACAINE

Ropivacaine hydrochloride (rINN)

Ropivacaine is an amide local anaesthetic and is the hydrochloride salt of 1-propyl-2'-6'-pipecoloxylidide. It belongs to the same group of drugs as mepivacaine and bupivacaine. Unlike the latter two drugs, which are presented as a racemic mixture, ropivacaine is the pure S-enantiomer. It is structurally identical to mepivacaine and bupivacaine, except that the former has a methyl group on the piperidine nitrogen atom whereas bupivacaine has a butyl and ropivacaine a propyl. Ropivacaine has a pKa of 8.07.

Ropivacaine was developed following concern about the cardiotoxicity of bupivacaine. This followed reports of maternal deaths in the USA resulting from the accidental intravenous injection of 0.75 per cent bupivacaine during epidural anaesthesia. In the United Kingdom, five deaths were reported following intravenous regional anaesthesia when bupivacaine was used, almost certainly due to faulty tourniquets. As a result, 0.75 per cent bupivacaine was banned from use in obstetric practice.

Pharmacology

Pharmacokinetics   Ropivacaine is highly protein bound, approximately 94 per cent, and has a lower lipid solubility than bupivacaine. In animals, clearance of ropivacaine is greater than bupivacaine, and this also applies in humans. The terminal elimination half-life (111 minutes) is also less than that of bupivacaine. Ropivacaine is largely metabolized in the liver and only about 1 per cent is excreted unchanged in the urine. The major metabolites are 3-OH and 4-OH ropivacaine, 2-OH methyl ropivacaine and 2'-6'-pipecoloxylidide (PPX).

Pharmacodynamics   Ropivacaine is an effective long-acting local anaesthetic. Most studies have indicated that ropivacaine has a slightly shorter duration of action than bupivacaine, but that there appears to be a greater degree of separation of sensory and motor block. The motor block of equivalent doses of bupivacaine and ropivacaine is slower in onset with the latter and of shorter duration. Increasing the concentration of ropivacaine increases the density of motor block. Ropivacaine is effective in a 1 per cent concentration for surgical anaesthesia via the epidural route. The lesser degree of motor block is a significant advantage for ropivacaine over bupivacaine during epidural analgesia in childbirth.

Toxicity

The toxicity of bupivacaine was the main stimulus for the development of another local anaesthetic agent. Animal work has consistently shown that ropivacaine is less toxic to the myocardium than bupivacaine. Studies have shown that ropivacaine lies between lidocaine (least) and bupivacaine in myocardial depressant activity. Bupivacaine produces more serious arrhythmias than ropivacaine in the isolated heart, whereas lidocaine produced none. In human volunteers, ropivacaine was 25 per cent less toxic to the cardiovascular and central nervous systems than bupivacaine following an infusion of 10 μg/minute up to 150–250 mg (Caderholm, 1997). Knudsen *et al.* (1997) found that the maximum tolerated dose in human volunteers for CNS symptoms was higher after ropivacaine during intravenous infusion of 10 μg/minute of ropivacaine or bupivacaine. The maximum tolerated unbound arterial plasma level was twice as high after ropivacaine while the time to disappearance of all symptoms was shorter after ropivacaine.

Caderholm, I. (1997) Preliminary risk benefit analysis of ropivacaine in labour and following surgery. *Drug Safety*, **16**, 391–40
Knudsen, K., Beckman-Suurkula, M., Blomberg, S., Sjovall, J. and Evardsson, N. (1997) Central nervous system and cardiovascular effects of i.v. infusions of ropivacaine, bupivacaine and placebo in volunteers. *British Journal of Anaesthesia*, **78**, 507–4

TETRACAINE (AMETHOCAINE)

Tetracaine hydrochloride (rINN)

Pharmacology

Tetracaine (amethocaine) is an ester local anaesthetic belonging to the procaine group. By subcutaneous injection it is effective in a 1:4000 solution. Its onset of action is slow (5 minutes or more) but its duration is 2–3 h.

Its pharmacological effects are similar to those of local anaesthetics in general; these include a stimulant and later depressant action on the CNS, a quinidine-like action on the heart, and a direct action on blood vessels causing vasodilatation. Like cocaine, it may cause sudden cardiac failure with asystole or ventricular fibrillation, which its quinidine-like action is not strong enough to stop. In contrast with procaine it produces excellent surface analgesia. The 1 per cent solution is approximately equivalent in potency to 10 per cent cocaine.

Detoxification takes place in the body, where it is hydrolysed by plasma cholinesterase, but it is eliminated at a much slower rate than the shorter acting local analgesics such as procaine and lidocaine. p-Aminobenzoic acid is a metabolite, and while present in the circulation will inhibit the action of sulphonamides.

Indications

Tetracaine is used for infiltration anaesthesia, regional, spinal and extradural block, and for surface analgesia. It is often mixed with procaine or lidocaine to combine the rapid action of the latter agents with its own prolonged effect.

Dosage and administration

Unless specifically contra-indicated, tetracaine should normally be used with epinephrine (adrenaline). Authorities vary considerably in the strength of solution and total dosage recommended for the different procedures for which this agent is employed. The following are effective and allow a reasonable margin of safety.

Infiltration and regional block Strengths of solution from 1:1000 to 1:4000 may be employed with epinephrine. Not more than 100 ml (100 mg) of the 1:1000 solution should be used; if a greater volume is required, a weaker solution must be given. The 1:4000 solution is reasonably effective and up to 500 ml may be used.

For nerve block a 1:1000 solution is used: up to 30 ml for brachial plexus block and up to 10 ml for individual nerve block, such as intercostal and pudendal.

Surface analgesia For the cornea, 0.5 or 1 per cent solutions are employed. For the pharynx, trachea and larynx, up to 8 ml of a 0.5 per cent solution may be used; stronger solutions should be avoided as they are relatively more toxic. The maximum dose is 40 mg. A 1:1000 solution is used for anaesthesia of the urethra, and a 2 per cent suppository for that of the rectum and anus. Anaesthesia of the mouth and pharynx can be effected by the sucking of a lozenge (65 mg). It should be started 20 minutes before operation and ejected as soon as analgesia is established. Solutions may be sterilized by boiling or autoclaving, but repeated sterilization by these methods causes deterioration. They are rapidly inactivated in the presence of alkalis and many antiseptic solutions.

Ametop is a formulation of tetracaine available for producing surface analgesia of intact skin containing 4 per cent tetracaine w/w of the base. It takes the form of a white, opalescent gel, each gram containing 40 mg of tetracaine base. It has the advantage of being faster in onset and of longer duration of action than EMLA cream and produces some vasodilatation (see page 206). Application for 30 minutes provides sufficient analgesia for venepuncture and 45 minutes for venous cannulation. The gel should be removed after 45 minutes, but analgesia persists for 4–6 h. It should not be applied to broken skin or mucous membranes.

Spinal block A 1 per cent solution in 6 per cent dextrose is used, 0.5–2 ml being injected according to the height of analgesia required. Alternatively, the calculated dose of tetracaine crystals (5–20 mg) may be dissolved in CSF and injected similarly.

For extradural block, a 0.15 per cent solution may be employed, 15–50 ml being injected according to the extent of block required.

Precautions

Precautions are as for local anaesthetics in general. Tetracaine is, however, a highly toxic agent and it is important that maximum doses are not exceeded. This applies especially to its use for analgesia of the respiratory passages.

Symptoms and treatment of overdose are discussed on page 209.

Other local anaesthetics

Chloroprocaine hydrochloride was introduced into USA practice in 1952, but has not yet been marketed in the United Kingdom. It has become increasingly popular in America for obstetric analgesia because of a very rapid rate of onset. However, it also has a similarly rapid rate of offset and is of relatively short duration. It is metabolized by plasma cholinesterase and claimed therefore to have minimal effects on the fetus.

The chief area of anxiety about the drug is related to reports of persistent or prolonged neurological deficit following its use, and some evidence of neurotoxicity.

Cinchocaine is a powerful local anaesthetic with a long duration of action which has been used for local infiltration, regional, spinal and extradural block, and for surface analgesia. It is no longer in use in clinical practice in the United Kingdom. Its main claim to fame is the fact that it is employed in 10^{-5} M concentration as a differential inhibitor which will distinguish between usual and atypical forms of plasma cholinesterase, under its original trade name of Dibucaine.

Etidocaine is a long-acting agent with a chemical structure similar to that of lidocaine and bupivacaine. It has been reported on quite widely but not yet introduced to the United Kingdom market. It has four times the potency of lidocaine but only twice the toxicity, thus giving it a better therapeutic ratio. It has a rapid onset of action and a prolonged action which is attributed to high plasma protein binding (94 per cent) and a high oil/water partition coefficient (141).

Its most characteristic difference from other agents is its ability to produce intense motor blockade which facilitates surgery. The small proportion which is unbound to protein may limit the amount that will cross the placenta. These two factors suggest a possible use in Caesarean section. It is used as a 1 or 1.5 per cent solution.

Mepivacaine has properties which place it somewhere between bupivacaine and lidocaine. It is a local anaesthetic of the amide type, with a rather more rapid onset and longer duration than lidocaine. Its chief advantage is an absence of any vasodilator effect on injection, so that the addition of a vasoconstrictor is unnecessary. Two or 3 per cent solutions are usually employed for nerve blocks; more dilute solutions are used for surface and infiltration analgesia. Solutions may be sterilized by autoclaving.

Procaine was first synthesized by Einhorn in 1905. It is a safe and effective local analgesic but it has been superseded by amide anaesthetics of various kinds and is no longer available in the United Kingdom. It has similar systemic actions to other synthetic local anaesthetics.

Local anaesthetics used in the eye

Oxybuprocaine is probably the most widely used topical agent in the eye. It is twice as potent as tetracaine and has twice the therapeutic ratio. It is less irritant to the conjunctiva in similar concentrations. One drop of 0.4 per cent is sufficient to render the conjunctiva anaesthetic.

Proxymetacaine causes less initial stinging and may therefore be particularly useful in children. It is used in a concentration of 0.5 per cent. Lidocaine (4 per cent) is also effective in this location as is tetracaine (0.5 per cent). Cocaine (4 per cent) is very effective but is no longer to be recommended for repeated use as it causes clouding and pitting of the cornea, as well as being a powerful mydriatic.

7

Drugs affecting mood

An improvement in mood, a stimulation of behaviour and other CNS functions can be induced by a wide range of drugs, and one or more of these effects may be complementary to a drug's main (therapeutic) purpose. For example even CNS depressants in small doses, such as ethyl alcohol, the barbiturates or benzodiazepines, may induce temporary stimulation because of their disinhibitory effects on behaviour.

However, several groups of drugs exist specifically to enhance mood in depressive illness (the *antidepressants*), increase alertness (the *psychomotor stimulants*) and heighten or distort mental awareness (the *psychotomimetics* or *hallucinogens*). One or more of these agents may fill a clinical need in some area of anaesthesia; more likely, their pre-admission use by a patient awaiting a surgical procedure may interact with the patient's responses to the drugs used by the anaesthetist.

Antidepressants

Depressive illness and related affective disorders are among the most common conditions that justify treatment with psychoactive drugs. Depressive illness is probably a collection of conditions sharing common (but not identical) symptoms.

By and large, two main groups of conditions are recognized. Firstly, *endogenous* (sometimes psychotic) depression, which does not appear to be precipitated by, or related to, specific life events. In its most severe forms, the illness alternates between depressive and manic phases (bipolar illness). Alternatively, depressive illness may be described as *exogenous* (or reactive) depression, which at least in its early stages appears to be linked to some recent life event, such as severe debilitating or life-threatening illness, redundancy at work, divorce, or the death of a loved one. Predictably perhaps, clinical depression often falls somewhere between these two forms. Fortunately, the antidepressant drugs currently available seem to be equally effective against both groups of illness, irrespective of the possible underlying causes.

It is estimated that perhaps a third to a half of all depression goes unrecognized or untreated; prolonged depression can become very resistant to drug treatment; and commonly, today's treatment requires prolonged medication lasting months or years. In the United Kingdom, some £200 million is spent on prescribed antidepressant preparations every year; further, the cost of other medical services and interventions is double this figure. Ultimately, the overall costs to society from the disruptive effects of a depressed family member are incalculable, but in the United Kingdom alone probably accounts for several billion pounds in social costs and loss of earnings. It has been estimated that 75 per cent of the United Kingdom's annual 4500 suicides may be suffering from a depressive illness, often unrecognized, immediately prior to taking their lives.

Antidepressant drugs, perhaps surprisingly, are often CNS depressants, at least following a single dose and during the early stages of treatment. The tricyclic antidepressants such as imipramine or amitriptyline, are chemically related to the phenothiazine neuroleptics and their introduction into clinical practice in the late 1950s followed serendipitously upon clinical trials of new anti-schizophrenic drugs when a number of agents were shown to improve depressive feelings. At the same time, chance observations of the stimulant side effects of certain experimental anti-tuberculosis drugs eventually led to the recognition of monoamine oxidase inhibition in the CNS, and it was suggested that the consequent enhancement of dopamine, norepinephrine (NE; noradrenaline) and 5-HT (5-hydroxytryptamine, serotonin) neurotransmitter functions might underpin an antidepressant action. Tricyclics and monoamine oxidase inhibitors (MAOIs) have proved to be effective clinical tools. They are, however, difficult to use. There is a high

Table 7.1 A classification of antidepressants based on chemical structure and pharmacological properties*

A. Neurotransmitter amine re-uptake inhibitors
NE/5-HT non-specific

Tricyclics	(tertiary amines)	Amitriptyline, imipramine, dothiepin
	(secondary amines)	Nortriptyline, desipramine
Non-tricyclic (SNRIs)		Venlafaxine

NE specific

Tricyclic	(secondary amines)	Maprotiline
Non-tricyclic		Tamoxetine†

5-HT specific

Tricyclics	(tertiary amines)	Clomipramine
Non-tricyclics (SSRIs)		Fluoxetine, paroxetine, sertraline, citalopram

B. Mono-amine oxidase inhibitors (MAOIs)
MAO-A&B non-specific inhibitors

Hydrazines (irreversible)	Phenelzine
Non-hydrazines (irreversible)	Tranylcypromine

MAO-B specific inhibitors

Irreversible	Selegiline (deprenyl)
Reversible	Brofaromine†

MAO-A specific inhibitors

Irreversible	Pargyline
Reversible (RIMAs)	Moclobemide

C: Antidepressants of miscellaneous structure and/or pharmacology

Pre-synaptic α_2-adrenergic receptor antagonists	Mianserin
Drugs acting on post-synaptic second-messenger systems	Rolipram†
GABA-ergic agents	Progabide†
Mood-stabilizing drugs	Lithium ions

* Since the underlying subcellular causes of depressive illness are only poorly understood, it is not possible to state with certainty which pharmacological properties initiate clinical improvement. It is assumed that any agent which raises the functional levels of CNS aminergic neurotransmitters will promote clinical improvement – argument continues, however, whether this is primarily a pre- or post-synaptic phenomenon. Drugs marked (†) are not licensed in the United Kingdom. NE = norepinephrine; 5-HT = 5-hydroxytryptamine; RIMAs = reversible inhibitors of monoamine-oxidase A; GABA = gamma-aminobutyric acid.

incidence of intrusive side effects and serious delays in therapeutic response following the start of medication. Consequently, the world's pharmaceutical industry has invested substantial sums to find better antidepressants.

Precious little advance has been made in understanding the biochemical basis of depressive illness, and many theories have been advanced following upon the introduction of the tricyclics and MAOIs in 1957. Most authorities today, whether they come from a clinical psychiatric or biomedical sciences background, accept that depressive illness is probably caused by an absolute or relative lack of function of one or more of the aminergic transmitters, namely 5-HT, dopamine or NE, a view continuously reinforced by the pharmacological properties of each new antidepressant class introduced. Controversy remains as to whether it is better to enhance aminergic function by a pre- or post-synaptic intervention, although recent work has revealed a deficiency in post-synaptic, post-receptor intracellular G-protein levels in untreated depressed patients, which is rectified following clinical improvement with antidepressant treatment. This might imply that the initial increased G-protein levels are themselves a consequence of post-synaptic receptor malfunction which has prompted compensatory G-protein synthesis.

The classification of antidepressants in *Table 7.1* is based upon a consideration of the drugs' chemical structures and their primary pharmacological properties, although in every case it remains to be proved whether the primary or alternatively some (unknown) secondary pharmacological action is ultimately responsible for the upswing in mood and the consequent clinical improvement. The fact remains that for all classes of antidepressant drug, clinical improvement is not manifest for some 3–5 weeks after commencing medication. The existence of concomitant intrusive adverse effects with many of these drugs is a serious impediment to achieving therapeutically useful (and tolerable) concentrations of these drugs in the body.

Neurotransmitter re-uptake inhibitors

Tricyclic antidepressants

The tricyclics, so called because of their phenothiazine-derived three-ring structure, are epitomized by imipramine and amitriptyline. These drugs possess a number of pharmacological actions both in the CNS and peripherally, with a consequential high incidence of parallel and usually adverse effects. Their primary pharmacological action is to inhibit the re-uptake of pre-synaptically released norepinephrine and 5-HT (there is little direct effect on dopaminergic synapses). Since re-uptake is by far the most important physiological route to inactivation for both neurotransmitters, it is assumed that re-uptake blockade is followed by an enhancement of transmission at noradrenergic and 5-HT synapses. Since this pharmacological action can be demonstrated in man within a few hours of starting medication yet is followed (if at all) by a clinical improvement that takes some 3–5 weeks to emerge, it is not unreasonable for many biologists and psychiatrists to assert that the eventual subcellular therapeutic action of the drug must lie in some secondary adaptive change, perhaps at a post-synaptic level. Possibilities include changes in post-synaptic receptor number or sensitivity, or in the secondary transmitter processes.

These delays in the appearance of a therapeutic response exist with all current groups of antidepressants, and many workers today accept that the development of a clinical improvement from depressive illness is inherently and unavoidably a slow process. This would be consistent with the illness being caused by a malfunction of one or more types of post-synaptic aminergic receptor, perhaps in their linkage to intracellular secondary transmitters such as G-proteins. However, where a patient is maintained in hospital and

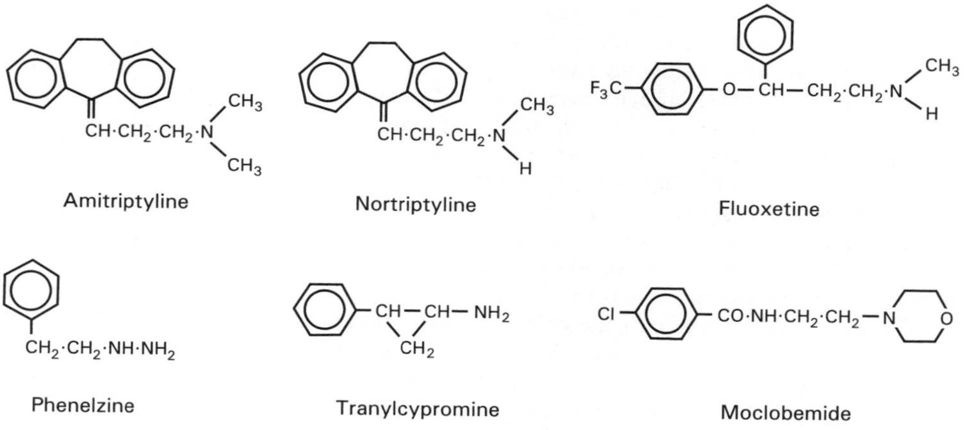

Figure 7.1 Structures of representative antidepressant drugs. *Amitriptyline* (tertiary amine) and its metabolite *nortriptyline* (secondary amine) are typical 'tricyclic antidepressants' (TCAs). The SSRI *fluoxetine* bears little structural resemblance to TCAs, and its spectrum of pharmacological properties differs markedly. *Phenelzine* (hydrazine) and *tranylcypromine* (non-hydrazine) are early irreversible, non-specific inhibitors of MAO (A and B) and are associated with dietary tyramine pressor effects (the 'cheese syndrome') – in contrast, the reversible MAO-A inhibitor *moclobemide* (RIMA) appears not to be

subjected to periodic, routine, objective mood assessment questionnaires, significant upswings in mood can be detected as early as the fourth day of treatment with an antidepressant drug, although, subjectively, that same patient will wait a further two or three weeks before 'feeling better'. Where tricyclics have been used alone or in combination with analgesics in the treatment of chronic or terminal pain, there is evidence of a much earlier onset of therapeutic effect, which may imply that it is the nature of the clinical condition rather than some delayed pharmacological action that determines onset of therapeutic effect.

Tricyclic antidepressants may be tertiary or secondary amines, according to the substitution on their aliphatic side chain (see *Figure 7.1*). Tertiary amines (e.g. imipramine, amitriptyline and clomipramine) are more potent inhibitors of 5-HT uptake than NE uptake, and are also significantly more sedative than their corresponding secondary amines (e.g. desipramine, nortriptyline, desmethylclomipramine) which favour NE uptake inhibition. This difference in sedative properties may be useful in calming agitated depressed patients (and has been exploited as a night-time anxiolytic to assist sleep even in patients not suffering from depressive illness): but this is unlikely to have a long-term therapeutic relevance, since the liver rapidly de-aminates the tertiary amines to their secondary amine equivalents (imipramine to desipramine, amitriptyline to nortriptyline). After 10–14 days of treatment, the plasma levels of the secondary amine metabolites often exceed those of the parent drugs.

Adverse effects

All tricyclic antidepressants induce a range of adverse effects. These include antimuscarinic activity, which impairs visual accommodation, salivation, gastro-intestinal movement, urination and sexual function. The enhancement of norepinephrine (and, peripherally, also epinephrine) function can lead to serious cardiovascular sensitization, and the tricyclics are contra-indicated in patients with impaired cardiac function. The tricyclics are also toxic following acute overdose, and overdoses are difficult to reverse.

Although the British National Formulary contains precise guidance on 'safe' doses for most tricyclic antidepressants, it must also be recognized that some psychiatrists believe that these doses fall below those required by many patients to achieve a clinical improvement. The guideline doses for tricyclics are therefore likely to be exceeded where depression is persistent. Most psychiatrists talk of a 'therapeutic window' which varies markedly between patients. This alludes to the need to exceed some tissue concentration if antidepressant activity is to be developed, and involves gently increasing the dose until side effects become almost too intrusive. Certainly many of the acute adverse effects can be avoided by giving the whole of the daily dose of a tricyclic at bedtime, when its greater sedative effects may also promote sleep. Higher doses may be accompanied by frank neuroleptic-type effects, emphasizing the pharmacological antecedents (the phenothiazine antipsychotics) from which the tricyclic antidepressants were developed.

In intensive care, the sedative tricyclics can be used to good effect as night sedation during 'ICU psychosis' which is often more manifest at night. They are effective and there is little hangover into the following day. The mood-elevating effect is usually also indicated, and can be regarded as an added bonus to the use of the drug for sedation. However, many patients in intensive care are prone to tachyarrhythmias, which are a relative contraindication.

Selective serotonin re-uptake inhibitors

Fluoxetine (also paroxetine, sertraline and more recently, citalopram) represent a new series of neurotransmitter uptake inhibitors. These exert a selective blockade of 5-HT presynaptic re-uptake: as a result, the term serotonin-specific re-uptake inhibitors (or SSRIs) has become an accepted generic title. They are not without significant adverse effects, but these appear to be better tolerated than in the tricyclics. As a consequence, patient compliance is higher and the incidence of clinical recovery is better. There also appears to be some gradation of clinically useful effects with increasing dose, in contrast to the tricyclics where the difference between an ineffective dose and an intolerable one is usually very small. A number of adverse effects related to the enhancement by SSRIs of central and peripheral 5-HT function can be troublesome. These include anorexia and insomnia, while peripherally the most significant effects are nausea and diarrhoea. However, SSRIs are considerably less toxic in acute overdose. Fluoxetine is currently the most commonly prescribed. The parent drug has a half-life of about 2 days, but is metabolized to a still active form, which has a half-life of about 5 days. The drug's effects are thus persistent, and before changing medication (e.g. before switching to a MAOI) a washout period of 5–7 days must be allowed.

Depression is common in the later stages of a prolonged period in intensive care, and in patients prone to tachyarrhythmias, fluoxetine (rather than a tricyclic antidepressant) is a rational choice. It is not sedative, but instead causes mild arousal and is thus best given in the morning.

That fluoxetine and other SSRIs are more expensive to prescribe may explain the continuing widespread use of the tricyclics, although compared with the wider and more substantial costs of depressive illness to society, differences in the costs of medicines should not be so influential. The potential value of a single dose of a tricyclic as a night-time sedative should not be overlooked where use of a benzodiazepine might be contra-indicated.

Serotonin and norepinephrine re-uptake inhibitors

Another recent sub-class of antidepressants that inhibit the pre-synaptic re-uptake of transmitter amines are the so-called SNRIs, the 'Serotonin and Norepinephrine Re-uptake Inhibitors', of which venlafaxine was possibly the first. Double blind studies have demonstrated that venlafaxine possesses antidepressant activity comparable to the tricyclics and SSRIs, with a similar 3–5 week delay in the appearance of clinical improvement. The major factor here in justifying another combined re-uptake inhibitor class of antidepressant is undoubtedly their structural differences from the earlier tricyclics. As a consequence, the pattern of adverse effects for SNRIs is both different and less intrusive, with no significant anticholinergic effects of note. Until the relative importance of serotonin- and norepinephrine-functional deficits in depressive illness have been elucidated, there seems merit in the development of new drugs which mimic the presumed desirable properties of the tricyclics, while avoiding their adverse effects.

While the belief continues that an actual or functional deficit of one or more neurotransmitter amines underlies the development of depressive illness, new drugs will continue to be introduced which enhance one or more of the trio of neurotransmitters, viz. norepinephrine, dopamine and 5-HT. Different profiles of re-uptake inhibition will feature among the pharmacological properties of new drugs. Moving away from the tricyclic structure has yielded a new clutch of drugs whose therapeutic potential is at least as good as that of the tricyclics, yet possess a totally different and generally far more acceptable spectrum of adverse effects.

Monoamine oxidase inhibitors (MAOIs)

Monoamine oxidase (MAO) is an array of subtly different enzymes, which can be partly classified according to their location (intra- or extracellular) and their main substrates. When the MAO inhibitory properties of iproniazid were first demonstrated in the middle 1950s, the existence of different MAO enzymes was only suspected. In the event, iproniazid, other hydrazine MAOIs and early non-hydrazine MAOIs such as tranylcypromine were irreversible inhibitors of all MAO enzymes. Undoubtedly their major and most notorious adverse effect was the precipitation of a serious (and often fatal) hypertensive crisis, subsequently shown to be caused by the ability of dietary tyramine (and related phenylethylamines present in some foodstuffs such as soft cheeses, red wine and yeast derivatives) to avoid gastro-intestinal and hepatic degradation by MAO which was blocked by the attendant MAOI. As a consequence, tyramine appeared in the systemic circulation where it exerted significant sympathomimetic activity through the release of adrenal and other endogenous sympathetic stores of epinephrine and norepinephrine. Today, MAO can be classified into two main types, MAO-A and MAO-B. Although MAO-A is found mainly intraneuronally and is believed to control available levels of neurotransmitters (principal substrates being dopamine, norepinephrine and serotonin), and MAO-B extraneuronally where it has mainly an elimination role (e.g. associated with glial cells in the CNS), in fact both isoenzymes have overlapping roles in man and are frequently found together. Recently, specific sub-type inhibitors have been introduced, for example selegiline (MAO-B inhibitor) and moclobemide (MAO-A inhibitor), the latter being a *reversible* inhibitor. Clinical experience with moclobemide suggests that it is devoid of interactions with tyramine-rich foods and drinks, due mainly to the reversible nature of its MAO inhibition. MAOIs have never been widely used as first-line treatment in primary care, but the selectivity, reversibility and increased safety of moclobemide may result in its wider use in the community. Selegiline is a selective MAO-B inhibitor used in anti-Parkinson therapy. It is not an antidepressant, but is included here for convenience. One possible mode of action is its ability to inhibit MAO-B found in glial cells, with a subsequent enhancement of nigrostriatal dopamine function. On a theoretical basis at least, tyramine-containing foodstuffs should be avoided by patients receiving selegiline treatment.

Miscellaneous antidepressants

Almost by definition, a 'miscellaneous' group will be different from the main categories of antidepressants, and perhaps have niche value or be used only in special circumstances. Four agents are worthy of note.

Amoxapine is a non-tricyclic antidepressant and has adverse effects similar to those of the tricyclics. While safer than the tricyclics in acute overdose, there are longer-term adverse effects such as extrapyramidal symptoms and tardive dyskinesia. It has a niche market, and is likely to be prescribed only in secondary care following referral for resistant depression.

Lithium salts, usually carbonate or citrate, are used to help control conditions such as manic-depressive psychosis or related, persistent bipolar disorders. Lithium is more a 'mood stabilizer' than an antidepressant. Its mode of action is a subject of much debate. One possibility is that Li^+ ions compete for NA^+/K^+ binding sites on ATP-ase in the axonal membrane, thus slowing axonal recovery following an action potential and stabilizing the axonal membrane. Among other effects, lithium inhibits adenylate cyclase (an intracellular enzyme widely involved in linking transmitter and hormonal agents) at many locations, and thus has wide toxic potential (see Monograph below).

Mianserin was introduced in the 1970s, against a background of tricyclic and older MAOI antidepressants with intrusive and dangerous adverse effects. On starting treatment, mianserin exerts a non-benzodiazepine type of sedation and tranquillity, which many depressed patients find comforting and indicative of useful drug activity. The drug is also much safer in acute overdose and has found particular use where suicidal thoughts are suspected. Its antimuscarinic effects are much less marked, and it does not interfere with neurotransmitter amine re-uptake either in the CNS or peripheral nervous system, and thus has a much lower propensity for interfering with anaesthesia, or inducing cardiotoxicity. It is profoundly sedative, and can be expected to enhance pre- and post-anaesthetic anxiolytics and analgesics and night-time sedatives. As with other antidepressant drugs, little is known of the pharmacological action which underpins its therapeutic effects, although chronic experiments in animals and man have revealed a progressive down-regulation in pre-synaptic α_2-receptors which normally regulate the availability of neurotransmitter amine. There is also some potentiation of brain 5-HT and attenuation of brain β-adrenergic function, but the relative importance of any of these properties in the clinical improvement is not known. Mianserin's main impediment to continuing widespread clinical use is its propensity for causing leucopenia, aplastic anaemia and agranulocytosis, and full blood counts must be carried out every 4 weeks during a patient's first 3 months of treatment.

Rolipram is an antidepressant not available in the United Kingdom or USA, but available in continental Europe. It is unique in possessing a site of action 'beyond' the synapse and post-synaptic membrane, where it is thought to be a selective inhibitor of cyclic AMP-dependent phosphodiesterase. It thus modifies (and at many sites promotes) secondary neurotransmission linked with the catecholamines norepinephrine and dopamine.

Antidepressant agents and anaesthesia

There are no pharmacological effects in this group of drugs that might usefully assist pre- or post-anaesthetic medication, or be of use during anaesthesia, that cannot more easily and safely be induced by other agents. However, the anaesthetist will meet these agents where patients are admitted for some procedure coincidentally suffering from a depressive condition for which they are receiving drug therapy. Most of the antidepressants have a propensity for interfering with agents used by the anaesthetist.

Whichever group of antidepressants has been prescribed, and whatever the current state or prognosis of a patient's depressive illness, sudden discontinuation of antidepressant therapy is likely to precipitate a resurgence or recurrence of the depression. Where a patient has been admitted to hospital as an emergency, the expectation must be of a continuation of antidepressant medication throughout their period in hospital. Where a major operation or procedure can be planned some weeks ahead, the possibility of discontinuing antidepressant treatment should be discussed with the patient's mental health physician.

The tricyclics have a wide range of pharmacological properties that extend into the peripheral nervous system and cardiovascular system. Because these agents are markedly protein bound, blood levels progressively rise and therefore length of previous treatment may be as important as dose. They have marked central and peripheral antimuscarinic activity: this interferes with visual accommodation (and pupillary signs of the depth of CNS depression), reduces salivation (giving possible difficulties in swallowing), and slows gastro-intestinal propulsion and transit times. Tricyclics thus also increase the antimuscarinic effects of atropine, hyoscine and certain neuroleptics, for example chlorpromazine, promazine and thioridazine. Since each member of the tricyclic antidepressants is also a CNS depressant, they are likely to enhance the effects of other CNS depressants. This would suggest care with doses of both pre- and post-anaesthetic anxiolytics or analgesics, and with night-time sedatives. Finally and importantly, tricyclics also inhibit the uptake, and thus enhance the effects of, circulating sympathomimetic amines, whether these be of adrenal or external origins. Hypertension and possible cardiac arrhythmias are adverse effects specifically highlighted, and special risks may be posed in the presence of certain β-blockers. Because tricyclics are protein bound (up to 90 per cent in some patients), they may displace other drugs and thus enhance their effects. Attempting surgery on a cardio-compromised patient concomitantly prescribed a tricyclic antidepressant will have special high risks. If it is decided to stop tricyclic treatment, a washout period of about 10 days is desirable because of their persistence in the body. Fluoxetine can interact with indirectly acting sympathomimetics, other amine agonists and opioid analgesics: hypertension with CNS excitation is a possibility, particularly in combination with levodopa (L-dopa) and 5-HT agonists such as sumatriptan.

The older, irreversible and non-selective MAOIs such as phenelzine and tranylcypromine have a wide range of interactions, notably either hypertensive or hypotensive reactions with some analgesics such as pethidine and perhaps also nefopam. MAOIs can delay the metabolism of other drugs, thus enhancing their effects. They enhance the effects of hypotensive and antihypertensive agents. They enhance the effects of all indirectly acting sympathomimetic amines, and many direct agonists at other aminergic receptor sites. With the newer MAOI moclobemide, which is both reversible and a selective inhibitor of MAO-A, the list of interactions is smaller: marked excitation or depression, with hypertension or hypotension, may occur with pethidine, codeine or fentanyl and there may be interactions with indirectly acting sympathomimetics and agonists at other aminergic sites. Moclobemide is a relatively new drug, for which marked caution is being observed. The list of cautions may be revised when the drug's marketing authorization comes up for its first review. Selegiline, a selective inhibitor of MAO-B, while not being an antidepressant, is included here for convenience: it interacts with pethidine to cause hyperthermia and CNS toxicity, with fluoxetine to cause hypertension and excitation and with non-specific MAOIs to cause hypotension.

Lithium ion levels may be increased to toxic levels by ACE inhibitors, NSAID analgesics and loop diuretics, all of which delay its excretion; in contrast, oral antacid preparations may reduce plasma lithium levels to a point where therapeutic effect is lost. In combination with lithium salts, anti-psychotic agents can cause extrapyramidal effects earlier and at a lower dose than normally expected. Although not inducing any overt change in plasma levels, antihypertensive agents such as α-methyl dopa may induce signs of lithium neurotoxicity. Lithium can also induce signs of glucose intolerance in susceptible patients.

Psychomotor stimulants

These agents may cause a useful increase in alertness, although this is often associated with unacceptable changes in mood such as increased anxiety, or in the development of lethargy and depressive symptoms after stopping the drug. Not surprisingly, the majority of psychomotor stimulants are subject to tolerance and eventually dependence with repeated use.

The amfetamines have been used both legitimately and illicitly for almost 70 years, but have now largely ceased to be used in bona fide clinical medicine. Classed as centrally-acting sympathomimetics, they are significantly lipophilic and thus cross the blood–brain barrier, but their spectrum of pharmacological effects includes significant peripheral as well as central actions. (+)-Amfetamine, methamfetamine, cocaine and methylphenidate (to name four important examples) enhance the actions of a number of aminergic pathways where norepinephrine, dopamine and 5-HT are primary transmitters. Their ability to increase aminergic function is due to a variety of sub-cellular events, ranging from an inhibition of neurotransmitter re-uptake (at modest doses), a direct release of amines from pre-synaptic stores (at higher doses) or even direct agonist actions upon post-synaptic amine receptors. Increased dopaminergic and noradrenergic activities in the brain are thought to underlie the stimulant effects of the amfetamines, while noradrenergic and serotonergic function are involved in the appetite suppression, employed therapeutically in the use of fenfluramine as an aid to weight reduction.

All of these interactions with aminergic function are repeated peripherally. The amfetamines are indirectly-acting sympathomimetic agents within the cardiovascular system and behave rather like tyramine, releasing epinephrine and norepinephrine from adrenal and sympathetic nerve stores producing tachycardia, vasoconstriction and/or hypertension. Unlike tyramine, the amfetamines prolong the effects of catecholamines by blocking re-uptake into stores. Higher doses may be associated also with hyperthermia and, after prolonged central and peripheral stimulation, with dehydration. Cocaine additionally exerts local anaesthetic activity at the site of administration. Methylphenidate is a synthetic piperidine derivative, whose CNS stimulant effects more prominently raise mental alertness than motor activities. This may be linked to claims that it has a preferential action upon the ascending reticular formation and sensory cortex, although at higher doses it becomes more typically 'amfetamine-like'. Methylphenidate is legitimately used only to treat attention-deficit hyperkinesia in children or to treat narcolepsy.

Wartime folklore suggested that the amfetamines were useful not only in delaying fatigue and lethargy, but also in increasing athletic or mental performance. There is no evidence for the latter; indeed the associated euphoria and over-confidence produced by these agents are associated with an increased frequency of simple errors, which thus actually reduce efficiency and motor skills. The amfetamines and cocaine are Controlled Drugs (see Chapter 1, page 58), which means that there are specified restrictions on synthesis, distribution, possession and availability. Cocaine as a local anaesthetic has been overtaken by a plethora of synthetic agents with more predictable pharmacological properties. Its illegal use as a 'social stimulant', however, continues to escalate.

Notwithstanding the legal restraints on the use of amfetamines and cocaine, human beings continue to seek out stimulants from other sources and use them for quasi-social purposes. Linked with this, and also the illegal trade in opiate drugs, a number of 'designer drugs' (a termed coined in the USA) have appeared, emanating wholly from illegal laboratories and remaining outwith normal protocols for drug development, licensing and commercial distribution. Because of their notoriety and widespread use, two are worthy of mention here.

'**Ecstasy**' (3,4-methylenedioxy-methamfetamine – MDMA; not to be confused with NMDA receptors) is structurally related to methamfetamine and mescaline. It was initially developed as an appetite suppressant and also found some use in psychiatry in that it was said to facilitate communication and increase self-esteem; it may also have euphoric effects. More recently, it has found widespread use as a drug of abuse, being used as a stimulant particularly by young adults. This also applies to the related 3,4-methylenedioxyethamfetamine ('**Eve**').

Because of its non-legal status, collecting objective data about the pharmacological properties of MDMA in man has proved difficult. Apart from observational analysis of young people under its influence, most of the data available comes from experimental animals, the human effects then being interpreted from this animal data. MDMA combines amfetamine-like stimulant effects with hallucinatory (psychotomimetic) properties. The former seem to be linked to a stimulation of brain dopaminergic and noradrenergic pathways, while the hallucinatory properties appear more related to agonist effects of MDMA at 5-HT$_2$ receptors. Its acute effects are dose related: in addition to the sought-after stimulant and hallucinatory effects, it produces tachycardia, muscle aches and muscle-locking (e.g. jaw clenching). As the dose of MDMA is increased or sequential doses are added, agitation, hyperthermia and panic attacks appear. Although no lasting neurotoxic effects have been proven in man, persistent low levels of CSF 5-HT metabolites, memory loss and neurotoxic effects in experimental animals all point to stepwise irreversible changes in some 5-HT pathways.

Overdose may present in emergency departments with a variety of symptoms, usually having been taken against a background of vigorous dancing in a hot environment with limited access to fluid. The subject may be comatose with seizure activity, accompanied by a high temperature and profuse sweating. There is a tachycardia, but the blood pressure may be increased or decreased. The pupils are usually dilated. Rhabdomyolysis is a feature and disseminated intravascular coagulation and organ failure will rapidly develop in the absence of treatment; metabolic acidosis is invariable.

Treatment is supportive, with general measures to reduce the temperature and maintain cardiovascular stability. Renal function must be closely monitored and specific measures taken to treat hyperkalaemia and metabolic acidosis if these do not rapidly resolve. Convulsions must be controlled and controlled ventilation is frequently necessary. Use of dantrolene remains controversial, as cases have been successfully managed without it. However, it would seem reasonable to use if temperature control is not rapidly achieved, since hyperthermia will lead to permanent organ damage. A dose of 1 mg/kg intravenously should be given initially and repeated according to the response.

MPTP (*N*-methyl-phenyl-tetrahydropyridine) was a contaminant of illicitly produced pethidine in the USA. Converted by substantia nigral MAO-B into a neurotoxic quaternary ion (MPP$^+$), it destroys dopamine cell bodies, and causes premature Parkinsonism in the young – although irreversible, this is amenable to palliative treatment with levodopa.

Khat is a preparation from vegetable sources popular with ethnic groups with northern African or Arabic origins. The active principle is (usually) cathinone, which has CNS stimulant properties similar to the amfetamines. Cathinone has been modified clandestinely, and the more potent methcathinone has had modest success as another designer stimulant.

Cyclizine is used recreationally, alone and in combination with other stimulants (see Chapter 8).

Caffeine (chemically a methyl-xanthine and related to both theophylline and theobromine) is a central stimulant present in a range of beverages such as tea, coffee and others, found around the world. Caffeine is the most potent stimulant of the naturally occurring xanthines, and beverages are designed to yield a dose of 50–75 mg, which is sufficient to reduce drowsiness and fatigue, and, it is claimed, increase mental alertness and thought processes. Larger doses of caffeine can cause insomnia, restlessness and even tremors. Unlike the amfetamines, caffeine and the other methyl-xanthines neither induce euphoria nor leave behind a sense of drug loss as the agent is cleared from the body. Daily doses in excess of about 1500 mg (say 20 cups of strong coffee) are associated with intrusive feelings of restlessness and anxiety, while there is also significant stimulation of the heart and cardiovascular system. In special care baby units, caffeine may be given intravenously (as the citrate) to patients of 33 weeks' gestational age or younger, who have exhibited apnoeas with or without bradycardias. Its use is prophylactic, to reduce the likelihood of further episodes. Compared with theophylline, which can also be used, it causes less tachycardia, less inhibition of gastric motility and less reduction in cerebral blood flow. Both drugs increase urinary calcium excretion in this setting.

Psychotomimetics (hallucinogens)

Illusions, hallucinations and other changes in thinking are among the adverse effects associated with a number of centrally-acting drugs, particularly the amfetamines in overdose or during withdrawal from the chronic use of opiates, ethyl alcohol and the benzodiazepines However, there is a range of chemically-diverse agents which elicit sensory illusions or, less commonly, hallucinations, sometimes at extraordinarily low doses, which are not accompanied by other central or peripheral direct pharmacological effects. These drugs are called the psychotomimetics.

The terms 'mind bending' and 'mind expanding' have been used to describe the state produced by these drugs. There is a heightened awareness of self, associated with unusually vivid sensory experiences and an inner appreciation of the clarity and meaning of one's own thinking. The psychotomimetic effects induced by these drugs in otherwise healthy individuals have been likened to the symptoms that may occur in psychotic patients, although the similarities are incomplete. Although described as hallucinogenic, the drugs' principal action is to distort existing images (whether these be visual, auditory or tactile in origin), rather than inducing bizarre or profound sensory experiences in the absence of relevant environmental cues or stimulation – as is seen in some of the more simple psychotic states.

Psychotomimetic drugs are also regulated by the Controlled Drugs Act, which limits their synthesis, distribution, possession and use. The agents appearing most frequently in Western and other urban cultures are D-lysergic acid diethyl-amide (LSD25), mescaline, psilocybin, phencyclidine, bufotenin, *N,N*-dimethyl-tryptamine (NNDMT), harmine and myristicin. They are chemically diverse, their effective doses varying perhaps a thousand-fold. LSD25 is hallucinogenic in man at a dose of 50 µg. What they do have in common is the ability to vigorously and rather specifically enhance 5-HT function in the brain; indeed, NNDMT is a potent and specific 5-HT$_2$-receptor agonist. Furthermore, in animal studies their behavioural and electrophysiological effects can be prevented or reversed by the specific 5-HT$_2$ antagonist, ritanserin. However, few believe this is the whole explanation for their hallucinogenic properties. As therapeutic agents, psychotomimetics were once used to assist in the behavioural treatment of certain mental disorders, including some types of drug dependency, but currently they find little use in therapeutics.

Dopamine as a neurotransmitter in the central nervous system

Increasingly, the major neurotransmitters acetylcholine (ACh), norepinephrine (NE), 5-HT, dopamine (DA) and γ-aminobutyric acid (GABA) are being associated with discrete neuronal pathways and areas of the brain. With the current developments in molecular pharmacology and successive cloning of neuronal receptors, an increasing array of receptor subclasses are being identified at which these transmitters act. Indeed, in the same pathway, a transmitter may have both stimulant and depressant properties according to the receptor subclass that dominates at any particular time. It is too early to be certain how many of these receptors are 'constitutive' and how many are 'induced' by physiological or pathological change, but differences in pharmacological responses to certain drugs between healthy individuals and patients might well be explained by changes in the *dominant* receptor subclass during (or as a cause of) illness. For example, in both central and peripheral 5-HT pathways, up to 14 discrete 5-HT receptors have so far been identified and assigned to seven main subclasses. Identifying the roles of the individual receptor subclasses should help to further our understanding of clinical conditions as diverse as depression, mania, schizophrenia and Parkinsonism.

In addition to the three pathways outlined below, dopamine-releasing neurones with very short axons are found in the retina, and also in interneurones within the hypothalamus and specific frontal areas associated with olfaction. *Table 7.2* lists the major dopaminergic pathways (i.e. neuronal pathways in which dopamine is a major neurotransmitter) found in mammalian brain. As with other neurotransmitters, dopamine is released to act upon a family of receptor subclasses. Two such families are currently recognized:

Table 7.2 Dopaminergic systems found in the mammalian brain

System	Nucleus of origin	Sites of termination
Nigrostriatal	Substantia nigra	Neostriatum (caudate and putamen)
Mesocortical	Ventral tegmental area and substantia nigra	Limbic system (including limbic cortex, amygdala, nucleus accumbens, septum and anterior perforated substance), and frontal cortex
Tuberohypophyseal	Periventricular and arcuate nuclei of the hypothalamus	Pituitary median eminence

- D_1 and D_5 are pharmacologically similar, and *stimulate* the intracellular synthesis of the second messenger cyclic AMP;
- D_2, D_3 and D_4 inhibit the synthesis of cyclic AMP.

(Four further isoforms of D_1 and three of D_2 have also been identified by molecular studies, but the pharmacological significance of these has yet to be determined.)

The physiological response of a given pathway will be determined by which of these receptor subtypes dominates (e.g. by receptor density or sensitivity). Receptors D_1 and D_2 are found associated with almost all brain areas in which dopaminergic neurones terminate (but particularly in the striatum), and appear to be the most important receptors in the development and alleviation of Parkinsonism. D_3, D_4 and D_5 are much less abundant and more discrete in their distribution. Large amounts of dopamine are found in the basal ganglia (especially the caudate nucleus), the nucleus accumbens, the olfactory tubercle, the amygdala, the median eminence and certain areas of the frontal cortex.

D_1 and D_2 receptors have been implicated in the pathophysiology of both Parkinsonism and schizophrenia. In Parkinsonism, it is believed that the loss of dopaminergic neurones leads to interference with both an excitatory D_1 and an inhibitory D_2 pathway, and successful treatment with, for example, levodopa involves the restoration of both pathways. In schizophrenia, an inverse correlation exists between the clinical doses of many current anti-schizophrenic drugs and their affinities for D_2 receptors. Long-term blockade of D_2 receptors by conventional neuroleptics is associated with the appearance of extrapyramidal (Parkinsonoid) symptoms.

Interestingly, it has been suggested that D_3 and D_4 receptors may represent promising new and more specific targets for the next generation of anti-psychotic drugs: both receptors are located in limbic areas of the brain involved in the control of cognition and emotion, where the symptoms of schizophrenia may originate. Selective D_3 and/or D_4 antagonists should also 'spare' D_1 and D_2 receptors, thus (theoretically) offering the advantages of minimizing extrapyramidal and endocrine side effects associated with the current phenothiazine anti-psychotics. Of the existing anti-psychotic agents, clozapine shows high affinity for the D_4 receptor, while there is some evidence from animal studies that the D_3 receptor may be associated with stimulant behaviour, thus offering a possible target for overcoming the inhibitory symptoms of schizophrenia.

Dopamine is a substrate for both MAO-A and MAO-B, and in the cerebral cortex roughly half of the dopamine metabolized by MAO is broken down by each isoform of the enzyme. Significantly, the picture is very different in the basal ganglia: in the caudate nucleus, for example, about 95 per cent of dopamine is broken down by MAO-B which is thought to reside extraneuronally (associated with glial cells). The inhibition of MAO-B using the MAO-B specific inhibitor selegiline (formerly deprenyl) makes a logical adjunct to levodopa in the treatment of Parkinsonism. Recently, the development of dyskinesias in Parkinsonism has been found to occur more slowly when selegiline is combined with levodopa, and it is widely believed that selegiline may slow the pathological development of Parkinsonism.

Other CNS stimulants: analeptics

Analeptics mainly exert their effects upon the brain stem, principally upon the respiratory and vasomotor centres from which benefit might be derived in profound anaesthesia. As doses increase, analeptics stimulate wider areas of the CNS and will eventually induce cortical convulsions. The analeptics are a chemically diverse group and little is known about their subcellular mechanisms of action. Although they initially lighten narcosis, a generalized central depression may follow which is resistant to further stimulation.

Analeptics which found a clinical use were of two types: those that were thought to act reflexly through carotid body receptors (e.g. doxapram), and those that acted directly on the medullary centres (such as nikethamide, picrotoxin and ethamivan). The drugs shared a similar inhibitory effect on the function of inhibitory transmitters such as γ-aminobutyric acid (GABA) and glycine. Analeptics thus differ from other stimulants such as (+)-amfetamine, which act to specifically raise aminergic transmitter function. The greater sensitivity of spinal cord and brain stem centres to analeptics is a reflection on the sensitivity of these areas to the drugs and drug access, rather than any selectivity: higher doses of analeptics are much more indiscriminate in the centres they affect.

Analeptics were once used routinely in cases of poisoning by CNS depressant drugs, notably the barbiturates: the effects were unpredictable and large doses were likely to precipitate convulsions. Furthermore, the duration of action of analeptics was frequently shorter than that of the original poisoning drug; thus, second and further doses of analeptic appeared justified, each became less effective and the final outcome was a still deeper generalized CNS depression. The stimulant effects of analeptics were also associated with an increased metabolic rate which itself could become dangerous in a patient already hypoxic following respiratory depression or arrest. Other common adverse effects included cardiac arrhythmias and vomiting. Specific antagonists are available to treat CNS depression secondary to benzodiazepines (flumazenil) and to opiates (naloxone), but in other cases of pathological drowsiness, drug therapy to reverse the drowsiness is not used. The term 'analeptic' is absent from the 1996 9th edition of Goodman & Gilman's *The Pharmacological Basis of Pharmacology*, as also are any mention of the former analeptics nikethamide and bemegride.

Today, analeptics have an extremely limited use in therapeutics and only a monograph on doxapram is thought worthy of inclusion.

MONOGRAPHS

AMFETAMINE AND DEXAMFETAMINE

Amfetamine sulfate (rINN)
Dexamfetamine sulfate (rINN)
For structural formulae see *Table 12.2*, p. 326

Pharmacology

Amfetamine is a congener of epinephrine, being racemic 2-aminopropylbenzene. The dextro-isomer (dexamfetamine) is twice as potent as amfetamine and four times as potent as the laevo-isomer. In general, its actions resemble those of ephedrine and, like it, it is an indirectly acting sympathomimetic agent, but it is more powerful on the CNS and less so at all other sites. It has both α- and β-effects and is an inhibitor of MAO.

It is a mild euphoriant. Fatigue is abolished, wakefulness is promoted and more work can be done. There is increased initiative rather than ability and mistakes occur more frequently. In the usual oral doses there is little cardiovascular effect, but the blood pressure is usually slightly raised. It causes less restlessness and apprehension than ephedrine. Tolerance is not accompanied by greater rates of excretion or destruction.

Because of its CNS-stimulating properties, it is a drug of illicit recreational use and is one of the 'dopes' that can be taken by athletes to improve their performance. Chronic abuse produces dependence and can induce a schizophrenia-like state. Dexamfetamine sulphate has identical but more powerful actions, with a similar dose range.

Amfetamine and dexamfetamine are among those drugs that may be lawfully in the possession of only a few authorized categories of user.

Indications

Owing to its tendency to cause addiction, therapeutic uses are now restricted to narcolepsy and treatment of hyperactivity in children. It has been used to treat post-encephalitic Parkinsonism. The official dose of the sulphate is 2.5–10 mg orally.

Fate in the body   About half of an oral dose is deaminated in the liver and the other half is excreted unchanged in the urine in slightly more than 2 days.

AMITRIPTYLINE

Amitriptyline hydrochloride (rINN)

Pharmacology

This agent, one of the original tricyclic antidepressants, is a potent inhibitor of both 5-HT and norepinephrine (noradrenaline) uptake. Although substantially protein-bound in the plasma, unbound drug readily crosses most cell membranes and is distributed into all compartments, including the brain. As a tertiary amine, it is also markedly sedative, and in high doses displays neuroleptic activity. It is an effective antimuscarinic (atropine-like) both centrally and peripherally, which contributes to the compound's many adverse effects. As with all current antidepressants, the manifestation of clinical improvement is slow and may take 3–5 weeks. Because of its adverse effects, the whole of a day's dose is commonly given at night, thus assisting sleep and avoiding the worst of its peripheral anticholinergic effects.

Indications

Amitriptyline is used to treat depressive illness, whether reactive or endogenous, especially when a sedative effect would also be useful. In small doses it can be useful as an adjunct to other treatments of chronic pain. It can be used as night sedation for patients in intensive care. Amitriptyline is also indicated for nocturnal enuresis in children (up to 20 mg daily in children aged 7–10).

Fate in the body   Amitriptyline is readily absorbed from the gastro-intestinal tract, with peak plasma levels occurring at about 6 h. The antimuscarinic activity of the drug may delay gastro-intestinal transit, so that absorption after overdose may be delayed. Because of plasma protein binding, amitriptyline has a long plasma half-life that varies between 9 and 25 h, leading to progressive accumulation of both parent drug and metabolite in the plasma. Both the half-life and actual plasma levels are markedly affected by the extent of plasma protein binding, which can be as high as 85 per cent of the drug. The active desmethyl metabolite, nortriptyline, is detectable in plasma within 1 h of administering the first oral dose, and after 2 weeks' continuous treatment plasma levels of the metabolite nortriptyline may be higher than those of the parent drug. As a secondary amine, nortriptyline is less sedative, and shows some selectivity for inhibition of norepinephrine uptake. Both amitriptyline and nortriptyline are further metabolized in the liver, eventually forming water-soluble glucuronides: elimination occurs via the kidneys as inactive glucuronides, parent drug and various metabolites.

Dosage and administration

Because of the 30-fold variability between patients in the plasma levels achieved following a standard dose, treatment starts with a low dose twice daily, increasing over a period of days until adverse effects become intrusive. Treatment should start with 25 mg 3 times daily by mouth – increasing over a period of about 10 days to 150 mg daily, when it may then be taken as a single dose at night. Doses should be lower in the elderly. In all patients, onset of therapeutic effects is delayed by 3–5 weeks, although adverse effects may occur within hours of commencing treatment, depending on the initial dose. Patients may require encouragement and psychological support during this delay. After a clear recovery has been established, treatment should continue for at least 3–6 months and then be discontinued slowly. Abrupt discontinuation may precipitate a recurrence of depressive illness.

Precautions

Amitriptyline may give rise to a number of intrusive adverse effects. Peripheral antimuscarinic effects present as dry mouth, loss of visual accommodation, aggravation or initiation of glaucoma, urinary retention, constipation and tachycardia. These effects are most intrusive at the start of treatment or following an increase in dose, and markedly reduce patient compliance. Central adverse effects may include ataxia, arrhythmia and (rarely) convulsions, decreased REM sleep and fine tremor. The incidence and severity of these effects are directly related to dose. Amitriptyline enhances the sedative and incapacitating effects of ethyl alcohol. Cardiovascular effects linked to both the atropinic and norepinephrine (and epinephrine) potentiating effects may occur at any time during treatment. Effects on cardiac function include arrhythmias such as ventricular flutter and atrial fibrillation. Even at comparatively low doses, the ECG may show prolongation of the QT interval, ST depression and a flattened T wave. Patients receiving tricyclic antidepressants must thus be observed with care before, during and after anaesthesia. Tricyclics are contra-indicated in cardiovascularly compromised patients, especially with heart block or recent myocardial infarction.

Amitriptyline (and other tricyclics) and MAOIs mutually potentiate one another. They are occasionally used conjointly in some forms of resistant depression: this involves commencing treatment with low doses of both drugs simultaneously (as opposed to adding a drug from the second group to treatment already established with the other), in hospital, and under constant monitoring. When switching from treatment with one group to treatment with the other, a washout period of at least 10 days should be observed because of the persistence of their pharmacological effects.

Accidental overdose may occur insidiously, especially in the elderly or with compromised hepatic or renal function. In common with all tricyclic antidepressants, amitriptyline may be lethal in accidental or deliberate overdose, and requires active intervention. This should consist of minimizing the quantity of drug absorbed by promoting vomiting and carrying out gastric lavage on admission to hospital. Subsequent therapy is symptomatic and supportive: cardiac and respiratory function and body temperature should be continuously monitored, and appropriate interventions carried out where necessary. Successive doses of i.v. physostigmine or other anticholinesterase drugs may, exceptionally, be of use in reducing some of the more severe atropinic actions.

Nortriptyline (the desmethyl metabolite of amitriptyline) is also available as a licensed medicine. The range of pharmacological effects is essentially similar to amitriptyline and it is used in similar doses and protocols. Its clinical use is not associated with a more rapid onset of actions or a reduced array of adverse effects. Typical of other secondary amine antidepressants in the tricyclic series, nortriptyline exerts significantly less CNS depression.

DOSULEPIN (DOTHIEPIN)

Dosulepin (rINN) and Dothiepin hydrochloride (BAN)

Pharmacology

Dosulepin/dothiepin is another widely-used tricyclic antidepressant. It is an uptake inhibitor of both 5-HT and norepinephrine (noradrenaline). As a tertiary amine, it is markedly sedative, but is rapidly metabolized to the active secondary amine, desmethyl-dosulepin, which is a more selective norepinephrine-uptake inhibitor and is less sedative. Its other pharmacological properties, both desirable and adverse, are also qualitatively similar to those of amitriptyline and imipramine. Primary drug and active metabolite have elimination half-lives of about 20 and 35 h, respectively. Once- or twice-daily medication thus leads to steadily rising plasma levels of the drug (and metabolite) which plateau at about 14 days.

Indications

Dosulepin is used to treat depressive illness, whether reactive or endogenous, especially when a sedative effect would also be useful.

Dosage and administration

An initial oral dose of 75 mg (25 mg 3 times daily or 75 mg at bedtime) is usual, increasing to a maximum of 150 mg daily. Doses in the elderly are usually reduced. In common with all current antidepressants, most patients will not experience any improvement in mood for at least 3–5 weeks after commencing treatment, and this delay may be extended if treatment is commenced with low doses. In contrast, adverse effects may be experienced within a few hours, and in common with all other tricyclic antidepressants, patients require psychological support pending the onset of therapeutic effects. Following recovery from depressive symptoms, treatment with dosulepin should continue for 3–6 months, and subsequent withdrawal should be progressive.

In the absence of depressive illness and where the use of a benzodiazepine is to be avoided, dosulepin may be used as a night-time sedative at a dose of 50–75 mg.

Precautions

The desirable and adverse pharmacological actions of dosulepin are qualitatively similar to those of amitriptyline: adverse effects arise from its antimuscarinic actions in the CNS and peripherally. Through its enhancement of norepinephrine and epinephrine, it may exert unwanted cardiovascular effects. As with other tricyclics, dosulepin's use where cardiac function is compromised and/or following a recent myocardial infarct, is contraindicated. Dosulepin may be lethal following accidental or deliberate overdose. Treatment of overdose is as outlined in the monograph on amitriptyline.

DOXAPRAM

Doxapram hydrochloride (rINN)

Pharmacology

In low doses doxapram stimulates respiration, mainly by an effect on the peripheral chemoreceptors, resulting in an increase in tidal volume with only a small increase in respiratory rate. This is usually accompanied by a small increase in arterial blood pressure and heart rate mediated by the vasomotor centre, resulting in an increase in sympathetic nervous activity, and can be attenuated by β-adrenoceptor blockade.

The ratio of convulsant to respiratory stimulant dose is 70:1. This comparatively wide safety margin has led to doxapram largely displacing nikethamide and other analeptics on the decreasing number of occasions when such drugs are used. With intermediate doses, side effects such as a crawling sensation on the skin, restlessness, warmth, nervousness and nausea may occur. There is a rise in 11-hydroxycorticosteroids as a result of a central action.

In patients with chronic airways disease in respiratory failure there is a significant increase in minute volume and arterial oxygen tension, and a decrease in arterial carbon dioxide tension. The slope of the ventilatory response to carbon dioxide is steeper and displaced to the left.

Rapid administration can cause an increase in cardiac output and a rise in arterial blood pressure, but this is less marked during a slow infusion. Side effects such as vomiting, coughing and apprehension are rare.

Doxapram has a half-life of 2.5–4 h and may be given by bolus injection or continuous infusion.

Indications

Doxapram should be used in the short term only during acute episodes of deterioration or when ventilation has been depressed by sedative drugs. It is no longer indicated as an analeptic to hasten recovery from anaesthesia, while it has been replaced by naloxone in the reversal of respiratory depression due to opiate overdose. An exception is buprenorphine whose firm binding to receptors renders naloxone relatively ineffective, and doxapram, which produces non-specific stimulation, can be useful. Unlike naloxone, it does not reverse the analgesia produced by opiates. When its action stops, the respiratory depression may return. Furthermore, there are many clinical situations when analgesia is required, but a reduction in the convulsive threshold would be undesirable. Another situation when doxapram has something to offer is in patients with chronic obstructive pulmonary disease in whom intensive care is thought inappropriate. An acute exacerbation is associated with respiratory depression secondary to hypercapnia, and stimulating the respiratory centre with doxapram may pull the patient back from this 'slippery slope'.

Doxapram increases alveolar ventilation in respiratory failure secondary to chronic pulmonary disease.

Dosage and administration

For the treatment of early respiratory failure, doxapram may be given as a 0.2 per cent solution in 5 per cent dextrose at a rate of 1.5–3 mg/minute. It can be given continuously for several days.

Precautions

Doxapram is contra-indicated in severe hypertension, thyrotoxicosis, status asthmaticus and significant coronary artery disease. It should be used with caution in patients with epilepsy. Its action is potentiated by MAOIs.

FLUOXETINE

Fluoxetine (rINN)

Pharmacology

Fluoxetine (well known in the lay press as Prozac, the 'happiness' drug) is pharmacologically and structurally dissimilar to the tricyclic antidepressants. It has seized a major share of both the North American and European markets for antidepressant drugs, this despite a very substantial price disadvantage.

It is a serotonin-specific re-uptake inhibitor (SSRI). As the description suggests, it singles out the pre-synaptic transport processes that take up neuronally-released 5-HT, exerting little or no effect on the re-uptake of either norepinephrine (noradrenaline) or dopamine. Since a deficiency or malfunction of 5-HT figures strongly in current theories of the underlying biochemical cause of depressive illness, fluoxetine's selectivity of action is thought to represent an advantage over the tricyclics. More important, however, is its different array of adverse effects. These do not include any significant atropinic action, widely believed to be responsible for poor compliance with tricyclic antidepressants such as imipramine. Fluoxetine's CNS adverse effects include appetite suppression and difficulty in getting to sleep, while peripherally an enhancement of 5-HT function is manifested as diarrhoea. Its interaction with catecholamine function is minimal.

Dosage and administration

Fluoxetine is given by mouth, 20 mg once, twice or thrice daily, with the last dose taken no later than lunchtime to reduce interference with sleep. The vast majority of patients do not experience any significant improvement in mood for at least 3 weeks, yet mild to modest adverse effects may be experienced soon after commencing treatment. The nature of the adverse effects are such that most patients can be encouraged to continue medication and await the onset of therapeutic effects. Following recovery from depressive symptoms, patients should continue with fluoxetine treatment for at least 3–6 months. Cessation of treatment should be gradual. The adverse effects profile of fluoxetine is such that the drug may be continued indefinitely at a lower dose as prophylaxis against recurrence.

Precautions

Fluoxetine should not be prescribed for children. It should not be used by nursing mothers, since the drug may appear in breast milk up to 25 per cent of its plasma concentration, when disturbances to infant feeding and sleep may be apparent. In underweight patients, fluoxetine may promote further weight loss. Interactions with MAOIs are predicted, and a washout period of at least 14 days must be allowed when switching from one form of therapy to the other. Care should be taken when fluoxetine is used simultaneously with lithium salts, anticonvulsants and opioid analgesics.

Patients with significant renal or hepatic impairment may show drug accumulation upon prolonged treatment, with increased incidence and severity of side effects. The drug's persistence in the body is such that alternate-day treatment is recommended if treatment must continue in the presence of renal or hepatic impairment.

On current evidence, fluoxetine is not significantly toxic in accidental or deliberate overdose, at least when it is the only drug so abused. Single doses up to 3000 mg have been recorded without fatal outcome. Restlessness, agitation, gastro-intestinal stimulation and convulsions may occur following significant overdoses, but should regress spontaneously. The anti-5-HT agent, cyproheptadine, may be a suitable antidote for peripheral effects.

Sertraline, paroxetine and **citalopram** are also SSRIs, although structural similarities with fluoxetine are difficult to demonstrate. Like fluoxetine, their principal pharmacological effect is to delay or hinder the transport process involved in the re-uptake of neuronally-released 5-HT, thus promoting the physiological effects of 5-HT at central and peripheral sites. Like fluoxetine, their adverse effects profile is fundamentally different from the tricyclic antidepressants such as imipramine and amitriptyline. The drugs are thus better tolerated, withdrawal rates appear to be lower, and they are effective at reduced doses in preventing disease recurrence. Their exact profiles of adverse effects show differences related to their chemical structural differences, although like fluoxetine they can delay sleep and cause gastro-intestinal disturbances. Each of them is subject to the same delays in onset of therapeutic action that is experienced with fluoxetine and other antidepressants.

IMIPRAMINE

Imipramine hydrochloride (rINN)

Pharmacology

This compound was the first tricyclic antidepressant. Originally tested for antihistaminic and anti-psychotic activity, clinical observation in schizophrenic patients revealed an underlying antidepressant action. As a tertiary amine, it is a potent inhibitor of both 5-HT and norepinephrine (noradrenaline) uptake, and exerts significant antimuscarinic activity. Its profile of pharmacological and clinical effects is remarkably similar to those already described for amitriptyline. Thus it is well absorbed following oral administration, protein binding extends its plasma half-life, and hepatic metabolism yields an active metabolite, desmethyl-imipramine (desipramine); as a secondary amine, desipramine is less sedative and, eventually, achieves plasma levels equal to or in excess of the parent compound. The kidneys excrete the parent compound, its metabolites and inactive glucuronides.

Indications

Imipramine is used to treat depressive illness, whether reactive or endogenous, especially when a sedative effect would also be useful. It is also indicated for nocturnal enuresis in children.

Dosage and administration

Like amitriptyline, imipramine is normally given orally, commencing with a low dose (25 mg 3 times daily) which is increased progressively to a usual maximum of 200 mg daily, all of which may be taken as a single dose at night. Appearance of a therapeutic action is usually delayed by 3–5 weeks, while the onset of adverse effects may occur within a few hours of commencing treatment. Patients may need encouragement and psychological support during this delay in the onset of beneficial effects. Doses should be reduced in the elderly.

Following upon recovery from the depressive illness, treatment with imipramine should be continued for at least 3–6 months, following which discontinuation should be gradual. For nocturnal enuresis, an oral dose at bedtime up to 50 mg is advised for children 8–11 years old.

Precautions

Imipramine can produce a range of adverse effects that are qualitatively similar to those of amitriptyline. These are related to marked antimuscarinic effects: in the periphery, they cause loss of visual accommodation, dry mouth, increased gastro-intestinal transit times, constipation and urinary retention. At a central level, effects include ataxia, arrhythmia, convulsions (rarely) and an altered balance between REM and non-REM sleep. There is also peripheral enhancement of norepinephrine and epinephrine which can initiate changes in cardiovascular function. Imipramine is contra-indicated in patients with compromised cardiac function and/or evidence of a recent myocardial infarct.

Imipramine may be lethal following accidental or deliberate overdose. Supportive measures, outlined under amitriptyline above, will be required.

Desipramine is desmethyl-imipramine, and is also licensed and available as an antidepressant. It is associated with significantly less sedative effects than imipramine, but in all major ways its pharmacology and therapeutic indications are the same.

LEVODOPA

Levodopa (rINN)

Pharmacology

Levodopa is practically inert: its main effects are produced by the product of its decarboxylation, dopamine. About 95 per cent of an oral dose is decarboxylated in the periphery but the dopamine that is produced, although responsible for side effects, does not cross the blood–brain barrier. Consequently, large doses need to be given to ensure that sufficient levodopa penetrates the brain. Levodopa is more commonly given in combination with carbidopa, which inhibits the peripheral decarboxylation of levodopa by an action on the enzyme L-amino acid decarboxylase. Carbidopa, however, does not penetrate the brain. By limiting only the extracerebral decarboxylation, more levodopa is available to penetrate the brain and the adverse side effects caused by systemic dopamine are reduced. The therapeutic use of systemic dopamine is described in Chapter 12.

Central nervous system   It is believed that levodopa produces its effects by enhancing the transmitter stores in the degenerating dopaminergic pathways between the corpus striatum and substantia nigra. This relieves the tremor, rigidity and akinesia. Levodopa also relieves the mental apathy associated with Parkinsonism and gives a sense of well-being. In a significant proportion of patients, psychiatric disturbances occur, ranging from agitation and insomnia to hypomania and frank psychosis. These symptoms tend to be dose dependent.

Cardiovascular system   The dopamine produced systemically exerts both α- and β-stimulating effects on adrenoceptors. This is largely abolished by the administration of carbidopa. Orthostatic hypotension is also a feature and is not so modified; it is believed to be a centrally mediated effect of CNS dopamine. Tolerance to these side effects tends to develop after several months.

Gastro-intestinal system   Nausea, vomiting and anorexia are common and are due to stimulation of the chemoreceptor trigger zone, another dopaminergic area of the brain.

Endocrine system   Levodopa inhibits the secretion of prolactin, but stimulates the production of growth hormone. Some effects on insulin and glucose metabolism are probably secondary to the increased levels of growth hormone.

Fate in the body   Levodopa is rapidly absorbed from the gut: the majority is decarboxylated in the gut and liver by L-amino acid decarboxylase, so that little unchanged drug reaches the circulation. This metabolism can be markedly influenced by the concurrent administration of the inhibitors carbidopa and benserazide hydrochloride.

Metabolism of dopamine is principally to 3,4-dihydroxyphenylacetic acid (DoPAC) and 3-methoxy-4-hydroxyphenylacetic acid (homovanillic acid or HVA). The metabolites are excreted in the urine.

Indications

Levodopa is used in the treatment of Parkinsonism; the majority of such cases are caused by idiopathic degeneration, but the disease can occur as a late consequence of encephalitis lethargica. It is not effective in the treatment of Parkinson-like extrapyramidal reactions to drugs such as the butyrophenones and some phenothiazines that have strong dopamine antagonist effects.

Dosage and administration

Initial dosage alone is 0.5–1 g daily in divided doses, gradually increasing to about 2.5–3 g daily in 2–3 weeks. Full benefit may not be reached for 3–4 months, when dose levels may range from 3–6 g daily. Given in combination with carbidopa in a ratio of 10:1, the total dose must be reduced by 75 per cent.

Precautions

The majority of patients experience side effects, but fortunately tolerance usually develops to most of them. The commonest early effects are nausea, vomiting and orthostatic hypotension. Cardiac arrhythmias occur, particularly in patients with pre-existing conduction defects. Psychiatric disturbance is a significant late consequence. Levodopa may interfere with diabetic management. It is contra-indicated in narrow-angle glaucoma. It should not be given to nursing mothers; even if lactation is not inhibited, it appears in the milk. There is animal evidence of teratogenicity. Stimulation of melanocyte-stimulating hormone may lead to growth of melanomas.

Pyridoxine (even in the amounts found in over-the-counter vitamin pills) increases peripheral decarboxylase activity and diminishes the amount of free levodopa available for penetration of the brain. Discontinuation of therapy for 6–24 h prior to anaesthesia is recommended, although no untoward reactions have been reported.

LITHIUM

Lithium carbonate (rINN)

Pharmacology

Although inherently toxic, lithium ions are useful 'mood stabilizers' and find a prophylactic and therapeutic use in manic and excited states, and in conditions where serious or rapid mood swings between extremes are a central feature. As a simple monovalent ion, Li^+ competes with Na^+ and K^+ in many physiological processes, notably in neurones and at other cell surface sites. In the tissues, lithium ions appear to be mistaken for sodium or potassium, but do not enter properly into cellular processes, for example the sodium pump. However, large concentration differences of lithium ions are not maintained either side of membranes, and thus they do not properly substitute for the physiological cations. Lithium is not a stimulant, sedative or euphoriant drug. It is best described as a 'neurotransmission modulator', and this property may form the basis of its mood-stabilizing effects.

Indications and dosage

Lithium is used in patients with acute mania, hypomanic episodes and for the control of aggressive and self-mutilating behaviour. In severe or endogenous psychotic depression, lithium is more effective in 'bipolar' than 'monopolar' conditions. Lithium carbonate is administered orally at 400–1200 mg daily, usually in divided doses, although under certain conditions the whole daily dose may be given before retiring or immediately on waking. In the elderly or those weighing significantly less than 70 kg, lower doses may be indicated. Importantly, serum lithium levels should be measured at about the fifth day after commencing treatment, and thereafter at 5–7-day intervals for as long as therapy continues, with a view to maintaining serum lithium levels between 0.5 and 1.5 mmol/litre. Although some control of mood swings may be apparent within 3–5 days of commencing treatment, continuing 'prophylaxis' of 6–12 months may be necessary to establish full control. The use of lithium carbonate in children and during adolescence is not recommended.

Precautions

The advised serum levels of lithium are important to maintain, the lower to ensure continuous clinical control, the upper to avoid toxicity. Toxicity is dose (or rather concentration) dependent: above serum levels of 1.5 mmol/litre, adverse effects include diarrhoea, weakness, thirst, drowsiness and ataxia. Above these levels, confusional states, convulsions and coma may ensue, leading to death. Lithium carbonate may induce modest hypothyroidism in up to 10 per cent of patients. It has also been linked with nephrogenic diabetes insipidus, through an interference with the effects of ADH. Lithium treatment is contra-indicated in patients with renal failure or renal tubular disease. It may interact adversely with muscle relaxants and anti-psychotic drugs. Simultaneous use of certain diuretics, steroids and NSAIDs can reduce lithium clearance or otherwise increase serum levels, thus precipitating toxic effects. Lithium is contra-indicated during pregnancy and lactation: if its continued use cannot be avoided, close monitoring of serum lithium levels and maintaining these levels between advised limits is vital.

METHYLAMFETAMINE

Methylamfetamine hydrochloride (rINN)

Pharmacology

Methylamfetamine is a derivative of amfetamine and has similar properties of increasing function of CNS pathways involving norepinephrine (noradrenaline), dopamine and 5-HT, but is more rapid in effect and acts for a longer period of time. It is an indirectly acting sympathomimetic drug that has both α- and β-effects. Its action on the cardiovascular system is more prolonged, but weaker, than that of amfetamine, whereas in equal dosage it has double the stimulant effect on the CNS.

Central nervous system   There is marked central stimulation and it produces an elevation of mood and general euphoria. It causes wakefulness and has some analeptic effect on the unconscious. Prolonged cerebral stimulation is followed by depression.

Cardiovascular system   As with epinephrine (adrenaline) there is an increase in cardiac output, force, rate and irritability. This is accompanied by peripheral vasoconstriction, although overall peripheral resistance may be increased or unchanged. Renal blood flow is increased. Systolic blood pressure is increased, but the rise in the diastolic pressure is less marked.

Respiratory system   There is no effect on bronchial musculature, but respiration is stimulated.

Gastro-intestinal tract   There is no inhibitory action on the plain muscle of the alimentary tract. Like amfetamine, it reduces appetite.

Fate in the body   Recovery from overdose may take several days, as it is excreted in the urine very slowly. Elimination can be increased by making the urine more acidic.

Indications

Methylamfetamine is a recreational drug with no medical indications.

Dosage and administration

Methylamfetamine is active by mouth, intramuscularly or intravenously. Recreational users often 'snort' a powdered form.

MOCLOBEMIDE

Moclobemide (rINN)

Pharmacology

Moclobemide is a MAOI antidepressant. It is a reversible inhibitor of the enzyme subclass, MAO-A, and thus represents the first of a new class of antidepressants. The introduction of an MAOI which targets only MAO-A, means that the body's natural defences to dietary amine absorption (oxidative deamination by gastro-intestinal and hepatic stores of MAO-A and MAO-B) are left effectively intact. For the time being, however, the possibility of food- or beverage-induced pressor effects in patients treated with moclobemide must be anticipated. Moclobemide in common with earlier MAOIs interacts with other drugs that modify aminergic neurotransmission at central and/or peripheral levels.

As a basis of its antidepressant actions, moclobemide is believed to delay the MAO-A-based intracellular destruction of 5-HT, an effect which is thought to lead to increased pre-synaptic stores of the neurotransmitter. While raising 5-HT CNS stores is consistent with theories of depression which invoke actual or functional 5-HT deficiencies, the drug is not CNS selective, so that peripheral 5-HT stores will also be raised. Furthermore, while 5-HT is a key substrate for MAO-A, the enzyme also metabolizes norepinephrine (noradrenaline) and dopamine. Levels of these transmitters in both CNS and peripheral stores therefore are also likely to be raised, and perhaps contribute to moclobemide's spectrum of desirable and undesirable effects.

Indications

Moclobemide is used to treat depressive illness, whether reactive or endogenous.

Dosage and administration

Moclobemide is administered by mouth, usually 150 mg twice daily. There is no general requirement to reduce the dose for the elderly or those with renal impairment. In hepatic disease, dosage may need to be halved. Its use in children is not currently recommended.

While moclobemide's pharmacological actions may be demonstrated within a few hours of commencing medication, signs of therapeutic recovery may take some days to appear, and substantial clinical improvement (as with all other current antidepressants) may take some 3–5 weeks to establish. Because of the reversible nature of its MAO-A inhibitory action, discontinuing moclobemide and substituting treatment with an alternative antidepressant does not require a washout period. As with the treatment of depressed patients generally, withdrawal of active medication should be gradual.

Precautions

Moclobemide should not be used in patients with phaeochromocytoma or other conditions associated with raised catecholamine levels. It is also likely to interact with other drugs where increased neurotransmitter function can lead to potentiation of effects, including therefore pethidine and related opioid analgesics, other antidepressants including both tricyclic antidepressants and other MAOIs. In animal studies, no risks to the fetus have been demonstrated during gestation, although the complete safety of moclobemide during pregnancy has yet to be established. On the other hand, only very small amounts of the drug pass into the milk if medication is continued or implemented during lactation.

In accidental or deliberate overdose, moclobemide is not seriously and immediately life threatening, but continuous supervision and preparedness to support vital functions is a treatment necessity.

8

Histamine, antihistamines; drugs affecting bronchial calibre

Histamine

Histamine is the oldest and most familiar of a group of substances that share the common property of being naturally-occurring agents with intense pharmacological actions, predominantly at the local site of release. This group also includes serotonin (5-hydroxy-tryptamine, 5-HT), 'slow-reacting substance in anaphylaxis' (SRS-A), the prostaglandins, angiotensin, and the various kinins. They have been referred to as local hormones, but the generic term, autacoid (Greek, *autos* – self, and *akos* – medicine) is now being applied to such substances. The more important of these (other than histamine) are discussed in Chapter 16.

Histamine is found in almost all mammalian tissues, (Greek, *histos* – tissue) particularly in the mast cells where, like heparin, it is present in high concentration. In allergic and anaphylactic reactions, both substances are liberated together. The structural formula of histamine is given in *Figure 8.1*.

It is an intensely active substance biologically, producing responses on suitable isolated tissues in concentrations much less than 1 part in 10^6. Histamine is present in an inactive form in intracellular particles, and is liberated from the tissues by trauma, certain drugs and other substances. It is found widely in nature, not only in animal tissues but also in plant and vegetable cells, in nettle stings, and in the stings of certain insects such as wasps.

The chief actions of histamine are contraction of plain muscle and dilatation and increased permeability of capillaries. It also stimulates secretions, especially of the oxyntic cells of the stomach, and causes secretion of epinephrine and norepinephrine from the medulla of the adrenal glands.

These actions are largely mediated by two types of receptors, which have been named H_1 and H_2, the actions being modulated by a third type of histamine receptor. H_2-receptors are involved in the release of acid in the stomach and in some of the cardiovascular effects of histamine. H_1-receptors mediate all the other actions of histamine discussed below. Both H_1- and H_2-receptors can be blocked by appropriate competitive antagonists. Recently discovered H_3-receptors appear to be involved in autoregulatory functions in both the CNS and the periphery.

The actions of histamine have been intensively studied, but even now its true physiological role is uncertain. In man, the highest concentrations are found in the skin, intestine and lung – parts in contact with the outside world. It has been suggested that the vasodilatation it produces may reduce the pathogenicity of invading organisms.

Action on plain muscle

Histamine was first isolated from ergot, and its action studied on the uterus, which it stimulates in most species whether this organ is isolated or *in situ*. It has a direct stimulant action on bronchiolar muscle which is unrelated to nervous innervation and usually

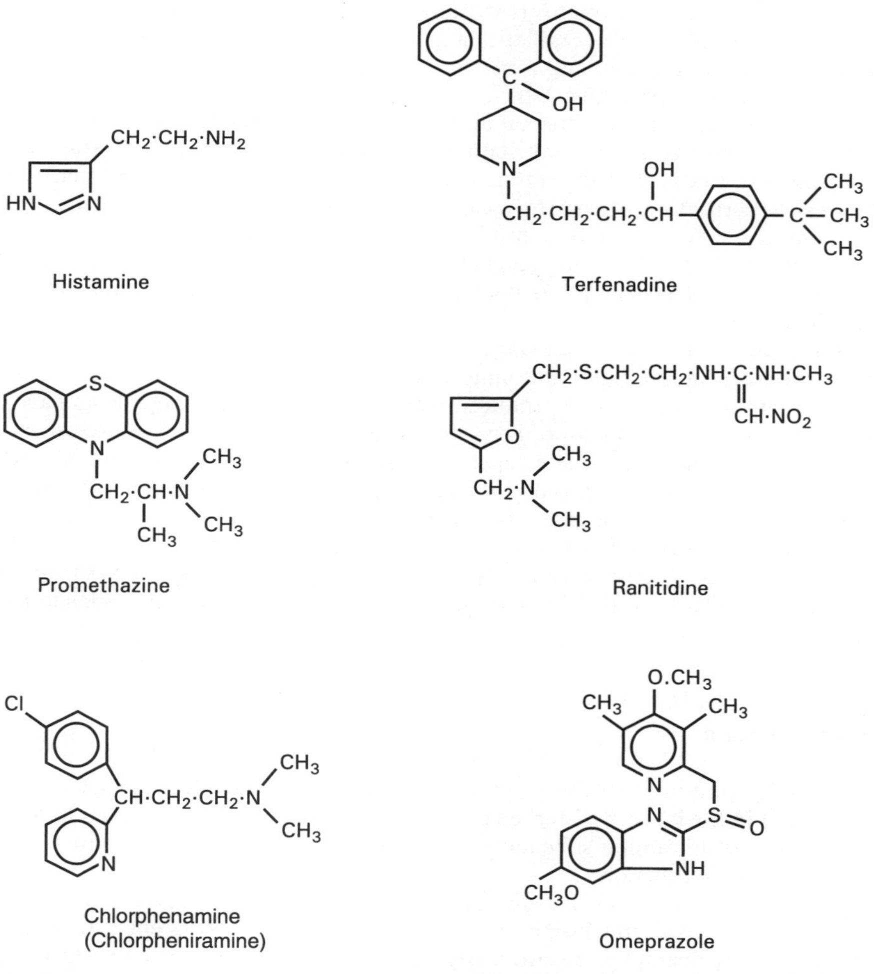

Figure 8.1 Structure of histamine and principal histamine receptor antagonists. Histamine is an agonist at H_1-, H_2- and H_3-receptors. Promethazine, terfenadine and chlorphenamine are antagonists at H_1-receptors, ranitidine an antagonist at H_2-receptors, while omeprazole is a proton-pump antagonist

not blocked by atropine. The guinea-pig is particularly sensitive to it, and as little as 0.1 mg will cause death from bronchoconstriction and oedema of the mucosa. This action of the drug is commonly used for testing the protective power of antihistamine drugs. In the normal human subject the bronchoconstrictor action of histamine is negligible, but patients with bronchial asthma, bronchitis, emphysema and even cardiac asthma (the wheeze associated with left ventricular failure) are much more sensitive to it as, in them, it exerts a bronchoconstrictor action. Its action on other plain muscle, except in the cardiovascular system, is of little importance.

Cardiovascular system

The action of histamine on the heart is not marked (although it can cause a bradycardia), but it is powerful on the capillaries and arterioles. An intravenous injection causes a severe fall in blood pressure and a rise in CSF pressure. This is followed by an intense headache of short duration, after which the pressure changes subside.

The action of histamine on the capillaries can be demonstrated in human skin if a scratch is made through a drop of histamine solution. The triple response which follows causes capillaries to dilate in the traumatized area, a weal due to increased permeability of the vessels permitting plasma to escape, and a flare consisting of dilated arterioles surrounding the weal. The flare is produced by an axon reflex through sensory nerves which can be blocked by local anaesthetics. If histamine is injected into the skin it causes itching, and pain if acetylcholine is injected with it. Both of these substances are found in the stinging nettle.

In some animals, histamine may cause a rise in the blood pressure through its vasoconstrictor action on the arterioles and almost complete absence of capillary effect as seen in man. Histamine shock can be produced readily in animals after large doses have been injected. The fall in blood pressure is pronounced and persistent due to excessive capillary dilatation, and much plasma escapes into the tissues, causing a diminished circulating blood volume and reduced cardiac output. Owing to haemoconcentration, haemoglobin estimations will give a falsely high reading.

The hypotensive effects of histamine are potentiated by anaesthetic agents that increase sympathetic activity. This is presumably due to histamine blocking the vasoconstrictor effects on the capillaries of the skin and mucous membranes, while the vasodilator effect on muscle blood vessels is unaffected.

Alimentary system

When given by mouth, histamine produces no pharmacological effects, probably because it is acetylated in the intestine. Marked stimulation of gastric secretion occurs in response to an injection of histamine subcutaneously, and 1 mg given this way is used as a test clinically for gastric function.

Peptic ulceration can be produced by continuous administration of large doses of histamine. Although gastrin and histamine are now known to be different substances, the former may act by liberating the latter. Histamine can cause an increase in salivary secretions and in those of the pancreas and intestine. These effects are not marked in man and seem to be cholinergic mechanisms as they are potentiated by physostigmine and abolished by atropine.

The plain muscle of the gut is not particularly affected by histamine *in vivo*, but it is a very powerful stimulant of mammalian intestine, especially guinea-pig ileum, in an isolated tissue bath.

Liberation of histamine

Histamine is released by a wide variety of drugs and physicochemical insults:

Physical and chemical damage Any mechanical, thermal or radiant injury, if severe enough to cause tissue damage, will liberate histamine. Some chemicals, such as bile salts and detergents, will also release histamine by direct injury.

Anaphylaxis and allergy These reactions have a basic mechanism in common. This involves an interaction between a specific antigen and a cell-bound antibody. The latter is an immunoglobulin of the IgE type in man. Antigens are usually proteins that are foreign to the individual, but may be other large molecules or complexes formed by the combination of a small reactive molecule with a protein. Many drugs can form such complexes and are then called haptens. The intensity of the anaphylactic reaction depends on the portal of entry of the antigen. If it enters parenterally, as with the case of a drug, a foreign serum or the saliva of a biting insect, systemic anaphylaxis supervenes and this is due to the explosive release of histamine from storage granules in a large number of tissues as well as other agents such as 5-HT, SRS-A and plasma kinins. If the reaction takes place at an exposed mucosal surface, the reaction is much milder and restricted to that tissue. Such restrictions give rise to hay fever, conjunctivitis, asthma, urticaria and gastro-intestinal upsets.

Drugs and macromolecules Apart from their potential for initiating an antigen/antibody response, many chemicals, including numerous therapeutic agents, have the capacity for eliciting histamine release directly. Among them are antibiotic bases, quaternary ammonium compounds such as tubocurarine, piperidine derivatives, and morphine derivatives. In the clinical situation it can be difficult to decide whether a drug releases histamine directly, or indirectly by a hypersensitivity mechanism.

Venoms and toxins Many sorts of venoms and toxins release histamine; this property so far transcends the other pharmacological actions that they have been called histamine liberators. The histamine released is that bound in the granules, and non-mast cell histamine is not depleted.

Synthesis, storage and metabolism

Ingested histamine is largely bound and subsequently destroyed by the liver and lungs or excreted in the urine. Tissue histamine is largely synthesized *in situ* by decarboxylation of histidine. In tissue mast cells and circulating basophils, histamine is synthesized and stored in a complex with heparin in membrane-bound storage granules. The turnover rate in this site is slow. Histamine is also found in substantial amounts in many tissues outside the mast cells where it undergoes a brisk turnover.

There are two main routes of enzymatic breakdown: (1) methylation, followed by oxidation to methylindoleacetic acid; (2) oxidation by diamine oxidase. The relative roles of these enzymes in the metabolism of endogenous histamine have not been established.

Histamine activity is increased by oxygen and oestrogens and is inhibited by cyanides, hydroxylamine, phenylhydrazine and isoniazid. Diamine oxidase activity increases during the first trimester of pregnancy and stays elevated until term. Its origin is the placenta but its function is not clear.

Antihistamines

The actions of histamine can be reversed or opposed in a number of ways. For example, an antagonism of the smooth muscle constrictor effects of histamine in the small intestine can be achieved with epinephrine (adrenaline), while histamine's constrictor effects on bronchial tone are reversed by β-adrenergic agonists such as salbutamol. (Histamine may also be its own antagonist, but see below). These effects, however, are brought about by the 'antagonists' acting through their own specific receptor systems, and are classical examples of physiological antagonism. In contrast, an 'antihistamine' is a substance that reverses or prevents the actions of histamine by exerting a competitive blockade at histamine receptors.

As with other neurotransmitters and autocoids, multiple histamine receptors have now been identified: to date, these are H_1, H_2 and H_3. Their different, even sometimes opposite, physiological roles are now largely understood, and specific antagonists with clear clinical indications have now been developed, at least for H_1- and H_2-receptors.

All three histamine receptors are G protein-coupled. Receptor occupation (whether by histamine or a related agonist) results in a decrease of Ca^{2+} influx into cells. H_1-receptors are the most prevalent, being located in the gastro-intestinal tract, on smooth muscle in the cardiovascular system and bronchial tree, and in many central sites where histamine is thought to act as a transmitter, for example in the hypothalamus. H_1-receptors are also found on brain capillaries and glial cells. On the other hand, H_2-receptors are primarily located in the stomach where they control basal (fasting) and nocturnal acid secretion, and are stimulated (to produce acid) by the presence in the stomach of food, by fundic distension and sham feeding. H_2-receptors are also found in peripheral capillaries (where they may exert an opposite physiological role to H_1-receptors) and in the heart. The most recently discovered receptors (H_3) appear to act primarily as feedback (autoregulatory) inhibitors of histamine acting at other (H_1- and H_2-) receptors in a variety of organ systems: in the CNS, H_3-receptors induce sedation by opposing the wakefulness effects of H_1-receptor stimulation; in the gut H_3-receptors can antagonize small intestine contraction induced by stimulation of H_1-receptors. H_3 receptors also down-regulate histamine (and thus gastrin) function in the stomach, and can antagonize the bronchoconstrictor effects of H_1-receptors. Via H_3-receptors, histamine may also reduce sympathetic nerve release of norepinephrine and can exert a negative chronotrophic effect in the heart.

H_1-receptor antagonists

These are the 'classical' antihistamines to which one refers when any subclassification of histamine receptors is omitted. First introduced in the 1940s, these antihistamines are used to control the principal effects of released histamine in allergic conditions such as hay fever, urticaria, certain dermatoses, serum sickness and idiosyncratic reactions to other drugs and blood transfusions. They belong to several different chemical groups:

CNS sedation and drowsiness have been prominent side effects, and these are notably more severe with the phenothiazine antihistamines such as promethazine. Indeed, the presence of sedative effects are either exploited clinically (e.g. in producing non-benzodiazepine sedation and sleep, particularly in children), or alternatively attempts made to eradicate sedative properties through chemical modifications that limit CNS penetration by the drugs.

All of the available H_1-receptor antagonists are reversible, competitive inhibitors of the interactions of histamine with H_1-receptors. As many as six pharmacologically slightly different subgroups of drugs can be identified according to their chemical structure:

Ethanolamines In addition to their predictable H_1-antagonism, this group also exert a significant dose-related sedative effect which is intrusive at usual clinical doses. Diphenhydramine is a typical example. The group also possesses a significant atropine-like (anti-muscarinic) activity: this manifests as a loss of visual accommodation, some hypersensitivity to bright lights and dry mouth, although effects upon the lower gastro-intestinal tract are minimal.

Ethylenediamines This group possesses more specific H_1-receptor antagonism and less atropinic activity. Tripelennamine is an example. CNS sedation is common and dose related, as are gastro-intestinal disturbances.

Alkylamines Drugs in this group, such as chlorphenamine (chlorpheniramine), are among the most potent antagonists at the H_1-receptor. They possess only minimal atropinic activity, while sedation is intrusive only at higher doses. They are thus more useful for daytime use where sedation is to be avoided. Some patients may be exceptionally susceptible to somnolent effects yet, conversely, stimulation may be observed in others.

Piperazines Relatively lacking in sedative effects, some members of this group (e.g. cyclizine, meclizine) have been used to combat motion sickness, although somnolence can be intrusive in higher doses and/or in certain patients. Some members of the group have a relatively prolonged duration of action, reducing the need for frequent administration.

Phenothiazines Promethazine is a powerful dose-related antagonist at H_1-receptors. At higher clinical doses it also possesses significant blocking activity at muscarinic, dopaminergic, serotonergic and adrenergic receptors. This wide spectrum of effects may be useful clinically or unacceptably intrusive. (The side effects of this group prompted the research which eventually led to the introduction of chlorpromazine and the phenothiazine class of neuroleptic/anti-psychotic drugs.)

Promethazine exerts a broad antagonism of allergic reactions, including those on skin and in mucous membranes; it is also anti-emetic, and is widely used as a non-hypnotic sedative in children. However, its central effects (which include some attention loss as well as somnolence) make it unsuitable for daytime use.

Piperidines These are very specific H_1-antagonists: the group includes astemizole and terfenadine, and in the vast majority of patients they are devoid of atropinic and sedative effects: indeed they are widely 'sold' as non-sedating antihistamines, due largely to their poor penetration of the CNS. Their side effect profile is both narrow and of low incidence, but their unrestricted sale over-the-counter has recently been curtailed because of some instances of *torsades de pointes* following their use in susceptible individuals. The effect is rare: a lengthening of the QTc cardiac interval is followed by polymorphic ventricular tachycardia.

As a generalization, sedation, gastro-intestinal and atropine-like effects plague the use of many of these agents, especially at higher doses and in susceptible individuals. In the past, several have been briefly associated with fetal developmental abnormalities, but without firm proof of a causal relationship.

Interactions with agents used in anaesthesia

H_1-receptor antagonists have a potential for interaction with a number of agents used in anaesthesia. Most interactions are predictable from a consideration of the drugs' main and subsidiary pharmacological properties. Thus, with the possible exception of the piperidine group of antihistamines, H_1-antagonists enhance the sedative effects of other CNS depressants, including the benzodiazepines and alcohol, and increase the effects of anti-muscarinic agents including the side effects of tricyclic antidepressants.

There is a need to exercise care when H_1-receptor antagonists are used concomitantly with agents which alter or control cardiac function, especially anti-arrhythmic agents such as amiodarone, disopyramide, procainamide and quinidine: in these circumstances, antihistamines generally may precipitate ventricular arrhythmias. Astemizole and terfenadine have been singled out and specifically contra-indicated in such combinations. Arrhythmias may occur when these agents are used in the presence of phenothiazine neuroleptics, or where hypokalaemia has been induced by certain diuretics, and when there is peripheral enhancement of circulating and sympathetic catecholamines because their re-uptake has been attenuated by certain antidepressants. Interactions also occur between astemizole or terfenadine and certain anti-fungal agents (e.g. ketoconazole) and anti-bacterial agents (e.g. clarithromycin and erythromycin). This is because these agents interfere with the metabolism of the antihistamines so that their plasma levels are raised and the likelihood of ventricular arrhythmias is increased.

The majority of the potential interactions between H_1-receptor antagonists and other drugs are dose related. All medication with H_1-receptor antagonists needs to be reviewed prior to general anaesthesia.

H_2-receptor antagonists

It had been known since the 1940s that histamine induced a gastric acid hypersecretion resistant to conventional (H_1) antihistamine drugs. The major objective of the development and introduction of H_2-receptor antagonists in the early 1970s was to control gastric hyperacidity and promote healing of peptic (gastric and duodenal) ulcers. Chemically, H_2-antagonists are histamine congeners that also contain a bulky side chain in place of histamine's ethylamine moiety (see *Figure 8.1*). Generally, they are more hydrophilic agents than the H_1-receptor antagonists, and their CNS effects are consequently minimal.

Cimetidine was the first H_2-receptor antagonist to be released for general clinical use. In a dose-dependent manner, it competitively inhibits the H_2-receptors of the stomach associated with basal and stimulated gastric acid secretion, reducing both the volume of acid secretion and its H^+ concentration. **Ranitidine** quickly followed and in many markets soon became the H_2-receptor antagonist of choice because of its lack of inhibition of cytochrome P-450.

The prolonged maintenance of gastric pH at a raised level is important in promoting healing. The stimulation of acid secretion by gastrin, by acetylcholine, by food, by sham feeding, by fundic distension and by various other pharmacological agents is also inhibited, a breadth of effect which clearly illustrates the pivotal role of histamine (at H_2-receptors) in controlling gastric acid secretion. In contrast, these agents have no consistent effect upon the rate of gastric emptying, the pressure of the lower oesophageal sphincter or subsequent pancreatic secretion.

H_2-receptor antagonists are used therapeutically for all those conditions in which a reduction of gastric acid secretion will promote an improvement in health. This includes gastric and duodenal ulcerations, reflux oesophagitis and the Zollinger–Ellison syndrome. At lower doses, cimetidine may be used as a non-prescription drug to treat episodic indigestion, epigastric pain associated with hyperacidity and acute gastritis.

In the case of cimetidine, its inhibition of cytochrome P-450 prolongs the half-life of a number of other drugs which may be used concomitantly. These include phenytoin, phenobarbital, certain benzodiazepines, carbamazepine, theophylline, propranolol, calcium channel blockers, sulphonylureas, warfarin and tricyclic antidepressants. Discontinuation of therapy with cimetidine and/or an appropriate reduction of dose of the other agents must be considered.

In the last decade, the role of *Helicobacter pylori* infection has also been recognized, and its eradication using appropriate antibiotics is important in preventing recurrence of ulceration when H_2-receptor antagonist treatment has been stopped. In the last two decades, elective surgical treatment of gastric or duodenal ulceration has all but ceased and the H_2-receptor antagonists have become one of the most widely prescribed categories of therapeutic agent.

Proton pump inhibitors

The so-called proton pump is the ultimate mediator of gastric acid secretion. The proton pump inhibitors covalently bind to the H^+/K^+ATP-ase system of the apical membrane of parietal cells in the stomach. Since this pump is unique to parietal cells, agents such as omeprazole and lansoprazole specifically inhibit gastric acid secretion to any extent required with minimal other pharmacodynamic effects. Their pharmacological actions and clinical use are discussed in more detail in Chapter 2.

Like cimetidine, both omeprazole and lansoprazole have a potential to interact with microsomal cytochrome P-450 enzymes, slowing the hepatic metabolism, and thus enhancing the effects of other drugs is a possibility.

H_2-receptor antagonists in the ITU

H_2-receptor antagonists may be contra-indicated in the severely ill patient. Gastric bleeding is a common sequel to serious illness, and it has been attributed to erosion of an unusually vulnerable gastric mucosa – so-called 'stress ulceration'. However, the routine administration of an H_2-antagonist prophylactically is no longer advocated.

Firstly, gastric acid secretion is already significantly impaired during life-threatening illness, and there is little merit in exposing the patient to the potential adverse effects of an additional and unnecessary drug. Secondly, in patients in whom gastric acid secretion is relatively normal, H_2-antagonist prophylaxis has been associated with an increased risk of ventilator associated pneumonia (VAP), in which the bacteria isolated from the infected lung have frequently been the same as those cultured from gastric secretions prior to the onset of pneumonia. If significant gastric bleeding does occur and then only if the gastric secretions are demonstrated to be acidic, is it reasonable to give an H_2-antagonist. The intra-gastric instillation of sucralfate (1 g every 4 h) or the introduction of gastric feeding without additional drugs are procedures at least as effective in preventing 'stress ulceration'.

The management of upper intestinal bleeding in an intensive care unit should involve assistance from a gastro-enterologist who can provide diagnostic and therapeutic manouevres through an endoscope. If, for example, the bleeding originates from the oesophagus, the use of a proton pump inhibitor such as omeprazole is indicated.

H_3-receptor agonists and antagonists

H_3-receptors are known to function as feedback inhibitors (autoregulatory) in a number of organ systems. In the CNS, agonist activity at H_3-receptors causes sedation and sleep by opposing wakefulness due to agonist activity at H_1 receptors. In the gastro-intestinal tract, H_3-agonists antagonize H_1-receptor-induced ileal contraction. There is also a down-regulation of histamine and gastrin levels, thus reducing gastric acid secretion by a non-H_2-receptor antagonism. Similarly, the bronchoconstrictor effects of H_1-receptor agonists may be opposed by a bronchodilatory effect instigated by H_3-receptor agonist activity. H_3-receptors have been found on sympathetic nerves where they appear to reduce sympathetic outflow and norepinephrine release.

Currently, H_3-receptor agonist and antagonist drugs are available only for research purposes. (R)-α-methylhistamine is a selective H_3-agonist, being some 3000 times more active at the H_3-receptor than the H_1-receptor. Antagonists in development and clinical trials include thioperamide and clobenpropit. As more potent and specific H_3-receptor agonists and antagonists become available, the pathophysiological roles of these receptors are expected to be better defined, and their potential therapeutic purposes identified.

Inhibitors of histamine release

Ideally, one would like to be able to inhibit the release not only of histamine, but also the other autacoids active in anaphylactic and allergic reactions. This is generally an unattainable objective at present. However, substances are now being developed which prevent the release of histamine and this is an important therapeutic approach in asthma and some other allergic conditions. The only drug of this type available at present is sodium cromoglicate, which is used prophylactically for both asthma and allergic rhinitis.

Bronchoconstrictors

A bronchoconstrictor is an agent that causes any degree of constriction of the smooth muscle of the bronchial tree. Some can bring this about via the nervous system, either by increasing vagal activity or by decreasing that of the sympathetic, and others affect the bronchial muscle directly.

Bronchoconstriction by drugs acting through the nervous system may be initiated at any link in the reflex arc. The important sites are at receptors (irritants), at the post-ganglionic vagal nerve endings (inhibitors of cholinesterase), and at the vagal centre in the medulla (morphine). The infiltration of local anaesthetic solutions to the relevant portion of the sympathetic chain would increase bronchial tone by removing the dilator action of the sympathetic, and bronchoconstriction is occasionally seen with high thoracic epidural blockade. A similar effect can be produced by β_2-adrenoceptor blocking agents which block bronchodilator receptors. None of these mechanisms produces severe bronchospasm in normal individuals, although it may cause measurable changes in airway resistance. They can be more serious in patients with existing abnormal bronchial tone.

Drugs that can cause bronchoconstriction by a direct muscular effect are theoretically all those that are general stimulants of plain muscle, but fortunately comparatively few have a marked effect upon bronchial muscle. The most important is histamine, which can be liberated in the body by a number of substances, as discussed above.

Bronchodilators

Bronchodilators are drugs that decrease the tone of the smooth muscle of the bronchial tree and so lessen resistance to airflow. Their importance lies in their ability to overcome bronchoconstriction and their efforts are usefully reinforced by drugs that diminish secretions, or which reduce mucosal engorgement by causing vasoconstriction, or which reduce inflammation (e.g. steroids).

The most important members act directly on the muscle to promote relaxation, or achieve this by potentiating the effects of norepinephrine being liberated normally at the sympathetic nerve endings. Powerful examples of the latter are sympathomimetic amines such as epinephrine, isoprenaline and ephedrine, and of the former theophylline is the most active of the xanthine derivatives The nitrites also exert a direct action but lower the blood pressure in effective doses; papaverine is ineffective. Ether in anaesthetic concentrations, although irritant, relaxes bronchial tone, although it is possible that it is the liberation of norepinephrine which is responsible for the bronchodilatation.

Since bronchial tone is the result of a balance between parasympathetic and sympathetic activity, specific antagonists of the muscarinic actions of the acetylcholine liberated at vagal nerve endings will act as bronchodilators. This is the mechanism of the bronchodilator activity of atropine and hyoscine; these drugs will also oppose the muscarinic actions of other choline esters upon the bronchial tree, but they are not very effective in bronchial asthma. However, more recent derivatives, deptropine and ipratropium (page 261), are effective in the treatment of this condition.

Competitive antihistamines will relieve bronchoconstriction caused by histamine. In the case of asthma, antihistamines fail to prevent bronchoconstriction. The reason usually advanced is that competitive inhibition by specific antihistamines is impossible because the histamine is intrinsic, which means that it is liberated directly in or on the effector cells of the tissue concerned and obtains immediate and intimate contact with receptors from a vantage point which a competitive antagonist cannot attain.

In this situation, however, universal β-receptor stimulating drugs, such as epinephrine and selective β_2 stimulators such as salbutamol and terbutaline, are effective, as are drugs acting directly on the bronchial smooth muscle.

In the treatment of asthma, drugs are best given by inhalation. Several types of inhaler system are available. To reach the bronchioles the drug should be delivered in particle sizes of 2–4 µm. Larger particles are deposited in the upper airway; smaller ones enter the alveoli or are exhaled. Pressurized inhalers deliver a metered dose of 25–100 µl suspended in a fluorocarbon propellant. Dry powder inhalers are less convenient but are sometimes preferred. In the intensive care situation various nebulizers, such as ultrasonic types, may be employed.

Mucolytic agents

In many clinical situations ventilation difficulties are caused not so much by bronchospasm as by tenacious secretions, and in such circumstances mucolytic therapy may be beneficial. Enzymes such as chymotrypsin can digest sputum *in vitro*, but their clinical use has not been satisfactory. Some preparations related to amino acids are available as aerosols or as oral preparations, such as acetylcysteine and carboxymethylcysteine. These principally affect sputum volume and viscosity. The volume of mucus may initially increase so greatly that endotracheal suction becomes necessary to maintain an adequate airway. The compounds, being related to proteins, may be attended by undesirable reactions such as fever when given by inhalation.

Another agent which has a specific action on sputum is bromhexine, an alkaloid derived from the plant *Adhatoda vasica*. This appears to break down mucopolysaccharide fibres and reduce sputum viscosity.

Although the effects of bromhexine are relatively easy to demonstrate *in vitro*, there are problems *in vivo*, and clinical studies have been conflicting. Whereas there may be an increase in sputum volume and a reduction in viscosity, improvements in ventilatory capacity are hard to demonstrate. No serious side effects have been encountered and most authors have felt that the drug was beneficial, and it has been occasionally tried in patients with postoperative chest infection and 'flail' chests.

Although drug therapy may prove to have a place in the therapy of viscid secretions, it must not be overlooked that adequate hydration of the patient and humidification of the inspired air have been shown to have a dramatic influence on sputum viscosity, and such simple non-specific lines of therapy should not be overlooked.

Drugs for hay fever

Antihistamines with H_1-receptor activity but minimal sedative properties are effective in the treatment of this allergic condition. Hay fever is a markedly seasonal reaction, usually to grass or other pollens. The same drugs are effective in perennial rhinitis and chronic idiopathic urticaria. The following preparations are on the market: acravistine, astemizole, cetirizine, fexofenadine, levocobastine, loratidine and terfenadine. The following are special points of difference:

Acrivastine is well absorbed from the GI tract and quick in onset, with noticeable activity at 1 h, peak effect at 2 h and lasting up to 8 h. Accumulation of the drug has not been recorded following continuous treatment, although care should be taken in patients with renal impairment.

Astemizole has a relatively slow onset and is more appropriate for regular use than symptomatic treatment. It is subject to the same important recommendations and potential interactions as terfenadine (below) but is still available over-the-counter (OTC).

Cetirizine dihydrochloride is an OTC medicine which is claimed to have an incidence of drowsiness indistinguishable from placebo. Dosage is 10 mg once daily, preferably in the evening. It is renally excreted.

Fexofenadine is an active metabolite of terfenadine but is not subject to the same problems of drug interactions.

Levocobastin is available as eyedrops and as a nasal spray. The latter is contra-indicated in the presence of significant renal impairment.

Loratidine has theoretical drug interaction problems centred on P-450 but these have not been noted clinically. It is an OTC medicine.

Terfenadine was introduced in 1982 and was regarded by many as the treatment of choice for hay fever sufferers. In a comparative study with cetirizine it was found to be as effective and even less sedating, given once a day in a dose of 120 mg. It became an OTC drug, but in 1997 reverted to being only available on prescription, following concerns about continuing reports of serious cardiac arrhythmias. In the avoidance of cardiac arrhythmias it is important not to exceed the recommended dose (120 mg daily in adults). It should not be given to patients with cardiac or hepatic disease. There are serious interactions with ketoconazole, itraconazole and related antifungals; erythromycin, clarithromycin and related macrolide antibiotics. It should not be taken with grapefruit juice which contains a psoralen which inhibits metabolism by the CYP3A subfamily of cytochrome P-450, resulting in higher plasma concentrations. (This restriction also applies to cyclosporin and calcium channel blockers other than amlodipine and diltiazem.)

MONOGRAPHS

CHLORPHENAMINE

Chlorphenamine maleate (rINN) (formerly chlorpheniramine maleate)

Chlorphenamine is a highly effective antihistamine, acting competitively at H_1 receptors with a rapid action and duration of effect lasting 4–6 h. Side effects are minimal, dizziness and drowsiness being rarely encountered. It is used in the prophylaxis and treatment of a wide range of allergic disorders and of drug and blood transfusion reactions.

Chlorphenamine is given by mouth in tablet form in a dose of 4 mg 3–4 times a day. In severe cases of allergic and drug reactions 10–20 mg may be given intramuscularly, or intravenously in an emergency. For prophylactic use in patients subject to allergic reactions, 10 mg may be injected intravenously immediately before a blood transfusion, or mixed with penicillin in the syringe prior to injection.

CIMETIDINE

Cimetadine (rINN)

Pharmacology

Cimetidine was the first H_2-receptor antagonist to be released for general clinical use. In a dose-dependent manner it competitively inhibits the H_2-receptors of the stomach associated with basal and stimulated gastric acid secretion. Cimetidine reduces both the volume of acid secretion and its H^+ concentration. Stimulated acid secretion, whether by gastrin, acetylcholine, food, sham feeding, fundic distension or various other pharmacological agents is also inhibited, a breadth of effect which clearly illustrates the pivotal role of histamine at H_2-receptors in controlling gastric acid secretion. In contrast, cimetidine has no consistent effect upon the rate of gastric emptying, the pressure of the lower oesophageal sphincter or subsequent pancreatic secretion.

Cimetidine is well absorbed following oral administration, with peak plasma levels obtained at about 2 h, and the elimination half-life is about 3 h. Although subject to hepatic metabolism, a substantial part of the cimetidine is eliminated in the urine unchanged. Thus renal impairment necessitates a reduction in dose.

Indications

Cimetidine is used therapeutically for all those conditions in which a reduction of gastric acid secretion will promote an improvement in health. This includes gastric and duodenal ulceration, reflux oesophagitis and the Zollinger–Ellison syndrome. The prolonged maintenance of gastric pH at a raised level is important in promoting healing. At lower doses, cimetidine may be used as a non-prescription drug to treat episodic indigestion, epigastric pain associated with hyperacidity and acute gastritis.

Dosage and administration

The normal dose is 1 g/day, that is 200 mg with each meal and 400 mg at night. The dose may be increased to 1600 mg/day.

Precautions

The incidence of adverse effects is low and dose related and the effects are generally of a minor nature. Among those reported are headache, dizziness and nausea, myalgia, and skin rashes. These effects may be slightly more common in the elderly due to minor renal impairment. Also reported have been interference with lactation, loss of libido, impotence and gynecomastia, especially after long-term therapy at high doses. These effects may be attributable to enhanced prolactin secretion or to interference with P-450 catalysed metabolism of oestradiol.

As a result of its inhibition of cytochrome P-450, cimetidine can prolong the half-life of a number of other drugs which may be used concomitantly. These include phenytoin, phenobarbital, certain benzodiazepines, carbamazepine, theophylline, propranolol, Ca^{2+}-channel blockers, sulphonylureas, warfarin and tricyclic antidepressants. Discontinuation of therapy with cimetidine and/or an appropriate reduction of dose of the other agents must be considered. The current view that routine gastric acid suppression is inadvisable in the critically ill is discussed above (page 253–4).

CROMOGLICATE

Sodium cromoglicate (rINN) and Cromolin sodium (USAN)

Pharmacology

Sodium cromoglicate has no direct action on bronchial smooth muscle, nor does it inhibit the direct action of bronchoconstrictor agents. Its mode of action is to prevent the release of histamine and SRS-A from mast cells in human lung as a consequence of

IgE-mediated allergic responses. Both histamine and SRS-A are potent bronchial spasmogens. It therefore prevents the immediate and late asthmatic response to allergens.

Cromoglicate does not inhibit the antigen-antibody reaction itself, but appears to suppress the release of histamine which is a consequence of this reaction. Moreover, this suppression of release is not universal. The actions of histamine liberators (page 249) are unaffected, and mast-cell mediated histamine release in other tissues, such as skin, is not blocked. The drug is, however, effective on the nasal mucosa.

Indications

Sodium cromoglicate is indicated in the prophylaxis of bronchial asthma, particularly where there is good reason to think that an allergic response to an inhaled allergen is implicated. It is also indicated for the prophylaxis of allergic rhinitis. The use of the drug is entirely prophylactic and not therapeutic.

Dosage and administration

For the prevention of asthma the drug is normally given as a powder by inhalation from a single-dose 20 mg cartridge ('Spincap') in a specially designed turbovibratory inhaler. This dose should be inhaled 4–8 times a day. It may be combined with a small dose of isoprenaline (0.1 mg) to counteract the immediate transient bronchospasm which may follow the inhalation of a dry powder. In the prophylaxis of allergic rhinitis it may be given as 2 per cent nasal drops. It is important for the patient to understand that the preparations must be taken regularly, and not in response to symptoms.

Precautions

There are no specific contra-indications. Cromoglicate powder may irritate the throat and trachea. Therapy may permit a reduction in concomitant steroid dosage; this should be reinstituted before sodium cromoglicate is withdrawn.

CYCLIZINE

Cyclizine hydrochloride and lactate (rINN)

Pharmacology

Cyclizine is a competitive antihistamine acting at H_1-receptors whose main action is on the vomiting centre, which it depresses. Its action is potent and prolonged and begins within a few minutes of administration. It is stated to cause side effects in only 5 per cent of cases.

Indications

It is used in the prevention of travel sickness, in the treatment of vertigo (Ménière's syndrome), and combined with analgesics and ergotamine to prevent the emetic side effects of these drugs.

Dosage and administration

Cyclizine is given intravenously as 25–50 mg over 5 minutes or by mouth in tablet form in doses of 50 mg up to 3 times a day. Children aged 6–10 years may be given half this dose.

Precautions

Bolus intravenous injection can result in tachycardia secondary to its anticholinergic properties. An intravenous injection of 25 mg will increase lower oesophageal tone.

Cyclizine should be used with caution in patients with severe heart failure, as it increases systemic and pulmonary arterial pressures, and right and left ventricular filling pressures, and negates the venodilatory effects of diamorphine (Tan *et al.*, 1988).

Recreational use of cyclizine has been reported (Bassett *et al.*, 1996), presumably to induce hallucinations, and often involving use of alcohol and illicit drugs. Tachycardia and systolic hypertension are frequently present in such cases. Tolerance to the drug occurs and, despite the fact that no clear-cut withdrawal syndrome is apparent, dependence upon cyclizine may also occur.

It has been suspected of producing teratogenic effects. Evidence is conflicting, and it should not be used during the early stages of pregnancy.

Tan, L.B., Bryant, S. and Murray, RG. (1988) Detrimental haemodynamic effects of cyclizine in heart failure. *Lancet*, **12**(1), 560–1

Bassett, K.E., Schunk, J.E. and Crouch, B.I. (1996) Cyclizine abuse by teenagers in Utah. *American Journal of Emergency Medicine*, **14**, 472–4

Dimenhydrinate is another competitive antihistamine of moderate potency acting at H_1-receptors which is also a powerful anti-emetic and is used almost entirely in the treatment and prevention of vomiting and vertigo.

In the prevention of vomiting associated with anaesthesia, 50 mg may be given by mouth 1 h before operation and repeated at the end of operation if necessary. A similar dose is given to prevent travel sickness, taken 30 minutes before departure, and it may be repeated 4-hourly if required. Larger doses are sometimes necessary. Vomiting associated with irradiation, toxaemias of pregnancy, carcinomatosis and drugs such as nitrogen mustard, morphine and its derivatives may be treated orally with 50–100 mg, repeated 4-hourly as required, the dose then being adjusted to control symptoms. A dose of 50 mg may be given intramuscularly if the tablets cannot be retained in the stomach. If a more rapid response is necessary, dimenhydrinate 50 mg in 10 ml of isotonic saline may be given slowly intravenously; if given rapidly it may cause venous irritation. Drowsiness is commonly associated with the administration of this drug, and the patient must be duly cautioned.

Diphenhydramine hydrochloride is a competitive antihistamine acting at H_1-receptors and has been used in all the common allergic conditions such as hay fever, urticaria and the dermatoses. It was one of the earliest available, clinically, and is one of the most sedative and least active antihistamines, lasting less than 5 h when given orally. The incidence of side effects is about 60 per cent, especially drowsiness, and it tends to be used now more as a sedative than an antihistamine.

The usual dose is 50 mg by mouth, repeated as necessary up to three or four times a day. A cream may be applied by local application in the treatment of skin conditions and pruritus.

Diphenhydramine is an inducer of hepatic microsomal enzymes.

IPRATROPIUM

Ipratropium bromide (rINN)

Pharmacology

Ipratropium is an antimuscarinic agent. These agents have traditionally been regarded as more effective in relieving bronchoconstriction in chronic bronchitis in patients who fail to respond to selective β_2-adrenoceptor agonists.

Indications

Ipratropium is used in the treatment of bronchoconstriction when this is thought to be due to vagal overactivity. It is used to produce bronchodilatation in patients taking β-blocking drugs and in the treatment of chronic reversible airways obstruction. It has been reported to be somewhat less effective than β_2-adrenoceptor agonist drugs such as salbutamol or fenoterol in patients with asthma, but at least as effective as these agents in bronchitis.

Dosage and administration

The drug is given by a metered inhaler, each metered dose containing 40 µg of ipratropium bromide or by nebulizer at a dose of 250–500 µg every 6 h.

It is also available with fenoterol in a combined metered dose aerosol, 40 µg of ipratropium with 100 mg of fenoterol. This combination is said to provide maximum bronchodilatation with minimal side effects.

Precautions

It can increase the viscosity of bronchial secretions, sometimes to the point of causing plugging of small airways.

RANITIDINE

Ranitidine hydrochloride (rINN)

Pharmacology

Ranitidine is a competitive antagonist at histamine H_2-receptors, inhibiting basal gastric acid secretion, reducing both volume and acid secretion, and reducing pepsin output. It is free from activity on all known H_1-receptors. Stimulated acid secretion, whether by gastrin, acetylcholine, food, sham feeding, fundic distension or various other pharmacological agents is also inhibited, a breadth of effect which clearly illustrates the pivotal role of histamine at H_2 receptors in controlling gastric acid secretion. In contrast, ranitidine has no consistent effect upon the rate of gastric emptying, the pressure of the lower oesophageal sphincter or subsequent pancreatic secretion.

It is rapidly and substantially absorbed by mouth, with peak plasma levels occurring at 2–3 h. Peak plasma levels are reached at about 15 minutes following intramuscular injection. The elimination half-life is 2–3 h, with up to 93 per cent of the drug excreted unchanged in the urine.

Ranitidine quickly followed upon the launch of cimetidine and in many markets soon became the H_2-receptor antagonist of choice, for a variety of reasons. There were reports that cimetidine might interfere with spermatogenesis.

More significantly perhaps, ranitidine was introduced at a dose level that minimized the number of doses required daily. Nor does ranitidine interfere with the cytochrome P-450 system, so that its potential for interactions with other drugs is dramatically less than that of cimetidine.

Indications

Clinically, ranitidine is active and non-toxic in a wide range of doses: it is available OTC without prescription for the treatment of mild acute conditions relating to episodic dyspepsia, hyperacidity and gastritis. At higher doses (on prescription) it is licensed to promote healing of gastric and duodenal ulcers, reduce reflux oesophagitis and control the Zollinger–Ellison syndrome. Raniditine may also be used to provide prophylaxis against, or treatment for, gastric irritation, ulceration and haemorrhage associated with treatment with NSAIDs and before general anaesthesia in patients believed to be at risk of acid aspiration, particularly obstetric patients during labour. As with cimetidine, permanent alleviation of peptic ulcer symptoms is best achieved in combination with an antibacterial regimen (e.g. amoxycillin and metronidazole) that eradicates the *Helicobacter pylori* infection present in about 90 per cent of patients with peptic ulceration.

Dosage and administration

Ranitidine is available as standard and effervescent tablets (150 mg and 300 mg), as syrup (150 mg in 10 ml) and injection (50 mg in 2 ml ampoules). Adult dosage is 150 mg, twice daily by mouth or 300 mg at night; or 50 mg by intravenous or intramuscular injection.

Precautions

No important adverse effects have been identified. It does not block androgen receptors or interact with cytochrome P-450. Since the drug is excreted by the kidneys largely unchanged, renal impairment may be associated with higher and prolonged plasma drug levels and the dose of ranitidine should be reduced accordingly. Long-term treatment for hyperacidity should not be considered unless a malignancy has first been excluded. Because of the drug's high specificity of action, no particular problems are encountered in overdose. Symptomatic and supportive therapy should be given as appropriate. The current view that routine gastric acid suppression is inadvisable in the critically ill is discussed above (page 253–4).

Famotidine and **nizatidine** are more recent H_2-receptor antagonists with pharmacologically identical properties. Like ranitidine, they do not interfere with microsomal cytochrome P-450, so that their propensity to delay the hepatic metabolism of other drugs is not significant.

SALBUTAMOL

Salbutamol (rINN) and Albuterol (USAN)

Pharmacology

Salbutamol is a selective β_2-adrenergic stimulant which has little or no action on β_1-receptors with normal doses. It belongs to a series of agents in which the -OH group in position 3 of isoprenaline is replaced by a -CH_2OH group. It resulted from research to find a β-adrenergic stimulant free from action on the heart. From a therapeutic point of view, it appears to have a highly selective action on bronchial musculature, lack of effect on the myocardium, and a long duration of action, when administered in the usual way by an aerosol inhaler. However, when given intravenously it has much less apparent selectivity. Its long action after inhalation may therefore simply indicate that absorption is very poor from the inhalation site, and thus the effect on the heart is slight. By the intravenous route the drug reaches both sites indiscriminately and thus its true nature becomes apparent. In all species so far tested, salbutamol is a more potent bronchodilator than isoprenaline when administered by aerosol or by mouth and about equally active intravenously.

Studies on asthmatic volunteers using a whole-body plethysmograph show that doses of 100 µg of salbutamol by inhalation produced a substantial and almost immediate reduction in airway resistance for several hours. In normal volunteers, doses of up to 400 µg by inhalation have no effect on heart rate, ECG or blood pressure. In the same subjects, 200 µg of isoprenaline has marked cardiovascular effects. Its duration of action is 4–6 h because it is not metabolized by catechol-o-methyl transferase, the enzyme which rapidly inactivates isoprenaline in the body.

Onset of action is rapid by inhalation, and near-maximal bronchodilatation occurs within 5 minutes. Side effects are not seen with normal therapeutic dosage. Doses greatly in excess of those needed for full bronchodilatation may cause short-lived secondary effects, such as peripheral vasodilatation, minor increase in pulse rate, and skeletal muscle tremor.

Indications

Salbutamol may be used in the treatment of asthma and all other types of bronchospasm. It is also used to inhibit uterine activity in premature labour (see Chapter 15).

Dosage and administration

Salbutamol is administered from a metered aerosol inhaler, delivering 100 µg at each inhalation. As the duration of action is at least 4 h, the number of inhalations should not exceed eight in any 24-h period. It can be given as a slow intravenous injection in a dose of 2–4 µg/kg, by mouth in amounts of 2–4 mg three to four times a day, or by nebulizer at 2.5–5 mg 4–6 times daily.

Precautions

If a previously effective treatment lasts for less than 3 h, diagnosis and therapy should be reconsidered. Like that of ephedrine when administered regularly by mouth, the bronchodilator effect of salbutamol gradually wanes after a period of 1–3 weeks of continuous therapy. As with other β-stimulants, therefore, it is advisable to reserve its use for the relief of acute asthmatic symptoms, and not to attempt to maintain continuous bronchodilatation.

All β_2-stimulants can cause tremor, palpitations, headache and muscle cramps. Angina is occasionally precipitated. Cardiac arrhythmias are a potential risk in patients with myocardial disease or hypokalaemia.

Salmeterol is a more recently introduced, longer acting β_2-specific agonist, which may be used to provide sustained long-term bronchodilatation. Powder and liquid forms are administered directly to the pulmonary tree, using specific devices. Salmeterol's principal difference from salbutamol is its prolonged action: after inhalation, onset of action is slow, some 10–20 minutes elapsing before appearance of clinical effects. These then, typically, last for up to 20 h following a single metered dose. Salmeterol is particularly useful in treating nocturnal asthma and in the prevention of exercise-induced symptoms. Salmeterol is not a replacement for corticosteroid or sodium cromoglicate treatment where these are already successfully used, and their use should be continued.

Paradoxical bronchoconstriction can occur, presumably a response to the propellant or dispersant which precedes the rather slower onset of the bronchdilatation produced by the drug itself.

Terbutaline is similar to salbutamol in that it selectively stimulates the β_2-receptors in the bronchial musculature while affecting the β_1-receptors in the heart to a lesser extent. Its action reaches a peak in 30 minutes after subcutaneous injection and in 2–3 h after oral administration. Its duration of action after a single oral dose of 5 mg is similar to salbutamol 5 mg orally and of the order of 5–6 h. The normal oral dose is 2–4 mg three times a day; by inhalation or aerosol or powder, 250–500 µg (1–2 puffs) 3–4 times daily, or by nebulizer 5–10 mg 2–4 times daily.

THEOPHYLLINE AND AMINOPHYLLINE

Theophylline (rINN) and Aminophylline (rINN)
Aminophylline is a mixture of theophylline and ethylenediamine

Pharmacology

Theophylline is a dimethylxanthine, sharing properties with caffeine and theobromine. In this group – the xanthine dertivatives – differences in action are of degree only, all being stimulants of the CNS and the heart, relaxants of smooth muscle, and diuretics by direct action on the kidney.

Central nervous system   The activity of theophylline is not great enough for it to be of use against central depressants. It does, however, have a stimulant action on the respiratory centre, which may be valuable in connection with its bronchodilator action. In overdose it can cause agitation and even convulsions.

Cardiovascular system   The force of the heart beat is increased and output rises. The rate is slightly raised, being the resultant of a direct effect offset by vagal stimulation centrally. Coronary vessels are dilated, but it is conjectural whether the increased blood flow is in excess of that demanded by the extra cardiac work. Central vasomotor stimulation acts against direct peripheral vasodilatation, which predominates in general, but cerebrovascular resistance increases and cerebral blood flow falls. The resultant of the various opposing cardiovascular actions upon blood pressure is usually a slight rise.

In common with other methylxanthines, theophylline is an inhibitor of the enzyme phosphodiesterase, and therefore allows tissue levels of cyclic AMP to increase. It therefore closely reproduces the effects of β-adrenergic stimulation which increase cyclic AMP levels by stimulating its production. A rise in cyclic AMP in lung tissue leads to bronchial smooth muscle relaxation. Its toxic effects in other tissues are probably related to a similar mechanism.

Extravascular smooth muscle   The most important site of action is bronchial smooth muscle, which is dilated, often in asthmatics refractory even to epinephrine (adrenaline). Biliary spasm is also relieved and there is a transient suppression of activity of the muscle of the small and large bowel.

The kidney   Renal blood flow is increased and this will increase urine output in conditions of poor renal blood flow. Probably of more importance is the direct depression of tubular reabsorption of electrolytes by an unknown mechanism. Tubular secretion of potassium is not affected.

Fate in the body   Xanthines are well absorbed following administration by oral, rectal or parenteral routes. They are irritant and some preparations attempt to overcome this disadvantage by combination with choline, glycine or other organic bases. When given by rectum or intramuscularly, effective blood levels are reached in 30–60 minutes. Appreciable blood levels remain for over 6 h, but its activity is over more quickly. Little unchanged theophylline reaches the urine, most of it being demethylated and oxidized to methyluric acid.

Indications

Aminophylline is used mainly in the treatment of asthma and bronchospasm. It possesses a combination of pharmacological actions particularly suited to geriatric patients.

Dosage and administration   Aminophylline may be given orally in a dose of 100–200 mg by tablet, in an elixir (containing about 80 mg/5 ml), or by rectum in the form of a suppository; these are available in at least five strengths and confusion about dose may lead to overdose. Suppositories should rarely be needed now that well-tested, oral, slow-release preparations are available. It may also be given slowly intravenously when a rapid response is required. It has been specifically recommended for the relief of bronchospasm associated with the carcinoid syndrome, by virtue of its ability to antagonize both 5-HT and histamine.

The dosage and rate of administration are crucial to obtaining a maximal therapeutic effect with the minimum of toxic side effects. Bronchodilatation can be first detected at a plasma level of about 5 µg/ml and increases as the plasma level increases to about 15–20 µg/ml. Toxic effects start to appear in this range. The optimum level appears to be 10–12 µg/ml and this can be achieved by giving a loading dose of 5–6 mg/kg over 15–30 minutes, followed by 0.9 mg/kg/h. Users of tobacco and alcohol need bigger doses to achieve the same serum concentration. Patients in heart failure need less.

Precautions

Rapid administration can lead to agitation, convulsions, tachycardia, hypotension and cardiac arrest. It has been suggested that if used in combination with a β_2-agonist, there is an enhanced danger of fatal cardiac arrhythmias.

9

Neuromuscular blocking agents

Muscle tone is thought to be maintained by a continuous train of nervous impulses originating in the anterior horn cells of the spinal cord. Complete muscular paralysis can be produced by blocking these impulses centrally by deep general anaesthesia, peripherally through nerve block by local anaesthetics, or by blocking myoneural transmission using certain specific drugs; these latter are known as muscle relaxants and myoneural or neuromuscular blocking drugs. Of these terms, neuromuscular blocking drug is to be preferred, being the term that most accurately describes the mode of action.

Some degree of muscular relaxation can also be obtained by drugs acting on the spinal cord, such as diazepam and chlorpromazine. The rigidity of Parkinsonism can also be relieved by drugs acting centrally.

Agents that act on the muscle itself are also now available and are of some value in relieving spasticity. Dantrolene is one such; this drug is not a neuromuscular blocking agent but is included in this chapter for the sake of convenience.

Physiology of neuromuscular transmission

At the junctional region between motor nerve and muscle there is a specialized portion of muscle membrane known as the motor end-plate. The structure of these active sites has been elucidated and consists of a group of five proteins (α, α, β, γ, δ) which traverse the lipid bilayer. The active site is on each α protein and when a molecule of acetylcholine (ACh) binds to each one, a conformational change takes place, opening a channel between the proteins for the passage of ions. This channel remains open for about 1 ms and then closes. Subsequently, the molecules of ACh dissociate from the receptor and are hydrolysed by acetylcholinesterase located in the junction. The receptor then reverts to its resting state. Under resting conditions selective permeability enables an unequal distribution of ions to be maintained between the inside and outside of the cell. The primary ionic disequilibrium is due to the active extrusion of Na^+ from the cell, a process that requires energy. The electrical gradient that results induces an unequal distribution of K^+ so that the intracellular concentration of this ion is higher than the extracellular. The net result of this ionic distribution is a difference of electrical potential across the membrane of the cell so that the inside is about -90 mV.

The arrival of a motor nerve impulse results in the release of acetylcholine from storage vesicles in the nerve terminal, but there is a delay of about 1 ms between the crest of the nerve action potential and the release of transmitter. The mechanism that couples depolarization to release is sensitive to the concentration of Ca^{2+} and Mg^{2+}. The released acetylcholine reacts with the α proteins in the receptor complex, allowing positively charged ions to flow through the protein pore.

When the membrane is at its resting potential the net driving force for K^+ is close to zero, since the voltage gradient almost balances the concentration gradient across the membrane. For Na^+, however, the voltage and concentration gradients act in the same direction, and the same is true for Ca^{2+}. In the latter case, however, the absolute extracellular concentration is so much lower than for Na^+ that it makes only a minor contribution to the inward current. About 30 000 Na^+ ions per channel pass during the 1 ms opening phase. This loss of polarization constitutes the end-plate potential, and the end-plate is said to be 'depolarized'.

The end-plate potential is produced by a ligand (or transmitter) gated receptor and is therefore a non-propagated potential. However, if its magnitude is greater than about 50 mV it 'short circuits' the adjacent muscle membrane, opening voltage-gated Na^+ channels in the membrane, allowing more Na^+ to enter. This further depolarizes the membrane and results in a self-propagating wave of depolarization, the action potential, which causes ion channels in the sarcoplasmic reticulum to open transiently and release Ca^{2+} into the cytosol. This causes the muscle fibres to contract.

When the acetylcholine dissociates from the receptor complex and the membrane returns to its resting state, impermeability is restored, Na^+ is extruded and replaced by K^+ and the end-plate and muscle membrane become repolarized.

The nerve potentials have a further important action which is pre-synaptic. Each impulse facilitates the release of acetylcholine by a subsequent impulse. It is thought that this is due to an action of acetylcholine on ACh_2 receptors on the nerve terminal which facilitates acetylcholine release.

Neuromuscular block

Interference with the mechanism described above will stop nerve impulses which arrive at the motor end-plate from causing contraction of the muscle fibre. The following main types of block are recognized.

Pre-synaptic deficiency block

Two types of deficiency block are theoretically possible: interference with synthesis of transmitter and interference with its release. Hemicholinium and triethylcholine act competitively on the synthesis of acetylcholine and are antagonized by choline. Their effects are slow in onset, being manifest only as the pre-synaptic store of transmitter is depleted. The toxin of botulinus, injected directly into muscle, will relieve spasticity by interfering with uptake of acetylcholine into the pre-synaptic vesicles. Many drugs, including local anaesthetics, aminoglycoside antibiotics (neomycin, kanamycin and streptomycin), as well as calcium deficiency and magnesium excess, diminish the quantal release of acetylcholine per nerve impulse, and may enhance clinical block produced by competitive receptor blocking drugs.

Competitive block

In competitive block the agents compete with acetylcholine for the end-plate receptors, but once attached to them they do not cause depolarization. They are often, therefore, referred to as non-depolarizing blocking drugs. This terminology is not to be recommended, since it merely describes what the drug does not do. Despite this, it is widely used. Once such a drug occupies a significant number of receptors, there are fewer receptors to which acetylcholine can become attached and consequently a lower end-plate potential follows a nerve impulse. If sufficient blocking drug is present, the end-plate potential will fail to reach the triggering threshold, and neuromuscular block occurs. Depending on the drug and the dose, this may last from a few minutes to three quarters of an hour.

Drugs that cause neuromuscular block by this mechanism include tubocurarine, pancuronium, vecuronium, atracurium, rocuronium and mivacurium. Their action can be opposed by increasing the local concentration of acetylcholine, and this can be brought about by giving anticholinesterases, such as neostigmine. Their action is enhanced when there is a diminution of the pre-synaptic quantal release of acetylcholine, as in myasthenia gravis, or in the presence of certain antibiotics. Competitive blockade is enhanced by volatile anaesthetics in a concentration-dependent manner, which differs from agent to agent. In general, the effect is in the order sevoflurane > isoflurane > enflurane > halothane.

Depolarization block

Drugs producing this form of block, such as decamethonium and suxamethonium, are agonists of acetylcholine at end-plate receptors but, unlike acetylcholine, the depolarization caused by these drugs persists for more than a few milliseconds. The initial depolarization causes a muscular contraction, seen as a short period of muscular fasciculation. This is the result of repetitive firing of the muscle fibres, a reflex initiated by the sudden depolarization of the muscle spindle.

If depolarizing drugs are applied for prolonged periods, partial repolarization of the end-plate takes place. However, long-continuing depolarization produces an area of reduced excitability of the surrounding muscle membrane which is associated with loss of potassium.

Other types of block

Several terms have appeared in the literature over the years to 'explain' abnormal reaction to depolarizing drugs:

- *Dual block* is a phenomenon in some species in which an initial contracture of muscle is followed by flaccid paralysis. It can be demonstrated in man only by decamethonium in the presence of myasthenia gravis.
- *Desensitization* and *receptor inactivation* were terms used to describe the consequence of maintaining a high concentration of a depolarizing drug at the end-plate, probably related to K^+ depletion.
- *Phase I* and *Phase II* block are terms borrowed from a two-phase action of decamethonium to describe a sequence of changes when suxamethonium is given in paralysing doses for long periods of time. In time, the block seems to take on characteristics of a competitive block, demonstrating post-tetanic potentiation and fade to train-of-four (TOF) stimuli and improvement with anticholinesterases when there is evidence of spontaneous recovery. Of several more or less fanciful explanations, impairment of prejunctional release of acetylcholine is most likely.

Monitoring of neuromuscular blockade

Direct monitoring is now almost universally employed, the commonest practice being to stimulate the ulnar nerve and record the response of the *adductor pollicis* or the muscles of the hypothenar eminence. The response to nerve stimulation can be assessed in two ways: either by recording integrated action potentials from surface or needle electrodes, or by measuring the muscle tension developed during the contraction. It is important to realize that these two measurements are not comparable because they do not measure the same thing. The action potential provides a measure of the electrical activity generated in a limited number of muscle fibres, whereas the tension measures the response of the whole muscle.

Although the introduction of direct measurements has enabled both qualitative and quantitative aspects of neuromuscular blockade to be recorded readily, the employment of a wide range of techniques of stimulation has led to a good deal of confusion. If the compound action potential is measured, it is essential to ensure that the electrodes cannot move and therefore the muscle must be tested in isometric contraction.

When muscle contraction is recorded, a force transducer is used. It is essential to ensure that the direction of movement of the transducer is aligned with the pull exerted by the muscle and that the resting tension is kept constant. The motor nerve may be stimulated with either needle or surface electrodes. The stimulus duration should be less than 0.2 ms; longer stimuli can result in double stimulation or repetitive firing of the muscle. The intensity of the stimulus must produce a maximal response. The pattern of stimulation also can influence the results: tetanus should be at a frequency of 30–50 Hz; single stimuli may be applied at intervals of 2–5 s. Tetanic stimuli should not be applied more frequently than at 5-minute intervals.

The chief clinical applications of such measurements is in monitoring the block and in the assessment of residual neuromuscular blockade. Because it is somewhat uncomfortable to obtain awake baseline measurements the technique of using four TOF supramaximal stimuli in 2 s, followed by an interval of 10–12 s has been developed. This technique of assessment has several advantages. Unlike tetanus, the stimuli do not alter the character or intensity of the block. Different types of neuromuscular block produce characteristic responses, and baseline values are not essential to the assessment.

During a competitive blockade (*Figure 9.1*) there is a progressive reduction in the height of the response to sequential stimuli. Four stimuli are used in practice because at this rate of stimulation the fourth twitch is always maximally depressed; a fifth, or any subsequent twitches, is the same height as the fourth. The ratio of the fourth twitch to the first is known as the T4/T1 ratio. The greater the intensity of the blockade, the smaller this ratio. With larger doses of relaxants, the ratio may be unmeasurable because the fourth, then the third and then the second twitches are progressively abolished by increasing doses, until there is no response even to a single twitch. At this stage, however, a burst of tetanus will temporarily improve responsiveness (post-tetanic decurarization, see below), so that the depth of block can still be roughly quantified by counting the number of post-tetanic twitch responses.

During recovery, the reverse sequence occurs. When the T4/T1 ratio reaches about 0.25–0.3 per cent, relaxation will be inadequate for abdominal surgery. When the ratio reaches 0.70–0.75, a single twitch (or the first of the four) will have returned to the control value (C in *Figure 9.2*) and tetanic fade (see below) will not be demonstrable. In contrast, a partial depolarizing block shows well-sustained twitches at all levels of block.

More recently, studies have shown that recovery from the effects of relaxants can be evaluated with 'double burst' stimulation. Two very short bursts of either two or three

Non-depolarizing neuromuscular block

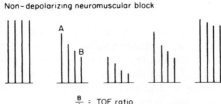

$\dfrac{B}{A}$ = TOF ratio

Figure 9.1 A diagrammatic representation of the response to train-of-four (TOF) nerve stimulation. The upper trace shows the response to a moderate dose of a competitive agent demonstrating a TOF ratio (see text) of about 0.4 at the height of the block. The lower trace shows the effect of partial depolarizing block with an unchanged TOF ratio of 1.0

Depolarizing neuromuscular block

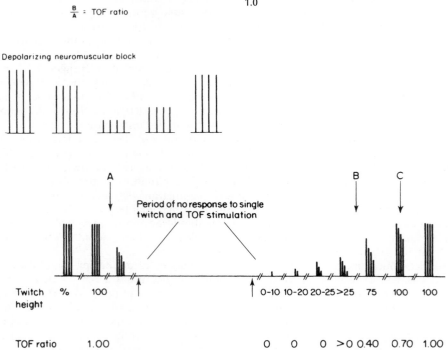

Figure 9.2 A diagrammatic representation of the response to TOF nerve stimulation during the onset and recovery from an intense competitive neuromuscular block. A = injection of relaxant; B = injection of neostigmine; C = control value

50 Hz square wave stimuli are separated by an interval of 0.6–0.8 s. The second burst should produce a stronger contraction than the first if the block is capable of reversal. If they are equivalent or the second is weaker than the first, more than 40 per cent of receptors are occupied by relaxant. This evaluation can usually be made by just sensing the strength of contraction with the operator's hand. All these phenomena are interpretable in terms of underlying mechanisms, some of which are related to the normal behaviour of muscle and some of which are pre-synaptic in origin. Some descriptive terms are used by different authors to mean different things and some precision is desirable.

Post-tetanic potentiation   An increase in twitch tension which occurs physiologically in normal muscle following tetanic stimulation. It is unassociated with any change in the muscle action potential, thus indicating that the effect is due to a change in the contractile properties of the muscle.

Post-tetanic 'decurarization'   This is associated with an increase in the compound muscle action potential as well as in the muscle tension, in response to a single stimulus following tetanic stimulation during partial competitive neuromuscular block. The increase in the muscle action potential indicates that more muscle fibres are firing; this is due to the effects of the tetanus on pre-synaptic mechanisms and is discussed below.

Tetanic fade   This occurs physiologically in fatigued muscle or when unphysiologically fast rates of motor nerve stimulation are used. It is, however, readily demonstrated in the presence of competitive blocking drugs at normal rates of stimulation because pre-synaptic ACh receptors are occupied by the drug. This prevents the mobilization of ACh from intraneural stores, a process which normally occurs when these receptors are stimulated by ACh.

Post-tetanic fade   This is the waning of the post-tetanic decurarization induced by a tetanic burst of stimuli.

Post-tetanic facilitation   This is a term used by some authors to describe both post-tetanic decurarization and post-tetanic potentiation. There is some logic in this, in that the phenomenon presumably is a summation of both processes. It should not be forgotten, however, that two different mechanisms underlie it. Post-tetanic potentiation is a physiologically normal event, whereas post-tetanic decurarization depends on a pre-synaptic action which is made obvious by the presence of a partial competitive neuromuscular blockade.

Under normal conditions the store of transmitter in the nerve terminal is sufficient for many thousands of impulses, but a considerable amount is not available for immediate release. The immediately accessible fraction is readily depleted by a sequence of impulses, and an early decline in end-plate potential size during a tetanic burst is the manifestation of this. However, since the end-plate potential is much in excess of threshold, this reduction does not produce clinical weakness. When the end-plate potential is reduced by the presence of a competitive blocking drug, a reduction in end-plate potential will result in it falling below threshold in some fibres, and increasing weakness or 'fade' will result.

There is, however, a further dimension to this pre-synaptic effect. During a tetanic burst, facilitation due to stimulation of ACh_2 receptors is proceeding to a marked extent, even though the exhaustion of the readily available fraction disguises it. Following the tetanus, the facilitation persists for a short period and single impulses during this time will release a larger number of quanta of transmitter, with a consequent increase in end-plate potential which may now reach threshold and trigger an action potential in a previously unresponsive fibre. There is thus recruitment of muscle fibres with an increase in the compound action potential and in the developed tension leading to post-tetanic decurarization. This facilitation of transmitter release is transitory and the response soon fades off again. The rapidity of the fade is enhanced by the fact that the facilitated release exhausts the readily available fraction even more quickly. These features are illustrated in the top panel of *Figure 9.3* which shows the characteristic electromyographic picture of a competitive block which exhibits fade and post-tetanic decurarization.

In the presence of depolarizing drugs a variety of responses may be seen. If the block is intense the end-plate will be insensitive and no transmission will occur. With incomplete blocking concentrations, however, the presence of the drug lowers the threshold for triggering an action potential and a smaller number of quanta of acetylcholine are adequate for transmission. As a consequence, even the reduced amount available during

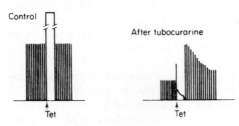

Competitive neuromuscular block

Control

After tubocurarine

Tet

Tet

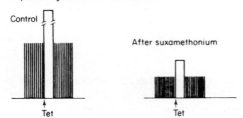

Depolarizing neuromuscular block

Control

After suxamethonium

Tet

Tet

Figure 9.3 A diagrammatic representation of the response to tetanic and post-tetanic single twitch stimulation. Upper panel, control and following a subparalysing dose of tubocurarine; lower panel, control and after a subparalysing dose of suxamethonium. Tet = a tetanic burst at 50 Hz for 5 s

repetitive stimulation maintains good tone in those muscle fibres whose end-plates have not been depolarized. The clinical manifestation, then, is either of complete block or of a weak response that is well sustained and unaffected by tetanic stimulation. This situation is illustrated in the lower panel of *Figure 9.3*.

Pharmacokinetics of relaxants

All the clinically used neuromuscular blocking drugs are quaternary ammonium compounds which are fully ionized at normal body pH. They are largely lipid insoluble, and therefore do not cross cell membranes, and are largely confined to the extracellular fluid. The distribution and metabolic fate differ from drug to drug. Suxamethonium and mivacurium are rapidly hydrolysed by plasma cholinesterase; the rate of decay of the pharmacological effect (twitch depression) is unaffected by the initial dose. Decamethonium is excreted unchanged in the urine.

The competitive relaxants undergo both renal excretion and hepatic metabolism, but the relative importance of these two routes differs from drug to drug. Atracurium and cisatracurium differ in that a significant proportion of the drug undergoes spontaneous (Hofmann) degradation. Gallamine is heavily dependent on renal excretion, but the other drugs currently available have sufficient hepatic metabolism to be usable in renal failure, at least with moderate doses. However, in renal failure, larger initial doses are needed, probably because of an increased volume of distribution. In this situation, atracurium and cisatracurium are the agents of choice; their activity is largely unaffected by the lack of renal excretion.

After intravenous administration the plasma drug concentrations decline in two phases: an initial rapid fall due to redistribution (described by the distribution half-life $t_{1/2\alpha}$) and a slower fall due to elimination (the elimination half-life $t_{1/2\beta}$). The relevance of the plasma concentration to the clinical action is, however, disputed, at least as far as recovery is concerned. Feldman (1993), mainly utilizing evidence from isolated forearm experiments, has summarized the evidence as follows:

1.   Recovery from neuromuscular block by two different non-depolarizing drugs with similar physical characteristics administered in similar doses, producing a similar degree of block at the same time, one in each arm, produce different, slow recovery rates when the tourniquet is released. This cannot be due to differences in plasma drug concentrations or blood flow.
2.   Simultaneous cross-over experiments in the isolated forearm demonstrate that at 50 per cent recovery from neuromuscular block in the isolated forearm sufficient drug remains in the biophase to affect markedly the recovery rate of a large dose of another drug. This effect is not seen following 100 per cent recovery in the isolated forearm.
3.   Letting down the tourniquet as soon as 50 per cent block is achieved in the isolated arm (at approximately 60 s) is followed in the next 2 minutes by increasing block to little short of that achieved when the tourniquet was kept in place for three minutes. This indicates that a higher concentration of drug is present in the biophase than at the receptor in the 60 s following administration.

Another feature suggesting the presence of biophase binding is the delay universally seen with competitive neuromuscular blocking agents between intravenous injection and the onset of block.

Feldman has proposed the existence of acceptor sites close to the acetylcholine receptor which result in binding within the biophase. This concept offers an explanation for features of the onset of, and recovery from, neuromuscular block which are difficult to explain. For example it explains: the similarity in the rates of recovery from block with atracurium and vecuronium despite their different rates of clearance and volumes of distribution; why block continues, for example, when mivacurium is rapidly metabolized and when the plasma concentration is rapidly lowered in an isolated forearm experiment; the inability to reverse a block with anticholinesterases when there is still a significant plasma concentration; why priming works; why weak blockers with a low affinity constant such as rocuronium and gallamine have a more rapid onset; and why the block in the isolated forearm continues to increase when the tourniquet is deflated prematurely.

There are important feedback mechanisms operating at the neuromuscular junction. There are nicotinic receptors on the prejunctional nerve terminals, activated by acetylcholine during normal transmission, which facilitate the release of further ACh during continuing neuronal activity. These receptors can also be blocked by neuromuscular blocking agents, although they differ in the extent of their pre-synaptic potency, tubocurarine being more active than pancuronium, atracurium and vecuronium. Some authorities believe that it is block of these prejunctional positive feedback receptors which is responsible for the phenomena of TOF fade and tetanic fade. There is, however, considerable experimental data to suggest that this is not a wholly satisfactory explanation. The origin of the fading remains to be fully elucidated (Wessler, 1993).

While such matters are the subject of intense debate, research and controversy, they have little bearing on how the various drugs are used in practice. Anaesthetists tend to have 'favourite' relaxants, for routine use, often unduly influenced by marginal factors such as predilection for histamine release. Special, rather rare, circumstances such as renal failure or liver dysfunction may rule out particular agents. In general, however, the variations in response are such that monitoring of effect is more important for safe usage than selection of the 'right' relaxant.

The newer shorter acting agents, vecuronium and atracurium, are increasingly being given by continuous infusion at a rate which matches the elimination rate. The volume of distribution at steady state ($V_{d(ss)}$) is small and varies from 200 to 450 ml/kg. These terms, plus a value for clearance (Cl, the volume of plasma from which all the relaxant is removed in unit time), are sufficient to describe the pharmacokinetics of any competitive relaxant.

Clinical use of relaxants

During the past 40 years muscle relaxants have come to be employed routinely in major surgery and to a considerable extent for even minor surgical procedures, the main advantage being that with their aid lighter levels of anaesthesia may be employed. Their widespread use has, however, led to the emergence of a new complication of general anaesthesia, namely awareness while paralysed. The use of nitrous oxide and oxygen with hyperventilation is now considered inherently unreliable in preventing this phenomenon, but even when potent inhalation agents are (allegedly) employed, unintended awareness is still occasionally reported. This may be due to faulty technique (improperly located vaporizer or incorrectly operated ventilator), but the essential safeguard is to monitor and maintain relaxation at a level which still permits some movement.

The competitive blocking drugs are more commonly used for major surgical operations as their duration of action is longer (20–45 minutes); suxamethonium is more often employed for short procedures, such as intubation, endoscopies, bronchoscopies and manipulations, when only a brief period of relaxation is required. Suxamethonium has also been used in repeated doses or by intravenous infusion for major operations, but this practice has largely ceased because a dual block usually develops which can be difficult to reverse.

The sensitivity of different muscle groups to relaxant drugs varies considerably; thus, the muscles of the eyelids are paralysed most easily, and then relaxation of the limbs and jaws, intercostals and abdominal muscles follows with increasing dosage, and finally the diaphragm will be paralysed. However, it is not uncommon to find that intubation can be performed when there is little effect on the muscles of the hand. There is considerable overlapping of these effects, and even small doses insufficient to produce abdominal relaxation may depress respiration. The muscles of the forehead tend to be resistant and wrinkling of the eyebrows may be an important sign of unintended consciousness in an otherwise fully paralysed patient.

Residual weakness due to competitive agents should be treated with neostigmine mixed with, or preceded by, glycopyrrolate or atropine. In the case of continued weakness due to depolarizing drugs, artificial respiration should be continued until ventilation is adequate.

It has been common practice in recent years to use suxamethonium for intubation, and later to give a competitive relaxant for maintenance of relaxation during operation. This practice rarely gives rise to complications but because of the inherent complications associated with suxamethonium administration, many anaesthetists' normal practice is to use a single (competitive) agent for both intubation and maintenance, the latter either by intermittent boluses or by infusion. Suxamethonium has also been given following the administration of a competitive blocking drug to provide relaxation for the closure of the peritoneum. However, this practice may lead to difficulties if neostigmine is given to reverse the competitive block before the suxamethonium has been metabolized or the end-plate regained its normal sensitivity, and is not recommended.

A fall in temperature enhances the effect of depolarizing relaxants, but diminishes the effect of competitive relaxants. As a consequence, higher doses of the latter may be necessary during hypothermia, and these will be excessive when the patient's temperature rises.

Apart from their use in anaesthesia for general surgery and obstetrics, muscle relaxants are used to minimize the convulsions in electroconvulsive therapy, and in the treatment of infective tetanus. They are occasionally used to aid controlled ventilation in intensive care units (see below).

Anaesthetists have long expressed a need for two properties which were not available in competitive relaxants for many years. One was a shorter duration of action; the other an agent with a rapid onset comparable to that of suxamethonium. Mivacurium is a competitive agent which is broken down by cholinesterase and is aimed at the first of these needs. Giving a large bolus of an agent such as vecuronium with virtually no side effects has been one approach to achieving a rapid onset, but this is likely to be superseded by the use of rocuronium which has been introduced as an agent with a more rapid onset of action. As with other agents, increasing the size of a bolus dose shortens the time to onset: with rocuronium a $3 \times ED_{95}$ dose will allow intubation in about 60 s, which is close to what can be achieved with suxamethonium. It has only minor cardiovascular side effects in these doses, although the duration is somewhat prolonged.

A different approach to this need is the technique of 'priming', which has generated a lot of controversy and investigation. The theory is that a small 'priming' dose of relaxant, not sufficient to cause any obvious effect but sufficient to occupy a reasonable proportion of the postjunctional receptors, should be given a short while before the main dose which then produces a much quicker onset of block. The priming dose does not necessarily need to be the same drug as the main dose. Investigations have largely centred on the best relative sizes of the two doses and the most effective interval between them. In general, the priming dose should be 10 per cent of the expected intubating dose and the interval between the two doses should be about 4–5 minutes. While 'priming' undoubtedly 'works', it is not without risks. A proportion of patients will experience unpleasant sensations and some may obstruct in the upper airway. The recent introduction of rocuronium is likely to consign this technique to history.

Reversal of competitive blockade

Residual muscle weakness is common after the use of long acting agents and may not be clinically detectable. A TOF ratio (T4/T1) of less than 0.7 may be found, even if reversal agents have been given. There is general agreement that long-acting and medium-acting agents must be reversed, although there is a school of thought which favours spontaneous reversal in the case of atracurium. Mivacurium may often be allowed to reverse spontaneously, but recovery may still be hastened with active intervention. A 'gold standard' of a TOF greater than 0.7 is now accepted. Clinically this equates with being able to sustain a head lift in the horizontal position.

There have been many studies of the best choice of drug, dose and timing, both of the reversal agent itself (an anticholinesterase) and the antimuscarinic agent which needs to precede its administration. The reversal agents, neostigmine, edrophonium and pyridostigmine, inhibit cholinesterase, leading to an increase in the concentration of transmitter ACh competing with the relaxant at the neuromuscular junction. In clinical practice, only neostigmine is routinely employed. The dose is 0.05 mg/kg (2.5–5 mg in an adult). The dose should not exceed this range without good reason: overdose with neostigmine can itself cause neuromuscular block.

Atropine has been the mainstay of antimuscarinic block, but glycopyrrolate is now widely employed because of its lesser penetration of the CNS and lesser effect on heart rate and blood pressure. The dose of atropine is 0.6–1.2 mg; that of glycopyrrolate is 0.2–0.6 mg.

Use in the intensive care unit

Many pathophysiological changes commonly occur in the acutely ill patient which may modify the response to relaxants, including acid-base and electrolyte disturbances, drug interactions, and muscular and neuromuscular disease. The ideal relaxant for use in the intensive care unit would have little effect on the cardiovascular system, not release histamine, not accumulate and not depend on good renal or hepatic function for its degradation. Rapid spontaneous termination of effect and ease of intravenous infusion would also be advantageous. No agent meets all these criteria, but cisatracurium comes closest to the specification because of its spontaneous breakdown and the lesser amounts of laudanosine produced compared with atracurium. If cisatracurium is not available, atracurium can be used with little additional risk.

Relaxants are rarely essential in intensive care unit and their use is avoided if possible because of the risk of awareness during paralysis. They are used in conjunction with heavy sedation to prevent coughing during bronchial aspiration in patients with raised intracranial pressure and to minimize oxygen utilization in severe adult respiratory distress syndrome (ARDS). It is important to monitor the level of block: an appropriate level is where the first twitch, or first and second twitches, of a TOF are present. Patients must be adequately sedated.

Abnormal reactions to relaxants

Neuromuscular blocking agents may give rise to atypical actions, both in pathological conditions and in previously normal patients. Some are not directly due to the action of the drugs themselves, but to the facility they have for disguising other errors of technique. Thus, in the absence of the usual indications, an overdose of centrally acting narcotic or anaesthetic agent may be given, leading to central depression. Likewise, hyperventilation may be imposed on the patient, leading to respiratory alkalosis. Thus, before a neuromuscular blocking drug is held responsible, myoneural block should be demonstrated with a peripheral nerve stimulator.

Possible causes of a continuing block should be considered in relation to the type of muscle relaxant employed; that is, competitive, depolarizing or a mixture of both.

After competitive muscle relaxants

Metabolic acidosis

Better management of fluid and electrolytes and the preoperative correction of metabolic acidosis has resulted in the virtual disappearance of a syndrome originally described as 'neostigmine-resistant' curarization. Three features dominated the clinical picture:

1. Inadequacy of respiration accompanied by a tracheal 'tug'.
2. Tachycardia, hypotension and raised central venous pressure.
3. Coma or semi-coma.

The onset of this syndrome in the immediate postoperative period led to the belief that penetration of the CNS by the relaxant might be involved. It seems more likely that the cause was metabolic acidosis complicated by a respiratory acidosis.

Inadequate respiration unresponsive to neostigmine, particularly if accompanied by coma and cardiovascular depression, calls for continued ventilation and assessment of acid-base state. Both intravascular and extracellular fluid and electrolyte therapy should be critically reappraised, with central venous pressure and ECG monitoring.

Myasthenia gravis-myasthenic syndrome

Latent myasthenia gravis may first be manifest by unexpected sensitivity to competitive relaxants, as may be the myasthenic syndrome, associated with carcinoma of the bronchus.

Antibiotics

Antibiotics of the 'mycin' variety (e.g. neomycin, streptomycin and kanamycin) can cause neuromuscular blockade which is similar to that produced by high concentrations of magnesium, or by calcium deficiency. It is thus pre-synaptic and is due to a reduction in the amount of transmitter released by each nerve impulse. The block is usually only clinically significant when the end-plate potential is simultaneously reduced by competitive blocking agents. Neostigmine may restore transmission. Calcium gluconate will produce further improvement.

After depolarizing agents

Overdose

The continuance of high circulating levels of depolarizing relaxants can lead to the onset of a dual block in some patients. This is rarely accompanied by apnoea, but may cause neuromuscular inadequacy lasting for up to an hour or more.

Low plasma cholinesterase

This can lead to a prolonged action of suxamethonium and mivacurium, but is unlikely to be clinically significant until the level falls to around 10–15 per cent of the normal level. This only occurs in severe liver disease, or in the presence of cholinesterase inhibitors.

Atypical enzyme

Complete apnoea for periods in excess of 5–10 minutes in fit individuals after a normal dose of suxamethonium or prolonged block with mivacurium indicate the probable presence of an atypical plasma cholinesterase. These are genetically determined variants which do not metabolize these agents. This was first demonstrated using as an enzyme inhibitor, the local anaesthetic Dibucaine (cinchocaine). In the presence of a 10^{-5}M concentration of this substance, the enzyme is about 80 per cent inhibited in 97 per cent of the population, who are believed to be homozygous for the 'usual' gene, which is responsible for the elaboration of the 'usual' enzyme. About 0.03 per cent of the population are homozygous for an atypical gene, and their enzyme is resistant to inhibition by

Dibucaine, being only about 20–25 per cent inhibited: 3 per cent of the population are heterozygous and have both types of enzyme in their serum. Their cholinesterase activity is about 60 per cent inhibited. The percentage inhibition of cholinesterase activity in the presence of a 10^{-5}M concentration of Dibucaine is called the Dibucaine Number (DN).

Sodium fluoride is also a differential inhibitor of cholinesterase variants, and the Fluoride Number (FN) can be similarly determined. By using this test, a subgroup of cases has been delineated within the atypical group which is unusually resistant to fluoride, but not particularly to Dibucaine. A 'silent' gene which fails to elaborate any enzyme has also been discovered and other even rarer variants have also been described.

Concurrent administration of cholinesterase inhibitors

Ecothiopate in eye drops can be absorbed in sufficient amounts to affect plasma cholinesterase levels, and prolonged apnoea after suxamethonium has been reported. Some cancer chemotherapeutic agents have also been implicated.

Patients suffering from poisoning by organophosphorus cholinesterase inhibitors would exhibit sensitivity to suxamethonium or mivacurium in addition to other derangements of neuromuscular and autonomic nervous system function.

Muscle rigidity and spasm

Muscle tone can be influenced by other mechanisms than blocking the neuromuscular junction. The rigidity and tremor of Parkinsonism can best be relieved by levodopa, which is believed to act by restoring the level of dopamine in certain motor pathways in the brain. This is discussed in more detail in Chapter 7. Symptoms can also be relieved by the use of anticholinergic agents that penetrate the brain.

There are now many centrally-acting drugs available for the relief of muscle spasm. Mephenesin, the oldest drug of this type, has been superseded by newer congeners such as orphenadrine, methocarbamol and metaxalone. In animals, these drugs diminish experimental hypertonia and protect against convulsive agents. In man, they can be employed to relieve spasticity, particularly associated with trauma and inflammation. They are all sedatives in large doses.

A third site of action for influencing muscle tone is the muscle itself. Dantrolene represents a class of muscle relaxant acting at this site. Its importance for anaesthetists is that it is effective in the treatment of malignant hyperthermia, an inherited condition associated with abnormal muscle calcium channel activity. It is also given orally in spastic conditions, such as those resulting from multiple sclerosis, spinal cord injury, stroke and cerebral palsy.

Muscle spasticity can also be relieved by local therapy via the neuromuscular apparatus. Very small doses of botulinum toxin A (20 ng) can be infiltrated which produce local paralysis by interfering with uptake of cytoplasmic acetylcholine into the pre-synaptic vesicles.

Feldman, S. (1993) Biophase binding: its effect on recovery from non-depolarising neuromuscular block. *Anaesthetic Pharmacology Review*, **1**, 81–7
Wessler, I. (1993) Pre-synaptic neuromuscular block. *Anaesthetic Pharmacology Review*, **1**, 69–76

MONOGRAPHS

ALCURONIUM

Alcuronium chloride (rINN)

Alcuronium is a derivative of calabash curare alkaloid C-toxiferine-I and is prepared from toxiferine by the substitution of an allyl radical in each of the two quaternary ammonium groups.

Pharmacology

It is a competitive muscle relaxant, about twice as potent as tubocurarine, but its duration of action is slightly longer. As with tubocurarine, hypotension may follow its use. Indeed, it is very difficult to distinguish between the cardiovascular effects of alcuronium and tubocurarine. There is usually a small fall in mean blood pressure and a slight rise in pulse rate. Alcuronium is bound to serum albumin.

Indications and dosage

Alcuronium can be used in any situation in which any other competitive relaxant could be employed and 10–20 mg may be given intravenously, depending on the site of operation and degree of relaxation required; further doses of 3–5 mg can be given as necessary. If an inhalational agent is being used for the maintenance of anaesthesia, smaller doses will be required. Alcuronium is effectively antagonized by neostigmine. Precautions are the same as for other muscle relaxants.

ATRACURIUM

Atracurium dibesilate (rINN)

Pharmacology

Atracurium is a highly specific, competitive, neuromuscular blocking agent which was designed to undergo spontaneous breakdown at body temperature and at physiological pH by 'Hofmann elimination', a spontaneous degradation into inactive fragments. Laudanosine is one of the breakdown products. It is also broken down by ester hydrolysis (see below).

Cardiovascular system There is normally little histamine release with recommended doses, although it has been reported. There is also little effect on autonomic ganglia. Bradycardia may, however, occur when vagotonic agents such as halothane and opiates are in use and no antimuscarinic premedication has been given because, like vecuronium, it has no intrinsic antivagal activity.

Respiratory system Effects are similar to those with other muscle relaxants. There is little risk of bronchospasm.

Muscular system Striated muscles are paralysed by a competitive action at the myoneural junction. The rate of onset depends on the size of the dose, as does the duration of action. A dose of 0.6 mg/kg will last approximately 30–40 minutes. The duration of action can be extended by further supplements in a predictable way. The blockade terminates spontaneously within about 20–30 minutes of the last dose. Recovery can be hastened by the administration of neostigmine, preceded by atropine or glycopyrrolate. Recovery from full blockade takes 10 minutes.

Placental barrier There is some placental transfer, but the quantities are not sufficient to produce clinical block in the fetus.

Fate in the body The mode of elimination varies between species. In man, Hofmann elimination is the principal mode of breakdown; the breakdown products are laudanosine and an acrylate ester (see below). There is also a breakdown pathway by non-specific esterases in man. The breakdown products of this reaction appear to be innocuous. Termination of action is thus unaffected by renal or hepatic failure and it has been used successfully in anephric patients.

Indications

Atracurium may be used in any situation in which other competitive muscle relaxants could be used, but is particularly indicated in the presence of renal failure. Its relative lack of cardiovascular effects would also appear to be an advantage in many clinical situations.

Dosage and administration

The initial intravenous dose lies between 0.3 and 0.6 mg/kg. The latter dose is necessary when the patient is to be intubated; a smaller dose can be used when the drug is given after intubation under suxamethonium. It has a relatively short onset of action, and intubation can be achieved in 1.5–2 minutes with doses of 0.6 mg/kg. The duration of action depends on the dose and lies between about 20 and 40 minutes for doses of 0.3–0.6 mg/kg. Supplementary doses of one-third as much extend the duration of action for an equal time. Such doses are not cumulative and have a similar effect.

The doses for children over the age of 1 year can be calculated on the same dose/body weight basis. Supplementary doses lie between 0.1 and 0.2 mg/kg, depending on the duration of action required. Dosage should be reduced by about one-third in the presence of hypothermia to 25°C. Changes in body pH within the physiological range seem to have little effect. The action is potentiated by halogenated anaesthetics and by aminoglycoside antibiotics.

Precautions

Laudanosine has been detected in plasma and has occasioned interest because it is a cerebral stimulant. The concentration of laudanosine required to produce convulsions in dogs is >20 µg/ml; the concentrations found after clinical use of atracurium have been between 2 and 14 µg/ml. Laudanosine is cleared by the liver and its clearance is not affected by concurrent renal failure. It is therefore safe for prolonged use in the intensive care unit although the situation in the presence of concomitant hepatic failure has not been studied.

It seems possible that the acrylate ester may also be of importance. This was not detected in pre-release testing in rodents, perhaps because there is rapid breakdown in these species, probably by esterases, leaving little for Hofmann elimination. Acrylate esters are likely to be cytotoxic to hepatocytes (Nigrovic *et al.*, 1990). That said, extensive post-marketing surveillance and two large prospective trials involving nearly 3000 patients have failed to detect any higher incidence of a wide range of serious side effects.

Nigrovic, V., Segal, F., Klaunig, J. E. and Fry, K. (1990) The site and mechanism of the cytotoxic effect of atracurium in vitro. *European Journal of Anaesthesiology* **7**, 123

CISATRACURIUM

Cisatracurium besilate (rINN)

Cisatracurium is the R-*cis*, R'-*cis* isomer of atracurium, preservative-free. It is a single isomer, one of the 10 isomers in commercial atracurium.

Pharmacology

Cisatracurium is approximately four times as potent as atracurium (ED_{95} of 0.05 mg/kg, compared to 0.23 mg/kg). Its action is at the neuromuscular junction where it blocks cholinoceptors. Its pharmacological properties closely resemble those described above for atracurium, which monograph should also be consulted.

Fate in the body The principal mode of breakdown is Hofmann elimination, a spontaneous degradation into inactive fragments. Laudanosine is one of the breakdown products. There is no direct metabolism by esterases. However, being more potent, much less cisatracurium is needed and therefore there is less laudanosine produced. Even in patients with renal failure or those receiving prolonged infusions, the highest plasma levels of laudanosine are well below the toxic threshold, about one-fifth of the level found with atracurium.

Cisatracurium does not cause histamine release, even after large bolus doses up to 8 $\times$ ED_{95}.

Cardiovascular system No significant changes have been seen in either heart rate or blood pressure, even with large doses.

Kidney and liver As breakdown is largely independent of renal excretion or hepatic metabolism, cisatracurium is particularly suitable in such conditions. The duration of action is, however, slightly prolonged in renal disease, suggesting that it may normally undergo slightly more renal excretion that atracurium.

The effect of cisatracurium is the same in patients with cirrhosis as in normal healthy patients.

Indications

Cisatracurium may be used for any indication requiring competitive neuromuscular blockade of medium duration. It is, however, particularly indicated in the presence of renal failure or hepatic dysfunction and seems likely to replace atracurium wherever the latter is particularly indicated.

Dosage and administration

The drug is presented in ampoules containing 2 mg/ml, but is also available as 5 mg/ml in vials. The usual dose ($2 \times ED_{95}$) allows intubation within 3 minutes and has a clinical duration of effect of 40–45 minutes. Large doses ($3 \times ED_{95}$) allow earlier intubation and have a longer duration of effect – 2 minutes and 55 minutes, respectively. For continuous infusion, an initial rate of 3 µg/kg/minute is recommended, falling to 1–2 µg/kg/minute for longer maintenance. The dose should be reduced by 40 per cent in the presence of isoflurane and ethrane anaesthesia. Dosage is not affected by age.

DANTROLENE

Dantrolene sodium (rINN)

The drug is presented as a dry orange-coloured powder, consisting of dantrolene 20 mg, mannitol 3 g, and sufficient sodium hydroxide to make a solution of approximate pH 9.5 when reconstituted with 60 ml of water. Unreconstituted, the powder can be stored indefinitely if kept below 30°C and protected from light. It is also available in tablet form.

Pharmacology

Dantrolene uncouples excitation–contraction coupling in isolated muscle preparations, probably by interfering with the release of ionic calcium from the sarcoplasmic reticulum. The malignant hyperthermia syndrome is an abnormality of muscle, inherited as an autosomal dominant, occurring in about 1 in 20 000 of the population. In those who have the syndrome, triggering agents, notably suxamethonium, halothane and other volatile inhalational agents, cause a rise in myoplasmic calcium, although it is not absolutely certain whether this is due to accelerated release from the sarcoplasmic reticulum or failure of this structure to re-accumulate it. This rise in myoplasmic calcium activates tropomyosin and sustains active contraction with consequent catabolism, heat and CO_2 production. The effectiveness of dantrolene in preventing and treating the condition in susceptible pigs (a syndrome that is believed to be the same as the human one) suggests that the main action is on the prevention of sarcoplasmic release of calcium.

Dantrolene has no action on neuromuscular transmission, the membrane action potential or muscle excitability. However, it diminishes the force of contraction of muscles stimulated via the motor nerve. Reflex contractions are affected more than voluntary ones.

Indications

The main therapeutic indication is the treatment of the malignant hyperthermia syndrome. The drug can also be given by mouth in spastic conditions such as those resulting from multiple sclerosis, spinal cord injury, cardiovascular accident and cerebral palsy.

Dosage and administration

Dantrolene is only one element in the management of malignant hyperthermia. As soon as the diagnosis is made, all anaesthetic agents should be discontinued, additional oxygen given, ventilation adjusted and cooling started. An initial dose of 1 mg/kg should be given rapidly intravenously and repeated if the physiological and metabolic abnormalities persist or reappear. The average dose needed is 2–3 mg/kg, but up to 10 mg/kg may be given. For the treatment of spasticity, 25 mg daily should be administered initially, increasing cautiously up to a maximum of 400 mg/day. Doses above 225 mg a day are rarely required to achieve the maximum therapeutic effect.

Precautions

The prognosis of untreated malignant hyperthermia is so poor that consideration of potential toxic effects is of no relevance when the drug is used acutely. As the solution is very alkaline, care should be taken to avoid extravasation.

Dantrolene is potentially hepatotoxic and liver function tests should be performed before starting chronic therapy and thereafter at intervals. Other common side effects are drowsiness, weakness, fatigue and diarrhoea.

GALLAMINE

Gallamine triethiodide (rINN)

Pharmacology

Gallamine is a competitive muscle relaxant, no longer available in the United Kingdom, where it has been superseded by agents with far fewer and less troublesome side effects. It is still in use in some developing countries.

Cardiovascular system   There is an inhibitory action on the vagal nerve supply to the heart which results in tachycardia. This increased heart rate is occasionally accompanied by cardiac irregularities. Blood pressure usually remains unchanged.

Respiratory system   Bronchospasm due to histamine release is extremely rare.

Placental barrier   Appreciable amounts of gallamine cross the placenta, but the infant's ventilation is not affected clinically after delivery.

Fate in the body   Negligible amounts of gallamine are excreted in the absence of renal function. Gallamine is bound to serum albumin, and the increase in potency in man with increasing pH which has been described is probably related to changes in this binding.

Indications

The indications for the use of gallamine are similar to those for any other competitive relaxant, but its briefer action has made it popular for short operations. However, if a full paralysing dose is still present at the end of the procedure, gallamine is in fact more difficult to reverse with neostigmine than an equipotent dose of tubocurarine or pancuronium.

Dosage and administration

An initial dose of 80–120 mg intravenously will produce full relaxation in 1.5–2 minutes. Duration of apnoea is variable but may last up to 10 minutes: inadequate ventilation lasts much longer. Supplementary doses of 20–40 mg are given as required.

Precautions

Gallamine should not be used in patients suffering from myasthenia gravis, in the presence of renal failure or when tachycardia is undesirable.

MIVACURIUM

Mivacurium chloride (rINN)

Mivacurium is supplied as a pale yellow aqueous solution containing 2 mg/ml, in 5 ml and 10 ml ampoules. Its pH is 4.5 and it should not be mixed with highly alkaline solutions (e.g. thiopental).

Pharmacology

Mivacurium is supplied as a mixture of three stereoisomers. The *trans-trans* isomer comprises 57 per cent of the mixture and the *cis-trans* isomer comprises 36 per cent of the mixture. These two isomers have similar very high clearances and small volumes of distribution, resulting in a half-life of elimination of about 2 minutes. The *cis-cis* isomer comprises only 4–8 per cent of the dose: its clearance is slow and its elimination half-life is 55 minutes. The manufacturers claim that this is of little importance, citing the fact that the recovery rate after a prolonged infusion is no different from that after a bolus dose. In cats, the *cis-cis* isomer has only one-tenth the potency of the other two isomers and is therefore thought to contribute little to the neuromuscular blocking action.

Mivacurium is a benzylisoquinolinium, the same class of compound as tubarine and atracurium, which has been specially designed with two ester linkages which can be hydrolysed by plasma cholinesterase. In this respect it has some similarities with atracurium but is not broken down by Hofmann degradation. It is thus a short-acting relaxant with a fast spontaneous recovery rate. Its actions can also be reversed more quickly than those of other blocking agents.

Its speed of onset is slower than that of suxamethonium, and comparable to that of atracurium and vecuronium. It is not suitable, therefore, for rapid sequence induction. The recommended initial dose (0.2 mg/kg) will allow intubation in 2–2.5 minutes. Mivacurium may show no TOF fade during onset, and intubation is possible before TOF is lost at the adductor policis. As with all competitive neuromuscular blocking agents, duration of effect depends on the size of the dose. A dose of 0.2 mg/kg can be expected to have a clinical duration of action of about 16 minutes.

Mivacurium's characteristic rapid spontaneous recovery rate depends on both the type of cholinesterase present and its concentration being 'normal'. A dose of 0.2 mg/kg will be associated with 95 per cent recovery in 25–30 minutes. The mean time to recover from 25 per cent to 75 per cent of the twitch response is 6 minutes. Recovery time is not affected by repeated doses or continuous infusion and is therefore considered non-cumulative. In common with similar agents, rapid injection of large bolus doses can result in histamine-induced cardiovascular responses, a rise in pulse rate and a transient fall in blood pressure. These are minor after recommended doses.

Kidney   The duration of action is prolonged in patients with chronic renal failure: in patients undergoing transplantation, the clinical effective duration is increased by 50 per cent. The reason for this is not clear.

Liver   If cholinesterase activity is reduced, as it may be in end-stage hepatic failure, the action of mivacurium will be prolonged. In patients in end-stage hepatic failure undergoing liver transplantation, the action has been reported as being increased three-fold.

Fate in the body   Mivacurium is hydrolysed by plasma cholinesterase by two pathways, depending on which ester bond is hydrolysed first. The rate depends on the concentration of drug in the plasma and so obeys first-order kinetics. The metabolites are inactive and excreted in the bile and urine.

Inhalation agents potentiate the effect, both in magnitude and duration, in the order sevoflurane > isoflurane > enflurane > halothane. In the presence of isoflurane, for example, the required dose may be reduced by 25 per cent. Alternatively, the action of an unchanged dose will be prolonged by 35–40 per cent. Halothane may prolong the duration of action by 20 per cent.

Indications

Mivacurium can be used in all situations requiring neuromuscular block, but is mainly indicated whenever rapid recovery is required, notably short surgical procedures of 5–20 minutes and in day-stay surgery. It can be used for longer procedures which nevertheless require rapid recovery by giving it as a continuous infusion.

Dosage and administration

The recommended initial dose in healthy adults is 0.2 mg/kg, given over 30 s. Slightly larger doses on a weight basis are needed in children to achieve similar effects. Doses may need to be less in elderly subjects. Top-up doses of half the initial dose can be given, approximately every 15 minutes.

Onset can be hastened by 'priming'. However, there seems little reason to use this technique (see page 275). If given by continuous infusion after an initial bolus, 10 µg/kg/minute is recommended as a starting infusion, but this can usually be reduced to 6–7 µg/kg/minute. Children require higher dose rates. Recovery can be hastened by standard doses of anticholinesterases preceded by a vagolytic agent. However, it may not be routinely necessary, since once spontaneous recovery is apparent it will be complete in 10–15 minutes.

Precautions

The dependence on plasma cholinesterase as the primary mechanism for inactivation raises some special problems. Mivacurium is not broken down significantly by atypical cholinesterases, so individuals homozygous for the atypical gene (phenotype $E^1_a E^1_a$) will have a very prolonged period of paralysis. As this occurs in roughly 1 in 3000 patients this is a rare risk which cannot be avoided, any more than it can with suxamethonium. However, the heterozygous condition occurs in 1 in 40 of the population and, unlike suxamethonium, the duration of action of mivacurium is obviously prolonged in such individuals, typically by about 10–20 minutes. In general, a dose of 0.2 mg/kg, which would produce total paralysis lasting 10–20 minutes in normal homozygotes, will last 25–60 minutes in heterozygotes and >60 minutes in atypical homozygotes. If the duration of the initial dose indicates a heterozygote, repeat doses should be reduced to about one-quarter (0.025 mg/kg).

In common with other similar neuromuscular blocking agents, the effect of mivacurium may be enhanced by aminoglycoside antibiotics and a wide variety of other drugs including propranolol, calcium channel blockers, diuretics, magnesium salts and ganglion blocking agents. Specific to mivacurium are other agents which enhance its action, including oral contraceptives and chronic administration of glucocorticoids, certain monomine oxidase inhibitors and irreversible inhibitors of cholinesterase.

PANCURONIUM

Pancuronium bromide (rINN)

Pharmacology

Pancuronium is a synthetic muscle relaxant, and is a bisquaternary aminosteroid without hormonal activity. Following its introduction it achieved wide popularity as a competitive muscle relaxant for routine use, with a duration of action comparable to tubocurarine.

Nervous system As with other relaxants of this type, the drug does not cross the blood–brain barrier. There is a mild vagolytic action on the heart but no evidence of ganglion blockade in normal doses.

Cardiovascular system Pancuronium causes a moderate rise in pulse rate of about 20 per cent, a rise in arterial blood pressure of 10–20 per cent, and an increase in cardiac output. There is no change in peripheral vascular resistance. None of these changes is seen in atropinized patients, thus indicating that the mechanism is due to a vagolytic effect of the drug.

Respiratory system Pancuronium appears to be free of histamine-releasing properties and has been used satisfactorily in patients with high bronchial reactivity, although bronchospasm and anaphylactoid reactions have been reported very occasionally. Respiratory muscles are depressed or paralysed, depending on the size of the dose.

Muscular system Relaxation of striated muscle follows a competitive blockade of the neuromuscular junction. The onset of paralysis is quicker than with tubocurarine; after a dose of 0.15 mg/kg it is usually possible to intubate within 1.5 minutes. Paralysis is readily reversed by neostigmine, except within 10–20 minutes of a paralysing dose. It increases the tone of the lower oesophageal sphincter.

Kidney Pancuronium can be used satisfactorily in cases of renal failure. It has been recommended for intubation and maintenance in renal transplantation, but has been replaced by atracurium for this indication.

Placental barrier Some pancuronium can be detected in the fetal blood, but no clinical effects on the fetus have been reported, and it may be used for operative obstetrics.

Fate in the body Eighty-seven per cent of a clinical dose is protein bound. The majority of the drug is broken down in the liver and excreted in the bile. It has been reported that some patients with liver disease show resistance to the drug, but the reason for this is not clear. Moderate degrees of hyperventilation do not affect recovery time, but a severe respiratory acidosis does slow recovery.

Indications

Pancuronium may be used for neuromuscular relaxation of fairly long duration. It can be used for any surgical procedure requiring muscle relaxation lasting more than 30 minutes. Because of its effects on the cardiovascular system it has been recommended as the relaxant of choice in poor-risk and emergency cases. However, most anaesthetists, given the opportunity, would use a newer agent with no side effects.

Dosage and administration

Pancuronium is only given intravenously. Dose–response curves show that the potency increases as the doses are increased. At the dose levels necessary to just produce total paralysis, it is seven times as potent as tubocurarine, and early reports of difficulty in reversing its action could have been due to relative overdose. Initial doses should not exceed 0.1 mg/kg.

Precautions

Pancuronium will trigger malignant hyperpyrexia in pigs, but there have been no cases reported in man. As with other relaxants of this type, it should be avoided in cases of myasthenia gravis; its actions can be antagonized by neostigmine preceded by an antimuscarinic parasympatholytic agent.

ROCURONIUM

Rocuronium bromide (rINN)

Pharmacology

Rocuronium is a competitive neuromuscular blocking agent, an aminosteroid analogue of vecuronium developed to have a more rapid onset. It is an agent of low potency and therefore given in higher doses: this is believed to be crucial to achieving rapidity of onset.

Fate in the body   As with other aminosteroids, rocuronium is mainly metabolized by the liver, but about 30 per cent is excreted unchanged in the urine. As it lacks an acetyl group in the 3C position, there is no accumulation of active metabolites during prolonged infusions in the presence of renal or hepatic disease. Rocuronium may liberate a small amount of histamine.

Kidney   In patients undergoing renal transplantation, onset and recovery times are similar to those in healthy patients with similar clearance values. A larger volume of distribution accounts for a longer elimination phase which, in patients with renal failure not undergoing transplantation, may account for longer recovery times. It seems unlikely that rocuronium will replace atracurium in such patients.

Liver   There is a decreased clearance in hepatic cirrhosis, leading to prolonged recovery time. It is unlikely that rocuronium will replace atracurium or cisatracurium in this condition.

Nervous system Rocuronium does not cross the blood–brain barrier and has no central action. It has no direct effect on intracranial pressure (ICP) but any cardiovascular effects will produce the predictable changes in ICP.

Cardiovascular system Larger doses (0.9 mg/kg) induce a small increase in heart rate and small rise in mean arterial blood pressure. These effects are due to a weak vagal blocking effect.

Eye The effects on intra-ocular pressure are minimal, although the mild cardiovascular effects of large doses may have a slight secondary effect.

Placenta Rocuronium does not cross the placenta.

Dosage and administration

The drug is available as solution in ampoules of 5 ml and 10 ml, both at a concentration of 10 mg/ml. The ED_{95} is close to 0.3 mg/kg. When doses of $2 \times ED_{95}$ (0.6 mg/kg) are given, mean onset time is 75 s and intubation is possible in about 1½ minutes. The onset times for $1 \times ED_{95}$ and $3 \times ED_{95}$ (0.3 mg/kg and 0.9 mg/kg, respectively) are about 3½–4 minutes and 1 minute. The dose required to maintain a 90 per cent block to twitch is about 0.15 mg/kg, given whenever block reduces to 25 per cent.

The duration of a 0.6 mg/kg dose is close to 35 minutes. There is some prolongation with isoflurane, enflurane and halothane. Sevoflurane, however, increases the duration by about 30 per cent. There is no accumulation on repeat dosing. Thus rocuronium has the most rapid onset of any currently available non-depolarizing agent, but its duration of action is as long as that of vecuronium when used in doses which enable rapid intubation to be performed.

Rocuronium may be given by continuous infusion, requiring about 0.6 mg/kg/h with a total intravenous anaesthetic technique, but only about 0.35 mg/kg/h when used with inhalational agents.

Indications

Rocuronium has been developed as an agent with a rapid onset. Several studies have compared it with suxamethonium for rapid sequence induction, and intubation is possible with large doses in broadly comparable times. However, it has still not been adequately evaluated for use for rapid sequence induction in emergency cases with a full stomach.

It is also of value as a relatively short-acting agent in moderate doses, the average duration of clinical effect of 0.6 mg/kg being 35 minutes.

Drug interactions There is potentiation of effect by some antibiotics. Prior administration of suxamethonium causes a more rapid onset and longer duration of action. Its action is rapidly reversed by neostigmine.

SUXAMETHONIUM SALTS

Suxamethonium bromide and chloride and Succinylcholine chloride (rINN)

Aqueous solutions of suxamethonium salts hydrolyse slowly with loss of potency; this hydrolysis takes place more rapidly at tropical temperatures and it is preferable that prepared injections should be stored in a refrigerator. The dry powders retain their potency for much longer periods. The rate of hydrolysis is markedly increased in alkaline media. It should not be mixed with intravenous induction agents.

Pharmacology

Suxamethonium is a short-acting depolarizing muscle relaxant, most commonly used as the chloride. When given intravenously it acts within 30 s, with duration of effect up to 3–5 minutes, depending on dose.

Nervous system   Suxamethonium has no action on the CNS. In spite of its chemical similarity to acetylcholine, its action on autonomic effector organs is not great, but muscarinic actions are sometimes observed.

Cardiovascular system   There is no direct action on the heart, but vagal stimulation may cause bradycardia and a fall in blood pressure. This is more likely to occur after large doses or when the dose is repeated. Arrhythmias and temporary cardiac arrest may also occur. Atropine given previously will prevent these effects and stop them when present.

Circulatory arrest has been reported when suxamethonium is used in burned patients. This is due to an acute rise in serum K^+. This rise is common in burned and injured patients and is maximal between the 21st and 26th day after injury.

Hypotension associated with a skin rash and other evidence of an anaphylactic reaction has also been reported not infrequently.

Muscular system   There is a rapid, profound and almost synchronous neuromuscular block of skeletal muscle, usually preceded by fasciculation, due to depolarization of the motor end-plate. The response varies widely between patients, even in the absence of detectable differences in plasma cholinesterase activity. Body surface area is more nearly related to the degree of block than either lean body mass or total body weight. Sometimes, especially when the drug is given repeatedly, the initial depolarizing block is followed by one with features resembling a competitive block, the so-called 'phase II' block. This may result in prolonged action and the block, when fully established, can usually be antagonized by an anticholinesterase, such as edrophonium or neostigmine. The onset is mainly dose (cumulative) dependent, not time dependent.

Suxamethonium has an abnormal effect in many muscular diseases, including myotonia (in which it may cause contracture) and polymyositis. It is also one of the drugs which trigger the malignant hyperthermia syndrome.

Respiratory system   Apart from paralysis of the muscles of respiration, there may be some increase in bronchial secretions. An anaphylactic response has occasionally been reported in which bronchospasm was a feature.

Alimentary tract   There is an increase in intragastric pressure and there may be some increase in bowel movement and in gastric and salivary secretions due to a muscarinic action. This may be inhibited by atropine.

Uterus and placental barrier   There is no change in intra-uterine pressure with either intermittent or continuous administration. Suxamethonium does not reach the fetal circulation.

The eye The administration of suxamethonium causes an abrupt and short-lived rise in intra-ocular pressure which returns to normal within 6 minutes. This is principally due to contracture (i.e. spasm) of the extra-ocular muscles and is a consequence of their multiple innervation. However, the rise does not occur in the majority of patients with glaucoma, which suggests that changes in arterial and venous pressure are also of importance.

Elimination Suxamethonium is hydrolysed by plasma cholinesterase into succinyl-monocholine and choline; the former is further broken down to succinic acid and choline and about 2 per cent is excreted unchanged in the urine. Suxamethonium is hydrolysed to the monocholine six times faster than the monocholine to succinic acid and choline. The monocholine therefore accumulates temporarily; it has some neuromuscular blocking action, but it is about one-twentieth of that of suxamethonium.

Low cholinesterase activity, which may be due to liver disease, malnutrition, pregnancy, particularly if associated with pre-eclampsia, poisoning with organophosphate compounds, or genetic factors, will cause delay in elimination of the drug and thus a prolongation of its action. Resistance to its effects occurs in mild myasthenia gravis and in the neonate. Longer periods of paralysis can be produced by combining it with reversible cholinesterase inhibitors such as edrophonium and tacrine.

Indications

Suxamethonium is used whenever profound relaxation of skeletal muscles is required for short periods. It is, therefore, particularly useful in endoscopies, manipulations and electroconvulsive therapy, and as an aid to tracheal intubation. It has been used for longer operations by repeated doses or by intravenous infusion, but this practice is no longer recommended.

Dosage and administration

Suxamethonium salts are ineffective by mouth, and although normally given intravenously they can be used intramuscularly. The latter method can be employed in infants and small children when suitable veins cannot be found.

The ED_{95} is around 0.5 mg/kg and therefore the average clinical dose of 0.75–1 mg/kg completely blocks motor activity in virtually all patients.

Doses recommended for neonates and infants vary considerably. Neonates may be given an initial dose of 1–2 mg as required. The total dose should not exceed 50 mg. A single dose of 2 mg/kg may be given intramuscularly for intubation, but should not be repeated owing to the danger of prolonged action. Children may be given 1 mg/kg intravenously; infants and small children may require an initial dose of 2 mg/kg.

Precautions

Suxamethonium is contra-indicated in severe liver disease, in burned patients, in those with large degenerating muscle masses, for example paraplegia of recent onset and major limb trauma, and in patients known to be liable to the malignant hyperthermia syndrome. Its use is best avoided in advanced myasthenia gravis. Premedication with atropine is advisable to prevent excessive bronchial secretions, bradycardia and other muscarinic effects. It is inadvisable in uraemic patients, particularly those with high serum K^+ in whom a further rise in K^+ may occur.

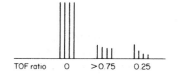

Figure 9.4 A diagrammatic representation of the development of a Phase II block with a TOF ratio changing from over 0.75 to 0.25

Suxamethonium should be used with circumspection in patients with a penetrating injury of the eye or while the globe is open. Suxamethonium is absolutely contra-indicated in patients with myotonia, who develop a rigidity which renders inflation of the lungs impossible.

Complications following the use of suxamethonium include muscle pains in the postoperative period and prolonged partial blockade or apnoea. Muscle pains similar in nature to the aches and discomfort following strenuous exercise, but sometimes much more severe, occur in the immediate postoperative period and may last for several days. There is usually little inconvenience to patients who are confined to bed after operation, but ambulant patients may suffer considerable discomfort, although this is said to be comparatively uncommon in pregnant women. These pains do not appear to be related to the size of the dose of suxamethonium given or the amount of fasciculation following the initial injection. The incidence can be reduced by giving small doses of a competitive relaxant just prior to the injection of suxamethonium. Thiopental given just previously also exerts a considerable protective effect. It is better to avoid the use of suxamethonium in outpatients and make sure that inpatients remain in bed for at least 24 h following operation. Muscle fasciculation is also associated with rises in serum creatine phospho-kinase, a muscle enzyme, and with rises in serum K^+. This rise also can be diminished by pretreatment with a small dose of a competitive muscle relaxant. The response is greater in traumatized and burned patients; the magnitude of the rise depends on the interval since injury.

Large doses or prolonged administration of suxamethonium lead to a change in the character of the block. The characteristics of a Phase II block appear gradually and not all of them develop simultaneously. The onset seems to be both time and dose depen-dent and the underlying mechanisms are still unclear. The development of Phase II block can be detected by TOF stimuli (*Figure 9.4*). A relatively well-sustained partial block with a TOF ratio of over 0.75 changes to a TOF ratio of much less. It seems clear from the examination of case reports that the administration of neostigmine in the early stages of a prolonged block was responsible for the very long apnoeas reported, but that when the block exhibited well-developed characteristics of a Phase II block, neostigmine restored normal function.

Decamethonium is no longer commercially available in Great Britain. It is a depolarizing muscle relaxant. Its action lasts for 15–20 minutes and is preceded by fasciculation. The dose is 2–4 mg. There is no action on the CNS, but depression of autonomic ganglia may cause a fall in blood pressure, bradycardia and dilatation of the pupil. Dual block and muscle pains may occur. It is excreted in the urine and it does not cross the placenta.

TUBOCURARINE

Tubocurarine chloride (rINN)
Synonym: (D)-tubocurarine chloride

History

Curare has been known since the beginning of the sixteenth century under the names of uiraery, urari, ourari, wourari and wourali. It was first obtained from the bark of various species of *Strychnos*, but more recently it has been extracted from *Chondrodendron tomentosum*, a member of the family Menispermaceae. It has been stored in a variety of receptacles – calabash, pot and tube (hollow bamboo canes) – hence the names under which it is described. Most of the experimental investigations have been carried out with tube curare, and it was from this source that the first purified extract and the active principle D-tubocurarine were first obtained.

Curare was first described as an arrow poison in 1516 by Ascorio Sforza in his history of the New World (*De Orbe Novo*), based on letters from explorers who had travelled in what is now Brazil. Similar observations were made by Sir Walter Raleigh in 1595 and Humboldt in 1807. In 1812, Charles Waterton described in detail the effects of curare on animals and his experiment in resuscitating a paralysed donkey with assisted respiration by means of a pair of bellows. Two years later he and Brodie suggested that this drug had a toxic effect on the myoneural mechanism, but it was not until some 40 years later that Claude Bernard proved by his classic experiments that this was in fact true.

The next landmark in the history of curare was in 1935 when King isolated the active principle D-tubocurarine but even this bore no fruit immediately although Palmer of the Middlesex Hospital used it in 1939 to control the spasms of electroconvulsive therapy. At about the same time, Gill returned to the USA from South America with a large quantity of tube curare, from which was extracted the commercial product Intocostrin. Bennet used this preparation in electroconvulsive therapy, and Griffiths and Johnson in Canada were the first to use it for the production of relaxation in anaesthesia in 1942. In Great Britain, much of the pioneer work concerning the use of this drug in anaesthesia was done by Gray and Halton of Liverpool.

Pharmacology

Tubocurarine is a competitive muscle relaxant with an onset time of about 3 minutes. Its effect lasts for 30–40 minutes.

Nervous system   Tubocurarine does not cross the blood–brain barrier and has little effect on the CNS. Autonomic ganglia can be affected in doses normally given to produce neuromuscular block, particularly the sympathetic ganglia, and a fall in blood pressure is common immediately following a bolus dose.

Cardiovascular system   There is no direct action on the heart. The 15–20 per cent fall in blood pressure produced by a bolus dose can be markedly potentiated by inhalational agents. Heart rate may decrease by 10 per cent, but there is no significant change in cardiac output.

Respiratory system   Bronchospasm may occur due to histamine release.

Alimentary tract   There is normally little effect on the gut.

Placental barrier   Tubocurarine does not cross the placenta.

Fate in the body About two-thirds of a dose is normally excreted in the urine, the remainder being metabolized in the liver. In the presence of renal failure, metabolic removal by the liver is able to deal with normal doses.

Larger doses of tubocurarine than those normally required are sometimes necessary when liver function is impaired, and this can be ascribed to the low albumin/globulin ratios which may occur and the ability of serum globulins to bind tubocurarine.

Sensitivity occurs in neonates, in the presence of electrolyte disturbance, myasthenia gravis, and of inhalational anaesthetics.

Indications

Tubocurarine is still used in many parts of the world and has played its part in balanced anaesthesia for many years, although it has been completely replaced by other agents, with fewer side effects, in developed countries. The tendency for the pulse rate and blood pressure to fall are not necessarily a disadvantage.

Dosage and administration

Tubocurarine is normally given in doses of 15–30 mg and supplementary doses of 5–10 mg when required. Tubocurarine can be used in neonates provided that the dose is carefully controlled.

VECURONIUM

Vecuronium bromide (rINN)

This compound is unstable in high concentrations and is presented as a freeze-dried, buffered powder, in vials containing 10 mg of the bromide salt with separate ampoules of water for mixing. The powder can be kept at room temperature without deterioration.

Pharmacology

Vecuronium is the 2β-monoquaternary homologue of pancuronium and is a competitive neuromuscular blocking agent of relatively short duration. The 3-acetyl group is also stereo-isometrically altered in position, resulting in a virtual absence of vagolytic and other cardiovascular effects. The removal of this acetyl group by the liver creates an active metabolite.

Nervous system Vecuronium does not cross the blood–brain barrier. Doses need to exceed 60 times the ED_{95} to produce any effect on the cardiac vagus or the autonomic ganglia.

Cardiovascular system Vecuronium is free of direct actions on the heart or vessels. However, the lack of cardiovascular effects will allow the vagotonic effects of other agents to be more pronounced. They can be prevented or treated with atropine or glycopyrrolate.

Respiratory system Vecuronium does not release histamine. Its effect on the respiratory muscles is as for any similar agent.

Muscular system Relaxation follows competitive blockade of the neuromuscular junction. The ED_{90} is between 40–50 μg/kg. A dose of about 80–100 μg/kg produces complete twitch suppression within about 2 minutes and lasts for 10–15 minutes, followed by recovery from 25 per cent to 75 per cent in a further 9–10 minutes.

Liver and kidney The duration of action of vecuronium is prolonged in the presence of renal failure; the time to 25 per cent recovery is nearly doubled, with clearance reduced by 40 per cent. This is due to the accumulation of an active metabolite. There is prolongation of action in hepatic failure.

Fate in the body Vecuronium is rapidly cleared from the plasma and repeated doses show very little accumulation. Continuous infusion rates to maintain a steady level of block show little change over time. This rapid distribution phase is due to rapid uptake by the liver, but it is not all metabolized; some 20 per cent is excreted unchanged in the urine.

Placental barrier Like pancuronium, the drug can be detected in the fetal blood. Despite its greater lipophilicity, vecuronium does not cross the placenta in clinically important amounts and it can be used for operative delivery.

Indications

Vecuronium can be used for any operation requiring muscle relaxation of any duration. However, because of its relative evanescence, it is highly desirable for the extent of the block to be monitored continuously.

Dosage and administration

Initial doses of 80–100 μg/kg (6–8 mg) are usually sufficient to allow intubation. Because of its lack of cardiovascular side effects, vecuronium can be given in larger doses which shorten the time to onset and extend the duration of action. When large doses are given, although the duration may be as long as after pancuronium, the rate of recovery from 75 per cent to 25 per cent block is significantly faster with vecuronium.

The block is enhanced by prior use of suxamethonium and by the concurrent use of inhalation agents, particularly isoflurane and sevoflurane. Repeat doses of 50 μg/kg given when the TOF ratio returns to 0.2–0.25 per cent will extend the block by 15–20 minutes. Neonates need approximately one-third more, on a weight basis, because of their much larger extracellular fluid volume.

Precautions

These are the same as for other competitive muscle relaxants. Anaphylactoid reactions have occasionally been reported.

Doxacurium is not available in the United Kingdom: clinical experience has been obtained in the USA. The drug is slower in onset (4 minutes to 90 per cent block after 40 μg/kg, which is 1:7 × ED_{95}) with a time to 25 per cent recovery of about 75 minutes. Larger doses (2.7 × ED_{95}) shorten the onset slightly but prolong the recovery time to 160 minutes.

The other feature of doxacurium is a relative lack of circulatory effects suggesting it may have a place in prolonged operations in patients with limited cardiovascular reserves and possibly in the intensive care unit.

Pipecuronium is a long-acting muscle relaxant, not available in the United Kingdom, which has onset times and duration of action similar to those of pancuronium when used in equipotent doses. Its pharmacokinetics are similar to those of pancuronium but it lacks the cardiovascular side effects of that agent. It is almost indistinguishable, therefore, from doxacurium. It may thus fill a useful niche of a 'clean' moderately long-acting muscle relaxant.

10

Parasympathomimetic and cholinergic agents; anticholinesterases

These are drugs which have a similar effect to that of stimulation of the parasympathetic system (fibres in the third. seventh, ninth and tenth cranial nerves, and sacral fibres from the spinal cord). Stimulation of this system may be expected to produce the following effects: constriction of plain muscle of the alimentary tract and detrusor muscle of the bladder; relaxation of sphincters; constriction of bronchial musculature; slowing of the heart and lowering of the blood pressure with dilatation of certain vessels; miosis; promotion of salivary, bronchial, gastric and mucous secretions; stimulation of the pregnant uterus; and contraction of the ciliary muscle of the eye (the lens is now set for near vision and by the opening of the canal of Schlemm intraocular drainage is improved, thus causing a fall in intraocular pressure, *Figure 10.1*).

A not uncommon error is to use the adjectives 'cholinergic' and 'parasympathomimetic' synonymously. Parasympathomimetic refers only to those effects of acetylcholine or cholinergic agents at parasympathetic effectors, whereas cholinergic can refer to acetylcholine reactions, be they muscarinic or nicotinic, and therefore includes actions upon all autonomic ganglia, sympathetic and parasympathomimetic, the neuromuscular junctions of striated muscle, and upon cholinergic sympathetic effectors such as sweat glands and the adrenal medulla.

Parasympathetic stimulation is an unwanted action during anaesthesia, as it increases salivary and bronchial secretions, slows the heart rate and increases myocardial irritability. Certain anaesthetics have this effect, for example chloroform and halothane, and it is usual practice to use an anticholinergic drug to block these muscarinic effects. Excess parasympathetic activity is only helpful in an emergency such as fainting or neurogenic shock, when it is of a protective nature.

Drug action

Cholinergic drugs act at receptors which normally respond to acetylcholine, the chemical transmitter of nerve impulses, at:

- the synapses in all autonomic ganglia, both sympathetic and parasympathetic, and the endings of the preganglionic sympathetic fibres in the adrenal medulla;

RELAXED

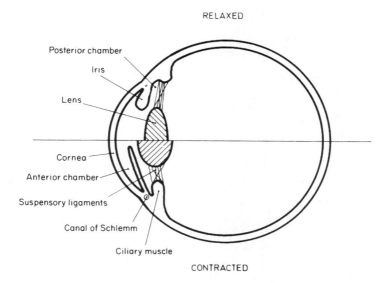

Figure 10.1 Muscarinic agonists contract the ciliary muscle, thereby relaxing the suspensory ligament, setting the lens for near vision. They also contract the circular muscle of the iris, thereby constricting the pupil and opening the canal of Schlemm

- all postganglionic parasympathetic nerve endings;
- postganglionic sympathetic nerve endings in the uterus and sweat glands;
- the end-plates of motor nerves to striated muscle;.
- many CNS synapses.

A variety of neurones, both central and peripheral, have muscarinic receptors which may be either excitatory or inhibitory. The excitatory receptors decrease potassium conductance by three mechanisms. They can close the channels which are responsible for the resting membrane potential, they can antagonize voltage-dependent channels, which leads to slow depolarization and facilitation of firing, and they influence a calcium-dependent channel that causes hyperpolarization after the action potential is generated. Inhibitory receptors cause hyperpolarization by opening potassium channels.

Acetylcholine also probably has actions as a 'local hormone', controlling the rhythmic activity of atrial muscle and of cilia. In tissues, at the relevant nerve endings, it is present combined as an inactive precursor from which it is liberated when a nerve impulse arrives. By its own direct action the acetylcholine then transmits the nerve impulse to postganglionic fibres, by stimulating the cell bodies of the postganglionic neurones; to the autonomic effector organ, by stimulating or depressing its cells directly; and to the motor end-plate of striated muscle, by depolarizing it. Immediately after a nerve impulse has taken effect, acetylcholine is hydrolysed by acetylcholinesterase into choline (which possesses only 1/500 to 1/1000 of the original activity) and acetate. The mechanism of this reaction is discussed in detail on page 300. Choline acetylase catalyses their resynthesis to acetylcholine, and further combination, probably with a protein, yields the precursor again. The effects of acetylcholine may be increased with anticholinesterases, such as neostigmine, which inhibit the hydrolysis of acetylcholine and thus allow it to

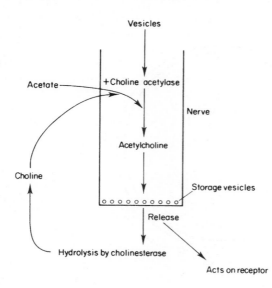

Figure 10.2 Acetylcholine is formed from choline and acetate. It is stored in vesicles and hydrolysed by cholinesterase

persist and to reach a higher concentration when liberated. There is no store of acetylcholine in the body comparable to that of epinephrine (adrenaline) and norepinephrine in the adrenal medulla.

Acetylcholine is stored in small vesicles in the terminal varicosities of cholinergic nerves. Each vesicle is thought to contain about 10^5 molecules of acetylcholine (*Figure 10.2*).

Two main classes of acetylcholine action are recognized – muscarinic and nicotinic – so called because they mimic the effects of muscarine and nicotine, effects which were known before those of acetylcholine.

There are at least three different types of muscarinic receptors, which have been categorized as M_1-, M_2- and M_3-receptors. They have been identified by using inhibitors which have different affinities at the various receptors. All three types of receptor are found in the CNS. Pre-synaptic feedback inhibitory receptors are M_2 type, as are cortical cholinergic nerve endings. The post-synaptic receptors are M_1 and possibly M_3. The cardiac conduction system and cardiac muscle have M_2-receptors, mediating bradycardia and decreased contractility. Vascular smooth muscle mostly has M_1-receptors. In the lung, the large airways contain M_3-receptors, but small airways also contain M_2-receptors. M_3-receptors are found in the gut, bladder and secretory glands.

This differentiation has not yet led to much in the way of development of specific therapeutic agents, although it has led to some clarification of existing drug actions. For example, gallamine and pancuronium have been shown to be specific inhibitors of the M_2-receptor, accounting for their antivagal effects. Bethanecol has a greater affinity for the M_3-receptor than for M_1- or M_2-receptors and this accounts for its selectivity in producing cholinergic effects mainly in the gut.

Carbachol, on the other hand, does not exhibit any selectivity and is now only used to reduce intra-ocular pressure by local application.

Muscarinic actions are antagonized by belladonna alkaloids and their synthetic substitutes and by a variety of agents such as pethidine, procaine, chlorpromazine and some antihistamines.

The nicotinic receptor is present in the cell bodies of autonomic postganglionic neurones, the adrenal medullary cells and the motor end-plates of striated muscle. Persistence of acetylcholine (or nicotine) at these sites finally produces depression there. The mechanism is probably receptor channel block. Antagonists of nicotinic actions usually act much more strongly at one of these types of site than at another. Thus, tubocurarine and other non-depolarizing (competitive) relaxants inhibit neuromuscular transmission in striated muscle in doses that have no demonstrable effect upon autonomic ganglia or the adrenal medulla. On the other hand, hexamethonium and pentamethonium salts have no effect upon neuromuscular transmission when used in doses that inhibit transmission to a high degree in autonomic ganglia.

When nicotinic effects are obtained from injected acetylcholine, it is those upon autonomic ganglia and the adrenal medulla which are mainly in evidence; the neuro-muscular effects, when evident, consist of fibrillary twitchings of striated muscle followed by a transient loss of power. Fortunately, when anticholinesterases are used their nicotinic effects are well in evidence at the neuromuscular junction of striated muscle, where useful clinical antagonism may be achieved against the effects of curare-like drugs. At muscarinic sites, excessive effects may then be counteracted by atropine, glycopyrrolate or hyoscine; the latter drug, however, has little effect on blocking the cardiac vagus in normal doses.

The actions of acetylcholine alone are too brief and too widespread for it to be of clinical use. Synthetic derivatives which are more stable and possess some specificity are used clinically.

Methacholine chloride has actions similar to the muscarinic effects of acetylcholine. It is more stable than the latter drug because it is a poor substrate for cholinesterase and thus more slowly broken down. It is 10–20 times more potent by subcutaneous injection; it simulates the stimulation of parasympathetic postganglionic fibres and opposes many effects of epinephrine. Its effect is mainly on the M_1- and M_2-receptors in the cardiovascular system: it slows the heart and dilates peripheral blood vessels, the combined effects lowering blood pressure. Intestinal tone is increased and the activity of the salivary and sweat glands is stimulated.

It is used to terminate attacks of paroxysmal tachycardia when these do not respond to usual measures, and in the treatment of Raynaud's disease and other vasospastic conditions. Untoward effects are due to excessive parasympathetic stimulation; nausea and vomiting are common with overdosage and precede flushing, sweating and increased salivation. Transient heart block is a rare occurrence, but care should be taken in hypertensive patients who may react to the drug by a sudden and marked fall in blood pressure. Overdose should be treated with atropine.

Bethanechol chloride is another choline ester which is resistant to cholinesterase and which has predominantly muscarinic actions on the M_3-receptor. In normal doses, therefore, it does not slow the heart or lower the blood pressure. It can be used for the treatment of urinary retention, ileus, gastric atony and megacolon. Optimal dosage lies between 30 and 60 mg daily in divided doses. Precautions are as for methacholine.

Pilocarpine is an alkaloid obtained from the leaves of a South American shrub, *Pilocarpus*. It acts primarily at the muscarinic receptors of autonomic effector cells, but also has some ganglionic action. Given systemically, it mimics general cholinergic stimulation, stimulating the smooth muscle of the intestinal tract, bronchi, bladder and gall bladder, and the secretion of sweat, gastric juice, saliva, tears and pancreatic juice. It has somewhat anomalous actions on the cardiovascular system because of its nicotinic actions at the sympathetic ganglia.

It is now used solely in the treatment of glaucoma. Pupillary constriction and spasm of accommodation lead to a fall in intra-ocular pressure after an initial transient rise. The miosis persists for several hours, although the ability to accommodate for near vision returns in about 2 h. It is given as 1–4 per cent eye drops. It is often combined synergistically with physostigmine.

Anticholinesterases

Cholinesterases are of two types: acetylcholinesterase, also known as true, specific, e-type, red cell cholinesterase, and plasma cholinesterase, also known as pseudo-, non-specific, butyro-, s-type cholinesterase. They differ in their location, behaviour towards substrates, and inhibitors. Acetylcholinesterase occurs in red cells and at the endings of all cholinergic neurones. Plasma cholinesterase is not only found in the plasma but also in the liver. Acetylcholine is a more specific substrate for acetylcholinesterase than plasma cholinesterase and the reverse applies to butyrylcholine.

Anticholinesterases are cholinergic in their action as they inhibit or inactivate cholinesterases which normally hydrolyse acetylcholine, and consequently they raise the concentration and duration of action of acetylcholine at all sites at which it is being released. The most noticeable effects are muscarinic ones, since these are evoked by lower concentrations of acetylcholine than are necessary for nicotinic actions. Nicotinic actions can usually be produced safely only when the patient is protected by atropine or glycopyrrolate from excessive muscarinic effects. A familiar example is the use of neostigmine to restore transmission at the neuromuscular junction after blockade with a competitive blocking agent, while atropine prevents untoward muscarinic effects upon the heart, bronchial tree and intestine. It should be noted that excessive amounts of acetylcholine persisting at the motor end-plates of skeletal muscle produce a persistent localized depolarization of the muscle membrane, analogous to that produced by blocking agents such suxamethonium salts. To understand the cholinesterase inhibitors, it is first necessary to understand the enzyme itself.

Acetylcholinesterase

Acetylcholinesterase is widely distributed in the body, and is found wherever acetylcholine is the chemical transmitter. The enzyme can be prepared in a purified form but has not been crystallized. It is a polymeric protein, each unit of which has a molecular weight of about 240 000 Da.

The active site on the enzyme is composed of two subsites, the anionic site and the esteratic site, which are so arranged that they are complementary to the natural substrate acetylcholine. The anionic site binds the N^+ of acetylcholine and this locates the ester linkage in the region of the esteratic site (*Figure 10.3*). Thus, the enzyme has an optimum substrate concentration, and is less effective against longer chain choline esters.

The steps in the hydrolysis of acetylcholine can be outlined diagrammatically (*Figure 10.3*).

Attraction between enzyme and substrate depends on electrical, intermolecular and hydrophobic binding forces. Hydrolysis begins with electron transfer at the esteratic site with the formation of an acetylated enzyme (the intermediate compound) and choline (first product). The half-life of the acetylated enzyme is only 42 μs, but until it is hydrolysed the active site is inhibited.

Although it has such an evanescent existence, the acetylated enzyme is of importance in understanding the action of acid-transferring cholinesterase inhibitors such as neostigmine, physostigmine and organophosphate compounds.

E	+	S	⇌	ES	→	E(Acid)	+	P₁	→	E	+	P₂

$$E \quad + \quad S \quad \rightleftharpoons \quad ES \quad \rightarrow \quad E(Acid) \quad + \quad P_1 \quad \rightarrow \quad E \quad + \quad P_2$$

Enzyme: | Substrate: | Enzyme–substrate complex: | Inter-mediate compound: | First product: | Enzyme: | Second product:

cholin-esterase | acetyl-choline | Michaelis–Menten complex | acetylated enzyme | choline | cholin-esterase | acetic acid

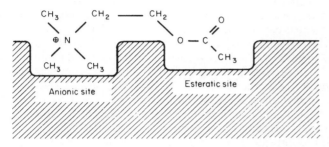

Figure l0.3 Anionic and esteratic binding sites of acetylcholinesterase. Acetylcholine bound to active sites. Initial binding to anionic site by ionic bond between charged nitrogen and ionized carboxylic group; also van der Waals' bonds. The esteratic site contains a glutamic acid–serine–alanine sequence. The serine hydroxyl is involved in the breaking of the ester linkage

Classification of cholinesterase inhibitors

Inhibitors of acetylcholinesterase can be classified as either prosthetic or acid-transferring inhibitors. Prosthetic inhibitors have an affinity for the anionic site on the enzyme, and by their presence impede the combination of enzyme and substrate. They may be regarded therefore as reversible competitive inhibitors of the enzyme. They contain a cationic group, usually a quaternary nitrogen. Examples include tetraethylammonium, edrophonium and tetrahydroaminacrine.

Prosthetic inhibitors form a relatively stable enzyme–substrate complex, the inhibitor molecule merely preventing enzyme and acetylcholine approximating correctly. The reaction between enzyme and inhibitor is in dynamic equilibrium, and the degree of inhibition depends on the concentrations of the three components and the binding affinity between enzyme and inhibitor.

In contrast, the acid-transferring inhibitors act as substrate substitutes for the enzyme. The initial formation of an enzyme–substrate complex (Michaelis–Menten complex) proceeds in the same way as the initial reaction between enzyme and acetylcholine. Likewise, the next stage of formation of an intermediate acid–enzyme compound and first split product also proceeds normally. However, at this stage the intermediate acid–enzyme compound cannot be hydrolysed to release the acid radical and reconstituted enzyme with the rapidity that the acetyl radical can be split off during hydrolysis of acetylcholine. The enzyme is thus inactivated, and the time course of the inhibition depends on the rate at which the hydrolysis takes place. With carbamates such as neostigmine and physostigmine this reaction takes place in a matter of minutes or hours, and such inhibitors used to be called 'reversible'. With the so-called 'irreversible' organophosphate inhibitors the hydrolysis takes days or weeks, but can be markedly speeded up by certain compounds such as pralidoxime iodide.

Acid-transferring inhibitors will also react with plasma cholinesterase. Prosthetic inhibitors, however, are relatively less effective, because this enzyme lacks an anionic site. Both classes of anticholinesterases exhibit excitatory and inhibitory actions on the CNS if given in suitable doses.

Organophosphate compounds

Organophosphate compounds, which have been developed in recent years for use in chemical warfare and as insecticides, are acid-transferring inhibitors of cholinesterase, the acid radical–enzyme complex formed having a negligible rate of hydrolysis. The insecticides, parathion, EPN and OMPA, differ from the nerve gases in that the active cholinesterase inhibitor is only produced as a consequence of metabolism. Malathion is a selective insecticide because it undergoes considerable metabolism in mammals and birds to an inactive compound by enzymes which insects lack. The nerve gases have extremely high lipid solubility so that absorption can occur from any site in or on the body, including intact skin. This high lipid solubility ensures that they cross the blood–brain barrier very easily and thus produce powerful effects on the CNS.

Treatment of poisoning requires atropine 2 mg intravenously, repeated every 30–60 minutes as required. This will relieve muscarinic effects such as bradycardia, hypotension, salivation and bronchospasm. Smaller doses at less frequent intervals may be necessary for several days in severe cases. Central actions, convulsions and nicotinic effects such as muscle weakness will be relieved only by specific therapy of the cholinesterase lesion. Hydrolysis of the acid radical–enzyme can be achieved, particularly with parathion, by pralidoxime iodide or the more soluble methanesulphonate. A dose of 1 g is given intravenously, repeated after 30 minutes if the condition has not improved. A maintenance dose may be given intramuscularly or subcutaneously if signs of poisoning persist. Such reactivators need to be given early because the phosphorylated cholinesterase undergoes 'ageing' and becomes refractory to reversal. Some organophosphate agents are inherently more difficult to reverse by this means. Barbiturates and benzodiazepines have also been employed to produce sedation and control convulsions. Artificial respiration may be necessary in the early stages of treatment.

The skin and clothing of patients poisoned by these agents may be highly contaminated and those handling them should wear gloves. The patient's clothing should be removed and destroyed and the skin washed with soap and water. If the agent has been ingested the stomach should be washed out with a solution of sodium bicarbonate.

Ecothiopate is the only organophosphate compound used medicinally. It is used as eye drops in the treatment of glaucoma, but systemic absorption has been reported to prolong the action of suxamethonium.

Myasthenia gravis

Myasthenia gravis is an auto-immune disease. In many cases antibodies to acetylcholine receptor protein are present in the patient's serum. It presents as a syndrome of increased fatigability of striated muscles.

For many years the principal effective drug therapy has been the regular use of an anticholinesterase which prevents the breakdown of the reduced quanta of acetylcholine, so that sufficient transmitter reaches the post-synaptic region of the neuromuscular junction. In recent years treatment has tended more towards immunosuppression with the use of prednisone and immunosuppressive drugs such as azathioprine. Plasmapheresis is also often effective. Many patients are now manageable on such a regimen without the use of anticholinesterases. The beneficial effects of such agents are associated with a fall in acetylcholine receptor protein antibodies.

When anticholinesterase therapy is employed, neostigmine 15 mg orally or 1 mg intramuscularly 3 times a day, increasing to 4 or more times a day, is the standard initial treatment. It may be convenient to change to pyridostigmine which has a longer duration of action; 60 mg orally is equivalent to 15 mg of neostigmine orally. Distigmine is also employed. On occasions it is necessary to determine whether muscle weakness is due to inadequate therapy or to the development of cholinergic crisis, and edrophonium 2–10 mg intravenously may be employed for this purpose.

The suppression of cholinesterase by these drugs is non-specific, and unwanted muscarinic effects in glands and smooth muscle also occur. Such parasympathetic excitation may give rise to colic, diarrhoea, nausea, salivation and miosis. If the dose is excessive, the drugs may cross the blood–brain barrier, giving rise to confusion and coma. The muscarinic effects can be prevented by atropine-like drugs, although in the presence of atropine it is even easier to give an overdose of anticholinesterase with its potentially dangerous cerebral effects. They also affect the miosis, and thus interfere with a useful index of anticholinesterase activity. With the exception of edrophonium, parenteral atropine should be given whenever anticholinesterases are given parenterally. For those on routine oral maintenance, 0.6 mg orally twice daily is usually sufficient to control muscarinic side effects.

Myasthenic syndrome

The myasthenic syndrome is most commonly found in a small proportion of patients with bronchogenic carcinoma. It may be due to defective release of stored acetylcholine and, as might be expected, anticholinesterases can give rise to some improvement. Guanidine, which acts by prolonging the action potential (due to its effect in delaying the time at which increase in sodium ion permeability is switched off), has been found of use also. It should be given in divided doses of about 20–30 mg/kg per day, a reasonable schedule being 250 mg 3 or 4 times a day. Full benefit may not occur until treatment has been continued for several days. No commercial preparation is currently available. Side effects, such as diarrhoea, restlessness or agitation, salivation, and tremor, can be corrected with atropine.

MONOGRAPHS

EDROPHONIUM

Edrophonium chloride (rINN)

Pharmacology

Edrophonium is a cholinergic agent which functions mainly by direct action but also as a prosthetic cholinesterase inhibitor. Its action on skeletal muscle is more marked than on ganglia and visceral effector organs. A small intravenous dose will cause fasciculation of muscle fibres, but excessive doses produce neuromuscular block, and death from peripheral respiratory paralysis will result. There is little effect on the cardiovascular system, and muscarinic actions in general are mild. Its duration of action is short, and is only effective for upwards of 10 minutes. It is rapidly destroyed in the body.

Indications

Edrophonium can be used to antagonize the effects of long-acting competitive neuromuscular blocking agents, for the diagnosis and assessment of therapy in myasthenia gravis, in the differential diagnosis between myasthenic weakness and cholinergic crisis, and to assess the progress of a dual block after depolarizing muscle relaxants such as suxamethonium.

Dosage and administration

Edrophonium, although normally given intravenously, can also be given intramuscularly or subcutaneously. As an antagonist to a competitive neuromuscular blocking agent, 10–20 mg may be given intravenously, preceded a few minutes previously by atropine 0.6–1.2 mg. As its effects are transient, further doses of edrophonium may be required at about 10-minute intervals if respiratory depression occurs.

In suspected dual block 10 mg is given intravenously (preceded by atropine). If the end-plate activation threshold has returned to near normal, muscle power and respiration will improve. If the block is still predominantly depolarizing, there will be either no improvement or actual intensification of the block, although deterioration may be preceded by a transient improvement.

In the diagnosis of myasthenia gravis, up to 10 mg is given slowly intravenously over a period of 30 s. In the presence of this condition there is a marked increase in muscle strength within 1 minute, which returns to its original state in 5–15 minutes. In the assessment of anticholinesterase therapy, and in differentiating inadequate therapy from cholinergic crisis, edrophonium 1 mg is given initially, and is repeated after 1 minute if no action is observed. Inadequate cholinergic therapy is apparent if there is improvement in myasthenic symptoms; patients in incipient cholinergic crisis, provided that they have not received atropine, exhibit marked muscarinic side effects and an increase in weakness.

In contrast to neostigmine, an overdose of edrophonium in normal individuals causes a preponderance of nicotinic effects, muscle fasciculation gives place to depression and peripheral respiratory failure will ensue. This will require controlled respiration while the effects of the drug, usually only transient, wear off.

NEOSTIGMINE

Neostigmine bromide, methylsulphate and methylsulfate (rINN)

Pharmacology

Neostigmine is an acid-transferring cholinesterase inhibitor (see page 301). It is a quaternary ammonium compound and is therefore poorly absorbed by mouth and largely confined to the extracellular fluid phase.

Nervous system By inhibiting normal hydrolysis of acetylcholine at the sites at which it is released, neostigmine raises its concentration and duration of action. This action thus excites or inhibits those parts of the nervous system where transmission is cholinergic. It also has pre-synaptic actions and increases the rate of repetitive firing following a single nerve impulse. This also contributes to the build-up of acetylcholine at the end-plates.

In normal doses there is no consistent action on the CNS, although the potentiation of narcotic analgesics may be such an effect. On the autonomic system its actions are clear-cut and both muscarinic and nicotinic effects are evident. The former result from stimulation of the effector organs of postganglionic parasympathetic nerve endings and of postganglionic sympathetic nerve endings in the uterus and sweat glands; the latter from stimulation after small doses and depression after large doses of all autonomic ganglia, cells of the adrenal medulla, and the motor end-plates of skeletal muscle fibres. Muscarinic effects predominate but can be blocked by atropine.

Cardiovascular system   Peripheral vagal stimulation will cause bradycardia, some degree of vasodilatation, and a fall in blood pressure. Cardiac arrhythmias and arrest may follow large doses, especially in the presence of hypercapnia. If atropine is given, blood pressure and pulse rate may rise as a result of stimulation of sympathetic ganglia and epinephrine release (nicotinic effect).

Respiratory system   There is little effect on respiration, but bronchi are constricted and secretions are increased.

Skeletal muscle   Neostigmine prolongs and intensifies local depolarization produced at the end-plate by acetylcholine. This is due mainly to the increased concentration of acetylcholine present, but also to the direct action of neostigmine itself. A small dose will increase the muscle contraction produced by a single maximal nerve stimulation; larger doses, or repeated stimulation, may cause depression. Fasciculation of groups of muscle fibres may also result. This is due to repetitive firing of the motor neurone. The various actions on skeletal muscle are increased by epinephrine, slightly reduced by atropine, and antagonized by competitive neuromuscular blocking drugs. In myasthenia gravis, the strength of muscle contractions is increased.

Smooth muscle   Neostigmine stimulates smooth muscle; peristalsis of the stomach, intestine, ureter and bile duct are increased and may give rise to colic. The bladder and the bowel may be emptied.

Other actions of neostigmine include sweating, salivation, and increase in mucous and other exocrine secretions. The pupil is constricted. There is evidence that neostigmine increases the intensity and duration of action of analgesics; how this effect is brought about has not yet been determined. Its cholinergic action is also beneficial when employed with analgesics as it prevents constipation and atony of the bladder.

Indications

Neostigmine is used to antagonize the effects of competitive neuromuscular blocking drugs and in the treatment of atony of the intestinal tract (paralytic ileus), atony of the bladder, myasthenia gravis, glaucoma and sinus tachycardia. It has also been employed to potentiate the effect of analgesics and the relaxation of muscle spasm.

Dosage and administration

Neostigmine is given by mouth as the bromide, and parenterally or intravenously as the methylsulphate. The poor lipid solubility accounts for the very high ratio (15:1) of oral to parenteral dose for comparable effects.

There have been several investigations directed at devising the safest way in which to reverse the residual paralysis of muscle relaxants. The prevailing view at present is that there is no advantage in giving atropine much before the neostigmine, and indeed this practice may in some circumstances precipitate both tachycardia and more serious arrhythmias. The recommended ratio of atropine to neostigmine is about 1:3. In Great Britain, doses below 2.5 mg are rarely used. The dose should not exceed 5 mg. Serious arrhythmias can occur in the presence of respiratory acidosis, and hypoventilation should be avoided during its administration. There is general agreement that the appropriate mixtures of atropine or glycopyrrolate and neostigmine should be injected slowly over about 60 s. The actions of neostigmine develop more slowly than those of atropine, and an initial moderate tachycardia may give way to a bradycardia because the duration of action of neostigmine exceeds that of atropine. Glycopyrrolate has a longer duration of action and is therefore preferred by many.

In the treatment of intestinal and bladder atony, 15–30 mg may be given by mouth, or 0.5–1 mg parenterally if a more rapid effect is desirable. In an emergency, 0.5 mg can be given intravenously. Oral and parenteral doses may be repeated every 4–6 h. A similar parenteral dose may be given to control sinus tachycardia.

The initial regimen for a recently diagnosed case of myasthenia gravis is neostigmine 15 mg orally 3 times a day, increasing up to two-hourly according to tolerance; 15 mg orally is approximately equivalent to 1 mg parenterally. Atropine or glycopyrrolate in appropriate dosage may be necessary to control muscarinic side effects. In the treatment of glaucoma, 1 drop of a 3 per cent solution may be instilled into the eye and repeated every 10 minutes for up to 12 doses.

Precautions

A parasympathetic antagonist should always be given prior to or with neostigmine when it is given intravenously, and when nicotinic effects only are required, as muscarinic actions are uncomfortable and can be dangerous when excessive. It should be repeated if bradycardia becomes marked (pulse rate below 50).

Neostigmine should be used with particular care in the presence of asthma and heart disease. It augments the action of suxamethonium and must not be used in an attempt to reverse its effects unless an unequivocal improvement has been demonstrated to a test dose of edrophonium (see suxamethonium, page 291).

Overdose of neostigmine may cause sudden death due to cardiac arrest, but otherwise is characterized by restlessness, weakness, muscular twitchings, dysarthria, pin-point pupils, nystagmus, sweating, salivation, nausea and vomiting, colic, defaecation, and a desire to urinate. The pulse is weak and rapid and accompanied by hypotension. Respiration is embarrassed by bronchospasm and excessive secretions, and death due to respiratory paralysis and pulmonary oedema may follow. Treatment with atropine or glycopyrrolate will antagonize the muscarinic effects and bronchospasm and excessive secretions are thus inhibited. Muscular twitchings are not affected, but may be relieved by small doses of a competitive neuromuscular blocking agent; if respiration is consequently depressed it must be assisted or controlled.

Care must be taken in the treatment of myasthenia gravis not to give an overdose, as this will increase muscular weakness rather than decrease it.

PHYSOSTIGMINE

Physostigmine salicylate, sulphate and sulfate (rINN)

Pharmacology

Physostigmine is an alkaloid obtained from the calabar bean, the seed of *Physostigma venenosum*, which is indigenous to West Africa, where it has long been used as an ordeal poison. It has been known to physiologists since the middle of the last century, when it was first introduced into England. It is an anticholinesterase whose properties resemble those of neostigmine. However, it is not a quaternary compound and, being lipid soluble, it crosses the blood–brain barrier, the placenta and penetrates the eyes. It is more potent than neostigmine and has a greater effect on the CNS and cardiovascular system.

It is destroyed in the body by hydrolysis and is eliminated in about 2 h.

Indications

Physostigmine was first used in the treatment of myasthenia gravis in 1931 because of the striking resemblance between this condition and the effects of curare, but has since been displaced by neostigmine and pyridostigmine. It is unsuitable for reversing neuromuscular blockade because of its widespread actions on other systems.

Physostigmine has been used (in increments of 0.5 mg) to reverse some of the sedative effects of CNS depressants, including atropine, hyoscine, the phenothiazines, benzodiazepines and tricyclic antidepressants. It is able to antagonize the psychotomimetic side effects of ketamine without reversing the analgesia, and shortens the recovery time. In postoperative patients, 1 mg physostigmine intravenously abolishes the somnolent effect of morphine and restores respiratory rate, without diminishing the analgesia. Pretreatment with *N*-butyl-hyoscine is necessary to prevent the peripheral effects of physostigmine and droperidol to prevent vomiting induced by physostigmine or morphine.

PYRIDOSTIGMINE

Pyridostigmine bromide (rINN)

Pharmacology

Pyridostigmine is a pyridine analogue of neostigmine. Compared with the latter it is 25–50 per cent less potent. It has less nicotinic action on voluntary muscle, although its onset and duration of action are longer. Its muscarinic action on viscera is weaker.

Indications

It may be used for similar purposes to neostigmine. It is less satisfactory as an antagonist to competitive relaxants, but it is more useful when a prolonged action is required, as in myasthenia gravis.

Dosage and administration

Pyridostigmine may be given by mouth, intramuscularly and intravenously. By mouth, 60 mg is approximately equivalent to 15 mg of neostigmine; by injection, 1 mg has a similar effect to 0.5 mg of neostigmine. As an antagonist to competitive muscle relaxants, an initial dose of 2–5 mg may be given intravenously, preceded by atropine 1.2 mg or glycopyrrolate 0.6 mg. At least 10 minutes should be allowed to elapse for the drug to take effect before a supplementary dose is given, and the total dose should not exceed 10 mg.

Distigmine bromide is an acid-transferring inhibitor of cholinesterase with a slow onset and prolonged duration of action. After a single intramuscular injection, inhibition of cholinesterase reaches a maximum in 9 h and persists for approximately 24 h. It may be used in conjunction with shorter acting but similar agents in myasthenia gravis, particularly to control morning weakness, in doses of 5–10 mg orally twice a day. It can also be used for urinary retention or ileus. Intramuscularly, the dose is 0.5 mg every 24 h. Muscarinic side effects are similar to those with other anticholinesterases, and can be controlled with atropine or glycopyrrolate; overdose should be similarly treated. Precautions and contra-indications are likewise the same as for neostigmine or pyridostigmine, and include all conditions in which acetylcholine potentiation would be undesirable.

Tacrine (tetrahydroaminacrine hydrochloride) is an anticholinesterase which crosses the blood–brain barrier and hence has central effects; it is also a mild analeptic. It gained some popularity among anaesthetists in the past as a method of extending the duration of action of suxamethonium. Because of its analeptic properties it was also combined with morphine, in the preparation Mortha, to allow larger doses of the opiate to be used in the treatment of chronic pain. The drug is no longer available in the UK, but in the USA it has been shown to have some benefit in the management of mild to moderate dementia in Alzheimer's disease.   .

Dopezenil is a specific and reversible inhibitor of acetylcholinesterase and was developed following the observations of the use of tacrine in Alzheimer's disease. It is about 1000 times more potent in inhibiting acetyl- than butyryl-cholinesterase, the latter being found mainly outside the CNS. To date there are no published case reports of prolonged apnoea after suxamethonium in patients taking dopezenil. The efficacy of the latter in Alzheimer's disease is still in doubt, but if proven an increasing number of patients are likely to present for anaesthesia who are taking the drug. It should also be borne in mind that the half-life of dopezenil is 50–70 h.

11

Parasympathetic antagonists and anticholinergic agents

The terms 'parasympathetic antagonists' and 'anticholinergic agents' overlap to a great extent, but not entirely. The anatomical and functional basis for the difference can be seen by reference to *Figure 11.1*. With the exception of some sympathetic postganglionic nerve endings (which are adrenergic), the transmitter at all preganglionic and postganglionic nerve endings is acetylcholine. Its action at ganglia is nicotinic and that on effector cells is muscarinic. Antagonists at the former are the ganglion-blocking drugs such as hexamethonium, and at the latter atropine and its derivatives. The transmitter at the neuromuscular junction is also acetylcholine and is antagonized at this site by competitive neuromuscular blocking agents. Acetylcholine is also a transmitter in certain pathways in the CNS.

Thus, any drug that interferes with the action of acetylcholine as a chemical transmitter can be classed as an anticholinergic agent. It may act by interfering with the release of acetylcholine, by competing with released acetylcholine for the cell receptors or, in the case of the motor end-plates of striated muscle and the nerve cell bodies of autonomic ganglia, by prolonged depolarization which renders them inactive.

Anticholinergic agents do not always inhibit transmission equally at the different sites of cholinergic activity and these differences are due to different degrees of penetration to

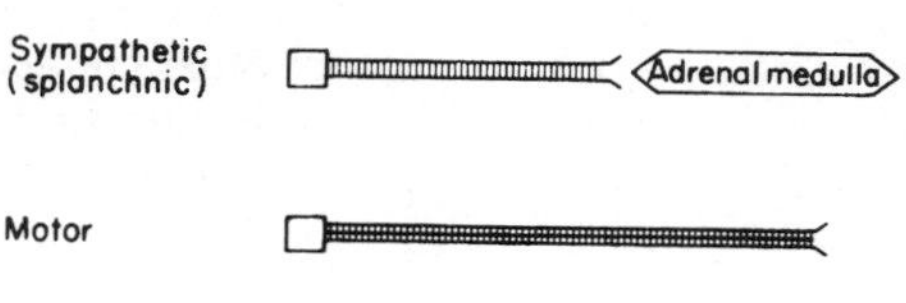

Figure 11.1 Chemical transmitters in cholinergic and adrenergic nerves. Medullated preganglionic fibres are indicated by double lines; postganglionic non-medullated fibres are indicated by single lines; cholinergic transmission is indicated by cross-hatching

different sites and different affinities for the various receptors. The most extreme examples are quaternary ammonium compounds such as tubocurarine and hyoscine butylbromide, which do not cross lipid membranes and therefore have no effect on the CNS or eye.

No class of drug is a pure parasympathetic antagonist. While the belladonna alkaloids (atropine and hyoscine) inhibit transmission at all parasympathetically innervated effector cells, they also block transmission to the sweat glands which, although cholinergic, are innervated by the sympathetic nervous system; they are antimuscarinic in action. They are used in premedication as anti-sialogogues, and to antagonize the unwanted muscarinic action of anticholinesterases when these are required for their nicotinic effect at the motor end-plates of striated muscles.

The parasympathetic pathway can also be blocked at the ganglia, but ganglion-blocking agents affect sympathetic ganglia as well, and antinicotinic action is marked.

Atropine-like action is found in many classes of therapeutic substances, which are considered in Chapters 3, 5, 6 and 7.

Synthetic atropine-like compounds

Synthetic atropine-like drugs usually have the basic structure shown in *Figure 11.2*. They may be divided into two types, tertiary amines and quaternary ammonium compounds. The former include many that are used therapeutically for their mydriatic and cycloplegic actions on the eye, for example homatropine. Others, such as dicyclomine, are used for their antispasmodic action on the gut. Such compounds, in addition to being muscarinic antagonists, have other non-specific relaxant effects with papaverine-like or local anaesthetic properties. Tertiary amines can cross the blood–brain barrier and thus have central actions. Quaternary amines, however, are ionized substances and cannot easily cross the blood–brain barrier. Examples are ambutonium, dibutoline, glycopyrrolate, ipratropium and tricyclamol.

Belladonna alkaloids

Belladonna alkaloids are widely distributed in nature, particularly in the deadly nightshade (*Atropa belladonna*) which yields mainly the alkaloids atropine and hyoscyamine, while hyoscine is found chiefly in the shrub henbane (*Hyoscyamus niger*). The naturally-occurring belladonna alkaloids consist of organic esters of tropic acid with organic bases such as tropine and scopine. The synthetic alkaloids contain mandelic rather than tropic acid, combined with a simpler organic base. Homatropine is a synthetic alkaloid consisting of a combination of tropine with mandelic acid.

Atropine is a racemic substance, DL-hyoscyamine, and owes its peripheral effects against the muscarinic actions of choline esters mainly to the L-hyoscyamine. The laevo-isomer of hyoscine is also much more active than the dextro-isomer. Atropine is closely related chemically to cocaine, and in fact has weak local analgesic actions.

Belladonna alkaloids are so called because of their mydriatic effect, which is seen especially when a solution is instilled into the conjunctival sac. This mydriasis is part of their action as antagonists of the muscarinic actions of acetylcholine and of other choline esters. Their other shared effects include various excitatory and depressant actions upon the CNS and an indirect vasodilator action upon the skin vessels, especially those of the blush area.

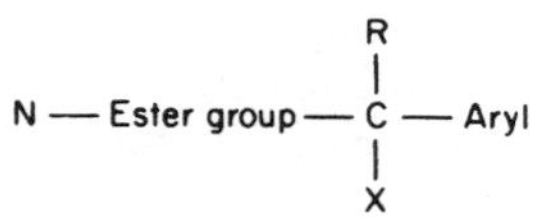

$$N — Ester\ group — \overset{\overset{\displaystyle R}{|}}{\underset{\underset{\displaystyle X}{|}}{C}} — Aryl$$

Figure 11.2 Structure of atropine-like compounds. N may be tertiary or quaternary; X may be alkyl,–H,–OH,–CN,–CONH$_2$, or –COOR; R may be hydroxymethyl, cyclohexyl, or phenyl; aryl group may be phenyl or a phenyl-containing polycyclic group

Hyoscine differs from atropine mainly in having central depressant actions of a sedative nature without causing any preliminary excitatory effects, except in rare instances. Peripherally, it is the more potent in antimuscarinic activity upon the ciliary muscle, the constrictor pupillae, and the gastro-intestinal, bronchial and sweat glands, whereas atropine is the more potent upon the bronchial and gastro-intestinal musculature and on the heart.

The usefulness of such drugs depends on their variability of action on different end-organs. Small doses which depress salivary secretion and palmar sweating do not necessarily accelerate the heart or slow micturition. The time course of these drugs varies with the different end-organs studied. The changes in heart rate, salivary secretion and sweating begin and end sooner than those affecting the pupil and accommodation. The peak effect on the heart rate and salivary secretion tends to occur sooner with increasing dosage, but that on the iris and ciliary muscle always occurs later, perhaps because the aqueous humour may be acting as a reservoir for these drugs.

Acceleration of the heart is frequently preceded by slowing, indicating that these drugs have a dual action and that the central effect seems to take place before the peripheral action. In healthy young adults, when vagal tone is greatest, the influence on rate is most marked.

Atropine and hyoscine usually increase the heart rate when given intravenously in sufficient doses, although both drugs decrease the heart rate in small doses.

Anti-Parkinsonian drugs

Anticholinergic agents were the mainstay of treatment for many years but have been relegated to a secondary role by levodopa (see Chapter 7). They are, however, still much more effective than levodopa for the control of drug-induced Parkinsonism and dystonias. Synthetic anticholinergic agents with selective central actions still have a place as supporting therapy when the side effects of levodopa prevent optimum dosage being used.

For many years benzatropine, which combines the chemical and pharmacological features of atropine and diphenhydramine, was the drug of choice. It reduces tremor and rigidity and depression, as well as secondary problems such as excessive salivation and hyperhidrosis. Peripheral cholinergic effects such as dry mouth, loss of accommodation, constipation and urinary retention usually limit dosage, even though these are less prominent than with the natural alkaloids. Overdose produces typical central symptoms of atropine intoxication. Newer drugs such as benzhexol and benapryzine produce milder side effects and are particularly suitable for combination with levodopa therapy.

Mydriatics

Antimuscarinic agents are used topically in ophthalmology to produce dilatation of the pupil (mydriasis) and to paralyse accommodation (cycloplegia). The latter requires higher concentrations or more prolonged application and so is invariably accompanied by pupil dilatation.

Atropine is prone to produce local irritation and tends to have too long an action for most purposes. Homatropine is shorter acting and its effects can be more readily reversed by physostigmine, although usually not completely. Cyclopentolate has mydriatic and cycloplegic actions, the effects of which can last for 24 h. If dilatation of the pupil only is required, eucatropine or tropicamide may be used. These drugs also have a much shorter duration of action. They can be supplemented by sympathomimetic agents such as phenylephrine. Mydriasis produced by the shorter acting agents can be effectively reversed by pilocarpine (4 per cent) drops; the effects of atropine and hyoscine are more difficult to reverse completely.

Mydriatics are contra-indicated in narrow-angle glaucoma. Systemic absorption of drugs after conjunctival application is minimal, although drugs reaching the nasal mucosa via the nasolacrimal duct are readily absorbed.

MONOGRAPHS

ATROPINE

Atropine, atropine sulphate and atropine sulfate (rINN)

Pharmacology

A full discussion of the properties and chemical aspects of atropine will be found under belladonna alkaloids (page 310), where comparison with hyoscine and hyoscyamine is made. Its main actions are on the central and autonomic nervous systems.

Central nervous system   Certain cerebral and medullary centres are stimulated and subsequently depressed by high dosage. An exception is apparent in Parkinsonism, where the ability to diminish tremor may be a purely depressant action as no initial stimulation occurs. In general, the central stimulant actions are elicited to a marked degree only by doses that have a pronounced antimuscarinic effect peripherally, but some authorities maintain that even small doses may produce an initial powerful vagal stimulation with obvious cardiac slowing. This does not occur after intravenous injection of doses exceeding 0.5 mg.

Autonomic system   The muscarinic actions of acetylcholine and other choline esters are inhibited. This is also true of nearly all cholinergic nerves and is the basis of the use of atropine in depressing important secretory activity, much smooth muscle, and the effect of the vagus on the heart. Sweating is prevented and body temperature rises; skin blood vessels are dilated, particularly in the blush area.

Cardiovascular system   The main action of atropine is on the heart rate, which it usually increases by inhibiting the cardiac vagus peripherally; occasionally central slowing occurs initially after subcutaneous injection, but not when adequate doses are given intravenously. Blood pressure is unchanged, but if already depressed by vagal activity due to reflex or drug action it will be raised.

Respiratory system   Minute volume is slightly increased due to central stimulation. Bronchial musculature is relaxed and secretions are reduced. There is an increase in both the anatomical and physiological dead space, but blood-gas tensions are not affected.

Absorption and fate in the body Atropine is rapidly absorbed from the gastro-intestinal tract, from the eye, and even slightly from the intact skin; it quickly disappears from the circulation and is distributed throughout the tissues. It is mainly broken down by enzyme hydrolysis in the tissues or liver to tropine and tropic acid; about 13 per cent (after oral administration) is excreted by the kidneys within 12 h. Traces appear in sweat and milk, which may affect a breast-fed baby. It crosses the placenta and reaches the fetus.

Indications

Atropine is used to diminish salivary and bronchial secretions during anaesthesia, to protect the heart from vagal inhibition, and to antagonize the muscarinic action of anticholinesterases, such as neostigmine, given to reverse the effects of the competitive muscle relaxants. It may be used to raise the blood pressure in hypotension associated with bradycardia due to vagal stimulation during operations on the neck, chest, upper and lower abdomen. It is also given to allay the pain caused by spasm in renal and other forms of colic and in the treatment of asthma, to control spasm of the pyloric and cardiac sphincters, and is given with vegetable purgatives to prevent griping. Its control of gastric secretion in cases of peptic ulcer is variable.

Atropine is also used locally in the eye where a prolonged action is required as a mydriatic and cycloplegic, in iritis to immobilize the iris and ciliary muscle and to prevent or break down adhesions. Dilatation of the pupil will occur in 30 minutes and lasts for about a week; paralysis of accommodation takes 1–2 h but wears off in half this time.

Dosage and administration

For premedication, 0.3–0.6 mg may be given subcutaneously or intramuscularly 0.5–1 h before operation, or intravenously immediately before induction of anaesthesia.

In the treatment of hypotension associated with bradycardia, atropine 0.3–0.6 mg may be given intravenously.

In the reversal of residual paralysis of competitive neuromuscular blocking agents, it is given prior to or with neostigmine to antagonize its muscarinic effects; 0.6–1.2 mg is given, in conjunction with neostigmine 2.5 mg. Oral doses of 0.6 mg are sometimes necessary to control the side effects of therapy with anticholinesterases in myasthenia gravis.

For the relief of pain due to renal and other forms of colic, atropine 0.6 mg may be given subcutaneously.

Precautions

Atropine as a premedicant is best avoided where there is marked tachycardia such as may occur in thyrotoxicosis, cardiovascular disease, and in cardiac surgery. Hyoscine or promethazine, which have little or no accelerating effect on the heart rate when given subcutaneously, may be substituted. Atropine premedication should also be avoided in hyperpyrexial patients when the operating theatre temperature exceeds 27.5°C; inhibition of sweating and increase in metabolic rate may give rise to hyperthermia and possibly to convulsions, especially in children.

When intra-ocular pressure is raised, as in glaucoma, atropine must not be used, but if mydriasis is necessary, one of the sympathomimetic amines such as ephedrine should be employed.

Atropine in overdose gives rise to dilatation of the pupils and blurred vision, dryness of the mouth, difficulty in swallowing, restlessness, a raised temperature and delirium;

convulsions followed by central depression may also occur. Treatment should include gastric lavage if the atropine was taken by mouth. Repeated small doses of thiopental (100 mg) or diazepam (0.1 mg/kg) may be given slowly intravenously to control convulsions; neostigmine, 1–2 mg intravenously, will antagonize the peripheral antimuscarinic effects of this agent. Central depression may require supportive therapy, including assisted respiration and the administration of pressor agents.

Atropine methonitrate has the same antispasmodic properties as atropine, but being a quaternary compound it fails to penetrate the CNS and the eye. It is accordingly less toxic. It is used mainly in the treatment of pylorospasm of infants and congenital hypertrophic pyloric stenosis.

GLYCOPYRROLATE

Glycopyrrolate (rINN)

Pharmacology

Glycopyrrolate is a potent long-acting muscarinic antagonist, five to six times as potent as atropine. Being a quaternary compound, it only weakly penetrates the blood–brain barrier, the placenta and the eye. In anaesthetized patients, intravenous glycopyrrolate is approximately twice as potent as atropine in producing a dose-related increase in heart rate. Thus it is possible to control secretions with doses that do not cause marked changes in heart rate. It has also been found to have less effect on blood pressure than atropine when used to reverse the bradycardia which is caused by large doses of vagotonic agents such as alfentanil. Because of its longer duration of action, and the fact that it does not penetrate the brain, it has been recommended for preventing the muscarinic actions of neostigmine.

Indications and dosage

Glycopyrrolate may be used for the reduction of secretions and other antimuscarinic effects. For premedication, 0.2–0.4 mg may be given intravenously prior to anaesthesia. The dose in children is 0.004–0.008 mg/kg. For reversal of competitive neuromuscular block, 0.2 mg with each milligram of neostigmine may be used, and repeated if necessary. Glycopyrrolate may be given either before or with the anticholinesterase. The availability of ready-mixed ampoules containing glycopyrrolate 0.4 mg with neostigmine 2.5 mg encourages simultaneous administration. It has been shown, however, that 5 µg/kg (approximately 0.4 mg for an adult) given 1 minute before edrophonium has the least effect on heart rate, causing less tachycardia than 10 µg/kg and less bradycardia than when the latter dose is given with the edrophonium.

Precautions and side effects

If dosage is excessive, anti-sialogogue action can be unpleasant. Overdosage produces peripheral rather than central atropine-like effects. As quaternary ammonium anticholinergics may block end-plate nicotinic receptors, it is contra-indicated in myasthenia gravis. Overdose may be relieved by small doses of neostigmine 1 mg per milligram of glycopyrrolate previously given.

HYOSCINE

Hyoscine hydrobromide (rINN) and Scopolamine hydrobromide (USP)

Pharmacology

Hyoscine is an alkaloid resembling atropine, found in the same group of plants, and with central and peripheral actions. These alkaloids are compared above (page 310). The peripheral actions of hyoscine resemble those of atropine. It blocks the action of acetyl-choline liberated at parasympathetic postganglionic nerve endings and, in fact, at any site where this exhibits muscarine-like effects. Its effect on the heart rate is variable: when given subcutaneously it tends to cause a decrease by central stimulation of the vagus; when given intravenously heart rate is decreased by small doses and increased by large doses. It is a powerful anti-sialogogue, requiring only one-third the dose of atropine to produce the same effect.

The central actions of hyoscine differ from those of atropine in that they do not produce initial stimulation and excitement, but depress the cortex from the start, especially the motor areas; it has, in effect, useful sedative properties. Hyoscine also affects other parts of the brain causing amnesia, which fact was used in the combination of hyoscine with morphine to produce 'twilight sleep'. When used as a premedicant for Caesarean section under ultra-light anaesthesia, there is a lower incidence of awareness than when atropine is used. It effectively controls motion sickness and diminishes the emetic effects of morphine-like drugs.

Hyoscine occasionally produces excitement and restlessness, chiefly in elderly patients. In therapeutic doses it usually causes drowsiness and dreamless sleep, amnesia and sometimes euphoria. In normal subjects it increases respiratory rate and volume, as does atropine, but when respiration is depressed with morphine, hyoscine is better in counter-acting this than atropine. When used in place of atropine in equivalent anti-sialogogic doses, there is less rise in pulse rate and blood pressure during surgical stimulation. In general, hyoscine tends to be used for its central actions, and atropine for peripheral ones.

Like atropine, hyoscine is rapidly absorbed and distributed throughout body tissues. It is almost entirely broken down in the body, only about 1 per cent appearing in the urine.

Indications

Hyoscine is used as a sedative and anti-sialogogue in premedication and in the treatment of motion sickness. It has also been used as a sedative in general medicine to calm the excited patient and induce sleep, especially in the acute mania of delirium tremens, and in the symptomatic treatment of paralysis agitans and post-encephalitic Parkinsonism.

Dosage and administration

For premedication, 0.2–0.4 mg may be given subcutaneously 0.5–1 h before operation, usually combined with pethidine or morphine or one of its derivatives. Hyoscine may cause depression or excitement in the elderly. Smaller doses may be given, but it is better to substitute atropine in those over the age of 60 years. Oral preparations are available for premedication in children, but they are less effective as drying agents than atropine by this route.

As a general sedative, doses up to 0.6 mg are given and repeated as required. In the acute mania of delirium tremens, 1.2 mg may be given alone or combined with morphine 20 mg.

Precautions

Precautions to be noted are the same as for atropine. Central stimulation prior to depression is, however, usually absent; drowsiness leading to coma ensues.

Hyoscine-N-butyl bromide (Buscopan) is a quaternary derivative of hyoscine which does not penetrate the CNS and eye. It is not well absorbed from the gut and oral doses have relatively little effect on the heart and salivary glands. Oral doses therefore have predominant effects on the intramural ganglia in the gut wall and the drug has been used for the symptomatic relief of abdominal pain associated with spasm of the gastro-intestinal tract. It is also useful by injection in a variety of radiological investigations of the gut, bile ducts, pyelography and endoscopy. Oral doses are 20 mg 4 times a day; intravenously, 20 mg may be given and repeated.

Other synthetic anticholinergics

A number of synthetic quaternary ammonium compounds have been shown to antagonize the muscarinic actions of acetylcholine. Their therapeutic efficacy depends to a considerable extent not only on their selectivity for the various muscarinic receptors but on the route of administration, since, being quaternary ammonium compounds, their lipophobic nature limits their distribution in the body. Most, like propantheline, block all types of muscarinic receptors unselectively; pirenzepine has some selectivity for the M_3-receptors in the stomach; ipratropium may have some selectivity for the M_2-receptors in the terminal airways. However, it is administration by aerosol which is the major factor in the selectivity of its action as a bronchodilator. The monograph on ipratropium is therefore located in Chapter 8 (page 261).

Anticholinergics all have the same spectrum of potential adverse side effects. They dilate the pupil and so are contra-indicated in glaucoma; hesitancy and retention of urine can occur when there is enlargement of the prostate; they raise the pulse rate and cause palpitations; they may cause constipation. Lesser effects include a dry mouth and blurred vision.

Propantheline is an anticholinergic which has been used for a variety of conditions in which parasympathetic overactivity is implicated, but chiefly in the gut. Its main use is for the irritable bowel syndrome, but it has also been used for pancreatitis, biliary spasm, pylorospasm, hyperhidrosis, enuresis and excessive salivation. Its former use with antacids for the treatment of peptic ulcer has given way to more specific therapy in that condition. The dose is 15–30 mg 3 times a day.

12

Drugs used for their effects on vascular tone and cardiac contractility

Cardiovascular control mechanisms

Before discussing in this and the next chapter the action of drugs on the cardiovascular system, the following brief physiological summary of the factors that control cardiac function and blood pressure is presented to indicate their possible modes of action. The major factors determining blood pressure are cardiac output and peripheral vascular tone. Other important factors are elasticity of the arteries and viscosity of the blood. Both cardiac output and peripheral vascular tone can vary in response to nervous stimuli.

Neurological control

In the CNS, autonomic cardiovascular representation occurs in the cerebral cortex, the hypothalamus, the medulla oblongata and the spinal cord, the most active motor control

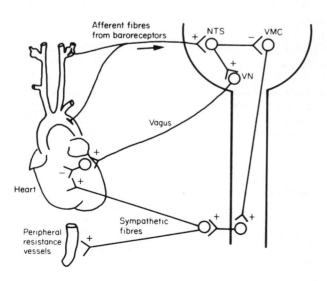

Figure 12.1 The baroreflex pathway. NTS = nucleus of the tractus solitarius; VMC = vasomotor centre; VN = vagal nuclei

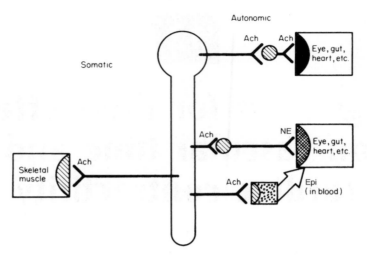

Figure 12.2 The peripheral nervous system. Ach = acetylcholine; Epi = epinephrine; NE = norepinephrine; ⊡ = nicotinic cholinoceptor; ■ = muscarinic cholinoceptor; ◰ = adrenoceptors

being from the medullary centres (vasomotor, cardio-accelerator and vagal). These are connected by catecholaminergic and serotonergic tracts. The nucleus tractus solitarius (NTS) in the medulla has an important role (*Figure 12.1*). Stimulation of neurones arising from this nucleus causes inhibition of the vasomotor centre; the transmitter here may be epinephrine (adrenaline). From the vasomotor centre, there is a facilitatory noradrenergic pathway to efferent sympathetic neurones in the spinal cord and, in addition, there may be a facilitatory serotonergic pathway.

All efferent autonomic fibres, including the cardiovascular, are relayed at synapses in the autonomic ganglia, except those fibres to the adrenal medulla. All these preganglionic fibres, including those to the adrenal medulla, are cholinergic. The acetylcholine that they release excites the cell bodies of the postganglionic fibres and so transmits nerve impulses; it also directly stimulates the adrenal medulla to liberate a mixture of epinephrine and norepinephrine (noradrenaline).

Postganglionic fibres may be cholinergic or adrenergic (*Figure 12.2*). In the cardiovascular system, postganglionic cholinergic fibres are parasympathetic (vagal); they slow the heart and dilate certain blood vessels. Postganglionic adrenergic fibres are sympathetic; they accelerate the heart, increase the force of contraction of cardiac muscle, and constrict or dilate blood vessels according to their site (vasoconstrictor to skin and mucous membranes, vasodilator in voluntary muscle). Sympathetic cholinergic vasodilator fibres have been reported; they could be involved in emotional responses like blushing.

Heart rate

Heart rate is reduced by the influence of the vagus, and therefore blockade of vagal transmission will increase the rate. Sympathetic tone opposes that of the vagus but is less influential at rest. If vagal and sympathetic influences are both blocked concurrently, the rate is increased. The 'intrinsic' heart rate so produced decreases progressively with age. The Bainbridge reflex is a function of intrinsic cardiac activity and mediates an increase in heart rate in response to increased venous return.

Blood pressure

In the reflex autonomic control of the arterial blood pressure, the most important afferent fibres run from baroreceptors in the carotid sinuses and aortic arch. Chemoreceptors in the carotid bodies are of much less importance in cardiovascular control but of major importance in respiratory regulation. Other receptors are present in the pulmonary circulation and the heart, but their significance in circulatory control is not yet clear. The aortic and carotid baroreceptors discharge afferent impulses to the CNS with increasing frequency as pressure rises. This results in efferent impulses via the vagi to slow the heart and probably inhibition of cardiac sympathetic activity as well. While constrictor activity from the vasomotor centre is inhibited, vasodilator activity may be applied instead. Carotid body chemoreceptors are stimulated by excess of carbon dioxide or lack of oxygen to produce a reflex increase in the cardiac rate and vascular tone.

Cardiac output

Throughout almost all of its functional range the force of contraction, and therefore the stroke volume, adjusts itself to the input load automatically (Starling's law). Sympathetic action on the heart affects the 'slope' of this relationship between venous return pressure and contractility. Cardiac output depends upon frequency of the heart beat and the stroke volume. Extreme changes in rate alone can cause output to fall, for severe bradycardia allows diastole to continue after maximum ventricular filling is completed, and marked tachycardia may allow too short a time for adequate ventricular filling. In heart failure the increase in stroke volume consequent upon an increase in venous return pressure only partially compensates for the loss of intrinsic contractile function.

Peripheral vascular resistance

In each vascular bed, arteriolar smooth muscle tone depends on local factors, such as the local pH (determined largely by the balance between carbon dioxide production and its removal) and local production of autocoids such as prostanoids and nitric oxide, and on global factors such as sympathetic activity and systemic catecholamine concentration. The measured resistance to flow of blood through the tissues depends not only on this smooth muscle tone, but also on the absolute number of arterioles and on the viscosity of the blood, which in turn is influenced greatly by the haematocrit.

Renin–angiotensin system

There are other control mechanisms that influence blood pressure and cardiac output, particularly over the long term. The most important of these is the renin–angiotensin system.

Renin is a protein (molecular weight about 40 000 Da) which is secreted from juxtaglomerular cells that are found in the walls of the afferent arterioles in the kidney in response to a fall in arteriolar pressure. Its plasma half-life is about 20 minutes. While in the bloodstream, it acts on plasma angiotensinogen, changing it to the decapeptide angiotensin I. This has little pressor activity. Angiotensin I is converted to angiotensin II by angiotensin converting enzyme (ACE) (*Figure 12.3*), the main site of conversion being the lung. Angiotensin II is not only an extremely potent vasoconstrictor but also induces the release of aldosterone. Angiotensin II has a plasma half-life of about 1 minute. Aldosterone, by causing salt retention, will tend to increase the interstitial fluid volume and thus the plasma volume, with which it is in equilibrium.

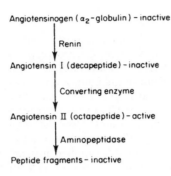

Angiotensinogen (α_2-globulin) – inactive

Renin

Angiotensin I (decapeptide) – inactive

Converting enzyme

Angiotensin II (octapeptide) – active

Aminopeptidase

Peptide fragments – inactive

Figure 12.3 Formation and degradation of angiotensin

Nitric oxide

Local control of smooth muscle tone in the medial layer of the blood vessel wall is effected by release of nitric oxide by the endothelium. This diffuses the very short distance from endothelium to medial layer and relaxes the vascular smooth muscles by activating guanylyl cyclase, which in turn increases cyclic 3'5-guanosine monophosphate. In the endothelium, nitric oxide is produced by an action on arginine by the enzyme nitric oxide synthase (NOS). The rate of synthesis is increased by shear stresses on the endothelial wall – in simple terms, this mechanism serves to limit the speed and turbulence of the blood flow within the vessel. Nitric oxide synthase exists in two forms: the endothelial one is termed ceNOS, constitutive endothelial nitric oxide synthase. The other form is found in a large number of sites in the body, not necessarily associated with blood vessels. It is normally present in very small quantities, but it is termed iNOS (inducible nitric oxide synthase), because in certain conditions such as sepsis, its levels can be increased by a factor of many thousand. Under these conditions, the majority of nitric oxide synthesis in the body is produced by iNOS, whereas under normal conditions, iNOS is responsible for a tiny fraction of the total synthesis. Arginine analogues can act as non-specific inhibitors of NOS (i.e. drugs which inhibit both types of the enzyme) and some of these have been tested in humans. Examples include Nw-monomethyl-L-arginine (L-NMMA) and Nw-nitro-L-arginine methyl ester (L-NAME). Specific inhibitors of iNOS, such as aminoguanidine or certain thiourea derivatives hold great therapeutic promise.

Edwards, R.M., Stack, E.J. and Trizna, W. (1998) Interaction of L-arginine analogs with L-arginine uptake in rat renal brush border membrane vesicles. *Journal of Pharmacology and Experimental Therapeutics*, **285**(3), 1019–22

Wolkow, P.P. (1998) Involvement and dual effects of nitric oxide in septic shock. *Inflammatory Research*, **47**(4), 152–66

The myocardium

The myocardium consists of the heart muscle of the atria and ventricles and their blood supply through the coronary arteries. Coronary blood flow is increased by some of the sympathomimetic amines, such as epinephrine, isoprenaline and, to a lesser extent, by norepinephrine and ephedrine. Drugs with a direct relaxant action on the plain muscle in the arterioles, such as the nitrites and calcium channel antagonists, can been used for this effect therapeutically in angina pectoris. Xanthines, particularly theophylline with ethylene diamine (aminophylline) have also been used. Coronary constriction may occur by the direct action of drugs on the plain muscle of the arterioles, such as when vasopressin is released by the posterior pituitary gland in neurogenic shock.

The heart muscle consists of an anastomosis of quadrilateral cells, joined longitudinally to form fibres, connected to neighbouring cells by short bridges. The muscle fibres in the right and left atria are continuous, so that an impulse will spread over both atria simultaneously, but these are separated from the ventricles whose muscle fibres are also continuous, by a fibrotendinous ring (A-V ring). The pacemaker of the heart is the sinoatrial node (S-A node), situated at the junction of the right atrium and the superior vena cava, and this can be influenced by an increase in vagal tone, which will cause slowing.

Heart muscle has the intrinsic property of rhythmical contraction, which originates in the S-A node, spreads over the atria, and stimulates the A-V node so that an impulse passes down the A-V bundle to the ventricles, causing their contraction. The A-V bundle, or bundle of His, passes across the A-V ring, enters the interventricular septum and divides into right and left branches supplying the ventricles. The bundle continues, as Purkinje fibres, forming a plexus beneath the endocardium of each ventricle. By this system, the number of atrial impulses reaching the ventricle is regulated, the maximum number possible in the mammalian heart being about 270 per minute. When the number is in excess of this, some degree of heart block will be present which can be greatly increased by the action of digoxin.

There are certain marked differences between heart muscle and other types of muscle. There is an 'all or none' response, so that above the threshold level an increase in the intensity of the stimulus does not cause an increase in the force of contraction. Conduction is delayed from atria to ventricles so that they always contract in the right order; the refractory period differs from that of skeletal muscle – it lasts much longer, as long as the phase of contraction, so that there is no summation of contractions or tetanus. Whether the heart rate is slowed by the vagus or increased by the sympathetic, the refractory period of the heart muscle gets shorter as the rate alters in either direction, which means it gets more excitable and conduction of impulse is more rapid through the myocardium. These three features – length of refractory period, excitability and rate of conduction – must always be influenced in the same direction owing to their inherent relationship.

Under normal physiological conditions, the heart beats regularly under the balanced influences of the parasympathetic and sympathetic systems. The mammalian heart has an inherent ability to retain its rhythmicity. This rhythmicity is determined by the spontaneous rate of depolarization of the cardiac cell membrane. Tachycardia will occur if the rate of depolarization is increased by inotropic agents, for example. If their effect is excessive, some arrhythmia may ensue. On the other hand, local anaesthetics, by stabilizing the cardiac cell membrane, reduce the rate of depolarization and tend both to slow the rate and reduce the number of ectopic beats.

The cardiac cycle commences with atrial systole (simultaneous contraction of both atria), then after a short pause, due to delayed conduction down the A-V bundle, ventricular systole (simultaneous contraction of both ventricles) follows; each chamber relaxes after contraction which constitutes diastole. At a rate of 72 beats per minute the cardiac cycle occupies 0.8 s, of which ventricular systole occupies 0.3 s and ventricular diastole 0.5 s. When the atria are not contracting, as in atrial fibrillation, the ventricles fill slowly. Ventricular filling depends on the difference between the atrial and ventricular pressures and on the length of diastole. Gravity may make a small contribution.

Hypothermia has a marked effect on cardiac function. The rate is slowed and irritability of the myocardium is increased. Ventricular extrasystoles commonly occur below 28°C, and below 25°C ventricular fibrillation and cardiac arrest may be expected. The cause of this increase in irritability has not been determined, but it has been suggested that hypoxia, hypercapnia, changes in electrolyte balance (calcium potassium ratio) or increased sensitivity to epinephrine and norepinephrine may be responsible.

Pressor agents and vasoconstrictors

Pressor agents are those which raise the blood pressure. They usually act by causing vasoconstriction, as with norepinephrine, thus increasing peripheral resistance, but some also increase cardiac output or act predominantly in this way, for example epinephrine.

Vasoconstrictors can act on the arterioles and small veins by several mechanisms: by stimulation of the vasomotor centre, by a central stimulant action releasing epinephrine and norepinephrine from the adrenal medulla, by direct action on the plain muscle in the arterioles, or by acting at vasoconstrictor nerve endings or receptors.

Central stimulants are not specifically employed as pressor agents, although several sympathomimetic amines that are used for their adrenergic action also have a central stimulatory effect. Stimulation is followed by depression and hypotension. Drugs that stimulate sympathetic ganglia are not suitable for producing vasoconstriction as they have undesirable side effects.

Vasopressin, which acts directly on the muscle of the arterioles, is a powerful pressor drug, but is no longer used as it causes constriction of the coronary arteries and cardiac ischaemia. Angiotensin amide, a synthetic agent, was thought not to have this effect. It is an extremely potent short-acting pressor agent, and is rapidly broken down by peptides in the blood. Arginine analogues such as L-NMMA and L-NAME (see above), which inhibit nitric oxide synthetase, have joined angiotensin amide as possible drugs of last resort in refractory septic shock, but as yet there is no scientific support for any of these drugs in this situation.

In practice, the drugs most commonly employed are the sympathomimetic agents (see below). They act by stimulating the heart, by causing vasoconstriction, or by a combination of both effects. The precise mode of action of some members of this group is still uncertain, experimental evidence is conflicting, and the effects of individual drugs often vary with the dose, the route by which they are given and the state of the circulation at the time.

It must be remembered that the action of these drugs is of little avail and is likely to be positively harmful in circulatory failure due to blood loss. This loss must first be replaced with intravenous colloid infusion. Pressor agents are most effective when hypotension is caused by vasodilatation due to central depression, spinal or ganglion block. In the former case, their use may be unnecessary if anoxia is prevented or removed. Patients under the effects of halothane or trichloroethylene anaesthesia should not be given pressor drugs that increase the irritability of the heart. Methoxamine and mephentermine are probably the safest.

Certain vasoconstrictors such as epinephrine and felypressin are also used locally with local anaesthetics to diminish their rate of absorption and increase their duration of action. They may be used alone locally to diminish bleeding and to decongest the nasal mucosa.

Adrenoceptors

Dale first suggested in 1906 that sympathetic nervous activity was mediated by two different receptors, when he showed that the normal pressor response of the cat to epinephrine could be reversed by ergot and that vasoconstrictor fibres were blocked while vasodilator fibres were unaffected.

Table 12.1 Types of adrenoceptors in various tissues

Tissue	Receptor present
Vascular smooth muscle (skin)	α_1
Vascular smooth muscle (splanchnic area)	α_1
Radial muscle, iris	α_1
Vas deferens	α_1
Intestinal smooth muscle	α_1 and β_1
Heart (myocardium)	β_1 (and some α_1)
Bronchial smooth muscle	β_2
Blood vessels to skeletal muscle	β_2
Uterus (relaxation)	β_2
Liver (glycogenolysis)	β_2
Pre-synaptic terminal sympathetic nerve	α_2

Ahlquist, in 1948, studied the relative potency of a number of catecholamines on different tissues. He noted that on some tissues, for example heart muscle, isoprenaline was more potent than norepinephrine, whereas in others, for example peripheral blood vessels, norepinephrine was more potent than isoprenaline. Using as a criterion the differential response to agonists, Ahlquist suggested that there were two types of adrenoceptor. These he called α-receptors and β-receptors. The development of selective antagonists has lent support to this subdivision. Since then β-adrenoceptors have been reclassified into β_1- and β_2-adrenoceptors, and α-adrenoceptors subdivided into α_1- and α_2- types. *Table 12.1* lists some sites where α-and β-adrenoceptors are found.

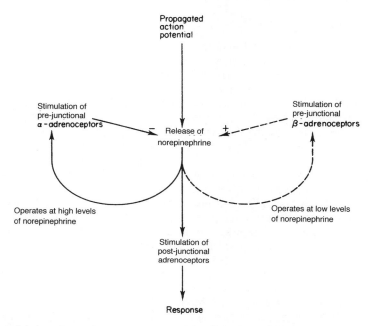

Figure 12.4 Modulation of norepinephrine release by feedback mechanisms operating upon prejunctional adrenoceptors

Following nerve stimulation, norepinephrine released into the synaptic cleft can inhibit further release from the nerve by acting on pre-synaptic receptors to cause pre-synaptic inhibition (*Figure 12.4*). These pre-synaptic α-adrenoceptors are referred to as α_2-adrenoceptors and post-synaptic α-adrenoceptors are referred to as α_1. However, α_2-adrenoceptors can also be found postsynaptically. α_2-adrenoceptors are now subdivided into α_2A, α_2B, α_2C and α_2D based on a range of specific antagonists. This subdivision has not, so far, translated into any change in clinical practice.

Control of contractility and rhythmicity of the myocardium depends predominantly on sympathetic tone involving β_1-receptors. However, there are also α_1- receptors, which mediate positive inotropism, but not positive chronotropism, and have an anti-arrhythmia effect. In hypoxic myocytes, there is an increase in the number of these α_1-receptors, because of sarcolemmal accumulation of long-chain acyl-carnitines. They cause activation of protein kinase C, which enhances production of inositol triphosphate, thereby increasing intracellular calcium and increased contractility.

The adrenergic supply to the coronary arterial bed, its effects, and the survival benefit of its effects are not as yet fully elucidated. There are post-junctional α_1-receptors (probably α_1A and/or α_1B) and pre-and post-junctional α_2-receptors. There are also β_1- and β_2-receptors (and acetylcholine receptors in the parasympathetic supply to the coronary arteries). All of these are vasodilator except the α_1-receptors, and the α_2-receptors on arteries of certain calibres. Coronary vasoconstriction is thought by some to cause myocardial ischaemia, and by others to prevent it by preventing coronary steal. This complex topic has been reviewed by Prys-Roberts.

Prys-Roberts, C. (1992) The changing face of adrenergic pharmacology. *Current Opinion in Anaesthesiology*, **5**, 113–24

Sympathomimetic drugs

Although drugs that stimulate adrenoceptors are often referred to as sympathomimetic amines, the effects are not completely identical with sympathetic stimulation because some postganglionic sympathetic fibres are cholinergic, notably those to the sweat glands.

Sympathomimetic agents, often referred to loosely as adrenergic agents, induce the same responses from various tissues as do epinephrine and norepinephrine. These tissues are those innervated by sympathetic postganglionic fibres whose impulses are transmitted at their nerve endings by the liberation of norepinephrine.

Two major classifications are in vogue at present. Drugs can be classified in relation to the receptors with which they interact. For instance, norepinephrine is a potent α-adrenoceptor agonist, whereas epinephrine is an agonist at both α- and β-adrenoceptors (see below). An alternative classification is to divide sympathomimetic drugs into two categories, labelled direct or indirect. Drugs that act by the release of norepinephrine from the pre-synaptic nerve terminal of the postganglionic fibres of the sympathetic system are then described as indirectly acting. Reserpine, a drug obtained from the plant *Rauwolfia serpentina*, can cause an almost complete loss of norepinephrine from adrenergic nerves. It releases norepinephrine from its bound stores in the pre-synaptic nerve ending into the cytoplasm, where most of it is broken down by monoamine oxidase (MAO). It can be shown that in reserpinized animals, in which almost complete loss of norepinephrine occurs, tyramine, amphetamine, methylamphetamine and mephentermine have very little action. Such results suggest that they are mainly indirectly-acting sympathomimetic agents. Moreover, indirectly-acting sympathomimetic agents have to penetrate the adrenergic nerve terminal to produce their effects. To do so they utilize the re-uptake process normally used by norepinephrine. Indirectly-acting sympathomimetic drugs will therefore have their action inhibited by re-uptake inhibitors such as imipramine, while the action of directly-acting ones will be potentiated. Destruction of the adrenergic neuron by postganglionic denervation or by immunosympathectomy will also inhibit the effects of indirectly-acting sympathomimetic drugs.

Using such techniques, sympathomimetic drugs fall on a spectrum from fully directly acting to fully indirectly acting. Norepinephrine, epinephrine, methoxamine and phenylephrine fall at the directly-acting end, amphetamine and tyramine towards the indirectly-acting end of the spectrum, whereas in between fall drugs like metaraminol and ephedrine.

The various sympathomimetic agents in common use include ephedrine, methoxamine, metaraminol, phenylephrine, isoprenaline and salbutamol, and their actions vary according to whether they produce a mainly α- or β-response or a mixture of the two. A mixed response such as that produced by epinephrine causes some degree of central stimulation, vasoconstriction in some blood vessels, dilatation in others, cardiac stimulation, bronchial dilatation, and intestinal inhibition with an increase in the tone of the sphincters. A sympathomimetic agent that appears to have no stimulant effect on the CNS in the dosage generally used is fenfluramine, which is used in the treatment of obesity. In addition to its anorectic effect, fenfluramine is claimed to increase the uptake of glucose by muscle and thus to reduce the glucose available for conversion to lipid.

Sympathomimetic drugs are used for the action or actions that mainly predominate; thus, those with strong pressor action are used to raise the blood pressure in the treatment of hypotension, and those with good bronchodilator action are used in the treatment of asthma and bronchospasm.

Symptoms of overdose with these drugs will vary with the predominant action of the individual drug concerned. They may be mainly those connected with central stimulation – anxiety, apprehension, restlessness and possibly convulsions; or hypertension and cardiovascular collapse – tachycardia, palpitation, cardiac pain and syncope. Treatment involves α-adrenoceptor blocking agents to control hypertension, and β-adrenoceptor blocking agents to control cardiac irritability and arrhythmias.

Catecholamines, a term also frequently used as synonymous with sympathomimetic, is in fact a classification on purely chemical grounds. It refers to those sympathomimetic amines that have hydroxyl groups in the 3- and 4-positions in the benzene ring (*Table 12.2*), since o-dihydroxybenzene is called catechol. Norepinephrine, epinephrine, dopamine and isoprenaline are truly catecholamines, whereas phenylephrine and metaraminol are not. As a group, they are basic substances forming salts. The structure–activity relationships of these compounds have been closely studied, and their actions can largely be determined from their formulae depending on the presence or absence of certain groupings (*Table 12.2*).

Drugs which, although they are closely related chemically to the catecholamines, are used predominantly for other purposes (e.g. salbutamol as a bronchodilator), are considered in their appropriate chapters.

The principal actions of sympathomimetic amines are summarized in *Table 12.6* (page 352).

Inotropic agents

Inotropic agents alter the force of the heart beat: those that increase it are used therapeutically or act physiologically and are generally beneficial, while those that decrease the force of the heart have not hitherto been much employed for such a purpose, as it is not often desirable to reduce cardiac output. However, β-adrenoceptor blocking agents are used to

Table 12.2 Basic structure and effect of replacing hydrogen atoms on the activity of sympathomimetic amines

Drug	Ring position				β-Carbon	α-Carbon	Amine
	2	3	4	5			
Dopamine		OH	OH				
Norepinephrine		OH	OH		OH		
Epinephrine		OH	OH		OH		CH_3
Isoprenaline		OH	OH		OH		$CH(CH_3)_2$
Orciprenaline		OH		OH	OH		$CH(CH_3)_2$
Terbutaline		OH		OH	OH		$C(CH_3)_2$
Salbutamol		CH_2OH	OH		OH		$C(CH_3)_3$
Phenylephrine		OH			OH		CH_3
Metaraminol		OH			OH	CH_3	CH_3
Methoxamine	OCH_3			OCH_3		CH_3	
Ephedrine					OH	CH_3	CH_3
(Dex)amfetamine						CH_3	
Methylamfetamine						CH_3	CH_3
Mephentermine						$(CH_3)_2$	CH_3
Notes*		b,c	c		a	d	e

* *a* An –OH group on the β-carbon atom favours direct action on receptors.
b An increasing number of –OH groups in the ring increases direct action on receptors. A decreasing number of –OH groups favours indirect (transmitter releasing) action.
c Drugs with –OH groups at both 3- and 4-positions can be metabolized by COMT (see page 355).
d Drugs *without* substitution on the α-carbon atoms can be metabolized by monoamine oxidase. Therefore, drugs *without* –OH groups on positions 3 and 4 in the ring, and *with* substitutions on the α-carbon atom, are either metabolized to an inactive compound before excretion (e.g. mephentermine) or excreted unchanged in the urine (e.g. ephedrine).
e Increasing size of substitution on the amine group increases action at α-adrenoceptors.

decrease myocardial work and oxygen consumption in angina pectoris. Use is also made of the fact that some of these, the anti-arrhythmic drugs, at the same time as reducing the force of contraction also lessen the excitability of the myocardium. All anaesthetics cause progressive myocardial depression, although this effect may be masked by sympathetic over-activity in the case of some agents.

In the normal heart, control in exercise is effected by the release of epinephrine and norepinephrine, which increase both the rate and force of contraction and produce a considerable increase in cardiac output. The opposite, or occurrence of excessive parasympathetic activity, occurs in the state of neurogenic shock when there is marked slowing of the heart through vagal stimulation and the cardiac output is greatly reduced. Initially the output per beat is not much affected until vasopressin is liberated from the posterior pituitary gland; this causes vasoconstriction of the coronary arteries, which, with the slowing, cause a profound drop in blood pressure leading to fainting and unconsciousness.

Drugs that stimulate myocardial contraction shorten the refractory period of cardiac

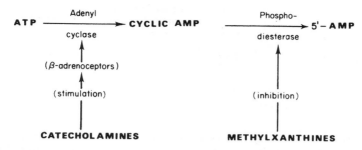

Figure 12.5 Influence of inotropic agents on cyclic AMP

muscle and increase its excitability, thus tending to promote irregular rhythm, which may predispose to ventricular fibrillation. When they are administered, the object is to employ them at a dose level that will give the desired therapeutic effect without running this risk. Thus, it is dangerous to inject epinephrine intravenously unless it is given diluted and very slowly; endogenous epinephrine and norepinephrine may be liberated in amounts sufficient to cause cardiac irregularities under conditions of stress and during anaesthesia. This can be particularly dangerous in the presence of vagal stimulation because, as the heart slows, it also becomes more excitable.

The sympathomimetic amines are the drugs that have been most widely employed for the production of a positive inotropic effect. Their potency depends on the extent to which the drug stimulates β_1- (cardiac) adrenoceptors. The effect on the blood pressure is, however, modified by the drug's action on other adrenoceptors. Stimulation of β_2-adrenoceptors causes vasodilatation, whereas stimulation of α-adrenoceptors causes vasoconstriction. The effects on force of contraction and blood pressure can thus be predicted if the pattern of receptor activation is known. For example, isoprenaline and dopamine are more powerful inotropic agents than norepinephrine.

A notable action of inotropic agents is to increase the intracellular concentration of cyclic AMP, an important energy substrate. Sympathomimetic agents such as the catecholamines do so by stimulating the enzyme adenyl cyclase via the β-adrenoceptor, and this in turn increases the conversion of ATP into cyclic AMP (*Figure 12.5*). The concentration of cyclic AMP can also be increased by inhibition of the enzyme phosphodiesterase, the enzyme responsible for the inactivation of cyclic AMP to 5'-AMP. The methylxanthines such as aminophylline are inhibitors of phosphodiesterase and owe their inotropism to this mechanism. These effects are additive to those of β-adrenoceptor agonists. Glucagon, the hormone secreted by the α-cells of the islets of Langerhans, also exerts positive inotropic effects that are not blocked by β-adrenoceptor blockade. It too increases adenyl cyclase activity. However, there is some evidence that, in the case of the catecholamines, stimulation of adenyl cyclase and positive inotropism are separate effects and so this aspect of their actions is still controversial.

Inotropic effects can also be produced by drugs that affect ion movements into myocardial cells. An important group of drugs with this effect is the cardiac glycosides, which facilitate calcium entry. They are most effective in congestive heart failure, in hypertensive and ischaemic heart disease involving the left ventricle, when the failure is mainly muscular, and when contractility is unimpeded by obstructed or incompetent valves. They are often ineffective in severe aortic valvular disease, certain types of cor pulmonale, and anaemic heart failure.

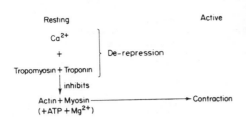

Figure 12.6 Effect of calcium ion on contractile processes. Ca$^+$ removes inhibition of actin–myosin complex

Calcium ions play a crucial role in excitation–contraction coupling in muscle, and many drugs fundamentally act by facilitating calcium transport across the cell membrane. Calcium ions are also, therefore, inotropic agents.

Cardiac muscle contraction

Although it was approximately 130 years ago that Sydney Ringer noted that the isolated heart would only contract if calcium was present in the medium, it is only relatively recently that the basis for this observation has been elucidated. Contraction depends on an interaction between two proteins, actin and myosin, which in the highly purified state contract in the presence of ATP and magnesium without requiring calcium ions. Normally, however, contraction is regulated by the presence of two regulating proteins, troponin and tropomyosin. Calcium interacts with troponin and prevents it from inhibiting the actin–myosin interaction (*Figure 12.6*). In cardiac muscle some of the calcium ions necessary to produce contraction may come from calcium bound to the sarcoplasmic reticulum but, in contrast to skeletal muscle, cardiac muscle has a very small calcium pool bound to the sarcoplasmic reticulum. Influx of extracellular calcium is therefore indispensable, even under normal conditions, in maintaining cardiac muscle contraction.

Cardiogenic shock

Acute myocardial infarction is the commonest cause of cardiogenic shock, although the syndrome can develop as a consequence of any procedure that produces arrhythmias, leading to impairment of myocardial function. Systolic arterial blood pressure can fall precipitously and associated with this fall there is reflex tachycardia, which can enhance the arrhythmia. Peripheral vasoconstriction occurs and the skin becomes pale and cold. Renal blood flow can be decreased. In many patients vomiting, decreased fluid intake and diuretics all contribute to hypovolaemia. Therapy is directed towards treating any arrhythmia with appropriate drugs (or by electrical pacing), replacing fluid loss, and administration of oxygen if hypoxaemia is present.

Norepinephrine, isoprenaline and glucagon have all been used to stimulate cardiac activity and raise the blood pressure. However, norepinephrine enhances peripheral vasoconstriction with the risk of kidney damage, and isoprenaline markedly increases myocardial oxygen consumption. Tachyphylaxis to glucagon can occur and, at least experimentally, it can produce lung damage. For these reasons, the usage of these drugs has declined and epinephrine, dobutamine and milrinone are now more frequently used. Dopamine, in former times a first-line drug, is used less often because of concerns about gastro-intestinal mucosal ischaemia, and effects on hormone production, notably growth hormone.

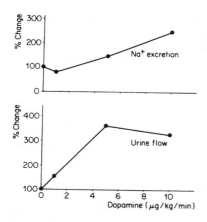

Figure 12.7 Mean percentage change in urine flow and sodium excretion produced by intravenous infusion of dopamine. Note the rise in urine flow and in sodium excretion

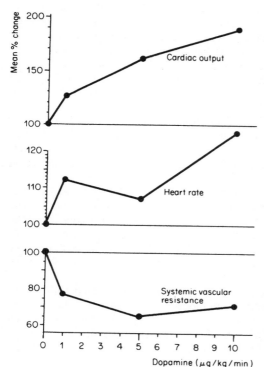

Figure 12.8 Mean percentage change in cardiac output, heart rate and systemic vascular resistance produced by *in vivo* infusion of dopamine. Note that between 1 and 5 µg/kg/minute there is a rise in cardiac output but heart rate is relatively unaffected

Dopamine is a naturally-occurring precursor of norepinephrine to which it is converted by the enzyme dopamine β-oxidase at various adrenergic sites. It is the natural transmitter at some synapses in the CNS. Dopamine increases cardiac output primarily by increasing stroke volume: it dilates vessels to vital organs such as renal, mesenteric and splenic beds, but constricts vessels in the skin and muscle. In responsive patients with the shock syndrome or with refractory congestive cardiac failure, dopamine improves the efficiency of the heart and increases cardiac output at lower cost in terms of excess myocardial oxygen consumption. In addition, it has specific dopaminergic effects on diuresis and natriuresis (*Figure 12.7*). The drug has been given at low infusion rates principally for its renal effects – so-called renal dopamine – but no beneficial effect has been shown in terms of survival or in terms of preservation of kidney function.

Dopamine has dual effects on the heart. There is a direct action via β-adrenoceptors and an indirect effect through the release of norepinephrine from myocardial storage sites. Both these effects are blocked by β-blocking agents. In the isolated heart there is little difference between inotropic and chronotropic effects. However, in the intact animal dopamine exerts a positive inotropic effect without changing the rate up to a certain dosage at which point the rate rises (*Figure 12.8*). This is probably related to the peripheral effects of dopamine. Dopamine has little effect on peripheral resistance, so that reflex tachycardia is not marked. In addition, unlike isoprenaline, it has a pre-synaptic effect, reducing norepinephrine release.

Dobutamine resembles dopamine chemically. It acts directly on β-adrenoceptors with some selectivity for $β_1$-adrenoceptors. Its other actions are slight. It therefore increases the force of cardiac contraction with a lesser effect on rate. Unlike dopamine, it does not produce renal vasodilatation and it does not cause release of norepinephrine. It also has some α-adrenoceptor activity such as increasing peripheral vascular tone, an effect that can be demonstrated by giving an infusion of the drug in the presence of a non-specific β-blocking agent.

The drug is ineffective by mouth and has to be given as a constant intravenous infusion. The half-life is about 2 minutes due to rapid metabolism by the liver to inactive conjugates. Dobutamine can produce arrhythmias, but the incidence is lower than with isoprenaline. It also raises the heart rate and blood pressure in a dose-dependent fashion if given at too high a rate of administration.

Dobutamine is used to produce a dose-dependent increase in cardiac output in patients with congestive cardiac failure. It may be of value in patients who have had cardiopulmonary bypass surgery. It has also been used to improve cardiac output in patients with acute myocardial infarction with congestive cardiac failure. It is given as an infusion at a rate of 2.5–20 µg/kg/minute.

Inhibitors of phosphodiesterase with selectivity for the 'Peak III' isoenzyme include milrinone and enoximone. These drugs are positive inotropic agents with little chronotropic activity. They are also vasodilators and improve left ventricular diastolic relaxation. The mode of action is similar to that of aminophylline, being inhibitors of phosphodiesterase, thus enhancing the intracellular concentration of cyclic AMP, but they are more cardioselective than aminophylline by virtue of their selectivity for the 'Peak III' isoenzyme in cardiac and vascular smooth muscle.

They can be used to treat a low cardiac output state when it is associated with a high peripheral vascular resistance. In this situation the blood pressure may well be normal. The aim is to use a vasodilator that also has positive inotropic activity. They may also be used for the short-term treatment of congestive heart failure, in which they improve haemodynamic performance without significant effects on heart rate or on myocardial oxygen consumption.

Hypotensive agents and vasodilators

Drugs that lower arterial blood pressure can do so theoretically in a number of ways (*Figure 12.9*), but only a few of these are exploited therapeutically. They either produce peripheral dilatation by central or peripheral actions that lower peripheral resistance and affect tone of capacitance vessels, or act by diminishing the force of cardiac contraction and output. The sites of action of these drugs are described in *Table 12.3*.

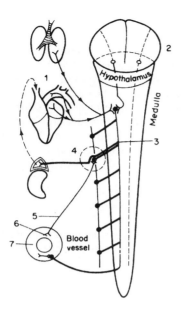

Figure 12.9 Sites of action of vasodilators. Preganglionic medullated fibres are shown in thick lines; postganglionic non-medullated are in thin lines; afferent fibres are drawn thinly with arrow marks indicating direction of impulse. The figures indicate the sites of action of drugs producing vasodilatation: (1) afferent receptors; (2) hypothalamus and medulla; (3) preganglionic fibres; (4) autonomic ganglia; (5) sympathetic neurones; (6) adrenoceptors; (7) vascular smooth muscle

When drugs are widely employed in therapy, the relevant Monographs are included in this chapter. Those relevant to spinal and epidural analgesia and the cholinomimetics are discussed in Chapters 6 and 10, respectively.

Stimulants of the depressor reflexes

The veratrum alkaloids act at afferent sites via receptors in the heart, lungs and great vessels, and also have a central action. Because of the undependable and mild nature of their action, they are rarely employed.

Table 12.3 Classification of vasodilators according to site of action

1. Afferent receptors in the heart, lungs and great vessels (veratrum alkaloids)
2. Hypothalamus and medulla:
    (a) general depression (anaesthetics and barbiturates)
    (b) α_2-adrenoceptors (clonidine, methyldopa)
3. Preganglionic sympathetic fibres as they leave the spinal cord (local anaesthetics used for spinal and epidural analgesia)
4. Nicotinic cholinergic receptors in autonomic ganglia (ganglion blockers)
5. Sympathetic neurones (guanethidine, bethanidine)
6. Adrenoceptors:
    (a) α-adrenoceptor blocking drugs (phenoxybenzamine, phentolamine, prazosin)
7. Vascular smooth muscle (see *Table 12.4*, page 336)
8. Inhibitors of angiotensin conversion
    (a) angiotensin conversion enzyme (ACE) inhibitors
    (b) angiotensin II receptor antagonists

Hypothalamic and medullary depressants

Clonidine, levodopa and methyldopa owe their hypotensive action primarily to the fact that directly or indirectly they stimulate α-adrenoceptors in the brain. Hypothalamic α_2-adrenoceptors are inhibitory and cause a decrease in outflow from the vasomotor centres. Medullary α-adrenoceptors are concerned with blood pressure control. The nucleus solitarius in the medulla is probably implicated. Micro-injections of norepinephrine, α-methylnorepinephrine and clonidine into this region result in a fall in blood pressure and heart rate; α-adrenoceptor blocking agents given into the same region can inhibit these effects.

Methyldopa also has peripheral actions in that it acts as a false substrate for norepinephrine elaboration, leading to the formation of a false transmitter (α-methylnorepinephrine). However, this mechanism, although generally adduced to be the mechanism of action, was always an unsatisfactory explanation because α-methylnorepinephrine was equipotent with norepinephrine as a vasoconstrictor. It was also not more tightly bound and thus released in smaller quantities by nerve impulses.

Levodopa is not used to produce hypotension, but may do so as a side effect because of its tendency to increase the availability of stimulators of α-adrenoceptors in the brain such as norepinephrine.

Ganglion blocking agents

Transmission through autonomic ganglia, both sympathetic and parasympathetic, is effected by means of acetylcholine. This is released when preganglionic nerve impulses reach the synapses, and it activates receptors on the cell bodies of the postganglionic neurones. Drugs that interfere with transmission at this site are known as ganglion-blocking agents.

Classification

A large number of compounds are capable of interfering with transmission through ganglia (although in some cases the ganglion blocking activity is small in comparison with the main pharmacological action). They can be divided into the following two main groups:

1. Substances that resemble acetylcholine and act by mimicking it, competing with it, or allowing it to accumulate. This group includes the following classes of substances:

(a) Substances whose properties must be very similar to acetylcholine, and which imitate its action at synapses. The depolarization produced is initially associated with increased excitability, but depolarization persists and so re-excitation of the neurone cannot take place and this constitutes a block. Such substances are tetramethylammonium, nicotine and decamethonium salts.

(b) Substances that compete with acetylcholine for ganglion cell receptors but do not stimulate them, such as tetraethylammonium, pentamethonium, hexamethonium and pentolonium.

(c) Anticholinesterases: the block produced by these substances is usually due to competition for the receptors between the anticholinesterase and acetylcholine, rather than to persistent depolarization by accumulation of acetylcholine.

2. Substances that do not resemble acetylcholine and probably act on preganglionic nerve endings or on effector cells, changing some of the properties essential for normal transmission. This group contains a large number of miscellaneous compounds whose ganglion blocking activity is small in comparison with their main

pharmacological action; examples of such compounds include general and local anaesthetics, barbiturates, many antihistamines, and atropine. This group also contains some highly specific ganglion blocking agents, such as mecamylamine (a diamine), trimetaphan (a thiophanium derivative) and phenactropinium chloride.

The ganglion blocking agents are non-specific and block both sympathetic and parasympathetic ganglia equally. The only practical method of blocking specific ganglia is by local infiltration with a local anaesthetic (as in stellate-ganglion block). Blocking of the sympathetic ganglia diminishes the number of impulses reaching the vasomotor fibres to the blood vessels, the accelerator fibres to the heart, inhibitory fibres to the smooth muscle of the alimentary tract, constrictor fibres to its sphincters, secretory fibres to the adrenals and to sweat glands, dilator fibres to the iris, inhibitory fibres to the wall of the bladder, constrictor fibres to its internal sphincter, and dilator fibres to the bronchial musculature.

Parasympathetic block similarly affects secretory fibres to the salivary glands, mucous glands of the bronchial tree and alimentary tract, decelerator fibres to the heart, constrictor fibres to the smooth muscle of the bronchial tree and the alimentary tract, constrictor fibres to the iris, and fibres responsible for the erection of the penis.

The overall effects on particular organs or systems depend on whether the autonomic activity of the system is predominantly sympathetic or parasympathetic. Thus, the overall effect on peripheral vessels is vasodilatation, due to release from predominant constrictor sympathetic control, while the effect on the alimentary tract can be so severe as to cause a paralytic ileus due to absence of parasympathetic motor impulses.

Uses of ganglion blocking agents

With the introduction of drugs that produce vasodilatation by specific action on sympathetic nervous transmission, or selective depression of the vasomotor centre, the use of ganglion blocking drugs in the treatment of hypertension has declined and they are now rarely employed for this purpose. The only ganglion blocking agent still available for the production of hypotension is trimetaphan which can be used with the aid of the gravitational effects of posture to produce a relatively ischaemic operative field during surgery.

Agents inhibiting norepinephrine release ('adrenergic neurone blockers')

These drugs interfere with the release of norepinephrine from stores in the adrenergic nerve axons, and so block nerve impulse transmission. They include reserpine, guanethidine and bretylium (which is no longer used in this context as tolerance to it may suddenly develop).

MAO inhibitors, such as pargyline, inhibit the intraneuronal metabolism of norepinephrine, and probably produce their action by causing a persistent depolarization of the adrenoceptor.

These drugs are no longer used in the treatment of hypertension. They were used alone or in combination with diuretics.

Adrenoceptor blocking agents

When Dale in 1906 showed that sympathetic nervous activity was mediated by two different receptors, and Ahlquist named them α and β (see page 322), the only blocking agents

available were those that blocked α-adrenoceptors. Since then, drugs that block β-adrenoceptors have been discovered, and those that produce blockade by interfering with the
release of norepinephrine from stores in adrenergic nerve axons. More recent developments include drugs that block some adrenoceptors selectively and some that block both
α- and β-adrenoceptors.

This has followed the recognition that the β-adrenoceptors could be divided into β_1
and β_2 groups. Heart muscle contains β_1-adrenoceptors; bronchi, arteries, uterus and
skeletal muscle contain β_2-adrenoceptors. It has been postulated that the enzyme adenyl
cyclase is the actual β-adrenoceptor, although it seems more likely that the enzyme just
has β-adrenoceptors on it. The evidence, however, is conflicting. In liver and fatty tissue,
adenyl cyclase mediates the responses of glycolysis and lipolysis to catecholamines.
Metabolic effects in liver due to this enzyme are also well established.

α-Adrenoceptor blocking agents

These drugs block the α-responses of epinephrine and other sympathomimetic amines.
General systemic effects produced include dilatation of peripheral vessels causing orthostatic hypotension with compensatory tachycardia, congestion of mucous membranes,
constriction of the pupil, and sometimes intestinal overactivity or colic due possibly to
preponderance of vagal action. In addition, each of these blocking agents can produce
side effects by direct actions either on effector organs or through the CNS, and these may
sometimes modify their main action.

In general, circulating epinephrine and norepinephrine are more easily antagonized
than are the effects of adrenergic nerve stimulation, a difference that has been attributed
to the more intimate nature of the contact between nerve and effector cell.

These drugs act as competitive antagonists for catecholamines and sympathomimetic
amines at α-adrenoceptors of the sympathetic nervous system. In most cases, both the
agonists and antagonists have a comparable affinity for the receptor, and increasing the
dose of either will overcome the action of the other. However, this is not the case with
phenoxybenzamine: once an adequate block has been established, a massive dose of a
sympathomimetic agent is ineffective until the effect of the blocking compound is terminated by metabolism.

There are four main groups of drugs that block α-adrenoceptors:

1. Imidazolines, such as tolazoline and phentolamine.
2. Benzodioxans, which are chemically related to epinephrine, such as piperoxan.
3. Chloroethylamines, which are chemically related to the nitrogen mustards. These
   include dibenamine and phenoxybenzamine.
4. Ergot alkaloids and their dihydro-derivatives, except ergometrine.

The ergot alkaloids are included solely for historical interest, as their direct actions on
the CNS and smooth muscle are so great that doses demonstrating adrenoceptor blockade in man cannot safely be used. Other drugs that block α-adrenoceptors include chlorpromazine and droperidol.

α-Adrenoceptor blocking agents may be employed in the diagnosis and treatment of
peripheral vascular disease in which there is increased sympathetic tone. They differ in
specificity, freedom from side effects, speed of onset and duration of action, so the
choice for any given purpose must be in the light of these factors. Except when used
in conjunction with other hypotensive drugs, they are of little use in the treatment of

essential or malignant hypertension or for the production of controlled hypotension. In the treatment of hypertension, a useful reduction in blood pressure cannot be obtained without causing unpleasant side effects. In addition, the action of many of these agents is transient. The development of labetalol shows, however, that α-adrenoceptor blockade, when combined with β-blockade, can be an effective treatment for hypertension. α-Adrenoceptor-blocking agents are, however, effective in the control of the hypertensive episodes that often occur during the removal of chromaffin tissue tumours.

β-Adrenoceptor blockers

β-Adrenoceptor blockers are not only employed to modify the force of contraction of the heart to control blood pressure, but are also commonly used to influence cardiac rate or rhythm; they are dealt with in Chapter 13.

Inhibitors of angiotensin conversion

Angiotensin converting enzyme (ACE) inhibitors

These compounds prevent the formation of angiotensin II, which is a powerful vasoconstrictor, by inhibiting the enzyme which converts angiotensin I to angiotensin II. They thus modulate a physiological mechanism, the renin–angiotensin–aldosterone system, which has an important role in the regulation of blood pressure. They must be given orally (there are no parenteral ACE inhibitors available) and the various alternative preparations mainly differ in the extent of uptake and first-pass metabolism. There is no loss of effect with long-term therapy and no rebound hypertension if they are suddenly stopped.

In suitable doses, ACE inhibitors are as effective as β-blockers and calcium channel blockers in reducing blood pressure. They are particularly effective in hypertension of renovascular origin: however, in this condition, there is a very high risk of suddenly worsening renal function on the affected side. They are also particularly effective in patients with congestive heart failure that is not controlled by diuretics. They help by reducing pre-load and after-load and raising cardiac output without producing reflex tachycardia. They have been shown to delay renal deterioration in diabetic microalbuminuria.

ACE inhibitors minimize the development of thiazide-induced hypokalaemia and hyperuricaemia. Such combinations enhance the hypotensive effect, and symptomatic hypotension is commoner in the presence of salt or volume depletion: these should be corrected before starting treatment. Hypotension occurring in patients treated with ACE inhibitors can be corrected by volume expansion.

These drugs have a tendency to elevate serum potassium, but this is only clinically significant when concomitant therapy includes potassium-sparing diuretics or potassium supplements. Other adverse factors include renal insufficiency and diabetes mellitus.

Angiotensin conversion enzyme is also known as kininase II and one of its functions is to metabolize bradykinin. High levels of bradykinin can result in oedema, fatigue and dry cough. All ACE inhibitors are prone to produce an intermittent dry cough; other side effects reported include headache, dizziness, fatigue, diarrhoea and nausea and are generally mild and transient. Urticaria is common and angioneurotic oedema occurs in about 1 in 1000 patients.

All ACE inhibitors are contra-indicated in pregnancy as they cause fetal abnormalities in animals and probably in man. They are probably also secreted in the milk. Compounds that contain sulphydryl groups (e.g. captopril) can cause membranous glomerulonephritis if given in large doses. The same compounds may cause a metallic taste. In patients taking ACE inhibitors, haemodialysis often provokes an anaphylactoid reaction. In diabetics, hypoglycaemia may occur secondary to enhanced insulin sensitivity.

Angiotensin II receptor antagonists

There is currently only one member of this group, losartan. Its effects and uses are the same as those of the angiotensin converting enzyme inhibitors, but there is no accumulation of bradykinin, and therefore a reduced tendency to fatigue, oedema and cough.

Direct-acting vasodilators

All of the drug groups mentioned above produce vasodilatation by their action on the vasomotor nervous or humoral mechanism at various levels. Other drugs acting directly on the smooth muscle of the arterioles, independently of its innervation or hormonal controls, are described in *Table 12.4*.

Several drugs are marketed for vasodilator actions in the treatment of intermittent claudication and other syndromes of peripheral vasospasm. They include derivatives of nicotinic acid, cinnarizine, cylandelate, naftidrofuryl and oxpentifylline. Only the last has

Table 12.4 Classification of direct acting vasodilators

1. Nitric oxide and nitric oxide donors:
   - (a) nitric oxide
   - (b) nitrites, e.g. amyl nitrite, octyl nitrite
   - (c) nitrates, e.g. glyceryl trinitrate, isosorbide mononitrate
   - (d) sodium nitroprusside
   - (e) nicotinic acid
2. Calcium channels blockers:
   - (a) blockers of L-type calcium channels
     - (i) dihydropyridine type (e.g. nifedipine)
     - (ii) phenylalkylamine type (e.g. verapamil)
     - (iii) benzothiazepine type (e.g. diltiazem)
   - (b) blockers of T-type calcium channels (e.g. mibefradil)
3. Phosphodiesterase inhibitors:
   - (a) xanthines, e.g. caffeine, theophylline, papaverine
   - (b) phosphodiesterase III inhibitors, e.g. milrinone, enoximone
4. ATP-ase-dependent potassium channel openers:
   - (a) diazoxide
   - (b) nicorandil
5. Adenosine and adenosine uptake inhibitors:
   - (a) adenosine
   - (b) dipyridamole
6. Unknown mechanism:
   - (a) hydralazine

much in the way of evidence for its efficacy. They can potentiate the hypotensive effect of other drugs. It should not be overlooked that vessels are maximally dilated in ischaemic vascular beds and vasodilators may create a 'steal' phenomenon. The direct-acting vasodilators may therefore be used to dilate blood vessels in a localized area, or to lower blood pressure by general vasodilatation.

Nitric oxide donors

Nitric oxide is released by endothelium in response to shear forces created by fast and/or turbulent blood flow (Moncada and Higgs, 1993). It reacts with the ferrous iron in the haem prosthetic group of the soluble guanylate cyclase in smooth muscle cells in the media of blood vessels, increasing the concentration of cyclic GMP and thereby causing relaxation. It also changes cyclic GMP levels in platelets, causing inhibition of aggregation. Interestingly, platelets are themselves able to generate nitric oxide and they do so when they become activated, causing negative-feedback regulation of the process. Nitric oxide also inhibits leukocyte activation.

The vasodilator effect of inhaled nitric oxide is evident only in the pulmonary vasculature. Inactivation by binding to haemoglobin occurs so rapidly that no systemic vasodilatation is seen. In this respect, nitric oxide is the only truly selective pulmonary vasodilator drug available. Gaseous nitric oxide dissolves in bronchial secretions to form nitric acid. Administration of inhaled nitric oxide to ventilated patients with severe lung injury causes a dramatic short-term improvement in oxygenation, but is not associated with a survival benefit. Conditions in which inhaled nitric oxide is associated with a survival benefit are those in which there is acutely raised pulmonary vascular resistance which is not secondary to severe lung disease, e.g. idiopathic persistent pulmonary hypertension of the newborn.

Systemic administration of various drugs which act as donors of nitric oxide, and which have longer durations of action than the native gas, results in generalized vasodilatation. Examples include various nitrites and nitrates. These are used in the relief of the pain of angina pectoris, in which their main mode of action is venodilatation with reduction in pre-load and thereby reduction in heart work. They produce coronary vasodilatation, but the extent that this mechanism contributes to the therapeutic effect is unclear. The muscle of the biliary tract may be strongly relaxed, but that of the bronchial tree, ureters and gastro-intestinal tract is less responsive.

For a rapid and transient effect, amyl and octyl nitrites are given by inhalation and glyceryl trinitrate by absorption sublingually. Orally administered nitrates undergo extensive but variable 'first-pass' metabolism in the liver. The major metabolite of isosorbide dinitrate is the mononitrate, and this is in fact the haemodynamically active agent. Isosorbide mononitrate tablets are available. Sodium nitroprusside is particularly potent because the 'nitro' and the 'prusside' portions of the molecule each act as source of nitric oxide. For unknown reasons, this agent appears to be somewhat selective for the arterial vasculature, i.e. it is predominantly an arteriodilator.

All nitrites tend to cause methaemoglobinaemia, but this does not occur to any extent except with sodium nitrite, or with excessive doses of glyceryl trinitrate used over a long period. In acute cases of methaemoglobinaemia, methylthioninium chloride (methylene blue) 1 mg/kg can be given intravenously together with the administration of oxygen. In the chronic condition, 300 mg/day by mouth and full doses of ascorbic acid are given.

Patients continually exposed to nitrates sometimes display tachyphylaxis. It is recommended that long-term treatment regimens include a four hour nitrate-free interval each day to prevent this.

Moncada, S. and Higgs, A. (1993) Mechanisms of disease: The L-arginine – nitric oxide pathway. *New England Journal of Medicine*, **329**(27), 2002–12

Nitrites in the treatment of cyanide poisoning

In cyanide poisoning, the induction of methaemoglobinaemia by sodium nitrite can, if given in time, be a life-saving measure. Methaemoglobin forms cyanmethaemoglobin and renders the cyanide ion less toxic by combination. This gradually dissociates, but by giving sodium thiosulphate, the cyanide ion is converted into thiocyanate. The dose of sodium nitrite for adults is 0.3–0.5 g dissolved in 10–15 ml of water, given by slow intravenous injection. While the solution is being prepared, amyl nitrite can be inhaled for 30 s every 2 minutes. After the injection of nitrite, but not with it, sodium thiosulphate 12.5 g in 50 ml of water should be given slowly intravenously, taking about 10 minutes over the injection. This procedure can be repeated if necessary with half doses of each drug. The administration of hydroxocobalamin (5 mg) has also been recommended for the treatment of cyanide poisoning.

If the fall in blood pressure is too profound, a pressor drug should be used. Oxygen and a blood transfusion may also be required.

Calcium channel blockers

Calcium ions are known to be involved in excitation coupling in skeletal, smooth and cardiac muscle. This ion also plays an important part in stimulus-secretion coupling in endocrine and exocrine glands and in transmitter release from neurones. Thus it can be seen that drugs which can modify calcium-dependent processes have potential in a wide spectrum of clinical applications. Calcium-dependent processes can be altered by affecting the influx or efflux of extracellular calcium or the binding of calcium to specific intracellular sites. Calcium channels exist in the membranes comprising the sarcoplasmic reticulum. Pharmacological manipulation of these is not available, although they can be blocked *in vitro* by ryanodine. The influx of Ca^{2+} ions across cell membranes is via calcium channels, which are closed in the unstimulated cell but open during excitation. Thus these ion channels may exist in several states – resting, open or inactivated. In cardiac muscle, the entry of calcium is responsible for the plateau of the action potential and is termed the 'slow inward current'. In smooth muscle, the Ca^{2+} channels can be opened by depolarization and are termed potential (or voltage) operated channels (VOCs). Other Ca^{2+} channels may be opened by activation of cell membrane receptors without change in membrane potential (e.g. norepinephrine on α-adrenoceptors of vascular smooth muscle) and are termed receptor operated channels (ROCs).

The voltage-dependent channels have been further subdivided according to location, duration of opening and sensitivity to inhibitors as the L-, N- and T-type channels. There are three major L-type (high-voltage) calcium channel blocker sites (a dihydropyridine site for nifedipine, a phenylalkylamine site for verapamil, and a benzothiazepine site for diltiazem) and one tetralol T-type (low-voltage) calcium channel blocker site. Calcium antagonists differ in terms of their tissue affinity and vascular selectivity resulting in different therapeutic applications. The initial disadvantage of a short half-life has been overcome with drug delivery systems that lower blood pressure over a 24 h period.

The classification of calcium antagonists has been confusing and the World Health Organization set up a committee whose classification is shown in *Table 12.5*. This classification is based upon differences in their profiles of pharmacological activity upon

Table 12.5 Classification of calcium channel antagonists (WHO classification)*

Selective for slow Ca²⁺ channels	

Selective for slow Ca^{2+} channels
Class I   Verapamil-like:
            verapamil, gallopamil (D600), anipamil
Class II   Dihydropyridines:
            nifedipine, nicardipine, nimodipine, nitrenipine, isradipine, amlodipine, felodipine
Class III   Diltiazem

Non-selective for slow Ca^{2+} channels
Class IV   Flunarizine-like:
            Flunarizine, cinnarizine
Class V   Prenylamine-like:
            prenylamine, fendiline, terodiline
Class VI   Others:
            perhexiline, bepridil, caroverine, etafenone

Vanhoutte, P.M. (1987) The expert committee of the World Health Organization on classification of calcium antagonists. The viewpoint of the raporteur. *American Journal of Cardiology*, 59, 3A–8A.

cardiac and vascular smooth muscle and their chemical structures. Specific binding sites associated with the L-channel have been identified for verapamil, dihydropyridines and diltiazem. Dihydropyridine binding is voltage dependent and the effectiveness of calcium antagonists is increased under depolarized conditions or when the channel is in the open or inactivated state. Verapamil displays a selectivity towards cardiac muscle and is frequency dependent. This is attributed to the increased probability of the channel being in the open or inactivated states. The L-channel has now been partially cloned and an α_1 subunit of 155–200 kDa identified which contains the dihydropyridine binding site.

The N-type Ca^{2+} channel is located on **N**eurones, its opening causing transmitter release. It is sensitive to blockade by α-conotoxin. T-type channels have **T**ransient opening, are found in smooth muscle and in the sino-atrial node and are opened by small changes in membrane potential. Both are relatively insensitive to the classical Ca^{2+} antagonists, but are acted upon by mibefradil.

Calcium antagonists are being used for the treatment of angina pectoris and hypertension. They have been used to treat cardiac arrhythmias. The beneficial effect in angina is due to a reduced myocardial oxygen requirement brought about by (a) reduced contractile force of the heart, (b) vasodilatation of arteriolar beds to reduce afterload on the heart and myocardial work, and (c) venous dilatation to reduce preload on the heart. In Prinzmetal's variant angina, the ischaemic pain is due to restriction of coronary flow, caused by coronary vasospasm. Calcium antagonists exert relief by an additional coronary vasodilator action.

Nimodipine, a dihydropyridine-type calcium channel blocker, is used to minimize vasospasm in the cerebral cortex secondary to sub-arachnoid bleeding. It is given for 3 weeks after the initial bleed, either by mouth or as an intravenous infusion.

The anti-arrhythmic effect of calcium antagonists constitutes part of their cardioprotective action. Verapamil and diltiazem have been used for the treatment of supraventricular arrhythmias including atrial fibrillation and flutter because they block the slow inward calcium currents in the S-A and A-V nodes. Depolarization is delayed and conduction velocity in the A-V node is depressed along with an increase in functional refractory period. The ventricular response to atrial fibrillation and flutter is thus reduced. These belong to the class 4 anti-arrhythmic drugs (see *Table 13.2, page 384*). Other aspects of the cardioprotective action of calcium antagonists include inhibition of Ca^{2+}-dependent platelet aggregation, prevention of ischaemia-related arrhythmias and protection from Ca^{2+} overload of the cells, which would impair mitochondrial oxidative phosphorylation and ATP production. The latter action has potential in the treatment of stroke. Other applications for calcium antagonists that are under investigation include Raynaud's phenomenon, epilepsy, migraine and intermittent claudication.

Class I calcium antagonists

Patients in whom β-adrenoceptor blockade may be inadvisable include asthmatics, in whom the resulting bronchospasm can be life-threatening, and diabetics, who rely on a sympathetic response to warn them of an impending hypoglycaemic crisis. In these patients, *and as long as there is no element of heart failure*, verapamil can be used to treat angina by slowing the heart and reducing myocardial contractility (although in most patients, diltiazem would be tried first because of its greater coronary vasodilator action, and because it is less likely to provoke heart failure). In patients with a contra-indication to β-adrenoceptor blockade who have hypertension, have no heart failure, and have a tendency to tachycardia with vasodilator therapy, verapamil can be a useful drug.

Verapamil has been used in the past to diagnose and treat supraventricular tachycardia and broad complex tachycardia, but this use of the drug has been superseded by adenosine.

Class II calcium antagonists

Nifedipine mainly acts on vascular smooth muscle. It dilates both coronary arteries and peripheral arterioles, reducing peripheral resistance and left ventricular after-load. There is a reflex baroreceptor-mediated rise in pulse rate. There is a moderate negative inotropic effect and this can cause heart failure, particularly if it is combined with a β-blocker. However, unlike class I calcium antagonists, nifedipine can normally be used in combination with a β-blocker to reduce the reflex tachycardia.

Nifedipine is used for the treatment of angina pectoris when there is no accompanying heart failure, and for mild to severe hypertension and Raynaud's phenomenon. As an antihypertensive it is usually a second- or third-line drug for patients refractory to treatment with β-blockers, diuretics, ACE inhibitors or other vasodilators. It can be used intravenously for the rapid lowering of blood pressure and to attenuate the hypertensive response to intubation and sternotomy. In the latter situation it has been found to be as effective as trinitroglycerin. The intravenous preparation requires rigorous protection from light, and is not commonly available in the United Kingdom.

Nifedipine can be used as a myocardial protecting agent during reperfusion after cardioplegia: it prevents accumulation of calcium in the cell, a process that inhibits ATP production by the mitochondria.

Nicardipine is a newer derivative of nifedipine which also inhibits calcium entry into arterial smooth muscle cells, causing vasodilatation, lowering peripheral vascular resistance, increasing cardiac output and lowering pulmonary capillary wedge pressure (Pansard *et al.*, 1990). It also dilates coronary arteries. It has negligible negative inotropic effects compared with other calcium entry blockers. It is well absorbed orally but undergoes extensive first-pass hepatic metabolism. This is saturable so that increasing oral doses may have a disproportionate effect. It is given for moderate to severe hypertension, particularly when there is normal plasma renin activity and for angina pectoris, in doses of 30 mg orally 3 times a day. For the control of intraoperative hypertension the dose is 0.02 mg/kg.

Amlodipine is another calcium entry blocker, acting predominantly on vascular smooth muscle. It has, however, a quite different pharmacokinetic profile to other calcium entry blockers acting at this site. It is slowly absorbed and metabolized, peak plasma concentrations occurring some 6–12 h after an oral dose, and also slowly metabolized, the terminal half-life being some 35–45 h. Thus once-daily dosing with 5–10 mg is effective in angina and hypertension. It has an affinity for both the dihydropyridine and diltiazem binding site (Burges *et al.*, 1989). Amlodipine lowers blood pressure in hypertensive individuals, but the slow onset of action minimizes any reflex rise in heart rate.

Class III calcium antagonists

Diltiazem is the main calcium entry channel blocker in this class and has a somewhat different spectrum of actions. Its principal effect is on coronary artery smooth muscle; it also has some effect on the A-V node, though much less marked than verapamil. It has little effect on systemic vascular smooth muscle and is therefore not of value in hypertension. Nor is there, therefore, any reflex tachycardia. Its actions are thus somewhere between those of nifedipine and verapamil. It is used for the treatment of angina pectoris and Prinzmetal angina. Dosage ranges from 180 mg to 480 mg a day divided into 3 doses. A slow-release preparation for twice-daily dosage is also available. It should be used cautiously in the presence of bradycardia and prolonged P-R interval and avoided in the 'sick sinus' syndrome and second- or third-degree heart block. It may increase the blood levels of digoxin.

Burges, R. A., Dodd, M. G. and Gardiner, D. G. (1989) Pharmacological profile of amlodipine. *American Journal of Cardiology*, **64**, 10

Pansard, J. L., Marty, J., Lancon, J. P., Barbier-Bohm, G. and Pastor, C. (1990) Nicardipine in the treatment of hypertension induced by sternotomy. *European Journal of Anaesthesiology*, **7**, 346

Blockers of T-type calcium channels

Experience in the United Kingdom with drugs in this class is limited to mibefradil, although it must be said that some blockade of L-type receptors also occurs with this drug. It has now been withdrawn because of an unacceptably high incidence of interactions with other drugs. It was used in angina and hypertension because it reduces smooth muscle tone in the peripheral and the coronary vasculatures, and causes a small reduction in heart rate, but has little effect on cardiac contractility. It is said not to be associated with a reflex rise in renin levels or in sympathetic activity.

Phosphodiesterase inhibitors

These drugs have peripheral vasodilator action, but in general this is an unwanted effect, and they are used for other purposes. The non-specific type, e.g. theophylline, is discussed in Chapter 8. The phosphodiesterase III inhibitors, e.g. milrinone, are discussed in this chapter under inotropic drugs. Papaverine is usually used by infiltration for a local vasodilator effect in anastomosis of small vessels such as in vascular grafts. Sildenafil is a selective inhibitor of the 'Peak V' isoenzyme of phosphodiesterase and is a novel oral therapy for erectile dysfunction. Its importance in anaesthetic practice relates to its potentiation of nitric oxide donors.

ATP-ase-dependent potassium channel openers

Nicorandil was introduced onto the market as one of the first of this class of drug, but it appears that a much older drug, diazoxide, which previously had had its hypotensive effect 'by an unknown mechanism' is also an example. Diazoxide has been used for the rapid control of malignant hypertension, but there is evidence that control of blood pressure in this condition is best achieved more slowly than was previously thought. Nicorandil is a nicotinamide ester. It opens ATP-dependent potassium channels but it also acts as a nitric oxide donor. Its effect on the myocardium is to ameliorate post-ischaemic stunning and this effect is mediated by the first of these mechanisms. Both mechanisms are involved in its vasodilator effect. It is used as a treatment for angina. Pinacidil is marketed as a pure ATP-ase-dependent potassium channel opener.

Adenosine uptake inhibitors

Dipyridamole inhibits adenosine uptake into cells. It decreases coronary vascular resistance and increases coronary flow and oxygen tension in coronary sinus blood. It has little effect on vascular resistance in ischaemic areas of the heart where small vessels are already maximally dilated, since adenosine, which is released from a hypoxic myocardium, is a coronary vasodilator. It can thus cause 'steal' and it is used for this purpose to identify coronary occlusive disease in a variation on the 'stress' ECG where the stress is produced by dipyridamole rather than by exercise (adenosine can be used for the same purpose). In therapeutic doses it does not usually cause marked changes in systemic blood pressure or peripheral blood flow, but in large doses it can produce hypotension. It can produce nausea, vomiting or diarrhoea, and occasionally headache or vertigo. It also has an inhibitory effect on platelets. This may be due to a potentiation of epoprostenol (prostacyclin) which in turn inhibits platelet function, or to an increase in platelet cyclic AMP by inhibition of platelet phosphodiesterase. It was used in conjunction with aspirin in the prophylaxis of thromboembolism in patients with prosthetic heart valves, until it was shown that the combination had no advantage over aspirin alone. It can be used to prevent pulmonary hypertensive crises in children with congenital heart disease. In patients taking dipyridanole adenosine has a dangerously prolonged action.

Vasodilators with an unknown mechanism

Hydralazine is a useful vasodilator in anaesthetic practice as it can be given by intravenous bolus. It is rarely used in the medium to long term, partly because of unpredictability of dose requirement, but mainly because of the lupus-like syndrome it can cause.

Drugs affecting coronary blood vessels

A number of drugs can cause coronary blood vessels to constrict. Among these are angiotensin II, vasopressin, 5-HT, histamine, L-NMMA, L-NAME and some prostaglandins. *In vivo* their effects can be modified by their other pharmacological actions. For instance, angiotensin II may increase coronary flow: although it constricts coronary vessels, it is less potent on such vessels than on arterioles elsewhere in the body and thus coronary perfusion pressure rises.

Bradykinin, adenine nucleotides, adenosine and prostacyclin dilate coronary vessels. Catecholamines like dopamine have a biphasic action, α-adrenoceptor stimulation causing constriction and β-adrenoceptor stimulation causing dilatation.

Coronary vasodilator drugs act in a variety of ways:

- By raising cyclic AMP concentrations, the concentration of free intracellular calcium ions is reduced; inhibitors of phosphodiesterase, such as papaverine and milrinone, or activators of adenyl cyclase, such as isoprenaline, can produce such effects.
- Drugs may block calcium ion transport into the smooth muscle vascular cell; verapamil and nifedipine and mibefradil have such actions, and an action on calcium channels is thought to contribute to the mechanism of action of volatile anaesthetics.
- The active transport into cardiac cells of adenosine, a potent vasodilator, can be inhibited by dipyridamole, lidoflazine and dilazep.
- Adenosine itself can be used for its coronary dilator effect.

It is important to appreciate that drugs that increase total coronary flow are not necessarily useful drugs for the treatment of angina. The coronary vessels in some patients with angina are atherosclerotic and thus unable to dilate in response to vasodilator drugs. Moreover, in the ischaemic area beyond the obstruction, the arterioles may be already dilated to their maximum capacity due to accumulation of vasodilator metabolites and reflex inhibition of sympathetic tone.

Under such conditions, vasodilator drugs may increase blood flow to other parts of the heart and actually divert flow away from the ischaemic area, the so-called 'coronary steal' phenomenon.

MONOGRAPHS

CAPTOPRIL

Captopril (rINN)

Pharmacology

Captopril was the first angiotensin converting enzyme (ACE) inhibitor and there has been more experience with it than its later competitors. ACE inhibitors prevent the formation of angiotensin II. There is no loss of effect with long-term therapy and no rebound hypertension if it is suddenly stopped. There is a tendency to elevate serum potassium, but this is only clinically significant when concomitant therapy includes potassium-sparing diuretics or potassium supplements. Captopril is excreted primarily through the kidney.

Indications

ACE inhibitors are effective in reducing blood pressure and in the treatment of congestive heart failure by reducing pre-load and after-load and raising cardiac output without producing reflex tachycardia. ACE inhibitors are indicated to delay renal deterioration in diabetic micro-albuminuria.

Hypertension, congestive cardiac failure and diabetic microalbuminuria are the principal indications for ACE inhibitors. Pretreatment with captopril has been shown to partially attenuate the hypertensive response to intubation.

Dosage and administration

Captopril needs to be given twice or three times a day, starting at 25 mg a day and rising to 100 mg a day if needed. For diabetic microalbuminuria, the dose is 75–100 mg/day in divided doses.

Precautions

All ACE inhibitors are prone to produce an intermittent dry cough; other side effects reported include headache, dizziness, fatigue, diarrhoea and nausea and are generally mild and transient. Urticaria is common and angioneurotic oedema occurs in about 1 in 1000 patients. All ACE inhibitors are contra-indicated in pregnancy as they cause fetal abnormalities in animals and probably in man. They are probably also secreted in the milk. Captopril (and other ACE inhibitors that contain sulphydryl groups) can cause membranous glomerulonephritis if given in large doses. The same compounds may cause a metallic taste. In diabetics, hypoglycaemia may occur secondary to enhanced insulin sensitivity. Captopril may cause a false-positive urine test for acetone.

Sensitivity is likely to be high in patients who are sodium or volume depleted. Some patients with renovascular hypertension, especially associated with bilateral renal blood flow restriction, will develop an exaggerated response to initial doses and may develop frank renal failure. Hypoglycaemia may occur in insulin-dependent diabetics. An anaphylactoid reaction may occur with haemodialysis.

Lisinopril has certain favourable characteristics. Its absorption is uninfluenced by food and there is no significant metabolism, 97 per cent being recoverable unchanged in the urine. Onset of action is about 2 h, reaching a peak effect in 4–6 h, and its effects continue for at least 24 h. It can therefore be given in a once-a-day dosing schedule. Because of the lack of metabolism, dosage needs to be modified in renal failure. The normal daily dose is 20 mg, but treatment should begin with 10 mg/day. The maximum dose so far needed is 80 mg/day.

Enalapril is a pro-drug, its metabolite enalaprilat contributing predominantly to its hypotensive effect. It is also recommended for once-a-day dosing and its bioavailability is unaffected by food. Doses start at 2.5 mg, rising to 10–20 mg/day. Its effect is definitely starting to wane after 12–14 h: a morning-only dose therefore may fail to protect against nocturnal hypertensive episodes. It is also excreted unchanged by the kidney.

Quinapril is another pro-drug, quinaprilat being the active metabolite. It is claimed to have a unique pharmacokinetic profile by way of a much higher binding potency to human ACE. It is also given once a day, starting with 5 mg, rising to 40 mg. It is claimed to produce fewer side effects, particularly excessive hypotension. As with other drugs of this group, it can be given alone or in combination with thiazide diuretics and β-blockers.

Losartan is an angiotensin II receptor antagonist. Its effects and uses are the same as those of the ACE inhibitors, but there is no accumulation of bradykinin, and therefore a reduced tendency to fatigue, oedema and cough.

CLONIDINE

Clonidine hydrochloride (rINN)

Pharmacology

Clonidine is an imidazoline derivative, chemically related to tolazoline and phentolamine, and causes a fall in blood pressure accompanied by bradycardia and a fall in cardiac output. The fall in systolic pressure is more marked than the fall in diastolic pressure. In patients on oral therapy, peripheral resistance is little affected.

Clonidine has complex actions, as yet not fully understood. Contributing to its hypotensive effect is postsynaptic stimulation of α_2-adrenoceptors in the adrenal medulla, and stimulation of pre-synaptic α-adrenoceptors, both centrally and peripherally. It may also interact with dopaminergic and tryptaminergic neurones centrally.

Clonidine probably owes its hypotensive action mainly to its ability to stimulate α-adrenoceptors in the brain. These receptors are inhibitory and cause a decrease in outflow from the vasomotor centre. Any interruption of the pathways from the vasomotor centre interferes with its action. With prolonged treatment, vascular smooth muscle develops a reduced ability to respond to catecholamines and angiotensin and this may contribute to the hypotensive action.

Following rapid intravenous injection, however, there is an initial rise in blood pressure due to direct α_1-adrenoceptor stimulant action, and this can be blocked by an α_1-adrenoceptor blocking agent, such as phentolamine. After oral administration, plasma levels reach a peak in 3 h and decline with a half-life of 20 h.

Clonidine is of interest because normal homeostatic cardiovascular reflexes are preserved, thus avoiding the problems of postural hypotension and hypotension on exercise. Diuretics given simultaneously act synergistically and enable the dose of clonidine to be reduced. Renal blood flow and glomerular filtration rate are maintained: there is a reduction in Na^+ and Cl^- excretion, but K^+ excretion is unaffected.

Clonidine has also been found to exert an analgesic effect when administered extradurally (Glynn et al., 1988). The mode of action may be post-synaptic activation of descending inhibitory pathways that synapse in the dorsal horn of the spinal cord. The onset is rapid, but the duration is less than with morphine. The effect has a ceiling due to competing α_1-effects of the drug. There is also an accompanying decrease in mean arterial blood pressure (Lund et al., 1989), which is due to an effect on α_2-receptors in the spinal cord. Clonidine has also been used to produce preoperative sedation, which is due to an effect on α_2-receptors centrally.

Indications

The principal indication for clonidine is in cases of essential hypertension when it is usually combined with a diuretic such as chlorthalidone.

It has also been found effective as a prophylactic in small doses in cases of migraine, particularly in those who give a history of migraine associated with particular foods, such as chocolate, cheese, alcohol and citrus fruits.

Dosage and administration

In the treatment of essential hypertension, the dose is 200–300 µg daily in divided doses. This dose is gradually increased on alternate days until a satisfactory reduction in blood pressure is achieved. Doses in excess of 1 mg/day may be required on occasions. For the prophylaxis of migraine, the dose is 25 µg twice daily, increasing up to 75 µg twice daily. Larger doses may cause hypotension.

Precautions

On withdrawal of the drug, metabolites of catecholamines increase markedly and this may be associated with rebound hypertension. The drug should, therefore, not be withdrawn abruptly prior to surgery. Patients on treatment are more sensitive to parenterally administered catecholamines. It should be used with caution in patients with Raynaud's phenomenon or thromboangiitis obliterans, who are unusually sensitive to any effects of endogenous or exogenous catecholamines. Clonidine would be expected to potentiate agents that lower blood pressure by ganglion blockade or direct action on the vessels and in which central vasomotor mechanisms normally act to try to limit the fall in blood pressure. Nevertheless, because of the danger of rebound hypertension it is normally inadvisable to stop therapy suddenly prior to giving an anaesthetic. Rebound hypertension due to sudden withdrawal of clonidine may be treated by administration of phentolamine or by reintroduction of clonidine.

Initially, sedation and dry mouth are encountered in a proportion of patients. The effects are seldom severe, usually subside in 2–3 weeks and the sedative effect may be beneficial in the early stages. It may aggravate depressive illness. In the early stage of treatment, there may be a little fluid retention and weight gain on occasions, which are usually transient and may be controlled with diuretics. It commonly causes skin rashes and constipation. Other occasional side effects include dizziness, headache, nocturnal unrest, nausea, euphoria, constipation and, rarely, impotence.

Glynn, C., Dawson, A. and Sanders, R. (1988) A double-blind comparison between epidural morphine and epidural clonidine in patients with chronic non-cancer pain. *Pain*, **34**, 123.

Lund, C., Qvitzau, S., Greulich, A., Hjorts, O. N-C. and Kehlet, H. (1989) Comparison of the effects of extradural clonidine with those of morphine on postoperative pain. Stress responses, cardiopulmonary function and motor and sensory block. *British Journal of Anaesthesia*, **63**, S16.

Guanfacine is an analogue of clonidine. There is evidence that like clonidine it stimulates α-adrenoceptors centrally. Bioavailability (measured by comparing the areas under the plasma level curves following oral and intravenous dosing) was close to 100 per cent, suggesting lack of first-pass effect and very good absorption of the drug. The elimination half-life after oral administration is about 21 h. Clinically the drug appears to be less sedative than clonidine and less likely to produce rebound hypertension. Tolerance to it can occur. For the treatment of essential hypertension, doses of 3–6 mg daily have been used.

DOBUTAMINE

Dobutamine hydrochloride (rINN)

Pharmacology

Dobutamine resembles dopamine chemically. It acts directly on β-adrenoceptors with some selectivity for β_1-adrenoceptors. Its other actions are slight. It therefore increases the force of cardiac contraction with a lesser effect on rate. Unlike dopamine, it does not produce renal vasodilatation and it does not cause release of norepinephrine (noradrenaline). It also has some α-adrenoceptor activity such as increasing peripheral vascular tone, an effect that can be demonstrated by giving an infusion of the drug in the presence of a non-specific β-blocking agent.

Dobutamine is ineffective by mouth and has to be given as a constant intravenous infusion. The half-life is about 2 minutes due to rapid metabolism by the liver to inactive conjugates. It can produce arrhythmias, but the incidence is lower than with isoprenaline. It also raises the heart rate and blood pressure in a dose-dependent fashion if given at too high a rate of administration.

Dobutamine is used to produce a dose-dependent increase in cardiac output in patients with congestive cardiac failure. It may be of value in patients who have had cardiopulmonary bypass surgery. It has also been used to improve cardiac output in patients with acute myocardial infarction with congestive cardiac failure.

Indications

Dobutamine may be used as an adjunct to general supportive therapy in the treatment of haemodynamic disturbance associated with myocardial infarction, open heart surgery, traumatic shock, endotoxin shock, renal failure, cardiac failure and circulatory decompensation. It may be of some value in improving perfusion of vital organs and in reversing hypotension due to inadequate cardiac output.

Dosage and administration

Dobutamine is available for intravenous use in ampoules containing 250 mg; it may be made up as 3 × [body weight] diluted to 50 ml (typically 210 mg for a 70 kg man). With the resulting solution, 1 ml/h is equivalent to 1 µg/kg/minute, and the standard range is 1–20 ml/h.

DOPAMINE

Dopamine hydrochloride (rINN)

Pharmacology

Dopamine is a naturally-occurring precursor of norepinephrine (noradrenaline) to which it is converted by the enzyme dopamine β-oxidase at various adrenergic sites (see page 351). It is the natural transmitter at some synapses in the CNS. Dopamine increases cardiac output primarily by increasing stroke volume: it dilates vessels to vital organs such as renal, mesenteric and splenic beds, but constricts vessels in the skin and muscle. In responsive patients with the shock syndrome or with refractory congestive cardiac failure, dopamine improves the efficiency of the heart and increases cardiac output at lower cost in terms of excess myocardial oxygen consumption. In addition, it has specific dopaminergic effects on diuresis and natriuresis. The drug has been given at low infusion rates principally for its renal effects – so-called renal dopamine – but no beneficial effect has been shown in terms of survival or in terms of preservation of kidney function.

Dopamine has dual effects on the heart. There is a direct action via β-adrenoceptors and an indirect effect through the release of norepinephrine from myocardial storage sites. Both these effects are blocked by β-blocking agents. In the isolated heart there is little difference between inotropic and chronotropic effects. However, in the intact animal dopamine exerts a positive inotropic effect without changing the rate up to a certain dosage at which point the rate rises (see *Figure 12.8*). This is probably related to the peripheral effects of dopamine. Dopamine has little effect on peripheral resistance, so that reflex tachycardia is not marked. In addition, unlike isoprenaline, it has a pre-synaptic effect, reducing norepinephrine release.

It can be started as an infusion soon after the onset of shock and as soon as hypotension or decreased urine flow become manifest. Adequate blood volume expansion is essential before dopamine therapy is initiated. Dopamine has a selective action on renal vessels at low doses. It has been combined with a peripheral vasodilator such as nitroprusside or glyceryl trinitrate to reduce after-load on the heart.

Because of concerns about gastro-intestinal mucosal ischaemia, and effects on hormone production, the administration of dopamine for its renal effects is now no longer practised, and the administration of dopamine for its cardiovascular effects has been replaced by the use of epinephrine (adrenaline) for this function.

Indications

Dopamine may be used as an adjunct to general supportive therapy in the treatment of haemodynamic disturbance associated with myocardial infarction, open heart surgery, traumatic shock, endotoxin shock, renal failure, cardiac, failure and circulatory decompensation. It may be of some value in improving perfusion of vital organs and in reversing hypotension due to inadequate cardiac output.

Dosage and administration

Dopamine is available for intravenous use as an aqueous solution in 5 ml ampoules containing 40 mg/ml; it may be made up as 3 × [body weight] diluted to 50 ml (typically 210 mg for a 70 kg man). With the resulting solution, 1 ml/h is equivalent to 1 µg/kg/minute, and the standard range is 1–20 ml/h. Up to 5 µg/kg/minute is termed 'renal dopamine'; 5–10 µg/kg/minute is termed 'cardiosupportive dopamine'; 10–20 µg/kg/minute is termed 'vasoconstrictive dopamine'.

Precautions

Dopamine should be administered via a central vein where possible, as extravasation may cause local ischaemia.

If any extravasation is noted, the area should be infiltrated immediately with 10–15 ml of saline containing 5–10 mg of phentolamine to prevent sloughing and necrosis. Overdose not responding to withdrawal of the infusion should be treated with phentolamine or another α-adrenoceptor blocking agent. Smaller doses and special care are necessary in patients who have recently been treated with monoamine oxidase inhibitors.

Adverse effects on myocardial performance have been reported in the presence of hypothermia, particularly with low doses, which were not seen with other inotropes (Heidelmayer et al., 1990).

Dopamine should not be given to patients with phaeochromocytoma or uncorrected cardiac arrhythmias. The use of cyclopropane or halogenated hydrocarbon anaesthetics is also contraindicated. Dopamine should not be added to sodium bicarbonate or other alkaline intravenous solutions.

Heidelmeyer, C. F., Schroeder, T., Hering, J. P. and Hellige, D. (1990) Dopamine in moderate hypothermia: a new and undesired myocardial effect. *European Journal of Anaesthesiology*, **7**, 337

DOPEXAMINE

Dopexamine hydrochloride (rINN)

Pharmacology

Dopexamine has a unique spectrum of actions at adrenergic and dopaminergic receptors. It is a potent agonist at β_2-adrenoceptors, thus producing systemic vasodilatation and lowering peripheral resistance. This is combined with positive inotropic and chronotropic effects on the heart. It is also (like dopamine) an agonist at peripheral vascular dopamine (D_1) receptors, which confers preferential dilatation of the renal, cerebral, coronary and mesenteric vascular beds. It has some indirect activity at β-adrenergic cardiac sites by inhibiting neuronal re-uptake of norepinephrine (adrenaline). Unlike dopamine, however, it has no action at α-adrenoceptors. One consequence of this is that it is less prone to initiate ventricular arrhythmias than dopamine or dobutamine, probably because it depresses the maximum rate of depolarization. There is also a tendency towards tachycardia with its use.

Indications

Dopexamine is used for the treatment of low cardiac output states, particularly after cardiac surgery. It reduces left and right ventricular after-load and thus increases stroke volume and cardiac index. Therapy aimed at increasing cardiac output is usually limited by the onset of unacceptable hypotension or tachycardia before the quoted maximum dose is reached. It is also suggested that it is effective in the prophylaxis of renal failure and in treatment of conditions involving low splanchnic blood flow.

Dosage and administration

Dopexamine may be made up as $3 \times$ [body weight] diluted to 50 ml (typically 210 mg for a 70 kg man). With the resulting solution, 1 ml/h is equivalent to 1 µg/kg/minute, and the standard range is 0.5–15 ml/h.

EPHEDRINE

Ephedrine hydrochloride (rINN) and Ephedrine sulfate (rINN)
For structural formula see Table 12.2, page 326

Pharmacology

Ephedrine is a sympathomimetic amine and is the active principle of the Chinese plant Ma Huang, known and used for centuries in the East. It was introduced to Europe in 1923 and is now produced synthetically. It has α- and β-effects and acts both directly and indirectly; as with amfetamine, tachyphylaxis is marked. It is an inhibitor of MAO.

Central nervous system   There is considerable stimulation of the cerebral cortex and medulla, but this is not as marked as with amfetamine, although wakefulness may occur and there is some analeptic effect on unconscious patients. Ephedrine stimulates the spinal cord and enhances spinal reflexes.

Cardiovascular system   Cardiac output and rate are increased and repeated frequent doses or a single very large dose may result in depression of the heart. In small doses, vasoconstriction is almost balanced by vasodilatation and overall peripheral resistance is little changed; diastolic blood pressure is increased, but less so than systolic blood pressure. There is also an increase in cardiac irritability. Vessels of mucous membranes are constricted following local application, but this action is not so marked after systemic administration. Cerebral blood flow is reduced, as is blood flow through the kidneys. Coronary vessels are stated to be dilated, but the increased blood flow through them may be due to the increase in cardiac output.

Respiratory system   There is dilatation of the bronchial tree due to inhibition of the smooth muscle of the bronchi and bronchioles. Respiration is stimulated, especially if drug-induced depression is present.

Alimentary system and urinary tract   There is inhibition of smooth muscle and increase in tone of the sphincters of the alimentary tract and the bladder. The drug may cause retention of urine, especially when there is an enlarged prostate.

Fate in the body   It inhibits MAO and is not destroyed by it. It is excreted unchanged in the urine within 24 h.

Indications

Ephedrine is commonly used for its pressor action, but it is still occasionally used in the prophylactic treatment of asthma. Many proprietary preparations contain ephedrine mixed with other bronchodilator drugs and are sold in considerable quantities. It may also be used as a local application to reduce congestion of the nasal mucosa during colds and hay fever, and prior to the passage of a nasal endotracheal tube to prevent bleeding from abrasions. If a vasopressor is needed in obstetric practice, it is the drug of choice as it does not reduce uterine blood flow. It has a limited place in a few cases of myasthenia gravis. Being an indirectly acting agent, some degree of tachyphylaxis can be expected due to depletion of stores or norepinephrine (noradrenaline). On the black market it is used by athletes, or mixed with caffeine and sold as amfetamine, or mixed with local anaesthetic and sold as cocaine.

Dosage and administration

For treatment of hypotension associated with spinal or epidural anaesthesia, 3–6 mg is given intravenously, repeated after 2 minutes if required, 15 mg may be given intramuscularly.
   Ephedrine is active by mouth, and may also be given intramuscularly; duration of action may be up to 1 h or more.
   The treatment of asthma is usually by the oral route in doses of 30–60 mg, repeated as required. Tolerance may be shown to repeated doses.
   For the relief of nasal congestion and the production of vasoconstriction to aid the passage of a nasal endotracheal tube, a 1 per cent solution in water or liquid paraffin may be used.

Precautions

Ephedrine produces a number of cardiovascular side effects that contra-indicate its use in myocardial or coronary disease. It should also be used with care in cases of even moderate hypertension. As it is apt to cause wakefulness, it should not be given late in the day.

Overdose causes anxiety, apprehension, restlessness, tachycardia, palpitations and hypertension. Treatment is limited to sedation to control the symptoms.

EPINEPHRINE (ADRENALINE)

Epinephrine (rINN)
Epinephrine bitartrate (rINNM), Epinephrine acid tartrate (rINNM) and Adrenaline acid tartrate (BP)
For structural formula see *Table 12.2*, page 326

Physical characteristics

Commercial preparations of epinephrine contain a stabilizer (potassium metabisulphate, 0.1 per cent); this enables them to be sterilized by autoclaving. Repeated autoclaving, however, causes deterioration.

Pharmacology

Epinephrine is a most important naturally-occurring hormone. It can also be synthesized. In the body it is produced from tyrosine by the following enzymatic processes:

Substrate	Enzyme
Tyrosine	
↓ ←	Tyrosine hydroxylase
Dopa	
↓ ←	Dopa decarboxylase
Dopamine	
↓ ←	Dopamine β-oxidase
Norepinephrine	
↓ ←	N-methyl transferase
Epinephrine	

There are other biosynthetic pathways, but the above is the main route. In the adult, epinephrine (adrenaline) forms about 80 per cent of the catecholamines in the adrenal medulla, the remainder being norepinephrine, but in infancy it is norepinephrine that predominates. There is evidence that epinephrine and norepinephrine are contained in different cells. They are liberated by acetylcholine, in its role of chemical transmitter, by impulses from the autonomic preganglionic fibres supplying the medullary cells. Thus, the adrenal medulla is essentially a sympathetic ganglion with postganglionic neurones replaced by a histologically different type of cell. This comparison is justifiable both on embryological and pharmacological grounds. In contrast, the mixture of catecholamines liberated at adrenergic nerve endings has a minute proportion of epinephrine and a large proportion of norepinephrine. Epinephrine accounts for less than 10 per cent of the catecholamines extractable from tissues other than the adrenal medulla, and probably occurs in them in scattered chromaffin cells. Epinephrine has both α- and β-effects.

In general, it is true to say that the effects of epinephrine, with the exception of sweating, are the same as those of sympathetic activity, but epinephrine may be thought of more

Table 12.6 Principal actions of some sympathomimetic amines

Drug	Receptors stimulated	Mode of action	Cardiac			Venous constriction	Total peripheral resistance	Blood pressure	Renal blood flow	Broncho-dilatation	CNS stimulation
			Out-put	Rate	Irrita-bility						
Norepinephrine	Mainly α	Direct	0/−*	−	+	+	+	+	−	0	0
Epinephrine	α and β	Direct	+	+	+	+	−	+	−	+	+
Isoprenaline and orciprenaline	Mainly β	Direct	+	+	+	+	−	−	?	+	+
Salbutamol	Mainly β₂	Direct	0	0	0	?	0	0	0	+	0
Phenylephrine	Mainly α	Direct	0/−	−	0/+	+	+	+	−	+	0
Metaraminol	α and β	Direct and indirect	+	−	?+	+	+	+	−	0	0
Methoxamine	α (β-block)	Direct	−	−	0	+	+	+	−	0	0
Ephedrine	α and β	Indirect mainly	+	+	+	+	+/−	+	+/−	+	+
Methylamfetamine	α and β	Indirect	+	+	+	+	+/−	+	+	0	+
Mephenteramine	α and β	Indirect	+	+/0	0	+	+	+	+	0	0/+

*In an *in vivo* situation, rate and force of cardiac contraction can be reduced by reflex inhibition consequent on rise in mean arterial pressure.

as an extra hormone mainly called forth from the adrenal medulla for use in physiological emergency. The ordinary requirements of sympathetic tone are controlled by norepinephrine liberated at adrenergic nerve endings. In the CNS, there is some evidence that there are adrenergic neurones as well as the more widely accepted noradrenergic neurones.

Mode of action   Epinephrine has an action both on the cell membrane and on intracellular metabolism by increasing the production of cyclic AMP. It does so by stimulating the enzyme adenyl cyclase, which converts ATP into cyclic AMP. Epinephrine causes sodium to leave the cell and reduces the sodium uptake of the cell. It also enters the cell itself and increases energy production. In the case of smooth muscle, most of this energy is taken up to stabilize the inherently unstable cell membrane, whereas with voluntary muscle, whose membrane is inherently stable, the energy is available for contraction. This explains how epinephrine inhibits intestinal muscle and enhances contraction of voluntary muscle.

Central nervous system   There is little effect in small doses. Larger doses have a stimulating effect on the cerebral cortex and medulla and may cause excitement, apprehension, headache and tremors. Compared with its congeners, ephedrine and amphetamine, its analeptic effect is minimal and of no use clinically.

The EEG spectrum is similar to that produced by attention, but the effect is more marked than that caused by caffeine or amphetamine.

Cardiovascular system   The action of epinephrine upon the circulation varies according to the size of the dose, the route by which it is given and the prevailing state of the circulation. The smallest effective doses raise the systolic blood pressure, but cause a slight fall in diastolic pressure. This latter effect is caused by a decrease in overall peripheral resistance, the vasodilatation of the vessels of the skeletal muscles and liver more than counterbalancing vasoconstriction of the vessels of the skin and mucosae.

In spite of this drop in peripheral resistance, the systolic pressure increases. This is due to the rise in cardiac output which results from increased heart rate and force of beat, caused both by the direct effect of epinephrine on the heart and by the increased venous return initiated by the constrictor action of epinephrine upon the veins (*Table 12.6*).

Large doses of epinephrine cause vasoconstriction even in skeletal muscle, and the overall peripheral resistance is then increased, so that both systolic and diastolic pressures rise. Pulmonary vasoconstriction occurs.

It should be noted that the degree of change in heart rate is a resultant of the opposing forces of the direct cardiac action of epinephrine and the depressor reflex evoked by the rise in mean arterial blood pressure. Rarely, reflex cardiac slowing may predominate and, conversely, the rise in heart rate and mean blood pressure will be much greater if the reflex arc is weakened at any point, as by block of the vagi or the autonomic ganglia. In complete atrioventricular block, epinephrine increases the ventricular as well as the atrial rate even if the block is not overcome by the improvement in conduction which epinephrine also achieves.

Wherever capillaries are constricted their permeability is decreased and the leakage of plasma protein into tissue fluids because of allergic reactions is opposed. Capillary constriction also retards the absorption of solutions containing epinephrine. Large doses of epinephrine, or the accidental intravenous injection of doses intended to be subcutaneous, can cause cardiac arrhythmias which may lead to ventricular fibrillation; acute pulmonary oedema may also occur due to left ventricular failure and to a direct action on the pulmonary epithelium. These complications may also occur from small doses if the heart is more sensitive than usual to epinephrine as the result of the action of certain other drugs, for example, halothane. Coronary vessels are said to be dilated by epinephrine, but the evidence is not conclusive. It appears that β_2-adrenoceptors mediating vasodilatation are present in the smaller arteries and arterioles, whereas α-adrenoceptors mediating constriction are present in the larger coronary arteries. Cocaine potentiates the action of epinephrine, and even on a mucous membrane the action of these two drugs together is not advisable.

Respiratory system Smooth muscle of the bronchi and bronchioles is inhibited by epinephrine and relaxes. The vascular action of epinephrine on the mucosa and the reduction of bronchial secretion will also improve the airway. The central action of epinephrine in causing respiratory stimulation is not great enough, in proportion to all its other actions, to be of use.

Other effects Epinephrine causes dilatation of the pupil and secretion of tears if it reaches the eye via the bloodstream, but not when instilled into the conjunctival sac, except in hyperexcitability of the sympathetic system in acute pancreatitis, in which it has been used as a diagnostic test (Loewi's), and in thyrotoxicosis.

The movements of the stomach and intestine are inhibited and the fundus of the bladder relaxed, but the ileocolic sphincter and that of the bladder are contracted. It increases the rate of recovery of skeletal muscle in fatigue, and will sensitize ganglion cells to the action of acetylcholine. The parturient uterus in women is relaxed, whereas in most other species the pregnant uterus is contracted.

Metabolism Stimulation by epinephrine is expensive in terms of tissue requirements of oxygen, as the usual doses of epinephrine can increase the body's total consumption by 20–30 per cent; cardiac efficiency is probably lowered, in spite of the fact that cardiac output is increased, since the extra oxygen uptake is out of proportion to the increased work done. Blood sugar is raised mainly by increased breakdown of muscle and liver glycogen, and glycosuria may occur. High levels of epinephrine in the blood can cause the release of corticotrophin (ACTH) and sometimes of histamine.

Antagonists The α-effects of epinephrine are antagonized by α-adrenoceptor blocking agents, such as phentolamine, tolazoline and phenoxybenzamine; the β-effects are antagonized by β-adrenoceptor blocking agents, such as acebutolol, oxprenolol and propranolol.

Fate in the body Epinephrine is rapidly inactivated by the enzyme catechol-O-methyl transferase (COMT; see Figure *12.10*) which replaces the hydrogen atom of the hydroxyl group in the meta-position with a methyl group. Oxidative deamination by MAO also plays a part, although a subsidiary one, in its inactivation. These two processes result in the appearance of 3-methoxy-4-hydroxymandelic acid in the urine (*Figure 12.10*). The level of this substance in the urine is a useful test in the diagnosis of phaeochromocytoma. Large amounts of epinephrine and norepinephrine also appear in the urine when this condition is present.

Indications

Epinephrine is employed to produce vasoconstriction in local anaesthesia, bronchodilatation in asthma, in the treatment of hay fever, and in the various forms of allergy

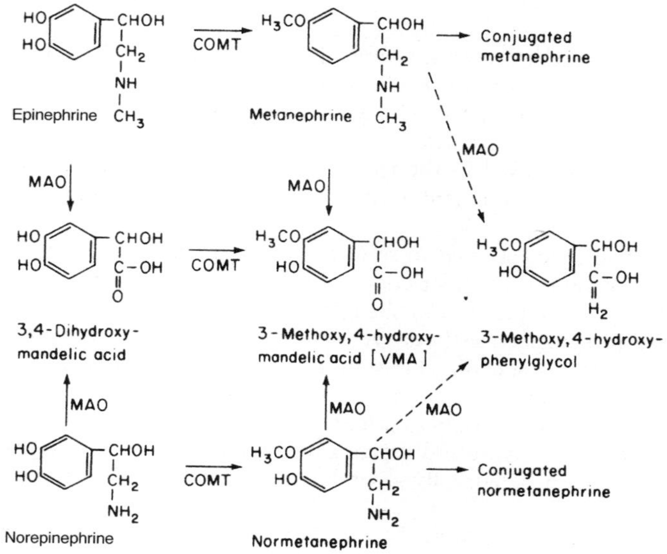

Figure 12.10 Pathways for metabolism of epinephrine and norepinephrine. MAO = monoamine oxidase; COMT = catechol-*O*-methyl transferase

including that following incompatible blood transfusion. It is an essential drug in the management of circulatory arrest.

Dosage and administration

In local infiltration anaesthesia and nerve block, a final strength of solution in the region of 1:200 000 is commonly used, although concentrations down to 1:500 000 are effective. A 1:200 000 solution may be obtained by adding 0.5 mg (0.5 ml of 1:1000 epinephrine) to 100 ml of the selected analgesic solution. For surface anaesthesia 0.05–0.1 mg epinephrine may be added to 1 ml of the anaesthetic agent: this concentration produces efficient vasoconstriction, but the rate of absorption of the anaesthesia is not retarded. It has been suggested that this effect can be achieved on mucous surfaces only by using epinephrine a few minutes before the local anaesthetic is applied.

In the emergency treatment of bronchospasm or in anaphylactic shock (see page 49) accompanied by severe hypotension the patient may be given a subcutaneous injection of up to 0.5 mg or 0.2–0.4 mg given slowly intravenously. In cardiac arrest, 1–5 mg may be given into a central vein or via the endotracheal tube.

In upper airway obstruction due to swelling, 2 ml of 1:1000 solution diluted to 3 ml with normal saline may be given by nebulizer. Remarkably, this dose is acceptable even in neonates with croup.

For the treatment of non-hypovolaemic shock with hypotension, epinephrine may be given by intravenous infusion into a central vein at a rate of 0.05–0.2 µg/kg/minute. In practice, 0.03 × [body weight] is diluted to 50 ml (typically 2.1 mg for a 70 kg man). With the resulting solution, 10 ml/h is equivalent to 0.1 µg/kg/minute, so the standard range is 5–20 ml/h.

Precautions

It is inadvisable to give an intravenous infusion of epinephrine without the use of invasive monitoring to assess and monitor its effect on blood pressure.

Great care must be exercised in its use in the presence of hypertension, hyperthyroidism and severe heart disease. It must not be given intravenously in strengths exceeding 1:250 000, and when used in the treatment of asthma and serum reactions and in conjunction with local anaesthetic the total dose given at one administration should not exceed 500 µg.

Epinephrine should not be used in solutions of local anaesthetics in ring block of the finger, as the consequent vasoconstriction is likely to cause gangrene of the tissues distal to the injection. The danger of impairing the blood supply to the cord also contraindicates its use in spinal anaesthesia. A concentration of 1:200 000 is permissible for epidural injections. It is best avoided in solutions used for local infiltration for the extraction of teeth as it may give rise to a 'dry socket'.

Overdose of epinephrine produces a feeling of anxiety and apprehension, pallor and tachycardia; circulatory collapse and syncope may follow. In mild cases, recovery is rapid, but cardiac arrest may occur usually secondary to ventricular fibrillation.

Epinephrine in the presence of anaesthetic agents   The interaction between epinephrine and volatile anaesthetics, which has been recognized since 1895, presents a common problem with agents such as halothane. It is seen clinically as barrages of multi-focal ventricular extrasystoles that can proceed to ventricular fibrillation.

The actual mechanism is believed to be an increased automaticity in the ventricular conducting system. Stimulation of β-adrenoceptors by the catecholamine can be inferred from the specific protective effect of β-adrenoceptor blockade. Hypercapnia and hypoxia have a potent aggravating effect, but the chief determinant is the effective dose of epinephrine reaching the heart. This depends on the total dose, the concentration, and the vascularity of the site, or route of injection. Epinephrine can be safely administered with halothane if the following points are observed:

- there should be no hypoxia or hypercapnia;
- solutions should be no stronger than 1:200 000;
- the total dose should not be more than the equivalent of 20 ml of 1:200 000 in 10 minutes, or 30 ml in 1 h.

The administration of epinephrine during anaesthesia with the more recent volatile agents is less hazardous than with halothane, but the advice to avoid hypoxia or hypercapnia still applies.

In the case of cyclopropane, however, the threshold seems to be lower and the combination of epinephrine with this agent should be avoided.

GLYCERYL TRINITRATE

Glyceryl trinitrate (rINN) and Nitroglycerin (USP)

Pharmacology

Glyceryl trinitrate (GTN) relaxes vascular muscle and is claimed to have a greater effect on capacitance vessels than on arterioles. Its mode of action involves conversion to nitric oxide, intracellularly, which stimulates guanylate cyclase conversion to cyclic GMP, which causes vasodilatation. Dilatation of post-capillary vessels, including large veins, results in peripheral pooling, reduced venous return and a fall in cardiac output. It is thus particularly of value in left ventricular failure, reducing pre-load rather than after-load.

Systemic vascular resistance, pulmonary vascular resistance and arterial pressure are all reduced: left ventricular end-diastolic volumes and pressures are reduced as well as myocardial wall tension and oxygen consumption. There may be an improvement in coronary blood flow: redistribution from normal to ischaemic cardiac muscle has been demonstrated.

The effects of GTN are apparent within 2–3 minutes of starting an intravenous infusion and are reversed within 5–10 minutes of discontinuing it. The metabolites are considerably less toxic in overdose than those from sodium nitroprusside but, this apart, the drugs are very similar. Both drugs increase intracranial pressure.

Indications

GTN can be used for the rapid control of hypertension during cardiac surgery or for inducing and maintaining controlled hypotension during anaesthesia. It has also been used to reduce pre-load in patients with unresponsive congestive cardiac failure, secondary to acute myocardial infarction.

It is used in the symptomatic treatment of angina pectoris by transdermal administration. This sustained therapy reduces the frequency of episodes of pain compared to oral treatment.

Dosage and administration

The drug is commercially available as a solution stabilized in 10 per cent alcohol, lactose and potassium monophosphate. It may be given by syringe pump or be diluted in an infusion of 5 per cent dextrose or isotonic saline. It is frequently diluted to a strength of 1 mg/ml, but it may be made up as 0.3 × [body weight] diluted to 50 ml (typically 21 mg for a 70 kg man). With the resulting solution, 1 ml/h is equivalent to 0.1 µg/kg/minute, and the standard range is 1–5 ml/h, and up to 20 ml/h in the short term.

Transdermal patches are available in two strengths, 25 mg and 50 mg. The average absorbed dose over 24 h from these patches is 5 mg and 10 mg, respectively. To minimize nitrate tolerance, patches should be removed for 6–8 h at night.

Precautions

The solution is incompatible with polyvinylchloride and should be administered after dilution only from glass or rigid polyethylene containers.

Side effects of nitrates include nausea and retching, headache, restlessness, muscle twitching, palpitations and dizziness. Overdose leads to hypotension which should be treated by elevating the legs, discontinuing the infusion or, if severe, by administering α-adrenoceptor stimulators such as methoxamine or phenylephrine.

Continuous administration can lead to tolerance. This is caused by a reduced availability of intracellular sulphydryl groups, which are essential for the conversion to nitric oxide.

GUANETHIDINE

Guanethidine monosulfate (rINN)

Pharmacology

Guanethidine is a hypotensive agent with a similar but not identical action to the peripheral vascular action of bretylium tosylate. Its chief peripheral action is the prevention of release of norepinephrine (noradrenaline) by nerve impulses from its storage sites in adrenergic nerves, thus leading to vasodilatation. Pooling of blood in capacitance vessels results in a fall in cardiac output, or a failure to raise cardiac output on exercise, and this causes hypotension. Indirectly acting amines will reverse its action. Adrenoceptors are unaffected. They behave as though denervated and are consequently considerably more sensitive to sympathomimetic substances. There is no action on the parasympathetic system, but the reduction in sympathetic activity may cause parasympathetic preponderance with overactivity of the bowel and consequent diarrhoea. Tolerance can occur. When the drug is withdrawn, several days may elapse before the blood pressure returns to its pretreatment level.

Indications

Guanethidine can be used distal to a tourniquet (so-called 'guanethidine Bier's block') to produce vasodilatation before microvascular surgery, after accidental intra-arterial thiopental and to improve angiographic pictures. This technique has been used in reflex sympathetic dystrophy (Sudeck's atrophy), but scientific evidence of benefit is lacking.

Guanethidine has been used in the treatment of hypertension, either alone or in combination with diuretics such as chlorothiazide.

Dosage and administration

For 'guanethidine Bier's block' 2 mg are dissolved in 20 ml of normal saline or 1 per cent lidocaine and this is held in place behind a tourniquet inflated to above systolic pressure for 20 minutes. As treatment for hypertension, guanethidine is given by mouth. It has a slow onset of action but its effects are prolonged. Treatment is commenced with a small dose of 10 mg/day in divided doses for the first week, increasing by 10 mg/day each week until 60 mg/day are given in the sixth week, by which time the majority of patients are under control. The drug does not appear toxic even in doses up to 500 mg/day, but with doses over 60 mg/day there is an increased likelihood of side effects and hypotension may become excessive. On a constant effective dose the blood pressure often falls progressively for about a week and then remains stable at the lower level unless the dose is changed. It can be given with chlorothiazide and its derivatives. Five per cent guanethidine eyedrops are used in the treatment of glaucoma.

Precautions

Guanethidine is contra-indicated in phaeochromocytoma as it increases the sensitivity of blood vessels to epinephrine and norepinephrine. It should be used with caution in coronary and severe renal disease. The blood pressure of patients who are under treatment with guanethidine may become markedly labile during anaesthesia. Excessive falls may arise from summation or even potentiation of the effects of treatment by the effect of anaesthesia. Acute rises in blood pressure may be due to hypersensitivity to circulating catecholamines released in response to a surgical stimulus. Premedication with atropine is advisable to prevent the potential risk of cardiac arrest. Stopping the drug the day before operation has little effect as its action lasts for more than a week. Excessive hypotension due to overdose can usually be controlled by keeping the patient recumbent.

If pressor agents are required, minimal doses should be used. Side effects of guanethidine are mainly due to postural hypotension. Myalgia, muscle weakness and blurring of vision have also been reported.

Bethanidine is related chemically to bretylium and guanethidine. It differs from guanethidine in that norepinephrine stores are not depleted so readily and its duration of action is considerably shorter. The drug is well absorbed after oral administration. Its action reaches its peak in 4–5 h and lasts about 12 h. It is mostly excreted in the urine within 12 h. Treatment is commenced at 5 mg 3 times daily, but the maintenance dose is typically 30–250 mg or more daily in divided doses. It is also contra-indicated in phaeochromocytoma.

Guanoxan and **guanaclor** are drugs with peripheral actions similar to guanethidine. Guanoxan is contra-indicated in patients with a previous history of liver disease, as some patients on treatment have developed jaundice. They have been shown to cause central as well as peripheral amine depletion.

Debrisoquine is another drug whose main action is the prevention of release of norepinephrine from storage granules. There is no depletion of norepinephrine stores on oral administration. Its chief advantage is its rapid onset and short duration of action, making it practicable to vary the intensity of dosage throughout the day and to minimize the inevitable orthostatic hypotension.

HYDRALAZINE HYDROCHLORIDE

Hydralazine hydrochloride (rINN)

Pharmacology

Hydralazine is a hypotensive agent that produces peripheral vasodilatation mainly by a direct action; it also has a mild α-adrenoceptor blocking action. Cardiac output and rate are reflexly increased by central sympathetic action. There are a number of side effects – headache, tachycardia, dizziness, nausea and vomiting. Renal blood flow is increased.

Indications, dosage and administration

It is used in the treatment of hypertension, often in conjunction with other drugs such as β-blocking agents or thiazide diuretics. It is of value in the treatment of hypertensive crises when 10–40 mg may be given intravenously. Otherwise, the usual commencing dose is 10 mg 4-hourly by mouth, increasing up to 200 mg daily if necessary.

Precautions

Tolerance may occur. A serious toxic effect, which can occur with prolonged use and large doses, is a condition resembling systemic lupus erythematosus. Note that there are fast and slow acetylators of hydralazine.

ISOPRENALINE SALTS

Isoprenaline sulfate (rINN), Isoprenaline hydrochloride (rINN), Isoproterenol sulfate (USP) and Isoproterenol hydrochloride (USP)
For structural formula see *Table 12.2*, page 326

Pharmacology

Isoprenaline is a catecholamine closely allied to epinephrine (adrenaline). It has powerful stimulant effects at all β-adrenoceptors, but only very weak actions at α-adrenoceptors.

Central nervous system   There is a mild stimulatory effect on the cerebral cortex.

Cardiovascular system   Isoprenaline has a powerful cardiac stimulating action and accelerates the heart rate. It produces marked peripheral vasodilatation. Effects on blood pressure are variable; usually there is a moderate fall in systolic and a greater fall in diastolic pressure. This results from the peripheral vasodilatation more than overcoming the β-effects of the increase in cardiac output. These observations also apply to therapeutic doses of isoprenaline given by aerosol. However, heavy users of isoprenaline aerosols are relatively resistant to the cardiac stimulant effects of isoprenaline. There is normally no vasoconstriction except when the drug is applied locally to mucous surfaces.

Respiratory system   There is a marked dilatation of bronchial muscle, even more effective than that of epinephrine. The rate and depth of respiration are slightly increased. Isoprenaline inhibits the release of histamine from passively sensitized human lung to a much greater extent than salbutamol, orciprenaline or sodium cromoglicate. This suggests that it is of particular use in bronchospasm associated with anaphylactic reactions. Isoprenaline, like orciprenaline, while improving airway resistance may cause a fall in arterial oxygen tension and raise the tension of carbon dioxide. This effect is thought to be due to an aggravation of the existing ventilation/perfusion inequality present in asthmatic subjects. Worsening of airway obstruction with prolonged use of isoprenaline in heavy doses and an improvement on withdrawal of the drug has been reported. It has been postulated that this could be due to the accumulation of 3-methoxy-isoprenaline, a β-blocking metabolite, although it has not been possible to produce demonstrable changes in respiratory function in man with this substance. However, it has been suggested that tolerance may also develop to other β-stimulants which do not form 3-methoxy derivatives, and may be a problem with all β-stimulant drugs. Prolonged heavy dosage may lead to decreasing response of the receptors, and this may also reduce the effect of the patient's own sympathetic nervous system and produce increasing bronchoconstriction.

Alimentary system   Ulceration in the buccal mucosa has been reported after sublingual absorption. There is some inhibition of peristaltic action and of the tone of the intestine.

Metabolism   Isoprenaline stimulates metabolism and increases oxygen consumption and carbon dioxide production.

Fate in the body   The metabolic fate of isoprenaline is similar to that of epinephrine.

Indications

Isoprenaline is chiefly used in the treatment of bradycardia and hypotension due to heart block. In the past it has been used in the treatment of bronchospasm, and for this purpose is administered as a metered dose from an aerosol spray. It can be used as an 'ino-dilator' to treat cardiogenic shock, but it causes more vasodilatation and more tachycardia than dobutamine.

Dosage and administration

For heart block, in emergency, 25 µg may be given intravenously. In practice, 2 mg is injected into a 500 ml bag of normal saline and aliquots of 5–10 ml are given.

For the treatment of extreme bradycardia or cardiogenic shock, isoprenaline may be given by intravenous infusion at a rate of 0.05–0.2 µg/kg/minute. In practice, 0.03 × [body weight] is diluted to 50 ml (typically 2.1 mg for a 70 kg man). With the resulting solution, 10 ml/h is equivalent to 0.1 µg/kg/minute, so the standard range is 5–20 ml/h.

In the absence of the more specific β_2-agonists, asthma may be treated with isoprenaline given by the inhalation of a 1 per cent spray from a nebulizer or proprietary pressurized spray delivering a metered dose.

Precautions

Side effects, which occasionally are severe, include tachycardia, palpitations and precordial pain, dizziness, faintness, headache, tremor, weakness, and sometimes nausea and vomiting.

The death rate from asthma increased in England and Wales in the years following the widespread introduction of pressurized isoprenaline aerosols for the treatment of this condition. In the age group 5–64 years the death rate in males doubled, and in the age group 5–34 years it trebled; in the age-group 10–14 years it increased eight-fold. A review of deaths certified as due to asthma showed that a high percentage of these patients had been using pressurized aerosols containing isoprenaline.

Possible mechanisms for this include cardiac stimulation causing arrhythmias, excessive doses causing increased airways obstruction, and cardiac depression under conditions of anoxia and right heart strain.

Isoprenaline should be used with the greatest caution in thyrotoxicosis and in the presence of serious cardiovascular disease.

Orciprenaline differs from isoprenaline only in having both the hydroxyl groups of its benzene ring in the meta-position instead of having one in the para-position. Its actions are similar, but it has a longer duration of action and it is active by mouth. It may be given as 20 mg tablets 3 times a day or by the inhalation of a 5 per cent spray from a nebulizer. It is chiefly used to provide prophylaxis against bradycardias in patients in intensive care with a recent high transection of the spinal cord.

METARAMINOL TARTRATE

Metaraminol tartrate (rINN)
For structural formula see *Table 12.2*, page 326

Pharmacology

Metaraminol has both α- and β-effects, and its action at adrenoceptors is mixed: both direct and indirect actions are demonstrable.

Cardiovascular system   Cardiac output and force are increased and there is an increase in peripheral resistance. The combination of these factors causes a well-sustained rise in blood pressure. Coronary blood flow is increased. The heart rate is slowed, especially after intramuscular injection.

Respiratory system   There may be moderate slowing of respiration with some increase in depth.

Indications

Metaraminol is used in the treatment of hypotension due to spinal anaesthesia and overdose of ganglion-blocking agents.

Dosage and administration

It may be given subcutaneously, intramuscularly or intravenously. When given intravenously, it acts in 1–3 minutes, and lasts for about 25 minutes. Intramuscularly it acts in 5–10 minutes and lasts for 1 h or more. Dosage is 2–10 mg given intramuscularly, and 1.5–5 mg intravenously. Administration should not be repeated until it is certain that the full effect of the previous dose has been produced.

Precautions

Metaraminol should be used with caution in patients with hypertension, severe heart disease or hyperthyroidism.

METHOXAMINE HYDROCHLORIDE

Methoxamine hydrochloride (rINN)
For structural formula see *Table 12.2*, page 326

Pharmacology

Methoxamine is a sympathomimetic agent whose agonist actions are mediated solely at α-adrenoceptors. It produces some blockade of β-adrenoceptors. Its action at α-adrenoceptors is mainly direct, but some degree of indirect action has also been demonstrated.

Central nervous system   There is no stimulatory action.

Cardiovascular system   Cardiac output is probably decreased, and there is no effect on force or irritability. Heart rate is slowed: this was originally thought to be due to vagal action initiated by baroreceptors, but is probably due to β-adrenoceptor blockade. Peripheral vessels are markedly constricted by direct action, and there is an overall increase in peripheral resistance. Consequently both systolic and diastolic blood pressures are increased; renal blood flow is reduced.

Other systems   There is no effect on bronchial musculature and respiration is not stimulated. Inhibitory action on the intestinal musculature is not marked.

Indications

Methoxamine is used in the treatment of hypotension associated with spinal anaesthesia, overdose with ganglion blocking drugs and in the control of blood pressure during anaesthesia in which hypotensive techniques are involved. It does not increase the irritability of heart muscle.

Historically, methoxamine has been used in the treatment of paroxysmal tachycardia.

Dosage and administration

Methoxamine may be given by the intramuscular or intravenous route. It acts within 2 minutes when given intravenously and lasts for about 1 h; when given intramuscularly it takes up to 20 minutes to act but lasts somewhat longer.

In the treatment of hypotension of moderate degree due to circulatory failure, 10–15 mg may be given intramuscularly; in more severe cases, 2–10 mg may be given slowly intravenously. Blood loss must, of course, be corrected.

In the treatment of paroxysmal tachycardia, 10-20 mg can be given intramuscularly.

Precautions

Methoxamine should not be given in severe myocardial or coronary disease or to patients on MAO inhibitors, and extreme care must be exercised when it is administered to patients with hypertension or hyperthyroidism. The effect of small doses should first be noted. If supplementary doses are considered necessary, they must not be given until the previous dose has had time to take full effect.

Overdose with methoxamine will produce an undesirably high blood pressure, excessive slowing of the heart, headache and projectile vomiting, a desire to empty the bladder and a marked pilomotor response. An α-adrenoceptor blocking agent such as phentolamine (1–5 mg) will relieve hypertension, otherwise treatment should be symptomatic.

METHYLDOPA

Methyldopa (rINN)

Pharmacology

Methyldopa has a powerful hypotensive action which is more marked in the hypertensive subject. The fall in blood pressure is most marked in the erect posture and during exercise. There is still uncertainty as to its mechanism of action. It provides an alternative substrate to dopa and is converted in the body to α-methylnorepinephrine, which replaces the normal transmitter, norepinephrine (noradrenaline), at storage sites in the nerve terminal. It was originally believed that this had a weaker action than norepinephrine and therefore functioned as a 'false' transmitter, but in fact its pressor properties are hardly less than those of norepinephrine. It is now clear that its principal site of action is centrally, where its metabolite, α-methylnorepinephrine, stimulates α-adrenoceptors, for instance, in the region of the nucleus solitarius in the medulla. These α-adrenoceptors appear to be inhibitory and cause a decrease in outflow from the vasomotor centre. No major redistribution of cardiac output occurs and renal blood flow and glomerular filtration are well maintained.

The laevo-isomer of methyldopa inhibits dopa decarboxylase activity and thereby diminishes synthesis and storage of norepinephrine. It is unlikely that this effect is of relevance to its clinical actions since other inhibitors of this enzyme fail to produce hypotension.

Normal sensitivity is retained to both directly and indirectly acting pressor amines.

Methyldopa regularly produces sedation and occasionally mental depression. Postural hypotension, although less frequent and less severe than with guanethidine or ganglion blockade, may occur on rare occasions: abnormalities in liver chemistry and granulocytopenia have been noted, but these conditions disappear on withdrawal of the drug. Autoimmune haemolytic anaemia has also been reported. The direct Coombs' test is positive. Rapid remission usually occurs when the drug is stopped or if steroids are given.

Indications

Methyldopa is used in the treatment of hypertension, either alone or in combination with diuretics.

Dosage and administration

Methyldopa is given orally in daily doses of 0.5–2 g. Commencing with 250 mg 3 times a day, the dose is gradually increased after 48 h until an adequate response has been achieved. If the blood pressure cannot be controlled by a daily dose of 2 g, or if tolerance occurs, a thiazide compound may be given in combination.

Precautions

Methyldopa is contra-indicated in phaeochromocytoma and active liver disease, and regular blood examinations should be undertaken in order to detect the onset of anaemia.

MILRINONE

Milrinone (rINN)

Pharmacology

Milrinone is a positive inotropic agent with little chronotropic activity, which is also a vasodilator and improves left ventricular diastolic relaxation. Its mode of action is similar to that of aminophylline, being an inhibitor of phosphodiesterase, thus enhancing the intracellular concentration of cyclic AMP. It is more cardioselective than aminophylline by virtue of a selectivity for the 'Peak III' isoenzyme in cardiac and vascular smooth muscle.

Its pharmacokinetic profile on intravenous administration is of a volume of distribution roughly equal to the extracellular fluid (0.4 litre/kg) with a terminal half-life of about 2–3 h and a clearance of about 0.13 litre/kg/h. The kidney is the primary route of elimination: about 70 per cent of the drug is bound to albumin.

Indications

Milrinone can be used to treat a low cardiac output state when it is associated with a high peripheral vascular resistance. It can also be used for the short-term treatment of congestive heart failure in which it improves haemodynamic performance without significant effects on heart rate or on myocardial oxygen consumption. It is not used as long-term oral treatment of heart failure because there is evidence that it increases mortality in this setting (Packer et al., 1991).

Dosage and administration

Milrinone is given intravenously: a loading dose of 50 mg/kg is followed by a continuous infusion of between 0.375 and 0.75 µg/kg/minute to produce a maximum response.

Precautions

In renal impairment, dosage must be reduced, depending on the creatinine clearance, ranging down to about 50 per cent when creatinine clearance is less than 10 ml/min in a standard 70 kg patient. Milrinone slightly enhances A-V node conduction, leading to the possibility of an increased ventricular rate in uncontrolled atrial flutter or fibrillation. Pre-digitalization is advisable in such patients. It may also cause an increase in the incidence of supraventricular and ventricular tachycardias. Because of its mode of action, there may be hypotension due to vasodilatation. As with other inotropic agents, milrinone is contra-indicated in outflow tract obstruction. Electrolytes should be closely monitored: an increase in cardiac output may induce a diuresis and lead to a fall in serum potassium levels, which is particularly undesirable in digitalized patients. Milrinone is precipitated by furosemide and bumetanide if mixed in syringes or in infusions.

Packer, M., Carver, J. R., Rodeheffer, R. J. et al. (1991) Effect of oral milrinone on mortality in severe chronic heart failure. The PROMISE Study Research Group. *New England Journal of Medicine*, **325**(21), 1468–75.

Amrinone and **enoximone** have similar properties to milrinone and can be used in the same way. Reservations have been expressed about the fact that enoximone is made up in ethanol, which itself has considerable cardiovascular activity.

NIFEDIPINE

Nifedipine (rINN)

Pharmacology

Nifedipine is a calcium channel entry blocking drug that mainly acts on vascular smooth muscle. It dilates both coronary arteries and peripheral arterioles, reducing peripheral resistance and left ventricular after-load. There is a reflex baroreceptor mediated rise in pulse rate. There is a moderate negative inotropic effect and this can cause heart failure, particularly if it is combined with a β-receptor blocker. However, unlike class I calcium antagonists, nifedipine can normally be used in combination with a β-receptor blocker to reduce the reflex tachycardia.

Almost all of an oral dose is absorbed, but first-pass metabolism accounts for 50–60 per cent of it. About 95 per cent is bound to albumin. Almost all is metabolized by the liver to inactive compounds. Elimination half-life after an oral dose (capsule) is about 3 h, but only 1 h after intravenous doses. The contents of one capsule can be administered sublingually for a more rapid onset, and to avoid first-pass metabolism, but this is a notoriously unpredictable means of administration. There are controlled release oral preparations available.

Indications

Nifedipine is used for the treatment of angina pectoris when there is no accompanying heart failure, for mild to severe hypertension and for Raynaud's phenomenon. As an antihypertensive, it is usually a second- or third-line drug for patients refractory to treatment with β-blockers, diuretics, ACE inhibitors or other vasodilators. It can be used intravenously for the rapid lowering of blood pressure and to attenuate the hypertensive response to intubation and sternotomy. In the latter situation, it has been found to be as effective as trinitroglycerin.

Nifedipine can be used as a myocardial-protecting agent during reperfusion after cardioplegia: it prevents accumulation of calcium in the cell, a process that inhibits ATP production by the mitochondria.

Dosage and administration

The maintenance dose for the treatment of hypertension and angina ranges between 20 and 40 mg 3 times a day. Ten milligrams sublingually prior to induction of anaesthesia attenuates the hypertensive response to intubation, but not the tachycardia. To control the response to sternotomy, an infusion of 1.5–2.0 µg/kg/minute is employed.

Precautions

Headache, flushing and dizziness occur in 20 per cent of patients and are probably a consequence of vasodilatation. Nifedipine reduces lower oesophageal sphincter pressure and decreases peristalsis. It also reduces platelet aggregation and can increase the bleeding time.

Parenteral solutions must be protected from light and administered within 1 h in daylight or 6 h in artificial light and only given through polypropylene catheters. Prefilled syringes in light-proof containers contain 0.2 mg for direct coronary injection.

NIMODIPINE

Nimodipine (rINN)

Pharmacology

Nimodipine is a dihydropyridine-type calcium channel blocker. It causes systemic and cerebral vasodilatation.

Indications

It is used to minimize vasospasm in the cerebral cortex secondary to sub-arachnoid blood. It is given for 3 weeks after the initial bleed, either by mouth or as an intravenous infusion.

Dosage and administration

By mouth, 60 mg 4-hourly. By infusion into a central venous catheter, 1–2 mg/h (which is 5–10 ml/h of the undiluted solution of 10 mg of nimodipine in 50 ml of diluent).

Precautions

PVC syringes and tubing should be avoided as the drug reacts with this. Renal function should be monitored closely if it is known to be abnormal prior to commencement of treatment.

NITRIC OXIDE

Nitric oxide (rINN)

Pharmacology

Inhaled nitric oxide reacts with the ferrous iron in the haem prosthetic group of the soluble guanylate cyclase in smooth muscle cells in the media of the pulmonary blood vessels, increasing the concentration of cyclic GMP and thereby causing relaxation. This increases blood flow in the ventilated part of the lung, tending to reverse the deleterious effects on the ventilation/perfusion relationship of severe lung disease. (This in turn is partly mediated by induction of large amounts of inducible nitric oxide synthetase in the diseased lung.) There is also a reduction in the pulmonary vascular resistance. It is degraded in the presence of oxygen and water to nitrogen dioxide, which is very toxic to lung tissue.

Indications

Conditions in which inhaled nitric oxide is associated with a survival benefit are those in which there is acutely raised pulmonary vascular resistance which is not secondary to severe lung disease, e.g. idiopathic persistent pulmonary hypertension of the newborn. It can be used as a 'last ditch measure' to improve oxygenation in severe acute-respiratory distress syndrome, but survival benefit has not been shown.

Dosage and administration

Nitric oxide is presented as 1 part per thousand nitric oxide in nitrogen. This is added upstream of a mixing chamber in the respiratory gases of a ventilated patient such that the inspired concentration is 0.5–50 parts per million. Humidification must not involve a significant amount of water, and condenser humidification is preferable to the hot water bath type of humidification.

NITROPRUSSIDE

Sodium nitroprusside (rINN)

Pharmacology

Sodium nitroprusside was first described in 1849 and its hypotensive action in 1929. It has a direct vasodilator action on the smooth muscle of the vessel wall, proportional to the blood concentration, and this action is independent of autonomic innervation. It thus causes a fall in peripheral resistance and an increase in venous capacity. Cardiac output, however, falls only when the pressure is lowered unduly. There is a marked increase in coronary blood flow with moderate falls in mean arterial pressure. Hypotension is more marked in elderly and hypertensive subjects, and is potentiated by ganglion blocking drugs. There is usually a moderate compensatory tachycardia; on discontinuing the infusion, the blood pressure rapidly returns to normal, usually within 2–5 minutes. Renal blood flow decreases, as expected, as the mean arterial pressure falls and there is a release of renin. Pulmonary artery pressure also falls, presumably due to dilatation of pulmonary vessels. Dilatation of systemic capacitance vessels is responsible for a fall in right atrial pressure. The effect on blood flow in other organs is uncertain.

Fate in the body Nitroprusside is rapidly broken down by haemoglobin non-enzymatically; electron transfer from haemoglobin (Fe^{2+}) yields methaemoglobin (Fe^{3+}) and an unstable nitroprusside which quickly breaks down to yield five cyanide ions. One of these then reacts with the methaemoglobin to form cyanmethaemoglobin. The remaining cyanide ions are converted into thiocyanate by an enzyme rhodenase, principally in the liver, but also in the kidney. Any cyanide not so inactivated causes biochemical toxicity by inactivating essential enzymes such as cytochrome oxidase. In sufficient doses this will result in cyanide poisoning. This syndrome has been reported clinically with large doses of nitroprusside and leads to a lactic acidosis, indicating anaerobic metabolism.

Indications

Sodium nitroprusside is used as an alternative to trimetaphan for the induction of hypotension during surgery. Its advantage over that drug is an absence of tachyphylaxis. However it does share the tendency to be associated with compensatory tachycardia. This may be controlled with a β-adrenoceptor blocking drug. It has also been used in the control of hypertension during the removal of a phaeochromocytoma. Disadvantages would seem to be a potential difficulty in reversing any overdose, the production of cyanmethaemoglobin and potential cyanide poisoning.

Dosage and administration

Although it can be given orally, sodium nitroprusside is now given only as a continuous intravenous infusion. It may be made up as 0.3 × [body weight] diluted to 50 ml (typically 21 mg for a 70 kg man). With the resulting solution, 1 ml/h is equivalent to 0.1 µg/kg/minute, and the standard range is 1–5 ml/h, and up to 20 ml/h in the short term. The total dose administered is related to the development of toxicity and should not normally exceed 3.5 mg/kg; 7 mg/kg is a lethal dose. The syringe and the infusion line must be protected from light.

Precautions

Toxicity is associated with increases in the blood concentration of both thiocyanate and cyanide but, for various reasons, neither is a reliable guide to the extent of toxicity. Evidence of increased anaerobic metabolism (rise in base deficit, elevated lactate and lactate/pyruvate ratios) is the most reliable indication of the onset of toxicity. Traditional treatment for cyanide poisoning has been the administration of nitrites to augment the antidotal effects of thiosulphate, which was thought to have too slow an onset. In the context of the metabolism of sodium nitroprusside this may not be true, and Krapez *et al.* (1981) have shown that dogs pretreated with thiosulphate, 75 mg/kg, maintained low cyanide concentrations even with high doses. They suggest that thiosulphate should be given prophylactically whenever doses of nitroprusside close to the toxic limit are likely to be used. Vitamin B_{12a} (hydroxocobalamin) is also a cyanide neutralizer, but only in very high doses. Reasonable doses undoubtedly have some beneficial effects, but there is disagreement as to whether these are synergistic with thiosulphate.

Sodium nitroprusside solutions are normally browny-pink; a change to blue indicates deterioration.

Ktapez, J. R., Vesey, C. J., Adams, L. and Cole, P. V. (1981) Effects of cyanide antidotes used with sodium nitroprusside infusions; sodium thiosulphate and hydroxocobalamin given prophylactically to dogs. *British Journal of Anaesthesia,* **53**, 793.

NOREPINEPHRINE (NORADRENALINE)

Norepinephrine (rINN)
For structural formula see *Table 12.2*, page 326

Pharmacology

Like epinephrine (adrenaline), norepinephrine is an important naturally-occurring hormone, and it can be synthesized artificially. In the body it is derived from the amino acid tyrosine via dopa and dopamine. In the adult it forms about 10–20 per cent of the catecholamines in the adrenal medulla, the remainder being epinephrine; in infancy the proportion of norepinephrine exceeds that of epinephrine. These hormones are contained in different cells, but both are liberated by acetylcholine, in its role of chemical transmitter, by impulses from the autonomic preganglionic fibres supplying the medullary cells. In the catecholamines liberated at adrenergic nerve endings, more than 90 per cent is norepinephrine, and a similar proportion is extractable from tissues other than the adrenal medulla, probably in scattered chromaffin cells. Norepinephrine has powerful α-effects and weak β-effects. It is the chemical transmitter released by postganglionic nerve fibres of the sympathetic system and is responsible for normal sympathetic tone, and the stimulation of effector cells. It is stored in granules in nerve axons and is also released by indirectly acting adrenergic agents such as mephentermine and methylamfetamine, whose pressor and other effects are due to this action.

Central nervous system   In contrast to epinephrine there is no central stimulation of the cerebral cortex.

Cardiovascular system   Cardiac output is unchanged, but the contractile force and the irritability of the heart are slightly increased, but not to the same extent as that produced by epinephrine. Heart rate is usually decreased, due to the effect of the increased blood pressure on the baroreceptors. There is constriction of all peripheral vessels and an increase in venous pressure producing an increase in overall resistance and consequent rise in systolic and diastolic blood pressures. Renal, hepatic and cerebral blood flow are reduced, but there is evidence, although not conclusive, that the coronary vessels are dilated. Muscle blood flow is reduced.

Respiratory system   There is little effect on bronchial muscle. Rate and depth of respiration are increased slightly.

Plain muscle Norepinephrine has a weaker inhibitory action on plain muscle than epinephrine, but it stimulates contractions of the uterus in late pregnancy and labour.

Indications

Norepinephrine is used in the treatment of hypotension due to excessive peripheral vasodilation, e.g. in septic shock and following operations for the removal of chromaffin cell tumours. It is impossible to determine clinically and reliably that hypotension is due solely to excessive vasodilatation; such an assessment requires the use of invasive monitoring such as pulmonary artery catheter.) Treatment of hypotension secondary to a low cardiac output state with norepinephrine alone causes harm rather than benefit.

Norepinephrine will overcome the hypotensive action of reversible adrenoceptor blocking agents, although not that of irreversible agents such as phenoxybenzamine. However, a direct α-stimulating drug without cardiac effects, such as methoxamine, is now regarded as more appropriate.

Fate in the body As with epinephrine, it is rapidly inactivated by the enzyme catechol-O-methyl transferase. Oxidation and deamination also play a part in its degradation.

Dosage and administration

For the treatment of septic shock with hypotension, norepinephrine may be given by intravenous infusion into a central vein at a rate of 0.05–0.2 μg/kg/minute. In practice, 0.03 × [body weight] is diluted to 50 ml (typically 2.1 mg for a 70 kg man). With the resulting solution, 10 ml/h is equivalent to 0.1 μg/kg/minute, so the standard range is 5–20 ml/h.

Precautions

It is inadvisable to give norepinephrine without the use of invasive monitoring to assess and monitor its effect on blood pressure.

If a norepinephrine infusion is abruptly stopped, severe hypotension will result. This is due to rapid relaxation after previous intense constriction causing the circulatory blood volume to become inadequate. Furthermore, the rate of offset of action is so fast that the physiological blood pressure control mechanisms will be 'taken by surprise'. Norepinephrine infusions must be discontinued slowly.

Norepinephrine must not be injected subcutaneously even in dilute solutions.

If norepinephrine is given by peripheral infusion the constriction of the vein will limit and render unreliable the passage of the drug to the central circulation. Furthermore, any leakage into the local tissues will result in gangrene of the skin. It is thus much safer to infuse into a central vein. Local treatment of extravasation is as for dopamine.

Five per cent glucose is the only solution commonly available that is sufficiently acidic to protect norepinephrine from oxidation. There is thus a theoretical advantage in diluting it with this, rather than with isotonic saline. In practice, either solution can be used.

Overdose of norepinephrine produces intense vasoconstriction and hypertension. These effects pass with the withdrawal of the infusion: α-adrenoceptor blocking agents antagonize its effects.

PHENOXYBENZAMINE

Phenoxybenzamine hydrochloride (rINN)

Pharmacology

Phenoxybenzamine is a chloroethylene derivative and is related to the nitrogen mustards. It is a powerful α-adrenoceptor blocking agent.

During administration, α-stimulating amines compete for the receptors, indicating that the initial attracting forces are of the same kind. However, once a block is established it cannot be reversed by other adrenoceptor stimulators (agonists) indicating the formation of a non-dissociating stable bond at or near the receptor. This is an example of a non-equilibrium blockade. This is clinically detected, however, only when the number of unblocked receptors has been reduced very considerably and with moderate doses sufficient receptors remain unblocked for some response of the tissue to normal agonists to be demonstrable. Onset of action is slow and it may take up to an hour for the drug to reach its full effect following intravenous injection. This delay is due to conversion of the drug into an active metabolite in the body. The block is very persistent, and decreases only slowly over 3–4 days. The major effects are on the cardiovascular system. In normal recumbent subjects there is a slight fall in diastolic pressure, but a marked postural hypotension occurs. The effect on blood pressure is greater in hypertensive subjects. Precipitous falls occur in the presence of even moderate hypovolaemia. Drugs such as morphine may have a similar effect.

Changes in blood flow depend on the existing pattern of α-adrenergic activity. Cerebral and coronary blood flows will be unchanged unless blood pressure falls below a critical level. Muscle and skin flows tend to be increased. If splanchnic flow is much reduced, as in vasoconstricted states, phenoxybenzamine will cause an increase, which will be limited only by unmasked hypovolaemia.

The chronotropic and inotropic effects of catecholamines on the heart are not blocked, but the drug exhibits a considerable anti-arrhythmic action, and will block cyclopropane/epinephrine-induced arrhythmias.

Side effects may be troublesome. An initial central stimulation on rapid administration may cause nausea and vomiting. With slow intravenous administration, sedation is usually seen. Postural hypotension and reflex tachycardia occur, but are limited if the circulatory volume is increased. Giddiness, nasal congestion and fatigue are common.

Indications

Phenoxybenzamine is used in the control of hypertension in phaeochromocytoma during preparation for the definitive treatment, surgery. After treatment for 2 weeks, sufficient α-adrenergic blockade is established to make safe the introduction of a β-adrenergic blocker such as metoprolol. After a further 2 days of combined treatment, the autonomic blockade will be sufficient to produce reasonable cardiovascular stability during surgical manipulation of the tumour.

In paediatric cardiac surgery, it can be given as a single intravenous slow bolus of 1 mg/kg during cardiopulmonary bypass to patients who are at risk of pulmonary hypertensive crisis in the postoperative period.

It has also been used in the treatment of peripheral vascular disease.

Dosage and administration

Phenoxybenzamine may be given by mouth or intravenously by infusion.

In the treatment of the above conditions, 20 mg by mouth 3–4 times a day is usually effective, but doses up to 120 mg may be required; 0.5–2 mg/kg may be given in 300 ml of 5 per cent glucose solution if the intravenous route is employed. In the preoperative preparation of cases of phaeochromocytoma, α-adrenoceptor blockade should be progressively induced over 2 weeks prior to operation.

Precautions

Ambulant patients being treated with this agent should be warned about its side effects and advised accordingly.

Patients treated intravenously need central venous pressure monitoring and facilities for active therapy. Since the block cannot be reversed pharmacologically, potentially lethal hypotension must be controlled by transfusion and posture.

Phenoxybenzamine therapy may lead to uncontrolled β-stimulation in a hypertensive crisis associated with an epinephrine-secreting phaeochromocytoma. This is undesirable but it is not as dangerous as the other possibility if this condition is mismanaged: β-blockade without concomitant α-blockade (i.e. negative inotropism in the face of unrelieved peripheral vasoconstriction) will precipitously and dangerously reduce cardiac output.

PHENTOLAMINE

Phentolamine mesilate (rINN)

Pharmacology

Phentolamine is a short-acting α-adrenoceptor blocking agent belonging to the β-imidazoline group. Onset of action is rapid, its full effect being reached within 2 minutes. It lasts from 10 to 15 minutes following intravenous injection. As well as producing a moderate catecholamine blocking effect, phentolamine also has a mild sympathomimetic action and a powerful direct vasodilator action on vascular smooth muscle. Following intravenous infusion it produces a reduction in peripheral resistance and blood pressure, an increase in cardiac output and heart rate, and a decrease in stroke volume and cardiopulmonary blood volume. Side effects that may occur include sweating, apprehension, palpitation, nausea, diarrhoea and nasal congestion.

Indications

Phentolamine is used in the control of blood pressure during surgery for phaeochromocytoma. It can also be used for the diagnosis of this condition if facilities for estimating catecholamines in the urine are not available. It is one of several drugs that can be used intravenously to control blood pressure in the early postoperative period after cardiac surgery. It has also been used for the treatment of peripheral vascular disease, for the relief of arterial spasm and as an antidote in the treatment of overdose of epinephrine (adrenaline) and other sympathomimetic amines. It may be of value in the treatment of toxic reactions between MAO inhibitors and tyramine-containing foods.

Dosage and administration

Phentolamine may be given by mouth, intramuscularly, intravenously or infusion.

For rapid control of blood pressure after cardiac surgery, 1–5 mg may be given every 10 minutes, with the effect being monitored through invasive blood pressure monitoring.

For the control of blood pressure during surgery for phaeochromocytoma, 5 mg may be given intravenously a few minutes, or intramuscularly 30 minutes, before induction of anaesthesia. This should ensure a smooth induction. Further doses of 5 mg are given during operation as necessary to control excessive hypertension, especially that likely to occur when the tumour is being handled by the surgeon.

When used for the treatment of vascular disease, 20–40 mg of the hydrochloride is given 3–4 times a day by mouth; alternatively, 5–10 mg can be given intra-arterially, intravenously or intramuscularly, repeated as required. Larger doses are sometimes necessary. For epinephrine overdose, 5–10 mg should be injected intravenously immediately. Speed is important.

For the diagnosis of phaeochromocytoma, 5 mg of the mesilate is given intravenously. The patient should be lying at rest and have had no sedation for 24 h. A fall of 35 mmHg (5 kPa) in systolic blood pressure and 25 mmHg (3.4 kPa) in diastolic blood pressure indicates a positive result. Blood pressure readings must be taken at 30-s intervals at first, as the fall may last only a few minutes. For several reasons, false results may be obtained and the estimation of urinary catecholamines should always be undertaken when possible.

Precautions

Ambulant patients should be warned about the side effects of this drug, and it should be avoided in serious heart disease and disorders of the gastro-intestinal tract.

PHENYLEPHRINE HYDROCHLORIDE

Phenylephrine hydrochloride (rINN)
For structural formula see *Table 12.2*, page 326

Pharmacology

Phenylephrine, like norepinephrine (noradrenaline), has strong α- and weak β-effects. Its action at α-adrenoceptors is direct.

Central nervous system   There is no effect on the cerebral cortex.

Cardiovascular system
There is little or no effect on cardiac output, force or rate, but irritability is slightly increased. The heart rate is slowed due to stimulation of the baroreceptors, an effect that can be antagonized by atropine. Blood pressure is increased due to vasoconstriction causing an increase in overall peripheral resistance.

Local application causes constriction of the vessels of mucous membranes. It is irritant and may cause local discomfort or even local necrosis if it leaks from the vein being injected.

Respiratory system   There is some degree of bronchial dilatation due to relaxation of the smooth muscle of the bronchial tree. It is considerably less effective than epinephrine (adrenaline) or isoprenaline.

Indications

Phenylephrine is used in the treatment of circulatory failure and of hypotension due to excessive doses of vasodilators. It has also been used in the treatment of paroxysmal tachycardia, as a local application for the relief of nasal congestion, and to produce mydriasis. It is effective in combating hypotension due to chlorpromazine. Because it has a lower β-agonist activity than norepinephrine, it is probably a safer agent to use to raise the blood pressure in patients given a halogenated anaesthetic.

Dosage and administration

Phenylephrine may be given intramuscularly or intravenously in the form of an infusion. By the intramuscular route, it takes 10–15 minutes to act and its effect lasts up to 1 h.

In the treatment of hypotension due to circulatory failure, 5 mg may be given intramuscularly, 0.5 mg intravenously, or an infusion containing 10 mg in 500 ml of 5 per cent dextrose may be set up and started at 40–60 ml/h and controlled in the same way as a norepinephrine infusion.

Solutions containing 0.5–1 per cent of phenylephrine are used to relieve nasal congestion, 2–3 drops being instilled into each nostril.

In the treatment of paroxysmal tachycardia, 5 mg is given intramuscularly. For the production of mydriasis, 2.5–10 per cent solutions may be employed; a suitable local anaesthetic should first be instilled into the eye to avoid irritation.

Precautions

Phenylephrine should not be given in severe myocardial or coronary disease, and special care is necessary when it is administered to patients with hypertension.

Overdose causes hypertension, palpitations, headache and vomiting. Treatment should be symptomatic; α-adrenoceptor blocking agents will relieve excessive hypertension.

PRAZOSIN

Prazosin hydrochloride (rINN)

Pharmacology

The exact mechanisms by which this drug produces its effects on the cardiovascular system are unknown. Probably its main action is that it blocks post-junctional α-adrenoceptors (α_1) while having little effect on pre-synaptic α-adrenoceptors (α_2). It is also a powerful phosphodiesterase inhibitor, being about 20 times as potent as theophylline. Despite the fall in peripheral resistance, there is relatively little increase in cardiac output or tachycardia. It has been suggested that prazosin impairs the baroreceptor reflex, possibly by an action on the carotid sinus impairing the afferent pathway response. Another suggestion is that it enhances the effects of the vagus by raising cardiac cyclic guanosine monophosphate (GMP) levels. This it does by inhibiting the phosphodiesterase responsible for breakdown of cyclic GMP. Cyclic GMP is a 'second messenger' involved in the cardiac effects of acetylcholine. Prazosin differs from hydralazine, another vasodilator, in that it appears to be less likely to produce tolerance and it does not raise renin levels. Unlike diazoxide, it enhances sodium excretion.

Indications

Prazosin is used as treatment for hypertension resistant to thiazide/β-blocker or ACE inhibitor therapy, or when these are contra-indicated. It is also efficacious in heart failure, although less so than ACE inhibitors.

Fate in the body   Prazosin is metabolized by the liver and there is a noticeable first-pass effect. Some of its metabolites also produce a fall in blood pressure and this may be why, in spite of its relatively short half-life ($t_{1/2}$ about 4 h), twice daily administration is usually sufficient.

Dosage and administration

For antihypertensive therapy the dosage range is 0.5–20 mg daily. The initial starting dose should be 0.5 mg 3 times a day, slowly increasing on the basis of the patient's blood pressure response.

Precautions and side effects

Orthostatic hypotension occurs infrequently. Headache, dry mouth, blurred vision, nasal congestion, pruritus and impotence have been reported, but are infrequent or mild. In some patients high initial doses (2 mg) can precipitate a severe fall in blood pressure and collapse. This is more likely to occur in patients treated with β-adrenoceptor blocking agents or sodium-depleted patients following diuretic therapy. Such reactions usually occur within 2 h of the initial dose. It is thus advisable to monitor the effects of the first dose for at least this period.

Doxazosin probably has a similar selectivity for α-adrenoceptors. It is less likely to cause precipitate hypotension with the first dose than is prazosin. It can be given in a once-daily regimen.

Indoramin is also an α-adrenoceptor antagonist. It causes sedation in a high percentage of patients. Dosage is 100–200 mg daily.

SILDENAFIL

Sildenafil citrate (rINN)

Pharmacology

Sildenafil is a selective inhibitor of the cyclic guanosine monophosphate (cGMP)-specific 'Peak V' isoenzyme of phosphodiesterase (also called phosphodiesterase type 5, or PDE5).

It is a novel oral therapy for erectile dysfunction. Penile erection involves release of nitric oxide in the corpus cavernosum, which activates the enzyme guanylate cyclase. This increases levels of cyclic guanosine monophosphate producing relaxation of vascular smooth muscle in the corpus cavernosum allowing increased inflow of blood. Sildenafil enhances the effect of nitric oxide (NO) by inhibiting 'Peak V' phosphodiesterase which is responsible for degradation of cGMP in the corpus cavernosum. Sildenafil is said to be 4000 times more selective for PDE5 than for PDE3, the phosphodiesterase inhibited by milrinone and enoximone. The recommended dose is 50 mg taken, as needed, approximately 1 h before sexual activity.

A single oral doses of sildenafil (100 mg) produces an average decrease in blood pressure of about 10 mmHg in normal subjects. Larger effects on blood pressure may occur in patients receiving concomitant nitrates. Mild, transient, dose-related impairment of colour discrimination (blue/green) was also detected. This finding is consistent with inhibition of PDE6, which is involved in phototransduction in the retina.

Fate in the body It is eliminated predominantly by hepatic metabolism (mainly cytochrome P-450 3A4) and is converted to an active *N*-desmethyl metabolite with properties similar to the parent drug. Both sildenafil and the metabolite have terminal half-lives of about 4 h in the young healthy population, but of somewhat longer duration with elderly subjects, those with renal or hepatic impairment and those taking drugs which inhibit cytochrome P-450 isoform 3A4, e.g. cimetidine, erythromycin, ketoconazole, itraconazole and mibefradil. Sildenafil is excreted as metabolites predominantly in the faeces (approximately 80 per cent of administered oral dose).

Precautions

Sildenafil has no effect on bleeding time when taken alone or with aspirin, but it potentiates the anti-aggregatory effect of sodium nitroprusside. It does not potentiate the hypotensive effect of moderate levels of alcohol in healthy volunteers. No interaction was seen with amlodipine in hypertensive patients. Other reported side effects include headache, flushing, dyspepsia, nasal congestion, urinary tract infection, diarrhoea, dizziness and rash. In overdose, adverse events are similar to those seen at lower doses, but incidence rates are increased. Standard supportive measures should be adopted as required. Renal dialysis is not expected to accelerate clearance as sildenafil is highly bound to plasma proteins and it is not eliminated in the urine.

TRIMETAPHAN

Trimetaphan camsylate (rINN) and Trimethaphan camsylate (USP)

Pharmacology

The drug is partly broken down by enzymatic hydrolysis and partly excreted unchanged in the urine. If the blood pressure is lowered so much that glomerular filtration ceases, excretion cannot occur, and this may account for the prolonged action that may follow.

Indications

It is mainly used for the production of controlled hypotension during anaesthesia, but has also been used to improve perfusion during and after cardiac surgery.

Dosage and administration

Trimetaphan can be given by repeated intravenous injection, but it is more usually given by continuous intravenous infusion. In either case the patient is first anaesthetized and positioned on the operating table. When the intermittent intravenous technique is used, an initial dose of 5–10 mg may be given, repeated at intervals of 3–5 minutes to maintain the desired level of hypotension.

For continuous intravenous infusion, a 0.1 per cent solution in 5 per cent dextrose or isotonic saline is used (e.g. 250 mg in 250 ml of diluent), started at a rate of about 60 ml/h. Frequent blood pressure readings are taken, and the rate of infusion is adjusted to maintain the blood pressure at the required level. Weaker solutions are recommended for the frail and the elderly, but children or infants, who are more resistant to this drug, may be given a 0.2 per cent solution.

Excessive hypotension can usually be controlled by reducing the rate of the infusion. If this fails, administration of fluid and lowering of the head of the operating table should be used; in emergency, a pressor drug such as mephentermine or methoxamine should be given.

Precautions

Trimetaphan is incompatible in solution with thiopental, gallamine, strongly alkaline solutions, iodides and bromides.

VERAPAMIL

Verapamil hydrochloride (rINN)

Pharmacology

Verapamil has a selective inhibitory effect on influx of calcium ions into cardiac cells, but particularly those of the S-A and A-V nodes. It depresses cardiac contractility and conduction.

Indications

In patients with a contra-indication to β-adrenoceptor blockade, *and as long as there is no element of heart failure*, verapamil can be used to treat angina by slowing the heart and reducing myocardial contractility (although in most patients, diltiazem would be tried first). In patients with a contra-indication to β-adrenoceptor blockade who have hypertension, have no heart failure, and have a tendency to tachycardia with vasodilator therapy, verapamil can be a useful drug.

Verapamil has been used in the past to diagnose and treat supraventricular tachycardia and broad complex tachycardia by slowing A-V node conduction, but this use of the drug has been superseded by the advent of adenosine.

Dosage and administration

Verapamil can be given orally and doses of up to 120 mg 3 times a day have been used in the prophylaxis of angina. Supraventricular tachycardias and ventricular arrythmias during anaesthesia can be controlled by 20 mg intravenously, but the hypotensive effect of this dose is significant. Acute hypertension can be controlled with up to 10 mg/h as an intravenous infusion. After intravenous bolus injection of therapeutic doses, the effect lasts about half an hour.

Precautions

Verapamil is contra-indicated in patients with heart block, bradycardia, sick sinus syndrome and uncompensated cardiac failure. It should also not be used concurrently with β-adrenoceptor antagonists, digoxin or quinidine. Verapamil can cause nausea and dizziness, flushing and constipation.

13

Drugs used for their effects on cardiac rhythm and rate

The cardiac electrical cycle

This is dependent on ionic movements of sodium, potassium and calcium (*Figure 13.1*). Prior to excitation, the resting potential is −80 mV; permeability of the cell membrane to the sodium ion is low, but permeability to the potassium ion is high. On excitation, there is a large increase in sodium permeability and sodium moves into the cell. The decrease in the external sodium concentration initiates calcium ion movement and calcium also starts to move inwards. At this plateau stage sodium permeability decreases. The calcium ions react with inhibitors (e.g. troponin) on the myofilaments. The removal of the inhibitor results in de-repression so contraction can occur. The rate of force developed is proportional to the rate at which calcium ions are delivered to the myofilament. The duration of action is related to the time the calcium ions remain in contact with the myofilament. Calcium is removed from the myofilament into the mitochondria, possibly by means of a calcium pump. It is also extruded from the cell, the sodium-potassium ATP-ase pump also being involved.

Cardiac action potentials

The heart is made up of a syncytium of cardiac cells. Cells that are part of a syncytium usually exhibit threshold behaviour. The cell membrane potential may vary in the absence of external stimuli and action potentials can arise spontaneously. The form and characteristics of the action potential can vary from place to place and this certainly occurs in the heart (see below).

A hypothetical action potential is shown in *Figure 13.2*. There is a spontaneous depolarization (called phase 4) which proceeds until a threshold transmembrane potential of about −70 mV is reached, at which point a rapid depolarization is triggered (phase 0) and this institutes the action potential. This is followed by an effective refractory period (ERP), which includes not only the absolute refractory period, but also a period during which the membrane is excitable but impulse propagation does not occur. Towards the end of phase 3 there is a relative refractory period when impulses can be transmitted at reduced velocity.

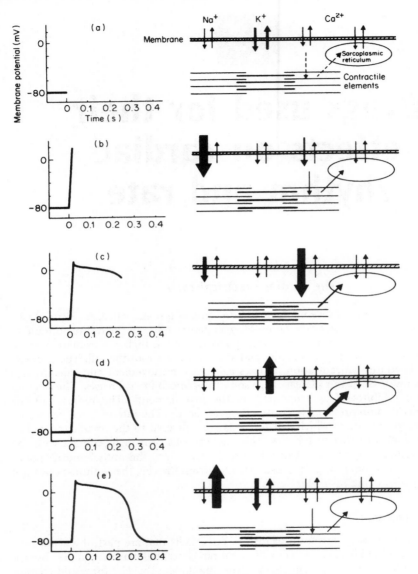

Figure 13.1 Ionic movements during the cardiac action potential:

(a) At rest, sodium permeability is low, potassium permeability is relatively high, and there is little calcium movement

(b) The rapid depolarization phase of the action potential is due to a large increase in sodium permeability. This reduces the potassium permeability and allows calcium entry to increase

(c) In the plateau phase, sodium permeability falls and massive calcium influx occurs, stimulating the contractile process

(d) Repolarization begins as the potassium permeability rises and sodium permeability falls towards the resting level. Calcium influx stops and sequestration of calcium leads to relaxation of the contractile elements

(e) At the end of the repolarization phase, passive permeabilities have fallen to resting levels, but active extrusion of sodium and uptake of potassium restores the ionic concentration gradients

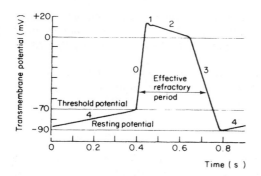

Figure 13.2 Transmembrane potential of a spontaneously firing Purkinje fibre (hypothetical)

Normally, excitation starts in the sinoatrial (S-A) node and an excitation wave is spread three-dimensionally over the surface of both atria and channelled into the atrioventricular (A-V) node. Here a dramatic slowing occurs. The wave then proceeds rapidly through the Purkinje fibres in the bundle of His and is distributed to the endocardial surface of both ventricles almost synchronously.

Sinoatrial node

This consists of a group of cells with special characteristics that are anatomically situated in the wall of the right atrium near the opening of the superior vena cava. Normally these cells are responsible for initiation of the cardiac excitatory process. They act as the pacemaker for the heart and receive impulses via both sympathetic and parasympathetic nervous systems.

A peculiarity of these cells is that they exhibit slow diastolic depolarization called the pacemaker potential. The pacemaker potential rises to a threshold and, when this is reached, the next action potential is fired off. The resting membrane potential, defined as maximum polarization between action potentials, is lower than in other parts of the heart (*Figure 13.3*). It is approximately –65 mV. In contrast, the atrial myocardium has a stable resting potential of approximately –85 mV. The action potential also has a different configuration, the down stroke being slow in comparison to the rising phase.

Atrioventricular node

The A-V node is also innervated by both the sympathetic and the parasympathetic parts of the autonomic nervous system. Anatomically, it is found on the right wall of the

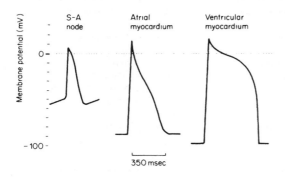

Figure 13.3 Comparison of cardiac action potentials of the S-A node, atrial myocardium and ventricular myocardium

septum. It is the origin of the specialized conducting cells, the Purkinje cells, whose fibres transmit the excitation wave from the atria into the ventricles. The A-V node has a similar pattern of activity to the S-A node. For instance, it shows slow diastolic depolarization and has a low resting membrane potential.

The A-V node normally acts as a filter to limit the frequency with which impulses are conducted from the atria to the ventricles, but it can take over from the S-A node and function as a pacemaker.

Bundle of His

This consists of Purkinje fibres, which originate in the A-V node. The bundle crosses the fibrous tissue that demarcates the atria from the ventricles and enters the ventricular septum. There it splits into two branches that ramify to the endocardial surface of each ventricle. Conduction through the bundle of His occurs at a faster rate (2.5 m/s) than anywhere else in the heart.

Ventricular myocardium

This has a resting membrane potential of about −90 to −100 mV and the resting membrane potential remains stable between action potentials. The shape of the action

Table 13.1 Effect of stimulation of cardiac autonomic nerves. β-Adrenoceptor agonists will mimic effects of sympathetic nerve stimulation, and muscarinic agonists that of vagal stimulation

Cardiac site	Effects of sympathetic nerve stimulation	Effects of vagal nerve stimulation
S-A node	Heart rate increases. Pacemaker potential slope steepens, thus interval between action potentials decreases	Heart rate slows. Pacemaker potential slope becomes shallower, thus interval between action potentials increases
Atrial myocardium	Force of contraction is increased: decreased refractory period and increased conduction velocity	Force of contraction decreased Note: due to reduction in action potential duration, there is also a decreased refractory period and an increased velocity
A-V node	Quicker transmission due to decreased refractory period and increased conduction velocity	Slower transmission due to increased refractory period and increased conduction velocity A-V block can occur if parasympathetic stimulation is very marked
Purkinje fibres	Marked stimulation can initiate pacemaker activity	Marked stimulation leading to A-V block may be followed by initiation of pacemaker activity Basis of vagal escape phenomenon
Ventricular myocardium	Increases force of contraction	No vagal innervation but force of contraction depressed by acetylcholine

potential is shown in *Figure 13.3*. The action potential shape in the Purkinje fibre is similar but the refractory period is longer and it has a faster conduction velocity.

The effects of sympathetic and vagal nerve stimulation on the heart are shown in *Table 13.1*.

Cardiac arrhythmias

The genesis of the cardiac action potential was discussed on page 379. Anti-arrhythmic drugs generally prolong the ERP as a proportion of the total action potential duration and they may suppress ectopic foci, either by reducing the rate of spontaneous depolarization (phase 4) but also by raising the threshold potential. Quinidine and procainamide, for example, exhibit all three properties. Lidocaine (lignocaine) and phenytoin do not lengthen the ERP but depress phase 4 depolarization in S-A cells, and particularly in Purkinje tissue. This action is particularly striking in digitalis-intoxicated hearts.

Anti-arrhythmic drugs may also act by decreasing the conduction velocity, which is related to the maximum rate of depolarization during phase 0.

β-Adrenoceptor blocking drugs have this action and are effective in reducing digitalis toxicity by the same mechanisms as phenytoin and lidocaine.

Disorders of impulse generation include extrasystoles arising in abnormal foci in atria or ventricles, supraventricular tachycardia, atrial flutter and fibrillation, and ventricular tachycardia and fibrillation. Despite many attempts, no common physiological mechanism has been assigned to these disorders and two different mechanisms, at least, must be considered.

1. Repetitive ectopic rhythms can occur when an extranodal site undergoes spontaneous (phase 4) depolarization at an intrinsic frequency greater than that of the normal pacemaker. It may also arise when there is an 'entrance' block due, for example, to complete A-V block; this may possibly occur as a local block due to disease, thus allowing extrasystoles to occur at any time during the non-refractory phase.

2. Re-entry due to a circus movement is commonly invoked to explain atrial flutter and fibrillation. It is believed that if impulse transmission is blocked in a particular direction by a refractory tissue, the impulse makes a circuit around the obstacle. If the circuit is long enough, or the ERP short enough, the impulse will return to find the refractory tissue now responsive. This mechanism is probably also responsible for many cases of paroxysmal supraventricular tachycardia.

Re-entry may also be a functional disorder due to local disease. When an impulse meets a block, the action potential and ERP of the fibres immediately proximal to the block are very brief. Pathological Purkinje fibres may conduct very slowly, and slow conduction accompanied by a brief ERP may allow very short circuit lengths between two mutually activating foci.

Anti-arrhythmic agents

Drugs used to reverse cardiac arrhythmias can be divided into a number of groups. Groups 1–4 correspond with Vaughan Williams's classification (1992):

Table 13.2 Classification of anti-arrhythmic drugs

Class 1	Class 2	Class 3	Class 4	Class 5	Class 6
(Slows rate of rise in phase 0, slows conduction and prolongs repolarization)	(Anti-sympathetic)	(Prolongs ERF)	(calcium antagonists)	(Cardiac glycosides)	(Increases vagal tone)
A. Quinidine Procainamide Edrophonium Disopyramide B. Lidocaine Mexiletine Phenytoin C. Flecainide Lorcainide Encainide	(a) Propranolol Metoprolol Esmolol Atenolol (b) Bretylium Guanethidine	Amiodarone Bretylium	Verapamil Diltiazem	Digoxin	Methoxamine Edrophonium

1A. Drugs that produce moderate phase 0 depression, slow conduction moderately and prolong the repolarization phase.
1B. Drugs with minimal phase 0 depression, slight effects on conduction velocity and which shorten the repolarization phase.
1C. Drugs which cause marked phase 0 depression and slowing of conduction but with little effect on repolarization.
2. Drugs that block sympathetic transmission such as: (a) β-adrenoceptor blocking drugs, whether or not they also possess quinidine-like action; (b) adrenergic neurone blocking drugs.
3. Drugs that prolong the action potential of myocardial cells by increasing the ERP.
4. Drugs that block calcium movement from the membrane into the conducting system.
5. Cardiac glycosides.
6. Drugs that increase or induce vagal tone directly or indirectly in supraventricular tachycardia.

Examples of drugs with these actions are given in *Table 13.2*. This classification is useful because, in any given patient, a drug in one class will have a similar effect on an arrhythmia to another drug in the same class. Its limitation is that, given a particular arrhythmia in a particular patient, it is seldom easy to predict which class of drug will be the most effective treatment.

Class 1 anti-arrhythmic drugs: sodium channel blockers

Class 1 anti-arrhythmic agents all have the property of blocking sodium channels in an all-or-none fashion. The division of class 1 anti-arrhythmic agents into 1A, 1B and 1C subgroups described above is based upon their effect on rate of propagation of the action potential (seen in the intact subject as an increase in duration of the QRS complex) and their effect on repolarization, which alters duration of the ERP. It has been suggested by

Vaughan Williams that the underlying mechanism for this division is differences in the rate of binding and unbinding of drug molecules to their binding sites on the sodium channel. This rate is fast in group 1B, moderate in group 1A and slow in group 1C.

Apart from this subdivision, some of the differences between the class 1 anti-arrhythmic drugs are based upon additional actions by some of the drugs on other channels, including 'slow' sodium channels, ATP-ase-dependent potassium channels and calcium channels. Other differences depend on actions at extracardiac sites (e.g. the rare occurrence of hypoglycaemia or bone marrow suppression with some class 1 drugs) or actions by metabolites (e.g. the anticholinergic effects seen with disopyramide).

Vaughan Williams, E.M. (1992) The relevance of cellular to clinical electrophysiology in classifying antiarrhythmic actions. *Journal of Cardiovascular Pharmacology*, **20**(Suppl 2), S1–S7

Class 2 anti-arrhythmic drugs: β-adrenoceptor blocking agents

Propranolol was the first drug to achieve widespread clinical use to antagonize the actions of catecholamines at β-adrenoceptor sites effectively. The therapeutic success of this agent has been followed by the introduction of numerous other β-blocking agents. Many have been claimed to have advantages and it is important to remember that the structural and pharmacological differences between these drugs are slight and the therapeutic distinctions between them somewhat inconsequential. Before describing the detailed effects of these drugs, it would be convenient to discuss briefly the differences that exist between the different members of the group.

Cardioselectivity

Some β-blockers are, to a greater or lesser extent, cardioselective and have a greater effect on the β_1-adrenoceptors of the heart than the β_2-adrenoceptors of the bronchioles and of the arterioles in skeletal muscle. They are, therefore, less hazardous to patients with respiratory diseases in whom bronchoconstriction would be dangerous. Atenolol, acebutolol, metoprolol, betaxolol, bisoprolol, celiprolol and esmolol are substantially safer than their non-selective alternatives; see *Table 13.3*, which is based on the classification of Fitzgerald (1972). Cardioselective β-blockers are also less likely to worsen intermittent claudication in patients with peripheral vascular disease. It is important to remember that cardioselective β-blockers are not *cardiospecific*. Thus, they will block β_1-receptors at non-cardiac sites, and at higher doses may exert some blocking effects at β_2-receptors – this is particularly true in asthmatic patients whose bronchioles may be extremely sensitive to any adverse effect. *Table 13.3* classifies commonly used β-adrenoceptor blocking drugs into (a) non-selective and (b) cardioselective drugs. The table also gives an indication of whether individual drugs possess any intrinsic sympathomimetic activity (ISA, see below) or membrane stabilizing activity (MSA, see below), and their durations of action.

Fitzgerald, J.D. (1972) Beta adrenergic blocking drugs. Present position and future developments. *Acta Cardiologica*, Suppl. 1S, 199

Intrinsic sympathomimetic activity (ISA) (partial agonist activity)

Many β-blockers reduce heart rate not only during exercise but also at rest. Propranolol is a prime example. The resultant bradycardia can be extreme and will be associated with

Table 13.3 Specificity of action of β-adrenoceptor antagonists*

Drug	Selectivity	ISA	MSA	Plasma half-life (h)
Nadolol	Non-selective	–	–	10–20
Oxprenolol	Non-selective	+ +	+/–	1–2
Pindolol	Non-selective	++	+/–	3–4
Propranolol	Non-selective	–	+ +	3–5
Sotalol	Non-selective	–	–	10–20
Timolol	Non-selective	–	–	3–5
Carvedilol†	Non-selective	–	–	5–8
Labetalol†	Non-selective	–	+/–	4–6
Acebutolol	Cardioselective	+	+	2–4
Atenolol	Cardioselective	–	–	5–8
Betaxolol	Cardioselective	–	+/–	16–20
Bisoprolol	Cardioselective	–	–	10–20
Esmolol	Cardioselective	–	–	10 minutes, i.v.
Metoprolol	Cardioselective	–	+/–	3–4
Celiprolol††	Cardioselective	See below	–	5–6

* The table lists a number of β-blockers according to their non-selective (β₁- and β₂-blockade) or cardioselective (β₁-blockade only) status. Also indicated are qualitative estimates of their intrinsic sympathomimetic activity (ISA) and their membrane stabilizing activity (MSA). Their plasma elimination half-lives give an indication of their useful durations of action.

Drugs marked † also possess α_1-adrenergic antagonist activity; the drug marked †† also possesses β_2-adrenergic agonist activity.

a considerable reduction in cardiac output. On the other hand, some drugs fail to reduce the resting heart rate, even though the tachycardia of exercise is controlled. This apparent 'failure' to reduce the resting heart rate appears to be due to a partial agonist action, or some intrinsic sympathomimetic activity (ISA). In reserpinized animals (catecholamine depleted), β-blockers with ISA produce a rise in heart rate. Drugs with ISA thus offer some advantages in patients whose heart rate is already slow or where heart failure is a distinct possibility. β-Blockers with ISA are acebutolol, oxprenolol and pindolol, (only the first of these, however, belongs to the cardioselective group).

Other cardiac actions

Some β-blockers are potent anti-arrhythmic agents because of a local anaesthetic or membrane stabilizing action (MSA). The effect is only slight and may be of little significance compared with the anti-arrhythmic consequences of their β-blocking actions on the heart. However, it is a fact that the drugs most likely to induce serious bradycardia and a tendency to heart failure are also those that possess MSA. Drugs with MSA should perhaps be avoided where serious bradycardia would be hazardous; examples of such drugs in the non-selective group are oxprenolol, pindolol and propranolol, and in the cardioselective group examples are acebutatol, betaxolol and metoprolol.

Among the newer β-blockers, the non-selective carvedilol and labetalol combine β₁- and β₂-blockade with an antagonist effect at α₁-adrenergic receptors, and the cardioselective celiprolol combines β₁-blocking effects with some β₂-agonist effects.

Metabolism

Most of the β-blockers are metabolized hepatically. Drugs that are rapidly metabolized, such as oxprenolol and propranolol, need to be given 3 times daily. Sotalol and atenolol are eliminated predominantly by renal excretion of unchanged drug. Esmolol is hydrolysed by arylesterases in erythrocyte cytosol.

Toxic effects

Most of the toxic effects are a consequence of their primary pharmacological action. Bradycardia and heart failure may be made worse, as may conduction block. Severe hypotension and fainting may also occur; there is the obvious risk of precipitating bronchoconstriction in asthmatic patients and of hypoglycaemia in diabetics.

Some other effects are, fortunately, rare although serious. A dry form of conjunctivitis involving the cornea, which may result in corneal ulceration, has been described frequently. Other reactions affect the inner ear or the skin, or both. Fortunately, these effects regress on stopping drug administration. The most serious reaction, however, was the induction of sclerosing peritonitis by practolol. This was a sterile inflammation of the peritoneum, resulting in widespread fibrosis and intestinal obstruction. It did not regress spontaneously. This reaction was only recognized after several years of usage of the drug and so far none of the other newer drugs has been reported to cause similar effects. Consequently, practolol is no longer available.

Therapeutic uses of β-blockers (Emilien and Maloteaux, 1998)

Angina pectoris

Propranolol has been used effectively for many years for the treatment of angina. The beneficial effect results from a reduction in the work of the heart and blockade of the sympathetic nervous system drive. The effect is most marked on exercise-induced angina when both pain and ECG signs are prevented. Any β-blocker is usually equally effective and results in improved exercise tolerance and reduction in the consumption of glyceryl trinitrate tablets. This improvement is associated with a reduction in the rate at which ventricular muscle contracts.

Hypertension

The antihypertensive effect of β-blockers is associated initially with a fall in cardiac output. In many patients, peripheral resistance remains unchanged, but in some it falls. In some patients, β-blockade results in a reduction in circulating renin activity, although there is no close relationship between initial renin levels and the responses to β-blocking therapy. The antihypertensive action, therefore, remains at least partly unexplained, although as our understanding of the central effects of such agents increases we may be nearer a solution. Some investigators have found that β-blockers lower blood pressure when injected into the cerebral ventricles of animals. Of interest is the finding that β-adrenoceptor blocking agents are not as selective as was once imagined. Many are potent inhibitors of 5-HT, both centrally and peripherally. The combination of a β-blocker with a thiazide diuretic provides satisfactory antihypertensive therapy, resulting in few unwanted effects such as postural hypotension. Labetalol has been promoted on the basis that it blocks peripheral α-adrenoceptors, thus lowering peripheral resistance, and at the same time has sufficient β-blockade to block excessive reflex cardiac stimulation induced by the vasodilatation. However, it seems likely that it is predominantly the β-blockade that is therapeutic. The potency ratio of α- to β-effect is about 1:5. The half-lives are respectively about 30 minutes and 90 minutes. Thus the α-effect is not only very much weaker but more evanescent. At present, in terms of long-term efficiency, there appears to be little to choose between various β-blockers in the treatment of hypertension. Once-a-day treatment obviously has an appeal.

Cardiac arrhythmias

Arrhythmias that are most dependent on sympathetic activity are the most responsive. These include supraventricular tachycardias, atrial fibrillation and ventricular ectopic rhythms. Arrhythmias associated with myocardial infarction or digitalis overdose respond less well and conduction abnormalities are usually made worse. Early after myocardial infarction, β-blockers are frequently contra-indicated because of either conduction block or heart failure, but on occasions, when excessive anxiety and sympathetic drive are responsible for ectopic beats, patients may benefit from them. Long-term therapy in coronary occlusive disease has a survival benefit.

The efficacy of these drugs is due to their intrinsic β-blocking action, although in addition in some cases membrane-stabilizing properties may also be useful. The D-isomer of propranolol has membrane-stabilizing actions but no β-adrenoceptor blocking action and is relatively ineffective.

Ventricular outflow obstruction

In conditions such as Fallot's tetralogy and hypertrophic cardiomyopathy, β-blockers are often beneficial since the degree of outflow tract obstruction is exacerbated by sympathetic over-activity, and reduced by β-blockade.

Other uses

Propanolol has been shown to exert a sedative effect in anxiety and now has a product licence for this indication. Its site of action for this effect is unclear: while a central action may contribute, so too do its effects upon autonomic signs of anxiety. Propranolol has also been used to reduce the effects of thyrotoxicosis and the stimulant effect of thyroid hormones in the treatment of myxoedema. β-Blockers are used in combination with α-blockers to antagonize catecholamines before and during surgery for phaeochromocytoma. They also reduce intra-ocular tension and the tremor of Parkinsonism. They are not drugs of first choice in the last two conditions.

β-Blocking drugs in the treatment of cardiac arrhythmias during anaesthesia

Extrapolation of data obtained from conscious volunteers to patients under general anaesthesia is not always valid, as the whole autonomic balance is disturbed. Currently used anaesthetic agents lack the sympathomimetic effects that were seen with agents such as ether and cyclopropane, and thus during general anaesthesia the cardiovascular system is likely to be depressed. The negative inotropic effects of β-adrenergic block could in such circumstances cause a marked deterioration in myocardial function. Considerable care must therefore be used if these drugs are to be given, or if the patient is receiving them preoperatively. Drugs with intrinsic stimulant activity (see *Table 13.3*) may be slightly safer in this respect than propranolol.

Surgical stimulation is known to cause sympathetic over-activity in lightly anaesthetized patients, although such stimulation is rarely, if ever, of any great importance. Hypercapnia also causes release of catecholamines, thus explaining its association with cardiac arrhythmias. It is in the field of cardiac arrhythmias occurring during anaesthesia that β-blocking drugs are most frequently employed by anaesthetists.

Arrhythmias occurring during cardiac surgery or in response to the injection of epinephrine (adrenaline) should be regarded as potentially dangerous. Whether arrhythmias occurring in the course of otherwise uncomplicated anaesthesia should be so regarded is debatable. Although they often cause concern, the majority disappear spontaneously or respond to a moderate increase in ventilation. The replacement of halothane by enflurane, isoflurane and sevoflurane, and the wider employment of ventilation and of analgesic supplementation, have been factors in a reduction in the number of arrhythmias seen in practice.

Emilien, G. and Maloteaux, J.M. (1998) Current therapeutic uses and potential of beta-adrenoceptor agonists and antagonists. *European Journal of Clinical Pharmacology*, **53**, 389–404

Adrenergic neurone blocking drugs

Of the few uses that these drugs currently enjoy, none is aimed at influencing cardiac activity. They are discussed in Chapter 12.

Class 3 anti-arrhythmic drugs

The main effect of class 3 anti-arrhythmic drugs is to delay repolarization. This increases the duration of the action potential of myocardial tissue and thus increases the refractory period of atrial, nodal and ventricular tissue.

Amiodarone is at present by far the most frequently used class 3 anti-arrhythmic drug. In high doses it also has a β-blocking effect. It has an elimination half-life of about 4 weeks. The drug is stored in muscle (including cardiac muscle) and fat. Cumulation occurs, and it is said that to achieve a satisfactory class 3 effect the patient must be 'loaded' with 15 g over a fortnight. However, when it is used intravenously to provide urgent treatment for life-threatening arrhythmias, the onset of action is in the order of 15–30 minutes, and it is less depressant of myocardial contractility than alternative anti-arrhythmic agents.

Amiodarone is effective treatment for acute tachyarrhythmias, whether these are supraventricular or ventricular, and including fast atrial fibrillation. It can also be used in the long-term treatment of supraventricular or ventricular arrhythmias and has proved beneficial in patients with the Wolff–Parkinson–White syndrome. The decision to institute long-term therapy with this agent is not to be undertaken lightly: unwanted effects are rare in the short term, but are relatively common with chronic therapy, and these include corneal deposits, skin photosensitivity, peripheral neuropathy, pulmonary fibrosis and hepatitis.

It is a particularly useful drug in intensive care, and in the early postoperative period after cardiac surgery. Fast atrial fibrillation is common in both settings and there is frequently a contra-indication to drugs with negative inotropic effects.

Class 4 anti-arrhythmic drugs: calcium channel blocking drugs

These drugs are usually used for effects other than those on cardiac rhythm or rate. In the past, supraventricular tachycardia could be treated with verapamil, but this has been superseded by adenosine. The calcium channel blocking drugs (including verapamil) are discussed in Chapter 12.

Digitalis glycosides

Digitalis was first used by William Withering in 1775, he having noted that foxglove was a constituent of an old family recipe recommended for dropsy. The main active principle of the powdered leaf of the purple foxglove (*Digitalis purpurea*) is the glycoside digitoxin, but this preparation, *Prepared Digitalis (BP)*, is now only of historical interest. Digoxin from *Digitalis lanata* is the most commonly used glycoside and all such preparations, used therapeutically, are loosely referred to as digitalis. The most important of these glycosides are digoxin, digitoxin, ouabain (from *Strophanthus gratus*), lanatoside C and proscillaridin A.

The basic structure of the glycosides is that of the steroid cyclopentenophenanthrene nucleus and they are chemically related to the bile acids and the sex hormones. They consist of two parts, a glycone and an aglycone portion. The glycone is a sugar, often glucose, but closely related sugars such as digitoxose are also found. They have no cardiac action in themselves, but make the glycoside more soluble, help transport and are essential for fixation to cardiac muscle, without which the drug has little action. In the aglycone portions reside the digitalis-like activity, but their actions alone are more transient and less potent as they do not remain fixed in the muscle; their power to cause toxic effects such as vomiting equals that of the glycosides. The intrinsic activity of these drugs resides in the double bond in the unsaturated lactone ring, and opening the ring or saturating the double bond causes loss of both therapeutic activity and toxic effects.

Digitalis has effects upon the Na/K-ATP-ase sodium pump and also on sarcoplasmic reticulum Ca^{2+}-release channels (McGarry and Williams, 1993; Jortani and Valdes, 1997). In therapeutic doses, it acts on the A-V bundle of His which results in slower conduction of impulses from atria to ventricles, a useful effect in patients in atrial fibrillation because this reduces the ventricular rate. The excitatory effect of the drug on heart muscle shortens the refractory period and the rate of fibrillating atria will be increased. Digoxin also stimulates the force of contraction of the failing heart independent of catecholamine stimulation.

The prime indication for the use of digoxin is in control of ventricular rate in atrial fibrillation. In the past it was widely used to treat congestive cardiac failure, and there is currently a recrudescence of interest in digoxin in 'third-line' treatment of congestive cardiac failure unresponsive to diuretics and ACE inhibitors (Armstrong and Moe, 1993).

Signs of toxicity include anorexia, headache, nausea, vomiting, diarrhoea, bradycardia (more marked in the presence of atrial fibrillation), and prolongation of the P-R interval in the ECG. Extrasystoles with atrial tachycardia and incomplete heart block, any form of supraventricular tachycardia, the occurrence of regular rhythm with loss of the usual ECG pattern and coupling in sinus rhythm are all signs of serious intoxication.

Armstrong, P.W. and Moe, G.W. (1993) Medical advances in the treatment of congestive heart failure. *Circulation*, **88**(6), 2941–52

Jortani, S.A. and Valdes, R. Jr. (1997) Digoxin and its related endogenous factors. *Critical Review of Clinical and Laboratory Science*, **34**(3), 225–74

McGarry, S.J. and Williams, A.J. (1993) Digoxin activates sarcoplasmic reticulum Ca^{2+}-release channels: a possible role in cardiac inotropy. *British Journal of Pharmacology*, **108**(4), 1043–50

Drugs that alter vagal tone

First-line treatment for supraventricular tachycardia remains carotid sinus massage and other physical means of increasing vagal tone. In the past, drug therapy has been used to produce this effect, either by using muscarinic agonists or by using vasoconstrictors to increase the blood pressure to provoke a reflex increase in vagal tone. These techniques are not currently used.

Chronotropic agents

Chronotropic agents influence the rate of the heart, which may be increased or decreased. They can be divided into two main groups, those that act directly on the heart and those that act indirectly. The two aspects of cardiac function, the force of the muscular contraction and the rate, are closely connected, and when the drug is one that acts directly on the heart, the force is often influenced as well.

For example, epinephrine (adrenaline) increases both force of contraction and rate, whereas norepinephrine (noradrenaline) has less effect on force and the rate may be unaffected or even slowed. The reason for this is that the reflex slowing from the rise in blood pressure produced by vasoconstriction tends to overcome the feebler action of norepinephrine on the heart, whereas with epinephrine the reverse occurs. It is seldom necessary to alter the rate alone except in conditions such as paroxysmal tachycardia, or hypotension due to bradycardia.

The rate of the heart is controlled through the vagus, which is inhibitor, and the sympathetic, which is accelerator. There is no parasympathetic supply to the ventricles, and therefore changes in vagal activity have no effect on contractility. The influence of drugs on the heart rate through indirect action is complex, and many that act on the CNS, such as atropine, halothane and digitalis, cause slowing. Those that have a stimulant action also usually cause liberation of epinephrine and norepinephrine from the adrenal medulla so that a biphasic effect may be seen, the central effect preceding the release effect. Vasodilator drugs, which cause a fall in blood pressure by a peripheral action, give rise to a compensatory increase in cardiac rate.

The main reflex involved (Marey's) is the depressor reflex with its afferent impulses from the baroreceptors of the carotid sinuses and the aortic arch. Other important receptors are in the lungs and the chemoreceptors of the carotid bodies.

In addition to blood pressure, further factors affecting heart rate include the oxygen tension of the blood, intracranial pressure, muscular exertion and cerebral arousal. Changes in rate can also be caused by drugs affecting the rate of conduction or refractory period of the myocardium in the presence of abnormal rhythms, or by acting directly on the pacemaker of the heart by intracellular mechanisms that are neither sympathomimetic nor parasympathomimetic, such as digitalis and quinidine.

The heart is slowed by parasympathomimetic agents such as methacholine and the anticholinesterases. Certain anaesthetic agents such as halothane also cause bradycardia through a central vagal action. Acceleration of the heart by sympathomimetic action is produced by drugs such as epinephrine, ephedrine, isoprenaline and cocaine. Drugs that block parasympathetic or sympathetic action will have the opposite effects. Atropine-like drugs will increase the heart rate by blocking vagal transmission and blockade of adrenergic β-receptors or fibres will decrease it. Atropine, when given subcutaneously and in low concentration, will initially cause slowing. This is due to a central stimulatory effect preceding its peripheral blocking action, which only develops later when blood levels are higher. The same effect occurs with hyoscine, but larger doses than are normally given are required to produce a peripheral effect and a consequent increase in heart rate.

Drugs that have chronotropic effects associated with their action on conduction or refractory period of the myocardium or pacemaker, or on intracellular metabolism, include procainamide, the cardiac glycosides, some xanthines and catecholamines. Their effects are complex and are described in their individual monographs.

Atropine and glycopyrrolate are used to antagonize or prevent the bradycardia produced by halothane, alfentanil and neostigmine, and conversely neostigmine can be used in the treatment of paroxysmal tachycardia.

Adenosine

This short-acting drug is a general vasodilator, a negative inotrope and a negative chronotrope. The negative inotropic effect is probably due to an activation of a potassium outward current, which shortens the action potential duration and hence reduces the force of contraction. The negative chronotropic actions are due to prolongation of A-V conduction by an activation of potassium channels or an inhibition of the slow Ca^{2+} inward current at the A-V node. Cardiac bradyarrhythmias in hypoxia have been attributed to an increased formation and release of adenosine. Vasodilatation is one of the most prominent effects of adenosine and was one of the first to be recognized, but its mechanism of action is not completely understood. In particular, there is conflicting information about the potential contribution of endothelial factors.

Adenosine can slow or terminate supraventricular tachycardias involving the A-V node and it is this quality which provides it with therapeutic value. It is used as second-line treatment of a fast re-entrant supraventricular tachycardia (first-line treatment being carotid sinus massage.) It is also useful in the management of broad complex tachycardia. If the cause is ventricular tachycardia, adenosine will have no effect; if the rhythm is actually a supraventricular tachycardia complicated by bundle branch block this will become obvious when the rate is slowed, but the complexes remain unchanged. Awake subjects given adenosine report various unpleasant subjective sensations including apprehension, discomfort, burning sensations, heaviness of the limbs, nausea and light-headedness. It can cause bronchospasm and asthma is therefore a contra-indication to its use. Its action can be dangerously exaggerated and prolonged in patients taking dipyridamole.

MONOGRAPHS

ADENOSINE

Adenosine phosphate, adenosine monophosphate (rINN)

Pharmacology

Adenosine administered by rapid intravenous injection slows conduction through the A-V node. This action can interrupt re-entry circuits involving the A-V node and restore normal sinus rhythm in patients with paroxysmal supraventricular tachycardias. Once the circuit has been interrupted, the tachycardia stops and normal sinus rhythm is re-established.

Fate in the body   Adenosine is a substance that is naturally present in some form in all cells of the body. The effect of a therapeutic dose is terminated by uptake by many different types of cell, either for re-use or for metabolism within the cell. Since neither the kidney nor the liver are involved in the degradation of endogenous adenosine, termination of the effect of exogenous adenosine is unaffected by hepatic or renal insufficiency.

Indications

Adenosine is used to achieve rapid conversion to a normal sinus rhythm of paroxysmal supraventricular tachycardias, including those associated with accessory bypass tracts (Wolff–Parkinson–White syndrome). It is also used as an aid to diagnosis of broad or narrow complex supraventricular tachycardias. Although adenosine is not effective in converting atrial flutter, atrial fibrillation or ventricular tachycardia to sinus rhythm, the slowing of A-V conduction makes atrial activity easier to evaluate from ECG recordings and therefore adenosine can aid the diagnosis.

Adenosine may be useful during electrophysiological studies to determine the site of A-V block or to determine, in some cases of pre-excitation, whether conduction is occurring by an accessory pathway or via the AV node.

Dosage and administration

Adenosine is available as a solution for intravenous injection provided in glass vials containing 6 mg of adenosine in 2 ml of normal saline. It should be administered by rapid i.v. bolus injection according to the ascending dosage schedule below. In order to ensure that the solution reaches the systemic circulation as a bolus, it is administered into an i.v. line situated as proximally as possible, followed by a saline flush.

Adenosine should only be used when facilities exist for cardiac monitoring. Patients who develop high-level A-V block at a particular dose should not be given further dosage increments.

The initial dose is 3 mg by rapid intravenous bolus. If this does not result in elimination of the supraventricular tachycardia within 1–2 minutes, 6 mg should be given also as a rapid intravenous bolus. If the second dose is not effective within 1–2 minutes, 12 mg should be given also as a rapid intravenous bolus. Additional or higher doses are not recommended. Effective doses for children are between 0.0375 and 0.25 mg/kg.

Precautions

Adenosine is intended for hospital use only, with monitoring and cardiorespiratory resuscitation equipment available for immediate use.

Adenosine is contra-indicated in patients with second- or third-degree A-V block or with sick sinus syndrome (unless they also have a functioning artificial pacemaker). It is also contra-indicated in asthmatic patients. Patients with atrial fibrillation/flutter and an accessory bypass tract may develop increased conduction down the anomalous pathway.

Facial flush, dyspnoea, bronchospasm, a feeling of thoracic constriction, nausea and light-headedness occur commonly. More rarely observed side effects have been: feeling of discomfort; sweating; palpitations; hyperventilation; head pressure; apprehension;

blurred vision; burning sensation; bradycardia; asystole; chest pains; headache; dizziness; heaviness in arms; arm, back and neck pains; metallic taste.

Severe bradycardia has been reported and some patients have required temporary pacing. The effects of adenosine are not blocked by atropine. At the time of conversion to normal sinus rhythm, the ECG may show premature ventricular contractions, premature atrial contractions, sinus bradycardia, sinus tachycardia, skipped beats, sinus pause and/or atrioventricular block. The induced bradycardia predisposes to ventricular excitability disorders.

Drug interactions

Dipyridamole is a known inhibitor of adenosine uptake: it may potentiate the action of adenosine. Asystole has been reported following concomitant administration. It is suggested that adenosine should not be administered to patients receiving dipyridamole; if use of adenosine is essential, dosage should be reduced by a factor of 4 (e.g. initial dosage of 0.5–1.0 mg). Theophylline and other xanthines such as caffeine are known strong inhibitors of adenosine. Adenosine may interact with drugs tending to impair cardiac conduction.

AMIODARONE

Amiodarone hydrochloride (rINN)

Pharmacology

This is a class 3 anti-arrhythmic drug whose main effect is to delay repolarization. It increases the duration of the action potential of myocardial tissue and thus increases the refractory period of atrial, nodal and ventricular tissue. In high doses, it also has a β-blocking effect. It has an elimination half-life of about 4 weeks. The drug is stored in muscle (including cardiac muscle) and fat. Cumulation occurs, and it is said that to achieve a satisfactory class 3 effect, the patient must be 'loaded' with 15 g over a fortnight. However, when it is used intravenously to provide urgent treatment for life-threatening arrhythmias, the onset of action is in the order of 15–30 minutes, and it is less depressant of myocardial contractility than alternative anti-arrhythmic agents.

It is an iodinated compound and some iodine is released when it is metabolized.

Indications

Amiodarone is effective treatment for acute tachyarrhythmias, whether these are supraventricular or ventricular, and including fast atrial fibrillation. It can also be used in the long-term treatment of supraventricular or ventricular arrhythmias and has proved beneficial in patients with the Wolff–Parkinson–White syndrome.

Dosage and administration

For rapid control of tachyarrhythmias, 150–300 mg (in 20 ml of 5 per cent glucose) can be given over 20–60 minutes, followed by 1200 mg (in 250 ml of 5 per cent glucose) over 24 h. When given orally, initial treatment is with 200 mg 3 times a day until full response is achieved, which is usually about 1 week, thereafter reducing to about 200 mg daily.

Precautions

It is contra-indicated in patients with advanced A-V block or with S-A block. It should be used with special caution in patients who are receiving β-blockers. The drug can cause micro-deposits of lipofuscin in the cornea of some patients; while not an indication to withdraw the drug immediately, such patients should be carefully watched and the dose reduced if visual haloes or photophobia occur. The corneal deposits can disappear a few months after stopping the treatment. Thyroid metabolism can also be disturbed. Iodine released from the drug can interfere with the protein-bound iodine test. Photosensitivity of the skin and blue pigmentation of it has been reported. Nightmares and vivid dreams can occur. Peripheral neuropathy, pulmonary fibrosis and hepatitis have been reported. The drug increases free plasma digoxin concentration and maintenance doses of digoxin may need to be halved. It will also potentiate the action of warfarin.

ATENOLOL

Atenolol (rINN)

Pharmacology

Atenolol is a β-adrenoceptor blocking agent with a cardioselective action. Its action is comparable to that of propranolol at cardiac receptor sites, but that at extra-cardiac sites is considerably less. It has no sympathomimetic action and no membrane-stabilizing effect on cardiac muscle. Heart rate is slowed and this is associated with a reduction in cardiac output. There is some reduction in blood pressure, but with considerable variation in its degree.

The action of atenolol on bronchial musculature is less than that of propranolol. Nevertheless, there is a risk of precipitating bronchospasm in asthmatics.

Fate in the body Atenolol is consistently but incompletely (40–50 per cent) absorbed by mouth. Peak plasma levels occur 2–4 h after oral administration. There is no significant first-pass hepatic metabolism. The plasma half-life is about 6 h. Renal excretion is the major mechanism of elimination, and the dose must be adjusted in patients with a creatinine clearance of less than 35 ml/minute.

Indications

Atenolol may be used in the treatment of hypertension, angina and cardiac arrhythmias. It may be used to limit infarct size in myocardial infarction.

Dosage and administration

Atenolol is normally given by mouth, 50–100 mg once daily.

Precautions

Caution is necessary in the treatment of asthmatics and bronchitics, as there is a danger of producing bronchoconstriction. Bradycardia and hypotension may occur with effective β-blockade in patients with recent myocardial infarction. The use of any β-blocker in diabetes mellitus will alter the requirement for hypoglycaemic drugs, and will make recognition of hypoglycaemia more difficult. Muscle pains and intermittent claudication may occur.

DIGOXIN

Digoxin (rINN)

Pharmacology

The mechanism of action involves inhibition of the ion-transport activity of a membrane-associated protein called Na/K-ATP-ase (sodium pump). Present theory holds that, at least for the effect on rhythm, the sodium pump is the principal molecular receptor for the digitalis drugs. However, digoxin also activates sarcoplasmic reticulum Ca^{2+}-release channels, providing a possible mechanism for the increased free intracellular calcium ion concentrations in the cell and the cardiac inotropy. Recent evidence indicates the presence of naturally-occurring digitalis-like compounds in mammals.

Cardiovascular system   In very low doses, digoxin reduces heart rate by vagally mediated inhibition. In therapeutic doses, it acts on the A-V bundle of His which results in slower conduction of impulses from atria to ventricles, and is reflected in a prolonged P-R interval in the ECG. This effect is greatest in patients who have atrial fibrillation with a rapid ventricular rate. Digoxin also facilitates entry of calcium into myocardial cells, which directly stimulates the force of contraction of the failing heart independent of catecholamine stimulation. There is evidence from both animal and human studies that cardiac glycosides do not significantly change myocardial oxygen consumption. The excitatory effect of the drug on heart muscle shortens the refractory period and the rate of fibrillating atria will be increased, and in cases of flutter the irregularity changes to fibrillation, although on withdrawal of the drug normal rhythm may be resumed. In the absence of cardiac failure, and in the presence of normal rhythm, heart rate is reduced by central stimulation and by depression of the S-A node. In congestive cardiac failure the heart rate is reduced, largely from the improvement in cardiac output. This slowing is mediated mainly through the vagus. Thus, when cardiac failure occurs with atrial fibrillation, slowing results because of at least two different mechanisms.

Central nervous system   Neurological effects are commonly seen early in cases of digitalis intoxication. Headaches, drowsiness and an ill-defined malaise are frequently encountered. Visual disturbances and facial neuralgia may also occur on rare occasions.

Diuretic action   Although digoxin can directly inhibit the ion transport system in the proximal renal tubule, high doses are necessary for this to occur, and it is unlikely that this direct action plays a significant role in the diuresis that accompanies the use of digoxin in congestive cardiac failure. This is almost entirely due to its effects on cardiac output and the consequent improvement in glomerular filtration pressure. A marked improvement in urinary output and reduction in oedema will usually follow full digitalization, but many cases will also require a diuretic such as chlorothiazide.

Gastro-intestinal tract   Digoxin is less irritant orally than the natural powdered leaf. Nausea and vomiting may follow overdosage, and anorexia may be the first sign that full digitalization is being approached; diarrhoea may also be present. Digoxin can be given intravenously if the drug is not well tolerated by mouth, or for a more rapid effect.

Absorption and fate in the body   Digoxin is given only by mouth or by intravenous injection. The oral bio-availability is high. Owing to its irritant nature, the injection by subcutaneous or intramuscular routes has been abandoned; apart from pain and discomfort, absorption of the drug from these sites is irregular.

Digoxin acts in 1–3 h and lasts 1–2 days. It is somewhat more rapidly effective by the intravenous route. The delayed onset of action of these drugs is due mainly to the time taken for them to be fixed in cardiac muscle; protein binding with serum albumin also plays a part. Digoxin is not selectively retained by heart muscle, which does not keep it longer than other tissues. Digoxin is excreted only by glomerular filtration and its accumulation in renal insufficiency makes dose reduction essential in this situation.

Indications

The prime indication for the use of digoxin is in control of ventricular rate in atrial fibrillation. In the past, it was widely used to treat congestive cardiac failure, but while there seems to be short-term relief of symptoms, the unwanted effects are manifold, and no survival benefit has yet been shown. There is currently a recrudescence of interest in digoxin in 'third-line' treatment of congestive cardiac failure unresponsive to diuretics and ACE inhibitors.

Dosage and administration

Full digitalization by digoxin requires an oral dose of 1.5–3 mg according to the weight of the patient. This is usually given as an initial dose of 0.5–0.75 mg, followed by 0.25 mg at 6-hourly intervals until the total estimated dose has been given or signs of toxicity occur. If more rapid digitalization is necessary, half of the total estimated dose can be given initially, followed by the remainder in 24 h at 6-hourly intervals, or the drug can be given intravenously commencing with a dose of 0.5–1 mg, followed by 0.5 mg 6-hourly. The usual maintenance dose is 0.25–0.75 mg daily. However, the elderly can often be maintained satisfactorily on 0.125 mg daily.

Whenever digoxin is to be given it is of the greatest importance to ascertain whether the patient has previously been given any digitalis or strophanthin preparation during the preceding 2 weeks in order to avoid overdosage.

Precautions

Digoxin should be given cautiously in angina pectoris, myocardial infarction, or ventricular tachycardia, or if heart block is only partial. Digoxin is usually contra-indicated soon after a myocardial infarction as it may cause conduction block and has a tendency to excite the myocardium. It is definitely harmful in hypertrophic obstructive cardiomyopathy and should be used in atrial fibrillation only if control of the ventricular rate is required. Where there is peripheral circulatory failure in shock or during the course of an acute infection, it may aggravate the condition by further decreasing cardiac output. Digoxin must be given with caution to patients with impaired renal function.

It is dangerous to give calcium during digoxin therapy, as it excites heart muscle and the effect of the two drugs is synergistic. The effect of potassium depletion is similar. This is particularly important if potassium-depleting diuretics are being given together with digoxin, and potassium supplementation will be necessary.

Digoxin intoxication

It is important to monitor the patient carefully during digitalization, especially when large doses are given to induce this state quickly. Being cumulative, it can be given safely only if the effects of overdose are immediately recognized and the drug is withdrawn until they subside. The margin between adequate therapeutic effect and overdose is small, the former being about 60 per cent of the latter. Signs of toxicity include anorexia, headache, nausea, vomiting, diarrhoea, bradycardia (more marked in the presence of atrial fibrillation), and prolongation of the P-R interval in the ECG. Extrasystoles with atrial tachycardia and incomplete heart block, any form of supraventricular tachycardia, the occurrence of regular rhythm with loss of the usual ECG pattern and coupling in sinus rhythm are all signs of serious intoxication.

Measurement of plasma digoxin concentration is useful both in maintaining a satisfactory clinical control and in the diagnosis of intoxication. Therapeutic levels lie in the range 1–2 ng/ml (1.3–2.6 nmol/litre). Levels of 3 ng/ml (4 nmol/litre) or more are usually toxic.

Treatment

Gastric lavage may be necessary if a recent oral dose of digoxin is still likely to be in the stomach. General supportive measures should be instituted, and serum electrolytes estimated. Potassium depletion is likely, although the level in the myocardial cells may not be reflected by that of the serum. If renal function is normal, a small intravenous dose of 2–5 mmol of potassium may be given slowly, regardless of the serum potassium. Potassium should not be given in the presence of A-V block as it increases the effective refractory period of the A-V node and enhances the block.

Drug treatment of a life-threatening arrhythmia depends on the nature of the disorder. If potassium is ineffective, the most effective drug is phenytoin, which will suppress digoxin-induced ventricular tachycardia as well as supraventricular arrhythmias. It also diminishes S-A and A-V nodal block by decreasing the conduction time at these sites. The recommended dose is 100 mg infused slowly every 5 minutes until the arrhythmia is reverted or ECG evidence of toxicity is noted. Lidocaine can also suppress ventricular tachycardia, but is less effective than phenytoin against supraventricular arrhythmias. β-Adrenoceptor blocking agents are effective in combating extrasystoles and tachycardia of both ventricular and supraventricular origin. They are, however, liable to depress myocardial contractility and are contra-indicated in the presence of A-V block because of the further decrease in nodal conduction velocity that they produce. Atropine can also be of value when there is a sinus bradycardia or vagal inhibition of a nodal pacemaker.

DISOPYRAMIDE

Disopyramide phosphate (rINN)

Pharmacology

This class 1A anti-arrhythmic drug has quinidine-like actions. It appears to be more potent in producing atrial or ventricular refractoriness and less potent on the Purkinje system. Therapeutic concentrations will decrease the slope of phase 1 depolarization in Purkinje fibres and decrease their spontaneous firing rate. The drug has a direct effect on the sinus node, slowing its rate of discharge. It also has antimuscarinic activity.

Fate in the body The drug is well absorbed following oral administration, and first-pass metabolism is not marked. About 50 per cent of a dose is excreted unchanged through the kidney. The elimination half-life is approximately 7 h.

Indications and dosage

Disopyramide is used for the treatment of ventricular or atrial arrhythmias and the usual oral dose is 100–200 mg 4 times a day.

Precautions

Disopyramide will reduce cardiac output and this effect is more pronounced in patients taking β-blockers or those with pre-existing ventricular failure. Unexpected hypoglycaemia can occur. An active metabolite, mono-N-alkyl disopyramide has anticholinergic properties, and may cause typical anticholinergic symptoms such as dry mouth, blurred vision and urinary retention.

ESMOLOL

Esmolol hydrochloride (rINN)

Pharmacology

Esmolol is an ultra-short-acting β-adrenoceptor blocker with a distribution half-life of 2 minutes and an elimination half-life of about 9 minutes. It is relatively cardioselective, with a selectivity for β_1-adrenoceptors comparable to that of metoprolol.

The therapeutic level is between 0.2 and 1.2 mg/litre. Like other β-adrenoceptor blockers, it is a class 2 anti-arrhythmic agent. Esmolol has no local anaesthetic activity and no intrinsic sympathetic activity in clinical doses.

Indications

Esmolol is effective in attenuating sympathetic responses to laryngoscopy and intubation, to sternotomy and to emergence from anaesthesia and extubation. It has been claimed to be more effective than sodium nitroprusside in controlling postoperative hypertension following coronary artery surgery, causing less of a fall in diastolic pressure. There is also a reduction in heart rate (nitroprusside tending to cause a reflex tachycardia) and minimal effects on PaO_2, and oxygen saturation.

Fate in the body Esmolol is hydrolysed by arylesterases in erythrocyte cytosol. The major metabolite also has weak β-blocking activity and has a half-life of about 4 h. Metabolism of esmolol is unaffected by serum cholinesterase deficiency.

Dosage and administration

Esmolol is given by continuous intravenous infusion. An initial bolus of 1 mg/kg may be followed by an infusion of 50–300 µg/kg/minute, depending on response.

Alternatively, using a concentration of 10 mg/ml, an initial infusion of 500 µg/kg given over 1 minute is reduced to 50 µg/kg/minute for 5 minutes and then progressively increased by 50 µg/kg/minute every 5 minutes, up to the maximum of 300 µg/kg/minute adjusted according to the therapeutic response. Higher rates of administration, up to 500 µg/kg/minute may be necessary to abolish hypertension and tachycardia associated with severe surgical stimuli.

Precautions and side effects

Esmolol extends the duration of action of suxamethonium by a few minutes by competing with cholinesterases. The most common side effect is moderate hypotension. Esmolol is incompatible with bicarbonate solutions.

METOPROLOL

Metoprolol tartrate (rINN)

Pharmacology

Metoprolol is a competitive β-adrenoceptor blocking agent with a cardioselective action. Its action is comparable to that of propranolol at cardiac receptor sites, but that at extracardiac sites is considerably less. Heart rate is slowed and this is associated with a reduction in cardiac output. There is some reduction in blood pressure, but with considerable variation in its degree.

The action of metoprolol on bronchial musculature is less than that of propranolol. Nevertheless, there is a risk of precipitating bronchospasm in asthmatics.

Fate in the body   Metoprolol is reasonably well absorbed by mouth, but its short half-life means that when it is given orally it must be given several times a day or must be in the form of a slow-release preparation. The plasma half-life is about 3 h. Hepatic metabolism is the major mechanism of elimination, and the dose must be adjusted in patients with significant hepatic dysfunction.

Indications

Metoprolol may be used in the treatment of hypertension, angina, cardiac arrhythmias and hyperthyroidism. It may be used to limit infarct size in myocardial infarction and it has a place in the prophylaxis of migraine.

Dosage and administration

Metoprolol may be given during anaesthesia by intravenous bolus of 2–4 mg to a maximum of 10 mg. During the early stages of a myocardial infarct, 5 mg boluses may be given at 2-minute intervals to a maximum of 15 mg. It may be given by mouth, 50–200 mg twice daily.

Precautions

Caution is necessary in the treatment of asthmatics and bronchitics, as there is a danger of producing bronchoconstriction. Bradycardia and hypotension may occur with effective β-blockade in patients with recent myocardial infarction. Heart failure may be made worse. The use of any β-blocker in diabetes mellitus will alter the requirement for hypoglycaemic drugs, and will make recognition of hypoglycaemia more difficult. Muscle pains and intermittent claudication may occur.

Oxprenolol is a cardioselective β-adrenoceptor blocking agent which is known to have some intrinsic sympathomimetic action and some membrane-stabilizing effect. It is normally given by mouth, 2 mg 2–3 times daily for the treatment of arrhythmias, 40 mg 2–3 times daily in cases of angina, increasing to 120–200 mg a day or more if necessary. Hepatic metabolism is the major mechanism of elimination.

Alprenolol has very similar actions to oxprenolol on cardiac function and bronchial musculature, and may be used for similar purposes. It is normally given by mouth in a dose of 200–400 mg daily in the treatment of angina. It has no particular advantages over oxprenolol.

Nadolol is a non-selective β-blocking drug that has been used to treat angina and hypertension. It may have an advantage over some other β-blocking drugs in that it can increase renal blood flow. It is available as a once-a-day preparation.

PROPRANOLOL

Propranolol hydrochloride (rINN)

Pharmacology

Propranolol was the first effective β-adrenoceptor blocking agent to stand the test of prolonged clinical use, and experience with it extends more widely than with any other member of this group. It blocks all β-adrenoceptors indiscriminately. By blockade of β_1-adrenoceptors, it effectively slows the heart rate. This effect may be pronounced in mitral valve disease, atrial fibrillation and phaeochromocytoma. The block is competitive and can be overcome by an adequate dose of isoprenaline. If vagal receptors are also blocked by atropine the heart rate increases, which indicates that the reduced rate produced by propranolol alone is due to blocking of normal sympathetic drive. Cardiac output is reduced in normal patients and those with cardiac impairment. By opposing the haemodynamic response to stress and exercise in ischaemic heart disease, it has an 'oxygen-sparing' effect and this is of benefit to patients suffering from angina of effort, but in cardiac insufficiency inhibition of normal sympathetic drive may induce failure.

In hypertensive patients there will be some reduction in blood pressure. Its mechanism of action in lowering the blood pressure of hypertensive patients is still uncertain. Besides its effects on the cardiovascular system, it inhibits renin release from the kidney. Propranolol also has central effects that may be important.

Propranolol slows the ventricular rate in atrial fibrillation but does not correct the arrhythmia. In flutter it may slow the ventricular rate or convert the irregularity to fibrillation. In both atrial and ventricular tachycardia, the ventricular rate is usually reduced and extrasystoles are either abolished or their frequency reduced, and it is of special value in the management of digitalis intoxication. Its effect on forearm blood flow is variable. It abolishes the vasodilator action of adrenergic β_2-fibres; within skeletal muscle, so blood flow may be reduced. Fatigue and aching of muscles during exercise is commonly reported by patients taking propranolol, especially, but not exclusively, in patients with peripheral vascular disease. Electron microscope studies suggest that propranolol, in common with other β-adrenoceptor blocking drugs, affects the ionic permeability of the muscle membrane to potassium.

During anaesthesia it abolishes arrhythmias occurring in patients with thyrotoxicosis, respiratory acidosis and phaeochromocytoma, and will prevent those that might be precipitated if catecholamines are infiltrated to reduce peripheral bleeding under halothane or cyclopropane anaesthesia. Blood pressure and pulse rate are also reduced, but these effects are abolished by atropine.

During ether anaesthesia, sympathetic over-activity is believed to maintain cardiac output, and propranolol might therefore be expected to cause hypotension. However, in small doses propranolol usually has only a moderate effect on blood pressure in these circumstances.

Propranolol now has a product licence as an anxiolytic. There are several pieces of evidence to suggest that β-blockers work through a peripheral mechanism rather than within the CNS, although propranolol is relatively lipophilic and does gain entry to the CNS. It is most effective in performance anxiety, but is also as effective as benzodiazepines in some patients with chronic anxiety with peripheral autonomic symptoms.

Fate in the body Propranolol is rapidly absorbed after oral administration. Metabolic degradation is through two pathways: (1) hydroxylation followed by conjugation with D-glucuronic acid; (2) side chain oxidation. The metabolites are excreted in the urine.

Indications

Propranolol may be used to control cardiac arrhythmias, such as those associated with digitalis intoxication and those that occur during anaesthesia. It may also be used in the control of tachycardia in the management of phaeochromocytoma before and during operation, the tachycardia that is induced by ganglion blockers when employed in controlled hypotension, and when the ventricular rate in atrial fibrillation is not adequately controlled by digitalis alone. It is of value in the treatment of angina and to control the β-adrenoceptor stimulating effects of thyroid medication if they hamper adequate therapy in the management of myxoedema. Its use may well be superseded by the more selective β-adrenoceptor blocking drugs, such as oxprenolol or alprenolol, which cause less cardiac depression and bronchoconstriction. Propranolol can control the tremor in cases of Parkinsonism, in which emotional stress and epinephrine (adrenaline) aggravate the condition.

Dosage and administration

Propranolol is normally given by mouth, but it can also be given intravenously. For the treatment of arrhythmias, 10–30 mg may be given 3–4 times a day. Larger doses are usually required for the treatment of angina, which may require up to 80 mg 4 times a day. When a rapid effect is required, 0.5–5 mg may be given slowly intravenously at a rate not exceeding 1 mg/minute.

Precautions

Propranolol should be used with the greatest caution in the presence of incipient cardiac failure and metabolic acidosis, and it should not be given to asthmatics or those subject to bronchospasm. It should also be used cautiously during ether anaesthesia and only after atropine premedication.

When given intravenously, propranolol must be administered very slowly with pauses so that its full effect can be ascertained. Should marked bradycardia or hypotension occur, atropine 0.5–1 mg should be given intravenously.

QUINIDINE

Quinidine sulfate, bisulfate and gluconate (rINN)

Pharmacology

Quinidine is an isomer of the alkaloid quinine. It has a potent anti-arrhythmic action and has been used for the control of cardiac arrhythmias for many years. Its actions are complex. It directly depresses cardiac muscle with consequent decrease in irritability, lengthening of refractory period and slowing of transmission. It also depresses transmission in the A-V node and bundle of His and decreases vagal tone. Usually the heart rate is decreased, but if vagal depression is marked, it may rise.

Indications

Quinidine is used in the treatment of some cardiac arrhythmias, such as extrasystoles and ventricular paroxysmal tachycardia. For many years, it was used to convert certain recent cases of atrial fibrillation into sinus rhythm, but d.c. shock conversion is now preferred. In atrial fibrillation, the patient should first be digitalized and a maintenance dose continued throughout treatment to prevent an increase in ventricular rate and also to prevent the occurrence of a 1:1 ventricular response when the fibrillating atria slow below 200/minute.

Dosage and administration

In a successful case, a maintenance dose of 300 mg 3 times a day may be continued for 1 month following conversion, and digitalis is discontinued. Similar doses are given for the treatment of paroxysmal tachycardia, but the daily dose is gradually reduced after the first week. Quinidine is of limited usefulness as it can only be given orally. It is rapidly cleared from the body; to extend its effectiveness, delayed absorption preparations are often employed.

Precautions

Quinidine is a potentially dangerous agent. It can cause sudden cardiovascular collapse in high doses. Partly because of this tendency and partly because of its unreliability, its use in converting atrial fibrillation into sinus rhythm has been given up in favour of d.c. shock conversion. Cinchonism is another side effect of quinidine therapy; symptoms include nausea and vomiting, blurred vision, headache, tinnitus and diarrhoea. Thrombocytopenia has also been reported.

Flecainide is a class 1 anti-arrhythmic agent whose predominant effect is to slow conduction through the bundle of His. Indications include Wolff–Parkinson–White syndrome and other syndromes with accessory conduction pathways and anterograde or retrograde conduction, A-V nodal reciprocating tachycardia, symptomatic sustained ventricular tachycardia and premature ventricular contractions resistant to other therapy.

The usual oral dose for maintenance is 200 mg twice daily. It may be given by injection, 2 mg/kg slowly over at least 10 minutes. It should not be given to patients with the 'sick sinus syndrome', second- or third-degree A-V block or bundle branch block unless emergency pacing is available. It affects endocardial pacing thresholds and should therefore be used with caution in all patients with pacemakers. The ECG may show prolongation of the P-R interval and widening of the QRS complex. The negative inotropic effect renders it potentially dangerous to patients in cardiac failure. It is contra-indicated in patients with a history of myocardial infarction or with severe ischaemic heart disease.

Mexiletine also has quinidine-like actions. It has been used to treat arrhythmias produced by cardiac glycosides and ventricular arrhythmias after myocardial infarction. A dose of 200 mg orally is given 3 times daily for at least 1 week. It is several days, usually, before a therapeutic effect is observed. The dose is then reduced weekly to a maintenance dose of 200 mg daily or on alternate days. Following the cessation of treatment, anti-arrhythmic effects persist for about 4 weeks. It may produce a bradycardia and a fall in blood pressure and can produce cerebellar toxicity, for example nystagmus and ataxia. There is also an intravenous formulation of the drug.

SOTALOL

Sotalol (rINN)

Pharmacology

Sotalol is a non-cardioselective β-adrenoceptor blocking agent with additional class 3 anti-arrhythmic activity.

Indications

It can be used for prevention or treatment of supraventricular and ventricular tachycardias. It should no longer be used for angina, hypertension, thyrotoxicosis or secondary prevention after myocardial hypertension.

Fate in the body   Sotalol is eliminated predominantly by renal excretion of unchanged drug.

Dosage and administration

By mouth, 80 mg/day in 1–2 divided doses, increasing gradually at 3-day intervals to 160–320 mg/day in 2 divided doses. Doses up to 640 mg/day are occasionally used under specialist supervision. By injection, for treatment of acute symptomatic arrhythmias, 20–120 mg is given over 10 minutes, at 6 h intervals.

Precautions

Sotalol may induce torsade de pointes arrhythmia in susceptible patients.

As with all β-blockers, and especially with the non-cardioselective ones, caution is necessary in the treatment of asthmatics and bronchitics, as there is a danger of producing bronchoconstriction. Bradycardia and hypotension may occur with effective β-blockade in patients with recent myocardial infarction. Heart failure may be made worse. The use of any β-blocker in diabetes mellitus will alter the requirement for hypoglycaemic drugs, and will make recognition of hypoglycaemia more difficult. Muscle pains and intermittent claudication may occur.

14

Diuretics

The composition of the body fluids, especially the blood, would vary widely unless the excretory mechanisms of the kidneys and lungs kept them in a constant state. The kidneys maintain the volume and composition of the extracellular fluid by excreting variable amounts of water and selectively eliminating Na, K, Cl, HPO_4 and SO_4 ions. Plasma concentrations of non-electrolytes such as urea, glucose and creatinine are also controlled, and waste products, drugs and toxic substances which enter the body are excreted.

With the assistance of the lungs, which eliminate carbonic acid as carbon dioxide, the kidneys maintain the hydrogen ion concentration of the blood by the excretion of non-volatile acid in the urine. By this mechanism they can normally dispose of 50 mEq of hydrogen ions a day. Renal tubular cells are also capable of synthesizing ammonia; this combines with hydrogen ions in the tubular fluid to form ammonium ions and can account for over 300 mEq of hydrogen ions a day.

Structure of the nephron

The kidney consists of units called nephrons which are composed of three functionally different parts, as follows:

1. the malpighian corpuscle, consisting of Bowman's capsule and the glomerulus, which acts as a filter;
2. the renal tubule, down which the filtrate passes, and which consists of three histologically different segments – the proximal tubule, the loop of Henle and the distal tubule;
3. the collecting tubule, which leads into larger ducts and thence into the pyramids.

The kidneys receive sympathetic innervation which is mainly distributed to the afferent arterioles in the cortex. No parasympathetic supply has been demonstrated.

The cortex is the site of production of renin, which is an essential component of the renin–angiotensin system which is concerned with sodium and water homeostasis. Renin is formed in the cells of the juxtaglomerular apparatus and is secreted whenever the perfusion pressure in the afferent arteriole falls and the arteriolar wall is not stretched.

The macula densa cells are well placed to sense the sodium and potassium content of the tubular fluid in the proximal end of the distal tubule and are thought to provide additional local input to the juxtaglomerular cells. The juxtaglomerular cells are also innervated by α-adrenergic sympathetic postganglionic fibres.

The blood flow to the cortex remains unchanged over a range of arterial blood pressure from 80 to 180 mmHg (10.7 to 21.0 kPa) in man. The much smaller flow to the medulla varies directly with perfusion pressure.

The glomerular filtrate

The renal blood flow, which under normal circumstances hardly varies, is considerable, and at about 1300 ml/minute may take as much as 25 per cent of the cardiac output. Plasma flow is in the region of 700 ml/minute and the glomerular filtrate is formed at a rate of about 120 ml/minute. The greater part of this large blood flow is required for the formation of urine; provided that the blood flow is not less than one-fifth of the normal (200–300 ml/minute), the oxygen requirements of the renal parenchyma are satisfied.

The glomerular filtrate has the same composition as the plasma except that substances with a molecular weight greater than 67 000 Da are retained so that, in health, minute amounts of serum albumin and no globulin are present. The volume of glomerular filtrate is dependent on the net effective filtration pressure. This is the difference between the positive hydrostatic pressure in the glomerular capillaries minus the sum of the oncotic pressure of the plasma proteins and the intratubular pressure. The intratubular pressure is 15–20 mmHg (2.0–2.7 kPa) in man, and for glomerular filtration to occur a net filtration pressure of approximately 55 mmHg (7.3 kPa) is necessary.

The effect of anaesthesia on various aspects of renal function is inconsistent; there is considerable variation both above and below control values, the most variable of all being the urinary output. In the postoperative period the usual finding is oliguria and this is due to the release of antidiuretic hormone by the posterior pituitary gland.

Modification of the glomerular filtrate

During its passage down the tubules the greater part of the filtrate is reabsorbed. Of the 170 litres produced in 24 h only 1.5 litres are excreted as urine. In order to excrete excess of acid from the body, carbonic acid in the tubular cell dissociates and the hydrogen ions are exchanged for sodium in the tubules and the sodium bicarbonate thus formed is returned to the blood; in states of alkalosis, however, large amounts of bicarbonate may be excreted. The glomerular filtrate, pH 7.4, resembles blood as it contains mainly dibasic sodium phosphate (Na_2HPO_4) but, through the action of carbonic anhydrase, hydrogen ions are exchanged for sodium and the urine thus becomes more acid as the amount of acid phosphate ($Na(HPO_4)_2$) increases and, for every hydrogen ion excreted, a bicarbonate ion is reabsorbed.

The kidney thus reduces the acidity of the blood both by the conversion of basic to acid phosphate and by forming ammonia from amino acids which combines with chloride ions in the tubules and is excreted as ammonium ions in the urine.

The pH of urine depends therefore on the pH of blood, which is controlled by the carbon dioxide : bicarbonate ratio, and this in turn is governed by the carbon dioxide tension in blood which regulates the rate of carbonic acid formation by carbonic anhydrase.

The proximal and distal tubules differ widely in their functions. About 80 per cent of the filtered sodium is reabsorbed actively (i.e. against an electrochemical gradient) in the proximal tubule; chloride ions are also actively absorbed. Water is passively reabsorbed as a result of removal of these ions from the tubular fluid. Ten per cent of the sodium is reabsorbed in the loops of Henle, and the remainder in the distal tubules and collecting ducts. The distal tubule effects an ion-exchange mechanism, sodium being exchanged for potassium and hydrogen ions. When there is a need to conserve sodium, this distal mechanism is so effective that the urine is virtually sodium free.

The passive reabsorption of 80 per cent of the filtered water is obligatory and occurs whatever the state of hydration of the patient. The isotonic fluid in the loops of Henle becomes hypotonic as a result of active reabsorption of sodium and chloride without water in the first part of the distal tubule, which is not permeable to water. If pituitary antidiuretic hormone is not acting on the distal tubules and collecting ducts, no further water is reabsorbed and hypotonic urine will result.

The action of antidiuretic hormone is to make the cells of the distal convoluted tubules and of the collecting ducts permeable to water. These parts of the nephron normally separate hypotonic tubular fluid from relatively hypertonic interstitial fluid; they behave as a waterproof membrane which is made temporarily permeable to water by the action of antidiuretic hormone. Extraction of water beyond that necessary to render urine iso-osmotic with plasma occurs in the collecting ducts which pass into the medulla. Medullary interstitial fluid is hypertonic due to accumulation of sodium and chloride derived by active transport from tubular fluid in the loops of Henle.

The control of the renal handling of the body's principal osmotically effective electrolytes, sodium and potassium, is to a great extent exerted by the adrenal cortico-steroid hormone, aldosterone. Numerous factors influence the release of this hormone – posture, the potassium content of the body, circulatory haemodynamics, and the sodium concentration of the blood perfusing the adrenal glands are among them. Aldosterone production and secretion are also stimulated by angiotensin, the level of which is determined by renin output from the juxtaglomerular cells. This mechanism is probably the most important controlling factor. Aldosterone has powerful sodium-retaining and potassium-excreting effects on renal tubular cells of the distal tubule. The daily output averages 200 µg and over 90 per cent of this is rapidly inactivated by the normal liver, the remainder appearing as a conjugate in the urine.

Action of diuretics

Diuretics are drugs that cause an increase in the output of urine. They are mainly employed in the treatment of hypertension and to reduce oedema and ascites in renal and congestive heart failure. They can produce a diuresis in five different ways:

1. by increasing the blood supply to the kidney;
2. by preventing tubular reabsorption of water by osmotic action;
3. by preventing the tubular reabsorption of sodium and, as a secondary effect of this, of chloride or bicarbonate ions which carry water with them;
4. by inhibiting the action of the hormones that play a part in the control of normal urine volume;
5. by inhibiting the production of aldosterone and cortisone by the adrenal cortex.

The commonly employed clinically useful diuretics all act at one or more of the sites where sodium is removed from the lumen of the nephron.

If the normal mechanism of urine formation, as outlined above, is studied it will be seen that little increase in output is possible by increasing blood flow, as it takes more than 100 ml of glomerular filtrate to produce 1 ml of urine. When the blood supply to the kidneys is impaired, however, as in congestive heart failure, a diuresis can often be produced by the use of digitalis alone. Aminophylline also produces a diuresis under these circumstances, but it is normally only a weak diuretic when used alone.

Various salts and crystalloids can produce an osmotic diuresis by retaining water in the distal tubules and collecting ducts. Present practice is confined to the use of mannitol, which is an undissociated crystalloid and is given intravenously. It can be given in sufficiently high concentration to cause a net water loss from the body. Such an osmotic diuresis can be induced despite the maximal operation of pituitary antidiuretic hormone, and mannitol will therefore produce large volumes of urine during and immediately after surgery. This type of diuresis is characterized by a high concentration and rate of excretion of the loading solute associated with a decrease in concentration of other solutes (chiefly sodium and potassium). However, the fall in concentration is more than offset by the increase in urine flow rate, so that other solutes tend to be lost from the body in slightly greater total amounts than would otherwise occur.

To be effective as an osmotic diuretic a substance should be rapidly and completely excreted in the glomeruli and not reabsorbed at all in the rest of the nephron. The smaller its molecular weight the more effective it will be: substances such as dextran 40 (1 mosmol = 40 g) cannot exert any significant osmotic effect even in very high urinary concentrations. It is also desirable that such a substance should be inert and not penetrate the body cells.

Mannitol is given in very hypertonic concentrations and therefore will cause extensive tissue necrosis if it leaks extravascularly. It causes a rapid expansion of the extracellular space with intracellular water, and therefore increases the plasma volume. Osmotic diuretics should not be used when this would be undesirable and, with the important exception of the use of mannitol to determine if intrinsic renal damage has occurred (see below), they should also be avoided whenever there is any doubt that the kidneys can excrete them.

The volume of water extracted from the body by these agents depends on many factors, but the urine osmolality resulting from their use is generally about twice that of plasma, that is, 500–700 mosmol/litre. In practice, the use of 100 g of mannitol in an adult who is normally hydrated will result in the excretion of approximately 1 litre of water more than would otherwise have been expected.

The most important group of diuretics is that which interferes with tubular reabsorption of sodium, chloride and bicarbonate ions. They belong to unrelated chemical groups and act at various sites in the tubular part of the nephron. They include mersalyl, acetazolamide, thiazides, loop diuretics and potassium-sparing diuretics. Of these, three groups are in general use:

1. The thiazides and other medium efficacy diuretics which act principally on the cortical diluting segment of the distal convoluted tubule causing a natriuresis equivalent to between 5 and 10 per cent of the sodium that is normally filtered.
2. The 'loop' diuretics, furosemide (frusemide), bumetanide and ethacrynic acid, which act principally on the ascending loop of Henle and have a high peak effect, equivalent to 30 per cent filtered sodium.
3. The potassium-sparing diuretics, spironolactone, amiloride and triamterene, which act on the distal renal tubule.

Although not used for the purpose, renal function can be affected by blocking the production of aldosterone and cortisone by the adrenal cortex with metyrapone.

An important side effect of all diuretic drugs is the alteration they produce in the renal excretion of potassium. The normal driving force for potassium secretion by the distal tubule is the transtubular electrical potential difference created by sodium reabsorption. Most diuretics allow higher concentrations of sodium to reach the distal tubule and this increased sodium reabsorption stimulates secretion of potassium. Thiazide diuretics cause a small loss of potassium; in terms of whole body potassium this loss is not important and serum potassium concentrations, although reduced, rarely fall below 3.3 mmol/litre. Hypertensive patients tend to lose more potassium than patients in cardiac failure, in whom it might be clinically more significant. Unless there are reasons for avoiding even mild hypokalaemia, there is no reason to give simultaneous oral potassium supplements. Spironolactone, amiloride and triamterene when added to a thiazide diuretic reduce the potassium loss to a considerable extent. Given alone they are thus associated with only a slightly lower loss of potassium than other diuretics. However, when other sodium-losing diuretics are given simultaneously, or when potassium loss is associated with increased aldosterone activity, the reduction in potassium loss is marked. The administration of potassium as Slow-K tablets (32 mEq, or 4 tablets daily) will reverse any deficits.

MONOGRAPHS

ACETAZOLAMIDE

Acetazolamide (rINN)

Pharmacology

Acetazolamide is an inhibitor of carbonic anhydrase. This results in diminished production of hydrogen ions by the tubules, which are therefore not available for exchange with sodium ions in the distal tubular fluid; there is an inverse association between hydrogen and potassium ion excretion in the distal tubules so that potassium is excreted in greater amounts together with bicarbonate ions.

The net result is a metabolic acidosis with retention of chloride ions. This is the opposite effect to that resulting from mercurial diuretics; consequently the two drugs were often given alternately.

Indications

This drug is now only used for its effects on intraocular pressure; it is used in the treatment of glaucoma and preoperatively to reduce intraocular pressure.

Dosage and administration

Acetazolamide is given orally or intravenously, 250 mg–1 g/24 h. As its action lasts about 12 h, it is best given in the morning. Overdosage may cause drowsiness or paraesthesia.

FUROSEMIDE (FRUSEMIDE)

Furosemide (rINN)

Pharmacology

Furosemide (frusemide), although a sulphonamide derivative and thus having certain structural similarities to the thiazides, does not resemble them closely either chemically or pharmacologically. Its action is to prevent sodium and chloride reabsorption in the proximal and first part of the distal tubule and in the ascending limb of the loop of Henle. An important consequence of this is that the osmolarity of the renal medulla is reduced. Thus free water clearance is almost always increased and unlike the thiazides it produces a hypotonic urine in which the sodium ion concentration is lower than that of the plasma. There is, therefore, less stimulus to the induction of hyperaldosteronism. It is unaffected by disturbances of acid-base balance, and in large doses will tend to produce a hypochloraemic alkalosis. The ion-exchange mechanism in the distal tubule is not affected and therefore potassium loss is increased, although to a lesser extent than with the thiazides; the natriuresis may be enhanced and the potassium loss diminished by the addition of spironolactone or amiloride.

The response to furosemide is proportional to the glomerular filtration rate (GFR) over a wide range, whereas the response to the thiazides is unaltered for GFR above 20 ml/minute. The GFR is transiently raised in cases of poor renal function by the former. Larger doses may, therefore, need to be given in the presence of low GFR, and large doses may be used in the diagnosis of suspected renal failure. The plasma uric acid level is increased and although it has been claimed that furosemide does not impair glucose tolerance, a few cases of diabetes have presented following therapy.

A mild hypotensive effect similar to that of the thiazides, affecting both supine and standing blood pressures, has occasionally been noted.

Absorption and excretion   The onset of action following intravenous injection occurs within 2–3 minutes, while oral therapy produces a peak diuresis in 1 h with a total duration of 4–6 h. Excretion occurs rapidly by filtration and tubular secretion.

Indications

Furosemide is particularly of value by intravenous injection in the emergency treatment of acute pulmonary oedema, and in the preparation of patients with congestive cardiac failure for surgery. In view of its potency, it is otherwise usually reserved for cases resistant to milder diuretics. It is effective in all forms of refractory oedema, whether of cardiac, renal or hepatic origin. It is of limited value in cases with poor renal function.

Dosage and administration

The initial dose is usually 40–80 mg given orally on alternate days or on 3 consecutive days a week. This may be increased to 120 mg daily. In cases very resistant to treatment, attempts have been made to produce a diuresis with amounts of up to 500 mg daily. The danger of electrolyte disturbances with low dosage is not marked, although in patients likely to be sensitive to even mild hypokalaemia, potassium chloride supplements and biochemical control are essential. The addition of spironolactone has resulted in a satisfactory diuresis in cases previously resistant to furosemide alone. As in the treatment of all cases of oedema, some restriction of sodium intake is important if benefit is to be gained.

For immediate response, 40 mg may be given intravenously or intramuscularly and repeated in 20 minutes.

Precautions

Apart from the occurrence of transient diarrhoea and the rare reports of reversible thrombocytopenia and leucopenia, the only side effects have resulted from electrolyte disorders.

These can be severe: the potency of this drug is such that 40 per cent of the glomerular filtrate can be excreted as urine, and severe water and electrolyte disturbances can occur. Contra-indications include anuria, hepatic coma and electrolyte deficiencies. It should only be used in early pregnancy with great caution. Large doses may be associated with ototoxicity.

Ethacrynic acid, although chemically unrelated to any other diuretic, has pharmacological actions closely resembling those of furosemide. It was originally thought that its cellular mechanism of action was a combination with sulphydryl groups in the kidney, blocking sodium transport. This, however, would not explain the inhibition of chloride absorption or the fact that furosemide and bumetanide do not share this property.

The indications and precautions are the same as for furosemide. The dose of ethacrynic acid is 50–200 mg daily, usually on 3 days of the week. The addition of a potassium-sparing diuretic or spirono-lactone will reduce potassium loss. In emergencies, 50 mg may be given by intravenous injection.

Bumetanide is another powerful loop diuretic, chemically unrelated to any other diuretic. Its site of action is also on the proximal convoluted tubule, ascending limb of the loop of Henle and the first part of the distal convoluted tubule, where active sodium and chloride absorption is inhibited. It thus closely resembles furosemide in its actions, differing only in its milligram potency, 1 mg being equivalent to 40 mg of furosemide.

MANNITOL

Mannitol (rINN)

Mannitol is an undissociated crystalloid alcohol and is an effective osmotic diuretic. It is completely filtered at the glomerulus and none is reabsorbed; it is inert in the body and does not penetrate the cells.

Indications

Mannitol is used to reduce the brain volume in cerebral oedema, and in the prevention of acute renal failure, for which purpose its use is now well established, and to increase the excretion of drugs. It is also believed to protect the kidneys against damage by certain nephrotoxins. Thus it is indicated in mismatched blood transfusions and in poisoning with carbon tetrachloride and ethylene glycol.

Dosage and administration

Mannitol is normally given intravenously in 10 or 20 per cent solutions in a dose of 0.5–1 g/kg. A 25 per cent supersaturated solution can be prepared, but there is little to be gained by using this as it has to be kept above room temperature to remain in solution. Its use in forced diuresis is discussed on page 91. The above dose of mannitol may be given during surgical operations to all cases in whom the risk of acute renal failure is known to be high. The most common instance of this is in operations for the relief of severe obstructive jaundice when mannitol should always be given.

Suspected intrinsic renal failure   One of the most difficult problems in intensive care units is to determine when extra-renal causes of oliguria have caused intrinsic renal damage.

When the urine volume is less than 20 ml/h and the provoking incident has occurred less than 48 h beforehand, the following regimen may be employed. Three doses of 100 ml of 20 per cent mannitol are given, each dose being given in 10–20 minutes and at 2-hourly intervals. If a urine volume of at least 50 ml/h is established, the oliguria is unlikely to recur; if no diuresis results, fluids must be restricted to 400–500 ml/day plus measured losses and no more mannitol given.

Precautions

As with all hypertonic solutions, care must be taken to ensure that there is no extravascular leakage. Giving sets should either be flushed with isotonic saline or changed when mannitol is followed by blood. Mannitol should not be given more rapidly than 3 g/minute.

Urea is another undissociated crystalloid and is an effective osmotic diuretic, but it is highly diffusible and has a small molecule so that over 60 per cent of urea filtered at the glomerulus is reabsorbed in the remainder of the nephron. Urea therefore recirculates and gradually penetrates the cells to equilibrate across the cell membrane. For this reason its use has been largely abandoned.

SPIRONOLACTONE

Spironolactone (rINN)

Pharmacology

Spironolactone blocks the action of aldosterone on the distal tubule and prevents the reabsorption of sodium and accompanying chloride at this site. Reabsorption of potassium is increased. It is not a powerful diuretic when used alone but acts synergistically with other diuretics. It is most active when aldosterone is present in excess. When used with diuretics that cause excessive loss of potassium, potassium supplements are usually unnecessary.

Indications

Spironolactone is used in oedematous conditions associated with congestive cardiac failure, ascites and the nephrotic syndrome. It is especially useful in the management of secondary aldosteronism.

Dosage and administration

Spironolactone is readily absorbed from the intestinal tract. It is normally given in tablet form, 25 mg 4 times a day. Larger doses are occasionally required. It has a cumulative action and may take several days to exert its full effect. It is usually given in conjunction with another diuretic.

Precautions

Side effects are infrequent. Drowsiness, mental confusion and erythematous skin eruptions have been reported on rare occasions. It should be used with caution in patients whose serum potassium levels are raised.

THIAZIDES

Pharmacology

Chlorothiazide was the first of a number of benzothiadiazine derivatives which have similar properties. Subsequently a number of other thiazide analogues have been introduced, but in optimal dosage they all have a similar effect on sodium excretion. Bendroflumethazide (bendrofluazide), cyclopenthiazide and hydroflumethiazide are at present the most commonly prescribed drugs in this group now on the market, largely on cost grounds. Other drugs with similar properties include chlortalidone, clopamide, mefruside, metolazone, indapamide and xipamide. These drugs all act on the cortical diluting segment of the distal convoluted tubule, causing a natriuresis of up to 10 per cent of the filtered sodium. They also have a weak inhibitory effect on carbonic anhydrase; this increases the bicarbonate and potassium excretion into the distal tubular fluid in the same manner as does acetazolamide.

The loss of potassium that occurs does not normally require a supplement to make up for the deficiency, although the serum level is usually reduced. However, relative to the body as a whole, the loss is not a major one. The loss of sodium and chloride results in an increase in urinary volume. Recently it has become recognized that thiazide diuretics reduce arterial blood pressure by a direct action independent of the long-recognized effects of sodium depletion and the resultant fall in circulating blood volume. This is thought to be due to a direct effect on peripheral circulatory tone. In consequence they may be sufficient to control moderate hypertension, particularly in the elderly. The dose necessary to produce this hypotensive effect is smaller than that required for the relief of oedema and does not usually result in potassium depletion.

Thiazide diuretics have a paradoxical effect on patients suffering from diabetes insipidus in whom they effectively reduce the urine volume. They reduce free water clearance and thus tend to lower serum osmolarity. It is thought that the effect of this is to lessen the sensation of thirst and so reduce the water intake.

Diabetes mellitus may be provoked by prolonged treatment with thiazide drugs in patients who are latent diabetics. These drugs also provoke a rise in serum uric acid and may precipitate gout.

Absorption and excretion   After oral administration, maximum effect is obtained in about 4 h, with onset of action within 2 h, and these drugs are rapidly eliminated by the kidney. The duration of action varies between 12 and 72 h, but all have the desired therapeutic action with once-a-day administration.

Indications

Thiazide diuretics are used widely in the treatment of hypertension and for the relief of oedema in mild cardiac failure; they are used less often in other oedamatous states, for nephrogenic diabetes insipidus, and for prophylaxis against renal stones.

Dosage and administration

These drugs are usually given daily. The various drugs differ on a weight-for-weight basis but as there is no significant difference between them, there is no reason not to give the cheapest. At the time of writing this is bendroflumethazide. The relative potencies are as follows:

Bendroflumethazide (bendrofluazide)	2.5–5 mg
Chlorothiazide	0.5–1 g
Chlortalidone	50–100 mg
Clopamide	20–40 mg
Cyclopenthiazide	0.25–1 mg
Hydrochlorothiazide	50–100 mg
Hydroflumethiazide	25–50 mg
Indapamide	2.5 mg
Mefruside	25–50 mg
Methylclothiazide	2.5–5 mg
Metolazone	5–10 mg
Xipamide	20–40 mg

Potassium loss can be reduced by combining thiazide and spironolactone or amiloride therapy.

Precautions

Side effects are infrequent, nausea being the commonest, and this can usually be overcome by taking the drug after food. Rarely a skin rash or purpura may be seen.

Thiazides, in common with other antihypertensives, may cause impotence. They tend to potentiate the action of digitalis, and the dose of digitalis may therefore need to be reduced should anorexia, nausea, vomiting or bradycardia occur. Metabolic abnormalities, hypokalaemia, hyperuricaemia, glucose intolerance, hypercalcaemia, raised serum cholesterol levels and reduction in high-density lipoproteins have been cited as potentially prognostically adverse, but the benefits of treatment seem to outweigh these theoretical hazards.

When used for the treatment of hypertension, the dose of other hypotensive drugs can often be reduced by 25–50 per cent. Although routine administration of potassium supplements is no longer regarded as necessary, it is important to identify patients in whom even moderate reductions may prove a hazard. These include those with arhythmias, myocardial infarction, severe ischaemic heart disease or chronic liver disease, and patients on a poor diet, or taking digoxin, corticosteroids, carbenoxolone or drugs that interfere with ventricular repolarization, such as tricyclic antidepressants and phenothiazines. Oral potassium may not be sufficient in these circumstances and combination with a potassium-sparing diuretic is to be preferred. Loss of potassium may cause malaise, apathy, weakness and loss of deep tendon reflexes.

TRIAMTERENE

Triamterene (rINN)

Triamterene is a pteridine derivative and is chemically unrelated to other diuretics. It increases the excretion of sodium and depresses that of potassium by a direct action on the distal tubule where it diminishes sodium absorption. Bicarbonate excretion is increased and the pH of the urine is raised. Uric acid excretion is also increased. Further evidence that it acts in a different way to the thiazides or spironolactone is provided by the fact that, when it is given with these drugs together in full doses, its effect is additive.

Triamterene has a weaker natriuretic action than the thiazides, but it can be usefully employed with them when it will mitigate the extent of the potassium loss which would otherwise occur.

The potassium-sparing action is probably an indirect one: the driving force for potassium secretion by the distal tubule is the transtubular electrical potential difference created by the sodium reabsorption which occurs at this site. This sodium reabsorption is inhibited by triamterene, but the effect is magnified when larger quantities of sodium are reaching the distal tubule as a consequence of diuretic action elsewhere in the nephron. It cannot, however, wholly prevent some potassium loss when potent loop diuretics such as furosemide are employed. Toxic effects appear to be minimal, but diarrhoea may occur following large doses. Nausea and vomiting have also been reported.

Absorption and excretion Triamterene is well absorbed after oral administration and can be detected in the urine in 15–20 minutes. It is excreted partly unchanged and partly in the form of metabolites. Excretion reaches a peak in 6–8 h.

Indications

Triamterene may be used in the treatment of oedema associated with congestive heart failure, cirrhosis of the liver, nephrotic syndrome, and idiopathic and drug-induced oedema. It is more commonly used with a thiazide diuretic, as it is less effective when used alone.

Dosage and administration

Triamterene 50 mg in capsule form twice daily is usually sufficient, but up to 200 mg a day may be required.

Amiloride hydrochloride is a potassium-sparing diuretic whose actions closely resemble those of triamterene. The primary action is on the distal convoluted tubule which results in a small increase in the excretion of sodium, chloride and hydrogen ions. There is either no or only a small loss of potassium. This effect is most striking when it is given in combination with another saluretic agent. Amiloride is incompletely absorbed from the gastro-intestinal tract. It achieves its peak concentration between 3 and 4 h after oral administration. The majority is excreted unchanged through the kidney.

Amiloride may be used for the treatment of all kinds of oedema. It is generally combined with a thiazide which enhances its potassium-sparing effect. The normal daily dose is 10 mg orally in divided doses, rising to a maximum of 2 mg daily. Potassium supplements should be avoided.

Side effects are usually minor. However, postural hypotension has been reported and occasionally hyperkalaemia. Rarely, liver function tests have shown changes.

15

Drugs acting on the uterus

Uterine muscle

Uterine muscle shows spontaneous intermittent activity throughout reproductive life. Unlike the heart there is no pacemaker and the contraction process spreads from one cell to another at a rate of 1–3 cm/s, usually starting in the cornual regions. A and B types of contraction have been designated, the former occurring frequently and with low amplitude and the latter being of higher amplitude and more infrequent. B waves are usually called Braxton Hicks' contractions and become more frequent as pregnancy advances. The contractions of labour result in a peak of intra-uterine pressure during the first stage of 40–60 mmHg (5.3–8 kPa), rising to 60–80 mmHg (8–10.7 kPa) in the second stage. The resting uterine pressure in labour is approximately 10 mmHg (1.3 kPa). The cervix has some muscle in it, but takes no part in the expulsive contractions.

Uterine stimulants

Uterine stimulants may be classified as general and specific. Of the general uterine stimulants the local hormones predominate, including bradykinin, histamine, acetylcholine, norepinehrine (noradrenaline) and 5-hydroxytryptamine. The depolarizing relaxants have no demonstrable action on the uterine muscle.

The specific uterine stimulants are the ergot alkaloids, oxytocin, and synthetic derivative prostaglandins E_2 and $F_{2\alpha}$.

Tocolytic agents

Tocolytic agents are substances that inhibit uterine activity. They are mainly used during premature labour to inhibit uterine contractions for a sufficiently long period of time to allow delivery of a viable baby. Occasionally during labour, uterine contractions are so intense as to seriously impair placental blood flow, with resultant severe fetal asphyxia. Under these circumstances a tocolytic agent may be given to inhibit uterine activity for sufficiently long to allow rapid delivery.

β_2-adrenoceptor agonists

All β_2-agonist drugs will relax the uterus, but attempts to find such agents that are specific to the uterus have so far failed. The commonest employed to cause uterine relaxation are ritodrine and salbutamol, but other drugs used for this purpose are orciprenaline, terbutaline, isoxuprine and feneterol. These drugs also act on the smooth muscle of the bronchioles and arterioles. By combining with β_2-receptors they activate the adenylcyclase system, increasing the levels of a cAMP. Increases in this reduce the level of intracellular calcium which diminishes myosin light-chain kinase activity resulting in a reduction in actin–myosin interaction and a consequent muscle relaxation.

Adverse effects

Because of their action at β_2-receptors other than at those in the uterus, these drugs are associated with a number of other effects that are unpleasant to the mother and some of which are potentially serious and even life-threatening:

- Vasodilatation, with widening of the pulse pressure, leads to a tendency to hypotension with a compensatory tachycardia.
- Fluid retention results from the vasodilatation with a possible decrease in colloid osmotic pressure.
- Stimulation of glycogenolysis increases the blood sugar and an increase in insulin secretion, which can cause fetal hypoglycaemia.
- Intracellular potassium increases because of effects on the sodium/potassium pump, and therefore hypokalaemia is invariable.
- Increasing the dose of β_2-agonist increases the degree of uterine relaxation, but β_1 effects also begin to appear. This results in increased myocardial contractility, heart rate and cardiac output, which is superimposed on the already raised cardiac output of pregnancy.
- Arrhythmias may occur and the increased myocardial oxygen demands can outstrip the oxygen supply with resultant angina and ST depression, even in previously healthy women.
- Pulmonary oedema has been reported on numerous occasions in women receiving β_2-agonist therapy to prevent premature labour and delivery. The cause is usually cited as myocardial failure secondary to fluid overload.

Anaesthestic procedures in these patients must avoid anything that might increase sympathetic activity, such as too light anaesthesia, administration of ketamine, pancuronium, ephedrine and any drugs that will increase heart rate such as atropine or glycopyrrolate.

General anaesthetics

All volatile anaesthetic agents, particularly halothane, relax the uterus in a concentration-dependent manner. Administration of general anaesthesia in labour in those with intense uterine activity or tetany will produce uterine relaxation and improve placental blood flow until the baby can be operatively delivered. General anaesthesia can also be used to produce uterine relaxation in the presence of contraction rings and to aid delivery of the placenta.

Ethanol

Ethanol was one of the first substances used in the prevention of premature labour. It acts centrally by inhibiting the release of oxytocin. There is a high incidence of headache, nausea and vomiting and hence has rarely been used for this purpose.

Magnesium

Magnesium sulphate acts by preventing an increase in intracellular calcium and hence relaxes uterine muscle. Although used in the management of pre-eclampsia, it is rarely used as a tocolytic agent.

Nitric oxide

Nitric oxide is being increasingly implicated in many physiological processes and as part of the actions of many drugs. Its smooth muscle-relaxant properties are well documented and release of nitric oxide is the mechanism by which the nitrite group of drugs elicit their action. Recently, use has been made of the smooth muscle-relaxant properties of nitric oxide in the management of premature labour. The nitric oxide binds to the haem moiety of guanylate cyclase and this causes an increase in cyclic guanosine monophosphate (c-GMP) which in turn decreases intracellular calcium concentration resulting in muscle relaxation.

The nitric oxide is usually administered in the form of a patch of glyceryl trinitrate applied to the abdominal wall. Investigations into this method of inhibiting uterine activity are at a very early stage and its eventual place in clinical practice remains to be elucidated.

MONOGRAPHS

ERGOMETRINE

Ergometrine maleate (rINN), Ergonvine maleate (USP)

Ergometrine was originally obtained from ergot (*Claviceps purpurea*). It is an amine alkaloid and is now prepared by chemical synthesis. It may also be combined in a dose of 0.5 mg with 5 i.u. of syntocinon to form syntometrine.

Pharmacology

Ergometrine exerts its action as a result of α-adrenoceptor stimulation and its main effect is to induce contraction of uterine smooth muscle. Its action is rapid, coming on within 2–3 minutes after intramuscular injection and within 30 s of intravenous injection. The contractile effect on the uterus is dose dependent, with a steep dose–response curve. The gravid uterus is much more susceptible to its effects. If given during the first stage of labour, it leads to violent, abnormal contractions and uterine tetany may result with no intervening periods of relaxation. During these contractions the spiral arteries are compressed, leading to a marked reduction in uterine and consequently placental blood flow. In the third stage of labour, ergometrine causes sustained uterine contractions with superimposed irregular contractions.

Ergometrine also causes a constriction of vascular smooth muscle which results in an increase in central venous pressure and systemic arterial pressure that may persist for several hours. Vomiting is common after intravenous use, probably due to a direct action on the vomiting centre.

Ergometrine is used to promote uterine contraction and hence to prevent or treat post-partum haemorrhage following delivery or abortion. It has also been given intramuscularly with delivery of the anterior shoulder in order to prevent post-partum haemorrhage. This should be done only under strict obstetric supervision and must not be used in the presence of multiple gestation except at delivery of the last baby.

Fate in the body Ergometrine is metabolized mainly in the liver by hydroxylation and glucoronidation; a small amount is excreted unchanged.

Dosage and administration

It is usually given in a dose of 0.2–1.0 mg intramuscularly or 0.25–0.5 mg intravenously. It may be given directly into the uterine muscle at Caesarean section, after delivery of the baby.

Precautions

Ergometrine must never be used before delivery of the infant as even small doses may result in a tetanic contraction of the uterus with a marked reduction in placental blood flow. It should be avoided in patients with pregnancy-induced hypertension from any cause and in those with, or with a prior history of, arteriovenous malformations. Ergometrine may cause spasm of coronary arteries and it must be avoided in patients with any evidence of myocardial ischaemia; it should be used with caution in patients with other types of heart disease. Prolonged use can cause signs of ergotism. Ergometrine should not be given intravenously to conscious patients after delivery under regional anaesthesia because of its propensity to cause vomiting. It should be avoided in patients with peripheral vascular disease. Great care must be taken if it is given together with other sympathomimetic drugs.

OXYTOCIN

Syntocinon (rINN)

Oxytocin is a naturally-occurring nonapeptide produced in the hypothalamus. Chemical name: 3-isoleucine-8-leucine vasopressin. All the amino acids are in the L-form. It can be extracted from the posterior pituitary of mammals, but nowadays is prepared commercially by chemical synthesis and is known as syntocinon.

Oxytocin is synthesized in nerve cells in the supra-optic and paraventricular nuclei of the hypothalamus. It travels in secretory granules along the axons to the posterior pituitary gland where it is stored. It is secreted independently of the antidiuretic hormone (argenine vasopressin). Early oxytocic preparations contained vasopressin as a contaminant and as a result there was contraction of smooth muscle and an increase in blood pressure; vasopressin also causes constriction of coronary vessels. Syntocinon, the synthetic preparation of oxytocin that is now used, contains no vasopressin. A unit of oxytocin is equivalent to 2 µg of the pure hormone.

Pharmacology

Oxytocin acts on specific receptors in the uterus, causing an influx of sodium and calcium ions, lowering the transmembrane potential, with resultant myometrial contraction. Whether or not oxytocin elicits a response depends on the presence or absence of pregnancy, the duration of the latter and the relative balance between oestrogen and progesterone. As the former level increases so do the number of receptors in the uterus and hence the sensitivity to oxytocin. Thus, as pregnancy progresses the uterus becomes increasingly sensitive to the action of oxytocin. Significantly greater doses of oxytocin are required to produce a response in early pregnancy. The contractions produced by oxytocin in the full-term uterus are indistinguishable from those of normal labour. High doses of syntocinon may result in the uterus failing to relax completely between contractions.

Suckling causes an immediate release of oxytocin which binds to myoepithelial cells in the breast, causing milk to flow in the larger ducts.

A bolus injection of syntocinon relaxes vascular smooth muscle and there is a resultant decrease in peripheral resistance with a slight fall in arterial blood pressure and central venous pressure, and a reflex tachycardia. Large doses may cause an increase in arterial blood pressure. Infusions of syntocinon have little cardiovascular effect.

Because of its structural similarity to vasopressin, oxytocin possesses weak antidiuretic properties.

Indications

Syntocinon is used by continuous infusion to induce labour or to augment spontaneous labour. It is given by continuous infusion with close monitoring of uterine activity and fetal heart rate. The dose varies from 0.1 to 8 units/h and must be titrated to effect. Its use is preferable to ergometrine for the prevention of post-partum haemorrhage after delivery under regional anaesthesia.

Syntocinon can also be administered as a nasal spray and a buccal form is also available. Absorption by these methods may be rapid but unreliable and their use not recommended. A combined injection of 5 units of syntocinon and 0.5 mg ergometrine is available which can be used to prevent post-partum haemorrhage. The preparation (syntometrine) contains the maximum recommended dose of each drug and care must be taken in its use.

PROSTAGLANDINS

Chemical structure: prostaglandin is a generic term for a group of polyunsaturated fatty acids (*Figure 15.1*). The molecule contains a cyclopentane ring and two side chains. The configuration of the five-membered ring (in dotted box) determines the group; subscript numbers (for example, E_2, F_1) indicate progressive degrees of unsaturation of the fatty acid side chain (1 = least, and so on). There are six major groups, designated E, F, A, B, C and D. Their synthesis from phospholipids is described on page 425.

Pharmacology

The biological activity of the prostaglandins was discovered by von Euler in 1936. They have diverse actions on many systems (see page 424). These include stimulation of smooth muscle and lowering of blood pressure. They affect blood clotting and intra-ocular pressure and play a role in the inflammatory processes. Prostaglandins are present in many human organs, with the highest concentration in seminal fluid; blood levels are very low. They are estimated by bioassay, but immunoassay for certain members of the group is now available and is more sensitive and specific.

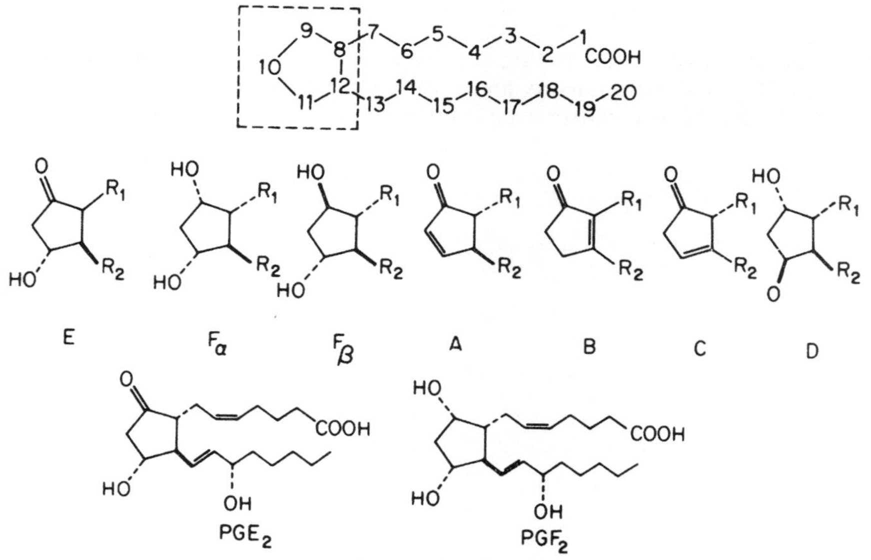

Figure 15.1 Basic ring structures of the prostaglandins series

PGE$_2$ and PGF$_{2\alpha}$ are now used clinically for their stimulant action on the uterus. As with oxytocin, the uterus in early pregnancy is less sensitive than at term. PGE$_2$ appears to be superior to PGF$_{2\alpha}$ as a stimulant throughout pregnancy, and has fewer side effects.

Intra-uterine administration has been used for induction of abortion without significant side effects and in greatly reduced dosage.

Ninety per cent of prostaglandins are believed to be inactivated in passage through the pulmonary circulation and this is the reason for the higher doses needed by the intravenous route.

Indications

PGE$_2$ and PGF$_{2\alpha}$, are used for the induction of abortion and for the induction of labour.

Dosage and administration

They may be given by the oral, intravenous or intra-uterine routes. The intra-uterine is the most effective and the oral the least effective route.

Labour may be induced at term by a single oral dose of 5 mg of PGE$_2$ or 5 mg of PGF$_{2\alpha}$. Contractions are stimulated in 5–15 minutes and continue for 2–3 h. In early pregnancy the oral route is ineffective in inducing abortion without significant side effects.

Labour can be induced by intravenous infusion of 0.5–2 µg/minute of PGE$_2$ or PGF$_{2\alpha}$ up to a dose of 600 µg. In early pregnancy, doses of 2–5 µg/minute up to a total dose of 2500–4000 µg may be needed.

By the intra-uterine route, smaller doses have been used to produce abortion in early pregnancy. This route is not used to induce labour at term.

Toxic effects

Significant nausea, diarrhoea, vomiting and fever, which are dose dependent, have been noted with $PGF_{2\alpha}$, and this limits its use in early pregnancy by the oral or intravenous route. Phlebitis has been noted in a high proportion of patients receiving intravenous infusions of PGE_2.

16

Chemical transmitters and enzymes

Chemical transmitters

To a considerable extent the functions of cells and tissues are controlled by a large variety of chemicals and specific receptors. Those that are secreted by specialized organs and exert their effects on various remote tissues are called hormones and are discussed fully in Chapter 17.

Much voluntary and reflex activity is controlled by the release of chemical substances in response to nerve impulses at nerve endings both within the nervous system and at blood vessels. The commonest of these are acetylcholine and norepinephrine (noradrenaline), which are discussed in Chapters 10 and 12, but within the CNS other agents such as γ-aminobutyric acid, dopamine, 5-hydroxytryptamine (5-HT), and probably many others function as transmitters at certain synapses.

Autacoids

An important group of chemical transmitters consists of those substances that act locally at the site of liberation in inflammatory or allergic reactions, and via the circulation may reach distant sites where they can also have important actions. A substance in this category is histamine which acts locally at its site of liberation in allergic reactions, and can reach the circulation and act at a distance to increase gastric secretion. When histamine is liberated by tissue injury, by drugs or by chemical transmitters such as epinephrine (adrenaline), heparin which increases the clotting time of blood is often also released. Histamine and its antagonists at various sites are considered in detail in Chapter 8.

Histamine, therefore, is an example of an autacoid (Greek, *autos* – self, and *akos* – medicine) or local hormone. Other substances that also have intense pharmacological actions at the site of release include the prostaglandins, 5-HT, angiotensin and the various kinins.

Prostaglandins

Prostaglandins (PGs) are a group of long-chain fatty acids derived from a 20-carbon compound, prostanoic acid. Their basic ring structures are shown in *Figure 15.1*, page 421. These substances are present in most mammalian tissues which have the capacity to synthesize them from precursors. They have numerous and diverse effects and the pattern

Table 16.1 Fatty acid precursors of prostaglandins

Precursor	Prostaglandin	
Dihomo-γ-linoleic acid	PGE_1	PGF_1
Arachidonic acid	PGE_2	PGF_2
Eicosapentaenoic acid	PGE_3	PGF_3

of their actions varies widely between the different members of the group. Generally they are potent vasodilators, although PGF_α is a vasoconstrictor of pulmonary arteries and veins. Capillary permeability is always increased. Prostaglandins have effects on most other types of smooth muscle. For example, PGFs contract bronchial and tracheal muscle in man, particularly in asthmatics. However, PGEs are potent bronchodilators with a potency greater than that of isoprenaline when given by aerosol. Their actions on uterine muscle are discussed in Chapter 15.

Gastric, pancreatic and intestinal secretions are inhibited by PGEs and PGA, probably by a direct effect on the secretory cells. This may prove to be of therapeutic use.

Prostaglandins are released by a wide variety of physicochemical insults; their role in acute and chronic inflammation, particularly in the eye and in arthritis, is well established. The ability of aspirin-type drugs to block the synthesis of prostaglandins seems to be crucial both to their effectiveness as anti-inflammatory agents and their adverse effects.

Prostaglandins are synthesized from 20-carbon polyunsaturated fatty acids present in the phospholipids of cell membranes. There are three precursors (*Table 16.1*), but those derived from arachidonic acid are by far the most important. Arachidonic acid in the cell membrane is derived from linoleic acid found in vegetables, or from arachidonic acid found in meat.

A key enzyme in arachidonic acid metabolism is phospholipase A_2. Chemical or mechanical stimulation of cell membranes activates this enzyme, which then releases arachidonic acid from membrane phospholipids. Arachidonic acid can then be converted via two distinct main pathways (*Figure 16.1*). Lipoxygenases, which have been found in platelets, lungs and white cells, can attack it, resulting in hydroperoxy-arachidonic acids. These are unstable compounds. In the other pathway, cyclo-oxygenase (present in cell membranes) catalyses the formation of an unstable cyclic endoperoxide, PGG_2. PGG_2 is converted rapidly into PGH_2 which in turn is converted to more stable prostaglandins PGE_2, PGF_2 and PGD_2. The half-life of both PGG_2 and PGH_2 is about 5 minutes at 37°C. The prostaglandin endoperoxides are also transformed by other enzymes, prostacyclin synthetase and thromboxane synthetase, into prostacyclin (PGI_2) (now called epoprostenol) and thromboxane A_2, respectively. These in turn are converted to 6-oxo-$PGF_{I\alpha}$ and thromboxane B_2.

Platelet aggregation

Thromboxane A_2 is a potent aggregator of platelets. In contrast, epoprostenol is a potent anti-aggregator of platelets, and is now used therapeutically in the prevention of clotting during haemodialysis. The explanation may lie in the fact that thromboxane A_2 reduces the concentration of cyclic AMP inside platelets, thereby increasing platelet adhesiveness, whereas epoprostenol increases cyclic AMP concentration. Aspirin and related NSAID

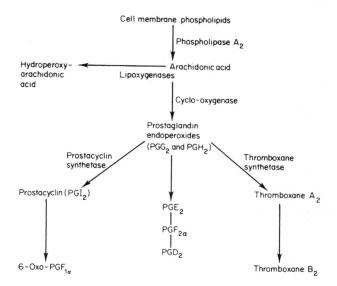

Figure 16.1 Arachidonic acid metabolism

analgesics inhibit cyclo-oxygenase and thereby should theoretically reduce both epoprostenol and thromboxane A_2 levels. Indeed, aspirin has been reported to reduce platelet thromboxane A_2 levels and epoprostenol formation in arterial intima. However, the dose required for each inhibition is different. Thus in theory selective depression of thromboxane A_2 formation is possible and this could have therapeutic potential in the prevention of thrombo-embolic disease. Another possible approach to this problem is the use of specific thromboxane synthetase inhibitors such as imidazole. However, this last drug is too toxic and not sufficiently specific; more specific and less toxic substances may appear in the next few years.

An alternative approach to the therapy of thrombo-embolism is to use epoprostenol or a derivative. Epoprostenol is crucial to maintaining the integrity of the vascular endothelium; the arterial intima synthesizes epoprostenol and this inhibits platelet aggregation. Platelets near the intimal wall may be the source of prostaglandin endoperoxide which the endothelial cells use to generate epoprostenol. When the intima is damaged, less epoprostenol is produced since the concentration of prostaglandin synthetase decreases as one moves from the intima to the adventitia. This would leave the prostaglandin endoperoxides available for conversion to thromboxane A_2 leading to aggregation (*Figure 16.2*). This local control of platelet aggregability could explain why thrombosis occurs in artificial grafts unless they become coated with endothelium which secretes epoprostenol. Lipid peroxides are known to inhibit epoprostenol synthetase and this might explain why thrombosis occurs on atheromatous plaques.

Epoprostenol is also synthesized by the lung and released into the circulation. This may be a mechanism for the dispersion of aggregated platelets trapped in fine vessels in the lung. Epoprostenol is a powerful vasodilator: it causes a fall in blood pressure and dilates coronary vessels. Epoprostenol also reduces the gastric acid secretion which is induced by pentagastrin.

Alprostadil (formerly know as PGE_1) and epoprostenol have many similarities, but are used in intensive care with very different treatment aims.

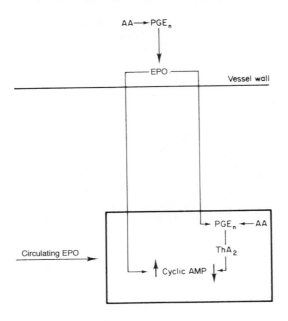

Figure 16.2 Regulation of platelet cyclic AMP. AA = arachidonic acid; PGE_n = prostaglandin endoperoxide; ThA_2 = thromboxane A_2; EPO = epoprostenol

Alprostadil is used mainly to maintain patency of the ductus ateriosus in neonates with congenital heart disease, in whom continued survival relies on blood flow through the duct. This is a short-term strategy, and is only used during transportation to a paediatric cardiac surgery centre and while emergency surgery is being organized. The most striking unwanted effect in this situation is apnoea, and intermittent positive pressure ventilation is indicated for babies receiving this drug. Other unwanted effects include bradycardia, haemorrhage, convulsions and necrotizing enterocolitis. After prolonged administration of alprostadil, thinning of the walls of the pulmonary artery and the ductus arteriosus have been observed. The use of alprostadil as an anti-hypertensive agent in pre-eclampsia has been described, the rationale being that the drug may have cytoprotective effects. Evidence for this remains anecdotal at present.

Epoprostenol is a vasodilator of the pulmonary and systemic vessels. It can be used in intensive care to treat pulmonary hypertension secondary to raised pulmonary vascular resistance. Therapy is limited by systemic hypotension due to generalized systemic vasodilatation, and evidence of improved survival is lacking. Its inhibitory effect on platelet stickiness has been exploited by using epoprostenol as a supplement to heparin in anticoagulant regimens for haemofiltration and haemodialysis. It has also been used in an attempt to minimize the size of the micro-infarcts of meningococcal septicaemia, but no formal clinical trial has investigated this. In animal models of sepsis, there is evidence of benefit both from prostanoids and also from *inhibitors* of prostaglandin synthesis (by NSAIDs). This contradiction has yet to be resolved.

Peptic ulceration

Another therapeutic use of prostaglandins has been in the treatment of peptic ulcers caused by treatment with NSAIDs. NSAIDs are ulcerogenic because they suppress prostaglandins both locally and systemically, thus compromising mucosal integrity. Misoprostol is a PGE_1 analogue specifically developed for the treatment and prevention of non-steroidal anti-inflammatory drug-induced gastro-intestinal ulceration but, unlike H_2-receptor antagonists, also stimulates bicarbonate and mucous secretion. It is a pro-drug: after oral administration it is rapidly converted to its free acid, which is the principal metabolite. Misoprostol inhibits both basal and nocturnal acid secretion as well as histamine and pentagastrin-stimulated gastric acid secretion. The elimination half-life is around 1.5–2 h but, despite this, doses at 6-hourly intervals are therapeutically effective. Misoprostol can be given prophylactically with NSAIDs to prevent the development of ulceration, erosion or haemorrhages. Healing of peptic ulcers secondary to NSAIDs has also been reported, even though NSAID treatment is continued. Divided doses of 800 µg of misoprostol a day are given with meals.

Enprostil is another synthetic prostaglandin E_2 analogue with gastric antisecretory and cytoprotective activity, currently undergoing clinical trials. These indicate that it also can heal peptic ulcers with minimal adverse effect.

Slow-reacting substance

As well as being the precursor of the prostaglandins and thromboxanes, arachidonic acid can be converted to substances known as leukotrienes (*Figure 16.3*). Their existence has been known since Feldberg and Kellaway in 1938 described a factor which appeared in the perfusate of guinea-pig lung treated with cobra venom and which they named slow-reacting substance (SRS). In anaphylactic conditions and allergic states, SRS is immunologically released from mast cells and is usually referred to as SRS-A. Leukotrienes such as LTC (leukotriene C) and LTD (leukotriene D) also possess SRS-A activity. The structure of SRS-A obtained from guinea-pig lung is shown in *Figure 16. 4* (Piper, 1989).

5-Hydroxytryptamine

5-Hydroxytryptamine (5-HT, serotonin, enteramine) occurs widely in the body, particularly in the chromaffin cells of the gastro-intestinal tract, and in the spleen, platelets and brain. Large amounts are found in carcinoid tumours of the intestine, ovary, testis and bronchus, and may be released from mast cells along with histamine in allergic conditions. Morphine and reserpine cause its release in animals, and the tissues in which it is found become depleted. It is synthesized in the body from tryptophan, broken down by

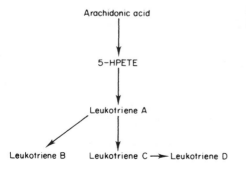

Figure 16.3 Formation of leukotrienes (5-HPETE leukotriene is 5-hydroperoxy-eicosatetraenoic acid)

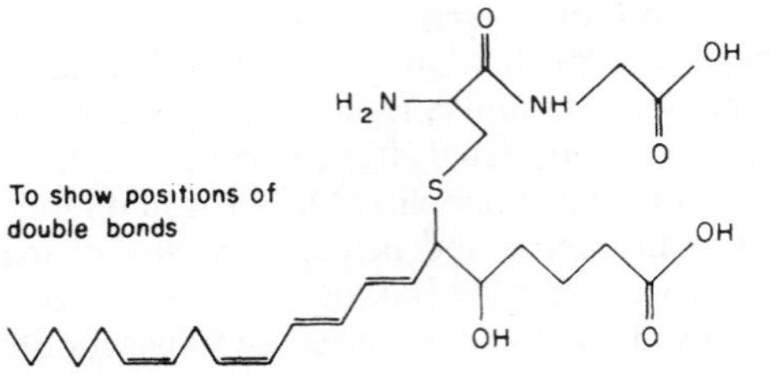

Figure 16.4 Reported structure for SRS-A from guinea-pig lung

To show positions of double bonds

monoamine oxidase, and excreted in the urine as 5-hydroxyindoleacetic acid (*Figure 16.5*).

Although our knowledge of its physiological significance is incomplete, it is known that 5-HT is a neurotransmitter in the CNS and its antagonists cause mental aberrations. It has been suggested that it might be important in the control of sleep, while a functional deficit may be responsible for depressive illness. It may also have a role in the maintenance of cardiovascular tone and intestinal gland activity. Although 5-HT is released from the platelets when blood clots, it has no action on the clotting process but may shorten the bleeding time as a consequence of its vasoconstrictor action. Its vascular effect when injected depends upon the dose administered, the existing level of vasomotor tone, and whether or not an anaesthetic is employed. The response also varies with different species. Often there is a transient fall in blood pressure, followed by a more prolonged rise. The fall is probably due to vagal reflex action, as it can be abolished by atropine and similar drugs. The rise is due to vasoconstriction, and will still take place in the presence of ganglion-blocking drugs. Other actions include hyperpnoea, antidiuresis and diarrhoea.

Carcinoid tumours may be of importance to anaesthetists; such patients may present preoperatively with cyanosis, raised jugular venous pressure, oedema, wheezing and right-sided heart murmurs, and thus mimic heart failure. An estimation of urinary 5-hydroxy-indoleacetic acid will confirm the diagnosis. Carcinoid tumours may also give rise to sudden and transient episodes of hypertension and skin blanching, alternating with hypotension during anaesthesia.

Many substances antagonize the actions of 5-HT by exerting receptor blocking effects. However, with fourteen receptor sub-types now identified, assigned to seven separate sub-classes of receptor, describing an antagonist's actions clearly and succinctly has

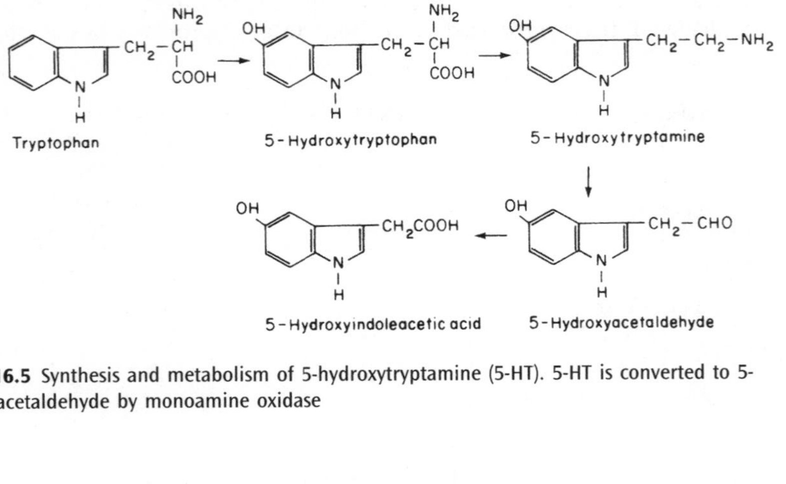

Figure 16.5 Synthesis and metabolism of 5-hydroxytryptamine (5-HT). 5-HT is converted to 5-hydroxyacetaldehyde by monoamine oxidase

become increasingly difficult. As the localized distribution and/or specialist functions of individual receptors become clearer, so will it be possible to explain the actions of existing 5-HT antagonists and develop more specific agents.

Of the long-standing 5-HT antagonists, the ergot alkaloids (and some related agents) are mainly non-specific antagonists: useful effects may be explained by actions upon certain receptors, while a myriad of adverse effects will be elicited by their effects at others. Ketanserin has been described as the prototypic $5HT_{2A}$ receptor antagonist. In some countries it has been used to lower blood pressure in hypertension and block 5-HT-induced platelet aggregation. Clozapine and risperidone are examples of new antipsychotic (anti-schizophrenic) drugs, and their mechanisms of action include antagonist effects at $5\text{-}HT_{2A/2C}$ receptors in the brain. Methysergide blocks $5\text{-}HT_{2A}$ and $5\text{-}HT_{2C}$ receptors, and in so doing inhibits the vasoconstrictor effects of 5-HT at peripheral sites but exerts a mix of agonist and antagonist effects centrally. It has been used to prevent migraine attacks but is of no use after an attack has already commenced. Cyproheptadine is a phenothiazine derivative which exerts antihistamine (anti-H_1), anti-muscarinic and anti-$5HT_{2A}$ effects. Cyproheptadine has been used clinically to control the pruritus and urticaria of certain skin allergies, to control the intestinal hypermotility of the carcinoid syndrome and provide migraine prophylaxis, although it is not the preferred agent for any of these conditions. Weight gain and increased growth in children treated chronically with cyproheptadine have been ascribed to its interference with growth hormone regulation, this too through a 5-HT receptor blocking action.

Predictably, the enhancement of 5-HT function also has useful clinical applications, but again the precise locations of action of individual drugs (and the 5-HT receptor subtypes involved) have yet to be clarified. Whilst the subcellular biochemical causes of depressive illness are still unknown, successive theories have invoked an absolute or relative deficiency of 5-HT in the brain. The majority of antidepressants *inter alia* enhance 5-HT function in the CNS. Most recently, serotonin specific re-uptake inhibitors (SSRIs), such as fluoxetine, have been introduced, which show useful dose-related improvements in mood, while the principal adverse effects (weight loss, sleeplessness and gastro-intestinal disturbances) also appear to be linked to the enhancement of 5-HT function.

There are also indications that opioid drugs critically require intact 5-HT function in the CNS to produce their analgesic effects. Thus, in experimental animals, agents which deplete 5-HT stores (e.g. reserpine) or block post-synaptic 5-HT receptors (e.g. cyproheptadine) antagonize opioid analgesics, including enkephalins. Opioid function is immediately restored on administration of small quantities of 5-HT directly into the brain. In man, tryptophan-free diets lead simultaneously to reductions in CSF metabolites of 5-HT (a measure of its turnover/functional level) and increase pain sensitivity, pain sensitivity being restored to normal by adding tryptophan to the diet. Drugs which enhance 5-HT function in man, for example certain antidepressants and MAOIs, can massively enhance the effects of certain opioids and may lead to toxic effects.

Angiotensin

This compound, which is formed *in vivo*, is the most powerful pressor agent known. It exists in the plasma as an inactive precursor, angiotensinogen, which is converted by renin into angiotensin I, a decapeptide which is also relatively inactive (renin is secreted by special juxtaglomerular cells in the kidney, located in the walls of the afferent arterioles as they enter the glomeruli). Angiotensin I is converted into the active angiotensin II, an octapeptide, by converting enzymes found in all tissues, but principally in the lung.

Angiotensin II is rapidly inactivated by peptidases. Angiotensin acts directly on receptors in smooth muscle independently of those reacting to norepinephrine (noradrenaline). It also depolarizes chromaffin cells in the adrenal medulla to release epinephrine; finally, it selectively increases the synthesis and secretion of aldosterone from the adrenal cortex (with little effect on other steroid hormone production), resulting in sodium and water retention.

The functions of the renin–angiotensin system are thus those of water and electrolyte balance: factors that tend to lower the blood volume, the perfusion pressure of the kidney or plasma sodium concentration stimulate the system to conserve sodium and water. Excessive secretion of renin is also a factor in the pathogenesis of some cases of hypertension.

Preparations of angiotensin amide are available and have been used for their pressor properties. Angiotensin has less tendency to provoke arrhythmias and does not cause venospasm or tissue necrosis. It does not, however, constrict capacitance vessels, and has no inotropic effect on cardiac muscle. Angiotensin-converting enzyme (ACE) antagonists are now available and have been developed into a class of important therapeutic agents in the treatment of hypertension.

Plasma kinins

There are two plasma kinins – a decapeptide called kallidin and a nonapeptide called bradykinin. Both are formed from an inactive precursor, kininogen, which is an α_2-globulin. This conversion is achieved by a variety of enzymes, including kallikreins, trypsin, plasmin, and proteolytic enzymes in snake and insect venoms. Of these, plasma kallikrein and the venoms produce bradykinin, whereas glandular kallikreins (in saliva, pancreatic juice, and so on) produce kallidin. It is notable that all of the ingredients for the production of kinins are present in the plasma. However, the kallikrein is present as an inactive precursor, prekallikrein. Its conversion into kallikrein is initiated by many of the same factors as initiate clotting, for example factor VII, the Hageman factor, and contact with glass and damaged tissues, and the process involves a 'cascade' of enzymatic reactions reminiscent of that which initiates coagulation. The half-life of kinins in plasma is less than 1 minute, being enzymatically degraded by peptidases and proteinases.

Like other autacoids, the plasma kinins are highly active, causing vasodilatation, increased capillary permeability and pain. They relax vascular smooth muscle and a fall in blood pressure can occur by this mechanism. However, they contract the smooth muscle of the bronchioles, the uterus and the intestine. They have no therapeutic applications at present. The kinins have been implicated in the pathogenesis of gout, acute inflammatory responses, hypersensitivity reactions and traumatic shock. Unfortunately there are no specific antagonists comparable to the antihistamines. However, there are inhibitors of kallikrein activation such as aprotinin which may be of benefit in certain situations (see below).

Substance P

This was discovered in 1931 and was first isolated as a powder, hence called substance P. It is now known to be an undecapeptide. Substance P and related undecapeptides have been called tachykinins. Substance P contracts gastro-intestinal smooth muscle. In contrast to bradykinin it has a fast onset of action but it has similar actions on smooth muscle, contracting bronchial smooth muscle and relaxing vascular smooth muscle. Its physiological role may be as a local hormone controlling peristalsis. It is also found in sensory nerves, in the brain for example, in the substantia nigra, and in the spinal cord, especially the posterior roots and columns. It thus may also be of importance in the control of pain pathways and in future a target for new analgesic agents. It is released in response to nociceptive stimuli and this is inhibited by opiates.

Enzymes

Another large class of specialized chemicals is the enzymes. Enzymes are formed by body cells. They may remain within the cell or may be secreted by it. Those secreted may circulate in extracellular fluids or be discharged externally such as into the alimentary tract. Their action is to break down, activate or inactivate other chemical substances in body tissues or the digestive system, and this may be brought about by oxidation, hydrolysis, deamination, or more complex processes. Thus, acetylcholine is hydrolysed by cholinesterase, epinephrine is oxidized by amine oxidase and catechol-o-methyl transferase, and proteins, carbohydrates and fats are converted into simpler products in the alimentary tract.

Although other substances play a part in their actions, those enzymes that have been purified are all of a protein nature. The proteins are composed of peptide chains and enzymes are globular, not fibrous, proteins. They can be composed either of single or multiple peptide chains. Ribonuclease has only a single chain of 124 amino acid residues; insulin is composed of two peptide chains, one of 21 and the other 30 amino acid residues. The activity of an enzyme is thought to reside in a certain part of it, which is called an active or catalytic site. This site probably consists of a small area of amino acid residues arranged in a very specific manner in such a way that it enhances the particular type of chemical reaction that the enzyme catalyses. It probably has also a geometrical arrangement of active groups which is complementary to that of the substrate on which it acts, so that only those substrates or compounds of a very similar structure can combine with the enzyme at its site of activity.

For an enzyme to act quickly in a particular reaction it must form, temporarily, an unstable complex with its substrate. Frequently the enzyme cannot act on the substrate alone and it requires a coenzyme to be present. Many of the vitamins play an important role, biologically, by acting in this manner.

It may be that most drugs act by accelerating or slowing some enzyme process, but until more is known about their action, not only on individual cells or organs but also on some of the vital contents of the cell, little will be understood about the mechanisms involved.

Amine oxidases

Monoamine oxidases

These are a rather non-specific enzyme group that are responsible for catalysing the destructive oxidative deamination of many different types of amine. These include epinephrine, many other sympathomimetic amines and 5-HT. MAO comprises two main groups of enzymes, MAO-A and MAO-B. Each group has a range of important locations and substrates. The former is important in the CNS aminergic neurones, while both

MAO-A and MAO-B play important roles peripherally. MAOs break down tyramine, phenylethylamine and phenylephrine, but ephedrine, amfetamine and mescaline are resistant to their action. They are also ineffective against histamine, which can be broken down by diamine oxidase. They are however, responsible for the second stage of the major metabolic degradation of histamine, converting methylhistamine into methylimidazoleacetic acid.

A physiological role of MAO is the intraneuronal conversion to inactive metabolites of any norepinephrine (noradrenaline) that leaks from storage granules. It is a mitochondrial enzyme which is present in the brain, kidney, lung, liver and intestine. The largest amount is found in the liver and it may be primarily concerned with the breakdown of certain amines formed by bacterial action in the gut.

Monoamine oxidase inhibitors (MAOIs) are rapidly active against the enzyme in the liver, but have less effect on the brain enzyme. Selegiline is a type B monoamine oxidase inhibitor and has been claimed to enhance the activity of levodopa in patients with Parkinson's disease. Non-specific MAO inhibitors include iproniazid, isocarboxazid, phenelzine, tranylcypromine and pargyline, but these are irreversible. This last substance has been used in the treatment of hypertension, whereas the remainder were employed in the treatment of certain forms of depression. Their usage, toxic effects and important interactions with certain foods and drugs are discussed on page 225. Moclobemide is a new reversible inhibitor of MAO-A (RIMA) and is licensed for the treatment of depression.

Although they are inhibitors of this enzyme, amfetamine and ephedrine owe their sympathomimetic action to their ability to liberate norepinephrine and dopamine from nerve terminals.

Diamine oxidase

This enzyme is commonly called histaminase. Experimentally it is effective, particularly with weak solutions of this substance. Histamine absorbed from the intestine may be inactivated in the intestinal mucosa where, together with the kidney, the enzyme is present in greatest amount.

Diamine oxidase plays a secondary role in the normal breakdown of histamine, 25–35 per cent of an injected dose appearing as metabolites attributable to its action. The remainder is methylated by imidazole-N-methyl transferase. The majority of the methylhistamine so formed is then oxidized by monoamine oxidase.

There is a marked increase in histaminolytic activity of plasma during normal pregnancy, which may be attributable to an increase in enzyme elaborated in the placenta. This increase begins at about the third month, reaches a maximum at the sixth and continues until term. After delivery it drops abruptly. Retained placental tissue is associated with a continuing high level. The significance of this rise is not known.

Carbonic anhydrase

Carbonic anhydrase catalyses the reaction $H_2O + CO_2 = H_2CO_3$. It is a natural enzyme, a zinc–protein compound found in the erythrocytes, whose function is to accelerate the transfer of carbon dioxide from the tissues to the red cells in the capillaries, and from the red cells in the lung capillaries to the alveolar air. Without the action of this enzyme, the transfer of carbon dioxide would be too slow to be effective.

It has been shown that in the stomach the enzyme is localized in the oxyntic cells and that they contain five to six times as much enzyme as the red corpuscles. Under appropriate experimental conditions it is possible to block secretion of gastric acid by enzyme inhibition, but these secretory processes are insensitive *in vivo* to ordinary doses of carbonic anhydrase inhibitors and this effect has no therapeutic use. The enzyme is present in the eye, where it probably plays a role in the secretion of the aqueous humour. Inhibitors are of value, therefore, in the treatment of glaucoma.

Carbonic anhydrase inhibitors affect renal tubular function (see page 409), but more than 99 per cent of the enzyme in the kidney must be inhibited before the effects become apparent. An inhibitor of carbonic anhydrase, dichlorphenamide, has also been used in the treatment of chronic respiratory failure. The mechanism of action is not clear, but it may be central, and due to a local increase in carbon dioxide tension in the brain affecting respiratory drive. The lowering of arterial P_{CO_2} brought about is usually not striking.

Cholinesterases

There are two main enzymes: acetylcholinesterase, also known as true cholinesterase, and plasma cholinesterase, often referred to as pseudo-cholinesterase.

Acetylcholinesterase

Acetylcholinesterase is widely distributed in the body and is found in erythrocytes and in the region of synapses and nerve endings wherever acetylcholine is the chemical transmitter. Inhibitors of this enzyme are important therapeutic substances; they are widely employed as insecticides and some are known to be the most toxic human poisons ever developed. The behaviour of the enzyme and its inhibitors is discussed in Chapter 10.

Plasma cholinesterase

This enzyme is elaborated in the liver, and the serum level closely parallels that of serum albumin, except in albumin-losing nephritis. The esteratic site does not seem to be closely related to an effective anionic site, and the enzyme readily hydrolyses other esters, including benzoylcholine, suxamethonium and procaine. Its physiological role is not known. Complete absence of the enzyme has been reported and was compatible with normal health. The serum level of enzyme may be low in advanced liver disease and malnutrition, and is reduced by about 30 per cent in pregnancy and a further 30 per cent by preeclampsia. It is depressed by many cholinesterase inhibitors including therapeutic agents such as ecothiopate eye-drops, some anti-cancer agents and organophosphate poisons, including many insecticides and the nerve gases. Prosthetic inhibitors of acetylcholinesterase have comparatively less action on plasma cholinesterase, although the relative effects in the body depend on additional factors such as lipid solubility. For example, hexafluorenium is a potent acetylcholinesterase inhibitor *in vitro*, but has no such action *in vivo*, and is used as an inhibitor of plasma cholinesterase.

The importance of this enzyme in anaesthetic practice depends on its essential role in the breakdown of suxamethonium, mivacurium and procaine-like esters. In practice, the action of suxamethonium is not clinically prolonged until the enzyme has been about 80 per cent inhibited.

Atypical enzymes, genetically determined, have been identified which have a limited capacity to metabolize suxamethonium. These atypical enzymes are resistant to the action of various inhibitors. The 'usual' enzyme is elaborated by the 'usual' gene which has been designated E_1, meaning that the 'usual' gene is found at the first esterase locus. An individual with the genotype $E_1^U E_1^U$ is homozygous for the usual gene, elaborating the usual enzyme. Genes E_1^A and E_1^F have been identified using 10^{-5} M Dibucaine and 10^{-5} M fluoride as inhibitors. E_1^S is a silent gene which does not elaborate any enzyme.

The pattern of inheritance is consistent with the view that plasma cholinesterase elaboration is largely under the influence of a pair of allelomorphic non-dominant autosomal genes. A second locus has, however, been identified, and has been named the C5 variant on the basis of its electrophoretic separation. Those who possess this additional activity (a small minority) do not show 'resistance' to suxamethonium. The clinical significance of abnormal cholinesterases is discussed in Chapter 9.

Choline acetylase

This enzyme catalyses the final step in the synthesis of acetylcholine. In the initial steps of this synthesis phosphorotransacetylase catalyses the formation of adenyl acetate from acetate and adenosine triphosphate (ATP) and then the transfer of the acetate moiety from this compound to coenzyme A (CoA). Choline acetylase now catalyses the reaction between CoA acetate and choline with the formation of acetylcholine.

Choline acetylase is found in the nervous system in any location in which cholinesterase and acetylcholine are also present, and is essential for the normal function of the acetylcholine mechanism. Hemicholinium prevents acetylcholine synthesis, and its configuration suggests that it inhibits choline acetylase by acting as a false substrate in place of choline.

Hyaluronidase

The accidental finding that aqueous extracts of normal testicle, when added to vaccinia virus and injected intradermally, produced unusually widespread lesions, led to the suggestion of the presence of a 'spreading factor'. This factor was later obtained from many sources, as widely diverse as streptococci and snake venom. Subsequent investigation showed that this spreading factor was an enzyme. It was named hyaluronidase, as it was demonstrated that its specific substrate was hyaluronic acid. It depolymerizes hyaluronic acid which is a mucopolysaccharide containing glycuronic acid and N-acetyl-glucosamine and is now regarded as the tissue cement or ground substance of the mesenchyme. Hyaluronidase is non-toxic and will produce a reversible reduction in the viscosity of the intercellular matrix. It also has mucolytic properties when applied topically to mucous surfaces.

Hyaluronidase can be used with local anaesthetics to spread their effect and increase the area of analgesia. It is advisable, however, to use epinephrine (adrenaline) to delay absorption which would otherwise be accelerated. It may also be useful in the reduction of inflammatory swellings due to trauma, and in the dispersal of irritant substances such as thiopental inadvertently injected into subcutaneous tissues. When it is impossible to administer fluids by intravenous or other routes, hyaluronidase may be used as an aid to hypodermoclysis. Its effect seems to be dependent upon the state of the subcutaneous tissue. When these tissues are loosely constructed, the rate of absorption of fluid is increased two-fold, but where the subcutaneous tissue turgor is high, the rate of fluid administration can be increased to a much greater extent.

For use with local anaesthetics various strengths have been recommended. The addition of 1000 i.u. to 20 ml of the anaesthetic solution is common practice and gives satisfactory results. To aid in the dispersal of thiopental injected perivenously 1500 i.u. may be dissolved in 5–10 ml of sterile water and injected into the surrounding tissues. For hypodermoclysis, 1500 i.u. are effective when mixed with 500–1000 ml of infusion fluid. As hyaluronidase is non-toxic and free from side effects, accurate measurement of dose is not essential.

Proteinases

Proteinases are enzymes that break down protein. They include trypsin, chymotrypsin, plasmin, thromboplastin activators and carboxypeptidases. Trypsin and chymotrypsin are important digestive enzymes produced in the pancreas; thromboplastin activators and plasmin, also referred to as fibrinolysin, are proteinases which are essential in the formation and removal of fibrin, processes which in health are normally in dynamic equilibrium.

Proteinases obtained from microbial and fungal sources have been used to dissolve clot, both in closed cavities and intravascularly to unblock haemodialysis shunts and dissolve emboli. They are discussed in Chapter 18.

Inhibitors of proteinases are multivalent and can inhibit kallikrein activation. Proteinase inhibition may thus be useful therapeutically. A naturally-occurring inhibitor, aprotinin, and a synthetic inhibitor, tranexamic acid, are available. They form a reversible complex with proteinases and are, therefore, competitive enzyme inhibitors. Other protease inhibitors (indiavir, ritonavir and saquinavir) are used in the treatment of HIV.

The main indications for proteinase inhibitor therapy are acute pancreatitis and certain cases of pathological bleeding. In acute pancreatitis, proteolytic and lipolytic enzymes escape from the pancreas and give rise to much of the systemic illness; present evidence suggests that the administration of proteinase inhibitors may be beneficial in alleviating pain and hypotension. Kallikrein inactivation has been recommended for the control of pathological bleeding, when, it is suggested, natural inhibitors are overwhelmed by a great increase in proteolytic enzyme activation (see Chapter 18).

References

Piper, P. (1989) Leukotrienes and the airways. *European Journal of Anaesthesiology*, 6, 241

17

Hormones

Endocrine disorders are unusual in human disease in several aspects. Many are characterized by deviations from normal, which often lie only just outside the range of normal physiology. More severe disease is characterized by changes that are recognizable as increases or decreases in physiological function. Endocrine glands are particularly liable to undergo neoplastic changes, often benign, and the tumour usually retains the capacity to synthesize the hormone produced by the parent tissue. The hormone output from most endocrine glands is controlled physiologically by a system of feedback modulation, but most hormone-secreting tumours escape from this control and excess secretion results.

The anaesthetist frequently encounters patients with either hormone excess or deficiency, either secondary to disease or pharmacologically induced, so that a basic knowledge of the effects of common hormones is essential.

Effects of anaesthesia

In general terms a carefully conducted anaesthetic, in the absence of surgery, is unlikely to alter hormone secretion greatly other than to decrease previously elevated values of stress hormones such as cortisol and epinephrine (adrenaline). The interaction between anaesthetic drugs and hormone secretion in response to the noxious stimuli of surgery is more complex.

The classic example of an anaesthetic drug which inhibits hormone secretion is the effect of etomidate on steroid synthesis in the adrenal cortex. Etomidate is the most potent inhibitor of adrenal steroidogenesis synthesized so far, and blocks cortisol and aldosterone secretion by inhibiting the enzymes, 11β-hydroxylase and cholesterol cleavage.

The effects of etomidate are seen most obviously when the drug is given by infusion, but even a single induction dose of etomidate has been shown to impair adrenocortical function for up to 8 h. The administration of potent opioid analgesics, such as fentanyl, inhibits the secretion of pituitary hormones in response to the stress of surgery. Although this action was originally described after the use of high-dose fentanyl (50 μg/kg), it has been shown that a dose as low as 15 μg/kg can still attenuate hormonal secretion in some patients. It is probable that this effect on pituitary function is found with all μ-opioid agonists and is mediated at the level of the hypothalamus (Hall et al., 1990).

Benzodiazepines also modulate the cortisol response to surgery, particularly midazolam at high doses. These drugs act by inhibiting ACTH secretion and the specificity of their effect is demonstrated by a paradoxical increase in growth hormone (GH) release. A similar effect is found with α2-agonists and in unstressed volunteers clonidine was shown to inhibit ACTH/cortisol secretion and enhance GH secretion. This phenomenon was not evident during surgery, although it is possible that more specific α_2-agonists, such as dexmetomidine, may modify stress-induced hormone secretion (Lyons *et al.*, 1997).

It is well recognized that regional anaesthesia which provides complete afferent neuronal blockade of the operative site, both somatic and autonomic, prevents the catabolic hormonal response to surgery. This can only be achieved for surgery of the pelvis, limbs and eyes, and results from the anaesthetic technique and not from a specific effect of the local anaesthetic.

Hall, G.M., Lacoumenta, S., Hart, G.R. and Burrin, J.M. (1990) Site of action of fentanyl in inhibiting the pituitary ñ adrenal response to surgery in man. *British Journal of Anaesthesia*, **65**, 251
Lyons, F.M., Bew, S., Sheeran, P. and Hall, G.M. (1997) Effects of clonidine on the pituitary hormonal response to pelvic surgery. *British Journal of Anaesthesia*, **78**, 134

Pituitary gland (hypophysis) and hypothalamus

The pituitary gland is the site of functional interaction between the CNS and the endocrine system.

The hypothalamic control of the anterior pituitary occurs by the secretion of releasing or inhibiting hormones which reach the gland via the portal venous system of the pituitary stalk. The five releasing and inhibiting peptides are thyrotrophin releasing hormone (TRH), gonadotrophin releasing hormone (GnRH), corticotrophin releasing hormone (CRH), growth hormone releasing hormone (GHRH) and somatostatin. These hypothalamic factors occupy specific receptors on the pituitary cells to stimulate or inhibit hormone secretion. The neurotransmitter, dopamine, exerts an inhibitory influence on prolactin secretion.

The regulation of pituitary function by the releasing and inhibiting hormones of the hypothalamus is complex. For example, ACTH secretion is stimulated by both CRH and arginine vasopressin (AVP or ADH) and the hypothalamic peptides are themselves influenced by the neurotransmitters norepinephrine (noradrenaline), acetylcholine and serotonin (5-HT). Further control can be exerted from higher centres through the hypothalamus to impose a normal circadian rhythm or to increase secretion in response to stress. ACTH secretion is inhibited by a feedback effect of cortisol at the level of the pituitary and the hypothalamus.

The posterior pituitary hormones, vasopressin and oxytocin, are classical neurohormones. They are synthesized in the supra-optic and paraventricular nuclei of the hypothalamus and transported as granules by axoplasmic flow to the nerve terminals in the posterior pituitary. From here they are released directly into the circulation to act as classical hormones on distant target sites.

Adrenal cortex

All the steroid hormones have the same molecular framework, sometimes called the steroid nucleus (see *Figure 17.1*). The structure of both rings and side chains can be modified and slight changes can cause major differences in biological activity. Many corticosteroids have been isolated, but in man only three compounds are released into the circulation in significant amounts and only two of these are of major physiological importance.

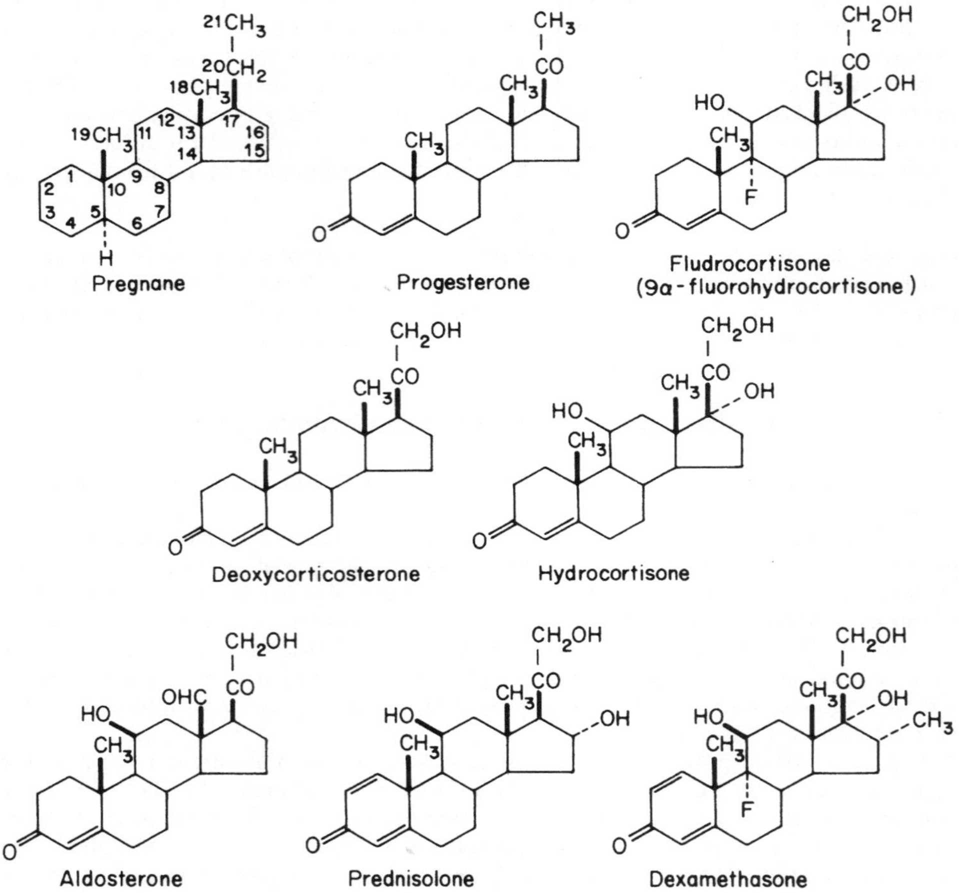

Figure 17.1 The steroid nucleus and structures of some common steroid hormones

Cortisol

The most important hormone produced by the adrenal cortex is cortisol, which is synthesized in the zona fasciculata and reticularis under the stimulatory influence of ACTH. The resulting increased circulating cortisol blocks ACTH secretion through feedback inhibition at both the hypothalamic and pituitary level. Synthetic corticosteroids used in therapy also suppress ACTH secretion.

Cortisol is a C^{21} compound with predominantly glucocorticoid actions, but with some mineralocorticoid effects. At physiological concentrations, more than 90 per cent of circulating cortisol is protein bound, mostly to corticosteroid-binding globulin (CBG) or transcortin and the remainder to albumin. Endogenous cortisol production is approximately 25–30 mg/day, circulating concentrations vary in a circadian pattern and the half-life of cortisol in the circulation is 60–90 minutes. The binding capacity of CBG is limited to about 700 nmol/litre cortisol. As total cortisol increases above this value, as often occurs during surgery, then the proportion of free cortisol rises.

Aldosterone

Aldosterone is synthesized by the zona glomerulosa of the adrenal cortex and the normal daily production rate is about 100–200 µg/day. It is only weakly bound to plasma proteins and so has a relatively short half-life of 20–30 minutes. The synthesis and release of aldosterone is controlled mainly by angiotensin II, although increased plasma potassium and corticotrophin concentrations also play a minor part. The production of angiotensin II is dependent on renin release from the kidney which, in turn, is regulated by arterial pressure, sympathetic tone and tubular sodium concentration. Aldosterone is a powerful mineralocorticoid and accounts for about 75 per cent of the total mineralocorticoid activity produced by the adrenal hormones.

Dehydroepiandrosterone (DHEA)

This compound is produced by the same synthetic pathway as cortisol and so is corticotrophin dependent. DHEA has weak androgenic and anabolic properties, but appears not to have an important physiological role, as replacement therapy is not required after bilateral adrenalectomy.

Metabolism

Only small amounts of free cortisol and aldosterone are excreted in the urine. Most of the corticosteroids are metabolized by the liver to a variety of compounds with low biological activity. These compounds are then conjugated, usually with glucuronic acid, and the resulting metabolites, without biological activity, are excreted in the urine. The measurement of urinary corticosteroids, other than free cortisol, is little used except for the investigation of complex defects of steroidogenesis.

Actions of corticosteroids

Corticosteroids can be classified as having glucocorticoid or mineralocorticoid effects. The primary mineralocorticoid effect is on the distal renal tubule with the reabsorption of sodium in exchange for potassium; long-term therapy results in hypertension. The glucocorticoid effects are mainly glucose intolerance, as a result of increased hepatic glucose production with impaired glucose utilization, muscle proteolysis, lipid synthesis and osteoporosis. Many synthetic corticosteroids have been developed in an attempt to separate the glucocorticoid and mineralocorticoid actions, because the glucocorticoid property is associated with a marked anti-inflammatory effect.

Synthetic corticosteroids

All synthetic corticosteroids when used in pharmacological doses for their anti-inflammatory properties produce undesirable side effects such as weight gain, muscle wasting, osteoporosis and suppression of the hypothalamic–pituitary–adrenocortical axis. However, at lower replacement doses a marked difference between the two main actions can be demonstrated for many synthetic steroids (*Table 17.1*).

Table 17.1 Relative potencies of commonly used corticosteroids

Steroid	Equivalent anti-inflammatory dose (mg)	Sodium retention
Hydrocortisone	100	++
Cortisone acetate	125	++
Prednisolone	25	+
Methylprednisolone	20	+
Betamethasone	4	±
Dexamethasone	4	±
Fludrocortisone	8	++++

Use of corticosteroids

Physiological replacement

For physiological replacement, oral hydrocortisone is given in a daily dose of 20–30 mg. This is usually given in two divided doses, the larger in the morning and the smaller in the evening, to mimic the normal diural rhythm. In hypopituitarism, aldosterone production is preserved so that hydrocortisone is the only replacement corticosteroid required. In Addison's disease or after bilateral adrenalectomy, a mineralocorticoid is usually needed so that oral fludrocortisone 50–300 µg/day is also given.

Pharmacological uses

Prednisolone is commonly used when an anti-inflammatory action is required, as its low mineralocorticoid activity reduces the likelihood of sodium and water retention and consequent hypertension. Corticosteroids are beneficial in a wide variety of inflammatory conditions such as the collagen disorders, some types of the nephrotic syndrome, asthma and ulcerative colitis. Doses may be as high as prednisolone 60 mg/day. Steroids are also used topically for various skin disorders such as uveitis and also injected intra-articularly.

Corticosteroids such as dexamethasone are frequently used to reduce cerebral oedema associated with head injuries and cerebral tumours, for example dexamethasone 8 mg intravenously as a bolus, followed by dexamethasone 4 mg intramuscularly every 6 h.

Previous treatment with corticosteroids

Perhaps the most common problem that anaesthetists meet in relation to hormone therapy is intercurrent surgery in patients who are having, or have had, treatment with corticosteroids. Three circumstances are commonly encountered.

Patients receiving treatment with corticosteroids

All exogenous glucocorticoids suppress ACTH secretion so that the response of the pituitary–adrenocortical axis to surgery is impaired. The suppression may be partial or complete and persists for some time after the drug has been discontinued. If the administration of corticosteroids has been prolonged, then the adrenal cortex will be hypotrophic so that the response to exogenous corticotrophin is also impaired.

The possible failure of steroid secretion during and after surgery resulted in the recommendation of empirical replacement regimens such as 300–400 mg hydrocortisone/day. Although undoubtedly safe in terms of providing adequate steroids, little thought was given to the deleterious side effects such as impaired wound healing and increased susceptibility to infection. In contrast, a low-dose substitution regimen based on the observation that total cortisol secretion during major surgery does not exceed 150 mg/24 h (e.g. hydrocortisone 25 mg i.v. at induction of anaesthesia, followed by hydrocortisone (100 mg i.v. infusion over 24 h)) reveals that even in patients identified as having impaired cortisol secretion by pre-operative corticotrophin stimulation, the regimen resulted in plasma cortisol values greater than the usual response to surgery.

Current recommendations for perioperative steroid supplementation are based on the use of a low-dose substitution regimen (Nicholson *et al.*, 1998):

1.   Patients receiving 10 mg or less of prednisolone/day have a normal response to testing of the hypothalamic–pituitary–adrenal axis and do not require perioperative steroids greater than their usual requirements.
2.   Patients undergoing minor surgery take their routine dose of glucocorticoids preoperatively, or receive 25 mg hydrocortisone i.v. at induction of anaesthesia, and resume oral replacement postoperatively.
3.   For moderate and major surgery, patients receive the usual glucocorticoid dose preoperatively, 25 mg hydrocortisone i.v. at induction and an infusion of 100 mg hydrocortisone i.v./day until oral therapy can be resumed. Occasionally, a hydrocortisone infusion may be necessary for several days.
4.   Patients taking high doses of steroids for acute immunosuppression have special needs. It is essential that the required dose is maintained in the perioperative period. For example, *Table 17.1* shows that prednisolone 50 mg/day is equivalent to hydrocortisone 200 mg/day and this equivalent dose of hydrocortisone should be given in these circumstances. Failure to maintain immunosuppression may cause acute deterioration in organ function.

Patients who have had treatment with corticosteroids in the past

Following the withdrawal of corticosteroid treatment, the hypothalamic–pituitary–adrenal axis slowly regains its usual sensitivity to stress-induced secretion. There is some dispute about how rapidly restoration of normal function occurs, but the available evidence suggests that steroid supplementation is only required for 3 months following cessation of glucocorticoid therapy (Nicholson *et al.*, 1998). During this 3 months, the low-dose substitution regimen should be used (see above).

Nevertheless, the possibility of adrenal failure should be considered in all patients who have received treatment with corticosteroids. If necessary, hydrocortisone should be given i.v., but only after a blood sample has been collected for estimation of the plasma cortisol concentration. This will enable the diagnosis to be confirmed or refuted in due course.

Patients receiving replacement doses of corticosteroids

These patients usually have Addison's disease or hypopituitarism and receive replacement doses of hydrocortisone together with fludrocortisone. They should be managed in the perioperative period with the low-dose substitution regimen (see above); fludrocortisone should be resumed as soon as possible postoperatively.

Nicholson, G., Burrin, J.M. and Hall, G.M. (1998) Peri-operative steroid supplementation. *Anaesthesia*, **53**, (in press)

Adrenal medulla

The three catecholamines released by the adrenal medulla – norephinephrine (noradrenaline), epinephrine (adrenaline) and dopamine – are described in Chapter 12.

Thyroid

The thyroid gland synthesizes two principal hormones: L-thyroxine (T_4) and L-triiodothyronine (T_3). The production of these hormones is controlled by thyrotrophin (TSH) secreted from the anterior pituitary. The release of TSH is stimulated by thyrotrophin releasing hormone (TRH), a tripeptide synthesized in the hypothalamus. Circulating concentrations of T_4 and T_3 exert a feedback control over TSH secretion by an action at the pituitary and possibly the hypothalamus, such that high values of circulating thyroid hormones suppress TSH secretion, whereas low concentrations stimulate TSH release.

Both T_3 and T_4 are synthesized from the amino acid, tyrosine, in the follicles of the thyroid gland. They are then stored in the colloid, bound to thyroglobulin, before release into the circulation. Although T_4 is formed exclusively in the thyroid, some T_3 is also produced by peripheral de-iodination of T_4 in the liver and kidney. The peripheral conversion of T_4 results in the formation of either active T_3 or the inactive optical isomer reverse T_3 (rT_3). In normal circumstances, active T_3 is the predominant product of peripheral de-iodination, but in a variety of 'stress states', such as after surgery, starvation and infection, more rT_3 is produced. This phenomenon is called the sick euthyroid syndrome, and its physiological significance is unclear.

T_4 and T_3 are mostly bound to plasma proteins in the circulation: thyroxine binding globulin, thyroxine binding pre-albumin and albumin. Normal circulating values of T_4 are 50–140 nmol/l total hormone and 9–24 pmol/litre free hormone; and for T_3 1–3 nmol/litre total hormone and 5–10 pmol/l free hormone. It is the concentration of free hormone that reflects the thyroid status and controls the metabolic rate. Estimation of free T_3 and T_4 values, together with circulating TSH concentration, enables a precise assessment of thyroid status to be undertaken. The determination of total T_3 and T_4 is influenced by thyroid hormone binding protein concentrations and this may lead to incorrect interpretation of the data.

Antithyroid drugs

Antithyroid drugs are used to make patients euthyroid before thyroidectomy. Those in common use are the thionamides, carbimazole and propylthiouracil. They act by preventing the incorporation of iodide into tyrosine to form mono- and diiodotyrosine, and also by blocking the combination of two diiodotyrosine molecules to form L-thyroxine. Potassium perchlorate is occasionally used if a patient is sensitive to the usual antithyroid drugs, but the risk of toxicity is greater. Perchlorate acts by inhibiting the concentration of iodide by the thyroid gland.

Since antithyroid drugs increase the size and vascularity of the gland, some surgeons administer iodine for 10–14 days before surgery, in combination with antithyroid drugs to reduce the vascularity of the thyroid. The usual preparation is aqueous iodine oral solution (Lugol's solution) which consists of iodine 5 per cent, potassium iodide 10 per cent in water, total iodine 130 mg/ml.

Propranolol is a useful adjunct to antithyroid drugs as it provides rapid control of the symptoms such as tremor and tachycardia. It has been suggested that only a β-adrenergic blocking drug is necessary for preoperative control in hyperthyroid patients, but conventional antithyroid treatment is preferred.

Pancreas

Most of the pancreas is concerned with exocrine function, and the islets of Langerhans constitute only a very small amount of the total mass of the gland. Three major hormones are secreted by the islets – insulin, glucagon and somatostatin – from the B, A and D cells, respectively.

The control of insulin secretion from the B cells of the pancreas is complex. The main stimulus is glucose, which has a sigmoidal shaped dose–response curve with threshold, half-maximal and maximal concentrations of 4.5, 8.0 and 25.0 mmol/litre respectively. Many other factors, such as pancreatic innervation, circulating catecholamines, glucagon, gut hormones and basic amino acids such as arginine, also modulate insulin secretion, particularly at low glucose values. The failure of insulin secretion to respond to the hyperglycaemia of surgery is usually attributed to the α-adrenergic inhibitory effects of circulating catecholamines. In the postoperative period insulin secretion increases, but insulin is less effective metabolically than usual. This period of 'insulin resistance' may be associated with the prolonged concurrent secretion of catabolic hormones such as cortisol. Thus the perioperative period is characterized by a state of absolute, or relative, insulin deficiency.

Insulin is the key anabolic hormone and not only alters glucose homeostasis but also modifies lipid and protein metabolism. It affects glucose metabolism at two sites, the liver and the peripheral insulin-sensitive tissues. The action of insulin on the liver is to decrease glucose output and increase its uptake and conversion to glycogen for storage. In the periphery, glucose uptake and utilization is increased so that large positive arteriovenous differences are found across tissues such as skeletal muscle. Insulin also inhibits lipolysis in adipose tissue so that circulating non-esterified fatty acid concentrations are decreased. This reduces the capacity for ketone body formation in the liver. Muscle protein synthesis is stimulated by insulin, an effect largely independent of nutritional status.

The main stimuli to glucagon secretion from the A cells of the pancreas are hypoglycaemia and β-adrenergic stimulation. Thus glucagon is an important counter-regulatory hormone when the blood glucose value is low. The main effect of glucagon is to increase glucose output from the liver by an action on preformed glycogen. Its effect is evanescent and does not occur if the liver is already depleted of glycogen, for example, by prolonged starvation. Although other metabolic effects of glucagon have been described, they are probably unimportant.

Somatostatin was originally isolated in the hypothalamus as a 14 amino acid peptide which inhibited GH and TSH secretion. Subsequently, somatostatin has been shown to inhibit the secretion of many other organs (*Table 17.2*), and is widely distributed throughout the body. It is also found in the CNS where its function is unknown, although

Table 17.2 Actions of somatostatin outside the central nervous system

Site	Inhibition of
Pituitary	Growth hormone
	Thyrotrophin
Pancreas	Insulin
	Glucagon
Gastro-intestinal tract	Gut peptides
	Gastric emptying
	Gall bladder emptying
	Pancreatic enzymes
	Intestinal absorption
	Gastro-intestinal blood flow

it may modulate sensory transmission in the dorsal horn of the spinal cord. In the pancreas, somatostatin acts as a paracine secretion, that is, it exerts local control over the secretion of adjacent cells such as glucagon, insulin and pancreatic enzymes. Other molecular forms of somatostatin have been isolated, including a 28 amino acid peptide, and a shorter analogue of eight amino acids (octreotride).

The main anaesthetic interest in the endocrine function of the pancreas is the management of patients with diabetes mellitus. The three important methods of obtaining glucose control in diabetic patients are diet, oral hypoglycaemic drugs and insulin. Of these three modalities, dietary control is an essential component of the management of all patients with diabetes. Many patients with non-insulin-dependent diabetes mellitus (NIDDM) can be successfully managed with the addition of hypoglycaemic drugs such as the sulphonylureas and occasionally biguanides. Patients with insulin-dependent diabetes mellitus (IDDM) obviously require the addition of insulin to maintain glucose control.

The management of patients with diabetes mellitus undergoing surgery has been reviewed in detail (Hirsch *et al.*, 1991; Milaskiewicz and Hall, 1992). IDDM patients should receive an intravenous infusion of insulin, together with adequate amounts of glucose and potassium. Initial recommendations were for the combined infusion of glucose, insulin and potassium in a single bag of 10 per cent glucose. More recently, concentrated solutions of insulin have been used (1 unit/ml) with a separate glucose + potassium solution through a single cannula. The enhanced flexibility of a concentrated insulin solution makes this the preferred method.

NIDDM patients undergoing minor surgery do not require an insulin infusion. It is usually sufficient to omit the oral hypoglycaemic drug on the day of surgery. The use of an insulin infusion in these patients increases the incidence of metabolic problems. All NIDDM patients undergoing intermediate or major surgery should be treated with a glucose–potassium–insulin regimen.

Hirsch, I.B., McGill, J.B., Cryer, D.E. and White, P.F. (1991) Perioperative management of surgical patients with diabetes mellitus. *Anesthesiology*, **74**, 346

Milaskiewicz, R.M. and Hall, G.M. (1992) Diabetes and anaesthesia: the past decade. *British Journal of Anaesthesia*, **68**, 198

Oral hypoglycaemic drugs

The oral hypoglycaemic drugs are the mainstay of treatment for NIDDM patients. The sulphonylureas are the most commonly used group of drugs and they exert an effect both on the pancreas and at extrapancreatic sites. They augment insulin secretion and so are only effective when there is some residual B-cell function. The sulphonylureas increase the sensitivity of the B cell to glucose so that more insulin is secreted at a given glucose concentration, but do not induce the synthesis of more insulin. A secondary pancreatic effect is to reduce glucagon secretion from the A cells. The extra-pancreatic effects of the sulphonylureas become more important with long-term administration and include an improved tissue sensitivity to insulin, either directly or indirectly, and reduced hepatic insulin extraction.

The biguanides are much less commonly used as oral hypoglycaemic agents than the sulphonylureas because of the high incidence of side effects. The only drug of this type in use in the United Kingdom is metformin. The mechanism of action is not clear, but its main effect appears to be the reduction of glucose output from the liver by the inhibition of gluconeogenesis. A secondary effect is, like the sulphonylureas, to increase glucose utilization peripherally. Metformin does not stimulate insulin secretion, but only acts in the presence of endogenous insulin so that some B-cell function must be preserved.

Early trials with a third group of oral hypoglycaemic drugs, the thiazolidinedione derivatives ('glitazones'), suggested that these drugs may be valuable clinically as they enhanced insulin sensitivity. Unfortunately, a high incidence of hepatic reactions and occasional deaths resulted in their prompt withdrawal in the UK.

There is little evidence for any difference in the effectiveness of the sulphonylureas, although the nature of the side effects varies. Three drugs in common use are tolbutamide, chlorpropamide and glibenclamide.

MONOGRAPHS

CARBIMAZOLE AND PROPYLTHIOURACIL

Carbimazole (rINN)
Propylthiouracil (rINN)

Physiology

Both drugs prevent thyroid hormone synthesis by inhibiting the incorporation of iodide into tyrosine and the coupling of iodotyrosyl residues to form iodothyroinines. Clinical changes are only seen after the existing stores of thyroid hormones have been depleted.

Indications

The antithyroid drugs are used to control hyperthyroidism either as long-term treatment or to make the patient euthyroid before thyroidectomy or ^{131}I ablation.

Dosage and administration

Carbimazole is used in a starting dose of 20–60 mg orally per day until the patient is euthyroid, often 4–8 weeks, and then reduced to a daily maintenance dose of 5–15 mg. Propylthiouracil is administered on a similar basis, with a starting dose of 300–600 mg orally per day, reducing to a maintenance dose of 50–150 mg daily.

Precautions

The early stages of treatment can be associated with further swelling of a large goitre. Overtreatment rapidly results in hypothyroidism. Rashes and pruritus are common with carbimazole, and propylthiouracil can then be substituted. Agranulocytosis is a rare complication of carbimazole treatment. Propylthiouracil dose should be decreased in patients with renal impairment.

CHLORPROPAMIDE

Chlorpropamide (rINN)

Pharmacology

Chlorpropamide decreases blood glucose by increasing insulin secretion from the pancreas and by improving tissue sensitivity to insulin.

Indications

Chlorpropamide is indicated for the management of NIDDM in conjunction with strict dietary control.

Dosage and administration

Chlorpropamide is given orally as a single dose of 100–250 mg daily, to a maximum of 500 mg. It has a duration of action of 24–72 h, with a mean elimination half-life of 33 h.

Precautions

Chlorpropamide has the highest incidence of serious side effects among the sulphonylurea drugs. The frequency of severe hypoglycaemia is 4–6 per cent, with an overall frequency of side effects of 9 per cent. Chlorpropamide should not be used in patients with renal impairment, as 20 per cent of the dose is excreted unchanged by the kidneys. An unpleasant facial flushing can occur in conjunction with alcohol. Although chlorpropamide does not have a diuretic effect, it can rarely induce severe hyponatraemia by virtue of its antidiuretic properties.

DEXAMETHASONE

Dexamethasone (rINN), Dexamethasone phosphate (BP), Dexamethasone sodium phosphate (BP)

Chemical constitution: This synthetic compound is derived from fludrocortisone (9α-fluorohydrocortisone) by the addition of a double bond between carbons 1 and 2, and a CH_3 -group at carbon 16.

Pharmacology

Dexamethasone is a very potent glucocorticoid with minimal effects on sodium retention (see *Table 17.1*, page 440).

Indications

Dexamethasone (and betamethasone) are used in conditions in which mineralocorticoid effects would be a disadvantage, for example cerebral trauma.

Dosage and administration

For cerebral oedema, 8 mg is given initially by intravenous injection, followed by doses of 8–16 mg/day by intramuscular injection in 4 divided doses. 1 mg dexamethasone $\cong$ 1.2 mg dexamethasone phosphate $\cong$ 1.3 mg dexamethasone sodium phosphate.

Precautions

These are the same as for prednisolone.

GLIBENCLAMIDE

Glibenclamide (rINN)

Pharmacology

Tolbutamide decreases blood glucose by increasing insulin secretion from the pancreas and by improving tissue sensitivity to insulin.

Indications

Tolbutamide is indicated for the management of NIDDN in conjunction with strict dietary control.

Dosage and administration

Glibenclamide is a so-called second-generation sulphonylurea and is about 100 times more potent than tolbutamide on a molar basis. The usual dose is 5–15 mg orally as a single daily dose; it has an effective duration of action of up to 24 h.

Precautions

The overall frequency of side effects and incidence of severe hypoglycaemia is intermediate between those of tolbutamide and chlorpropamide. Glibenclamide does not have an antidiuretic effect, so that severe hyponatraemia does not occur.

GLUCAGON

Glucagon (rINN) and Glucagon injection (BP)
Chemical constitution: glucagon consists of a straight-chain polypeptide of 29 amino acid residues; molecular weight 3483 Da

Physiology

Glucagon is secreted from the A cells of the islets of Langerhans in the pancreas in response to hypoglycaemia. Its major metabolic effect is to increase hepatic glycogenolysis, with a resultant increase in blood glucose concentration.

Indications

Glucagon is used for the treatment of hypoglycaemia.

Dosage and administration

A dose of 0.5–1.0 mg given by either subcutaneous, intramuscular or intravenous injection (1 mg is equivalent to 1 unit).

Precautions

Glucagon is ineffective in increasing the blood glucose concentration in patients who have a low hepatic glycogen content, such as in starvation or chronic alcoholism. If there is no response in 10 minutes after injection of glucagon, glucose should be given intravenously. Glucagon is contra-indicated in the endocrine tumours glucagonoma, insulinoma and phaeochromocytoma.

HYDROCORTISONE

Hydrocortisone (rINN), Hydrocortisone acetate (BP and USP), Hydrocortisone sodium succinate (BP and USP), Hydrocortisone sodium phosphate (BP)
Chemical name: 11β,17α,21–trihydroxypregn-4-ene-3,20-dione. For structural formula see *Figure 17.1*, page 438

Pharmacology

Hydrocortisone is a naturally-occurring adrenal hormone with mainly glucocorticoid effects. These include anti-inflammatory properties, impairment of glucose tolerance and muscle proteolysis. The mineralocorticoid properties are less pronounced, but become troublesome with prolonged therapy.

Indications

Hydrocortisone may be used for physiological replacement when the endogenous supply of cortisol is inadequate. It may be used to provide additional hormone in the perioperative period when the ability of the adrenal gland to respond to surgical stress is impaired.

Dosage and administration

As a physiological replacement, hydrocortisone tablets are given in a daily dose of 20–30 mg, with the majority given in the morning to mimic the diurnal pattern of secretion. Hydrocortisone for injection is given as the sodium phosphate or sodium succinate salts although the former may cause perineal irritation following i.v. injection. Steroid cover for surgery can be achieved by the bolus administration of 25 mg intravenously at the start of surgery, followed by an infusion of hydrocortisone 100 mg/24 h (see above).

Precautions

The use of systemic hydrocortisone in large doses for a few days is free of obvious side effects, but can lead to deleterious effects on wound healing and resistance to infection. Prolonged use of large doses causes iatrogenic Cushing's syndrome (see prednisolone, below).

INSULIN

Chemical constitution: insulin consists of two polypeptide chains containing 21(A) and 30(B) amino acids, respectively, and linked by two disulphide bridges. Most diabetics in the United Kingdom are now treated with human insulin produced by recombinant DNA technology. Human insulin can be synthesized by several different methods.

The enzymatic modification of porcine insulin to produce human insulin – insulin (emp) – has been a major method but is becoming less popular. Human insulin is also synthesized from proinsulin by using DNA technology in yeasts – insulin (pyr) – and from proinsulin in *Escherichia coli* (prb). A human insulin analogue – insulin lispro – has been introduced recently which has a shorter duration of action than soluble insulin.

There are only three formulations of insulin in common use (*Table 17.3*), but these are presented as a vast array of commercial preparations.

Physical characteristics

Soluble insulin is a clear solution, whereas all longer acting preparations are cloudy.

Table 17.3 Preparations of insulin in common use

	Peak activity (h)	Duration of action (h)
1. Short-acting, soluble neutral insulin	2–5	5–8
2. Isophane insulin (NPH)*	4–12	12–18
3. Insulin zinc suspensions (IZS)	6–14	18–24

* NPH is neutral protamine, Hagedorn.

Physiology

Insulin lowers blood glucose, inhibits lipolysis and promotes protein synthesis.

Indications

The only indication for insulin is in the treatment of diabetes mellitus.

Dosage and administration

Insulin is only available in a concentration of 100 unit/ml, and is given by injection. Soluble insulin is the only preparation that can be given intravenously.

Soluble insulin is administered intravenously in diabetic patients undergoing surgery. It is given by continuous infusion, often mixed with glucose and potassium (see above), and the dose adjusted according to the blood glucose concentration. Soluble insulin has a short biological half-life of 5 minutes when given intravenously.

Precautions

Hypoglycaemia is always a hazard in patients taking insulin. It has been suggested that there is a greater risk from hypoglycaemia in patients taking human insulin compared with the old porcine and bovine preparations.

METFORMIN

Metformin (rINN)

Pharmacology

Metformin acts on the liver to reduce hepatic glucose output and also improves insulin sensitivity in peripheral tissues.

Dosage and administration

Metformin is given orally, 500 mg every 8 h, to a maximum dose of 2 g/day. It has a plasma half-life of 2–4 h and is eliminated solely by the kidney. Metformin rarely causes hypoglycaemia. It can be given either alone or in conjunction with sulphonylureas.

Precautions

Gastro-intestinal side effects are common, but they are usually transient. A rare but serious side effect is lactic acidosis. The use of metformin is contra-indicated in patients with renal impairment because of the risk of toxic accumulation of the drug, and in those who are pregnant or who have liver disease, alcoholism and heart failure. It has been suggested that lactic acidosis with metformin treatment only occurs when excess drug is given or arises in patients in whom the drug is contra-indicated.

OCTREOTIDE

Octreotide (rINN) Octreotide acetate (BP)

Chemical constitution: octreotide is a long-acting synthetic analogue of somatostatin, consisting of eight amino acid residues. It is more stable than the natural somatostatin-14 and has a biological effect lasting several hours

Physiology

Octreotide inhibits the secretion of hormones in the pituitary and pancreas, as well as blocking gut hormone secretion and decreasing splanchnic blood flow (see *Table 17.2*, page 444).

Indications

For symptomatic relief of gastro-enteropancreatic tumours (carcinoid tumours, VIPomas and glucagonomas) and pituitary tumours.

Dosage and administration

Ocretotide is given by subcutaneous injection in a dose of 50 µg once or twice a day, up to 200 µg 3 times daily.

Precautions

Octreotide may cause abdominal symptoms. Diabetic patients may require smaller doses of hypoglycaemic agents. If carcinoid tumour patients do not show a response within 1 week, then octreotide should be discontinued.

PREDNISOLONE

Prednisolone (rINN), Prednisolone acetate (BP and USP), Prednisolone sodium phosphate (BP and USP)
Chemical constitution: Prednisolone is derived from hydrocortisone, by the single change of inserting a double bond between carbons 1 and 2 (see *Figure 17.1*, page 438)

Pharmacology

Prednisolone is more potent in its glucocorticoid actions than hydrocortisone, but has only weak mineralocorticoid effects (see *Table 17.1*, page 440).

Indications

Prednisolone is used very commonly when the pharmacological effects of steroid therapy are required because it is cheap and has relatively minor effects on sodium retention.

Dosage and administration

For systemic use the dose of oral prednisolone is in the range of 10–60 mg/day in divided doses. Maintenance doses of less than 10 mg/day are unlikely to be associated with serious side effects.

Precautions

All patients receiving systemic corticosteroids should carry a card indicating the drug, dose and other relevant clinical details. Systemic corticosteroid therapy at high doses produces iatrogenic Cushing's syndrome (diabetes, hypertension, muscle weakness, localized fat deposition, osteoporosis, mental disturbances and peptic ulceration) and suppresses the normal pituitary–adrenocortical response to surgical stress. Local applications of corticosteroids and inhaled corticosteroids are unlikely to lead to sufficient systemic absorption to cause significant physiological impairment.

Particular care should be exercised in using these compounds in patients with peptic ulceration, hypertension, osteoporosis, infection, diabetes mellitus and pregnancy.

SOMATOTROPIN

Synonyms: Synthetic human growth hormone
Chemical constitution: somatotropin is a polypeptide consisting of a single chain of 191 amino acids cross-linked by two disulphide bridges. Human growth hormone is produced using recombinant DNA technology

Physiology

Growth hormone exerts an effect on growth by increasing the proliferation of cartilage at the end of the long bones. This is an indirect action of somatotropin mediated by the synthesis of somatomedin C (insulin-like growth factor −1) in the liver. Somatotropin also affects metabolism by increasing protein synthesis, mobilizing free fatty acids from adipose tissue and impairing glucose tolerance.

Indications

Somatotropin is given for growth failure in children due to deficiency of endogenous growth hormone, including short stature in Turner's syndrome. It is also used in adult growth hormone deficiency, although this is controversial.

Dosage and administration

Somatotropin is given by either subcutaneous or intramuscular injection, daily or 3 times weekly. The weekly dose is up to 1 unit/kg in children and 0.25 unit/kg in adults.

Precautions

Care should be taken in the presence of intracranial lesions, diabetes, hypothyroidism and a history of malignant disease.

THYROID HORMONES

1. Levothyroxine (rINN) and Levothyroxine sodium (USP)
    Chemical name: Sodium 4-O-(4-hydroxy-3,5-di-iodophenyl)-3,5-di-iodo-L-tyrosinate
2. Liothyronine sodium (BP and USP)
    Chemical name: Sodium 4-O-(4-hydroxy-3-iodophenyl)-3,5-di-iodo-L-tyrosinate
Synonyms: L-tri-iodothyronine sodium

Physiology

The thyroid hormones increase metabolism in most responsive tissues and increase growth in the young. T_3 has a much faster onset of action than T_4 and is several times more potent than T_4 on a molar basis. The half-life of T_4 is several days, whereas that of T_3 is about 12 h. It is probable that T_3 is the more important compound physiologically.

Indications

Both T_4 and T_3 are used in the treatment of hypothyroidism.

Dosage and administration

Thyroxine sodium is the standard preparation and is usually given in a single oral dose. The starting dose is around 50 µg/day, but may be lower in the elderly, and most patients can be maintained on a daily dose of 100–200 µg. The effectiveness of replacement therapy is assessed by the clinical response, and circulating thyroid hormone and TSH values.

Precautions

Cautious administration is essential in the elderly and those with cardiovascular disease.

Liothyronine sodium has an identical effect to T_4 but is more active. It is commonly used in severe hypothyroid states to achieve a rapid response in a dose of 5–20 µg by slow intravenous injection. This may be repeated at intervals of 12 h until the desired clinical response has been obtained.

TOLBUTAMIDE

Tolbutamide (rINN)

Pharmacology

Tolbutamide decreases blood glucose by increasing insulin secretion from the pancreas and by improving tissue sensitivity to insulin.

Indications

It is used in the management of NIDDM in conjunction with strict dietary control.

Dosage and administration

Tolbutamide is given orally 500 mg 2–3 times daily to a maximum of 2 g/day. It has an effective duration of action of 6–10 h.

Precautions

Tolbutamide has a low incidence of serious side effects; it can be used in patients with renal impairment. The frequency of severe hypoglycaemia is very low (< 1 per cent) and the overall frequency of side effects is about 3 per cent. Tolbutamide has a weak diuretic effect and occasionally hyponatraemia arises from an antidiuretic action. Transient skin rashes usually occur in the first weeks of treatment.

VASOPRESSIN (AVP)

Vasopressin injection (rINN), Lypressin injection (BP) (Lysine vasopressin), Desmopressin (BAN)
Synonyms: Antidiuretic hormone (ADH)
Chemical constitution: Vasopressin is an octapeptide

Lysine vasopressin is identical to vasopressin except for the substitution of lysine for arginine. Desmopressin is 1–desamino-8-D-arginine vasopressin, that is, there is the loss of an amino group from the cystine at position 1 and the substitution of D-arginine for L-arginine at position 8.

Physiology

The major physiological role of vasopressin in man is as an antidiuretic. Vasopressin acts on the distal renal tubule and collecting duct of the nephron to increase their permeability to water; this results in a decreased volume and increased concentration of the urine. The release of vasopressin from the posterior pituitary is controlled by changes in the osmotic pressure of the plasma and by changes in arterial pressure and atrial filling pressure.

Indications

The main use of vasopressin is in the treatment of diabetes insipidus, but it may also have a role in the control of abnormal bleeding such as oesophageal varices and after cardiac surgery.

Dosage and administration

Vasopressin analogue is usually administered by nasal spray in diabetes insipidus, 10–20 μg, once or twice daily. If lysine vasopressin is used, then it must be given more frequently.

For the treatment of bleeding oesophageal varices, vasopressin 2 mg may be given intravenously, followed by 1–2 μg every 6 h for up to 72 h.

Precautions

Vasopressin analogues may cause vasoconstriction at the site of injection and nasal administration may similarly cause mucosal damage. Abdominal pain and nausea may occur due to splanchnic vasoconstriction. Vasopressin should be used with caution in patients with hypertension and ischaemic heart disease because of the associated arterial vasoconstriction.

Oxytocin although being a pituitary hormone, is used mainly as a uterine stimulant; it is discussed in Chapter 15.

18

Anticoagulants, antithrombotic, thrombolytic and haemostatic agents

The arrest of haemorrhage from a damaged vessel depends on several mechanisms which comprise the haemostatic system. Clot formation is normally confined to the site of injury and spread to intact vascular endothelium is avoided. Platelets act as the first line of defence by forming a plug to close breaches in capillaries, small arterioles and venules. Exposure of subendothelial collagen stimulates adhesion of platelets to form a platelet monolayer along the breach. This requires calcium, von Willebrand factor and platelet membrane glycoprotein – GP1b. During this adhesion process the platelets are activated and the release of several mediators stimulates further platelets to aggregate and form the platelet plug.

Anticoagulants delay or prevent the clotting of blood or plasma. There are several stages at which they can exert this action, both directly and indirectly. Anticoagulants, however, have no effect on thrombus once it has been formed. Antithrombotic agents influence the natural incidence of thrombus formation, usually by an effect on platelet function. Substances that have fibrinolytic activity, or that enhance the body's fibrinolytic system, are thrombolytic agents. Haemostatic agents enhance platelet adhesiveness or strengthen capillary cement substance by enhancing resistance to lytic agents.

To understand the mechanism of action of these agents, it is necessary to appreciate the normal clotting process and the means by which the fluidity of blood is maintained.

The normal clotting process

The primary haemostatic plug is relatively unstable and is easily dislodged if not consolidated by the formation of a meshwork of fibrin clot. Blood coagulation is a complex process involving a series of enzyme steps in a biological amplification system, the end result of which is the formation of fibrin from fibrinogen. The various clotting factors are listed in *Table 18.1*.

The original cascade theory of coagulation separated the activation of the system into the extrinsic pathway and the intrinsic path which converged at factor X. In this system the intrinsic path was initiated by the contact activation of factor XII with blood vessel

Table 18.1 Blood clotting factors

Factors	Synonyms
I	Fibrinogen
II	Prothrombin
III	Thromboplastin
IV	Calcium ions
V	Accelerator globulin (AcG)
VII	Proconvertin
VIII	Antihaemophilic globulin (AHG)
IX	Christmas factor
X	Stuart–Prower factor
XI	Plasma thromboplastin antecedent (PTA)
XII	Hageman factor
XIII	Fibrin-stabilizing factor

Note: Factor VI is no longer considered to be a separate entity.

endothelium. In the extrinsic path, factor X was activated directly by plasma factor VII in the presence of tissue thromboplastin (tissue factor). Clinical observations that patients deficient in factor XII do not have a bleeding diathesis and that deficiency of factors VII, VIII and IX do cause significant bleeding has led to the conclusion that coagulation is initiated mainly via factor VII and tissue factor (TF) and that factors VIII and IX are essential to sustain coagulation (Gailani and Broze, 1997). Tissue factor is a transmembrane protein expressed widely in the body: subendothelially in vessels, the epidermis, organ capsules, gastro-intestinal and respiratory tract, the brain, monocytes and renal glomeruli. Factor VII circulates in the plasma, is synthesized in the liver and is dependent for its synthesis on vitamin K. Factor VII can be activated to factor VIIa by tissue factor, factors IXa, Xa, XIIa, VIIa, and thrombin.

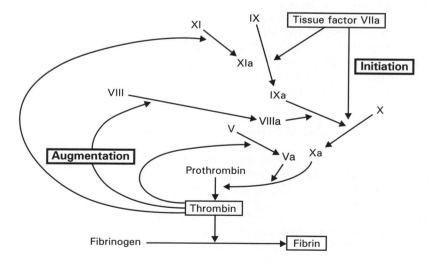

Figure 18.1 The clotting sequence

Thus, in the initiation stage of coagulation when plasma factors VII or VIIa come into contact with tissue factor, they form a complex which rapidly activates factor Xa which, along with factor Va as cofactor, converts prothrombin to thrombin. This in turn converts fibrinogen to fibrin (*Figure 18.1*). The tissue factor/factor VII complex, along with factor Xa, is rapidly inactivated by tissue factor pathway inhibitor. The augmentation stage now occurs in which the thrombin generated in the activation stage activates factors V, VIII and XI, and factor IXa with its cofactor FVIII activates factor X which ensures the continued activation of the coagulation cascade (Cameron *et al.*, 1996, see *Figure 18.1*).

The final part is the activation of prothrombin to thrombin by factor Xa, which requires calcium phospholipid and factor V as coenzymes, and this in turn cleaves fibrinogen to fibrin monomers. These monomers rapidly form dimers and then more slowly polymerize to fibrin. This results in the formation of an unstable clot. Factor XIII, which is also activated by thrombin, stimulates cross-linking and stabilization of the fibrin clot in a reaction which is also calcium dependent.

Cameron, E., Kolsto, A.B. and Prydz, H. (1996) Cell biology of tissue factor, the principal initiator of blood coagulation. *Thrombosis Research*, **81**, 1–41

Gailani, D. and Broze, G.J. (1997) Regulation of coagulation by tissue factor pathway inhibitor. In *Recent Advances in Blood Coagulation* (eds: L. Poller and C.A. Ludlam), pp. 1–17, Edinburgh: Churchill Livingstone

Control mechanisms

Several local mechanisms prevent spontaneous activation of platelets and other coagulation processes. Vascular endothelial glycosaminoglycans (which include heparans) and prostacyclin inhibit platelet adhesion to intact endothelium. The ADP released by activated platelets is catabolized by ADP-ase and thus inhibits ADP-induced platelet aggregation. Plasminogen activator stimulates fibrinolysis at the onset of coagulation and overcomes the stimulus to coagulation at the periphery of the lesion site, thus preventing further spread of fibrin deposition.

A series of circulating proteins act as inhibitors of the coagulation cascade. The most important is antithrombin III (AT III) which binds to the active sites of VIIa, IXa, Xa, XIa and thrombin. Thus thrombin is bound to AT III and to thrombomodulin from normal vascular endothelium which also renders it inactive. Thrombomodulin-bound thrombin activates the vitamin K-dependent natural anticoagulant protein C which, with its cofactor, free protein S, inactivates Va and VIIIa (*Figure 18.1*).

Sites of action of anticoagulants

In the light of *Figure 18.1*, the sites of action of these drugs can be outlined.

The **coumarin drugs** reduce or prevent the production by the liver of prothrombin and at least three other factors (VII, IX and X) which require vitamin K for their elaboration. They have no effect on clotting if added to whole blood, but must be absorbed and metabolized by the liver. They are discussed in greater detail below.

Heparin (and **protamine** if given alone) acts at several stages. It potentiates the activity of antithrombin III and inhibits particularly factors IIa, and Xa, but also XIa and XIIa. Thus, prevention of the formation of thrombin is probably its primary effect. In addition, it interacts with any thrombin present to prevent it catalysing the conversion of fibrinogen to fibrin.

Inhibition of platelet aggregation can be achieved by **aspirin**, which prolongs the bleeding time. It is being employed in the prevention of coronary and cerebral artery thrombosis; it is not likely to be of great value in the prophylaxis of venous thrombosis. **Dextran**, which also interferes with the function and aggregation of platelets has, however, been shown to be an effective prophylactic against venous thrombosis. This may be because it also coats erythrocytes and forms complexes with plasma proteins, thereby preventing rouleaux formation and sludging, both of which may contribute to the antithrombotic effect (see page 464–5). Newly available Clopidogrel is another orally active inhibitor of platelet aggregation which is a selective ADP receptor antagonist. It irreversibly inhibits ADP from binding to its receptor on the platelet cell membrane and thus blocks a fundamental step in the cascade of thrombus formation.

Tissue factors that inhibit platelet aggregation include **epoprostenol** (prostacyclin). This is synthesized by microsomal enzymes in arterial walls from prostaglandins G_2 and H_2 and has a powerful action against platelet aggregation as well as being a powerful vasodilator. This property has now been turned into a therapeutic tool and prostacyclin is given alone (or with heparin) to prevent clotting during renal dialysis and haemoperfusion.

Arvin is extracted from the Malayan pit viper and has been used to produce a different kind of anticoagulant effect, namely defibrination. Arvin breaks down fibrin which is rapidly phagocytozed by macrophages. All circulating fibrinogen is consumed in this way.

Calcium ion chelating agents, such as citrate, oxalate and ion-exchange resins, interfere with coagulation at several key points; they are suitable only for *in vitro* usage. For storage of blood that is to be transfused, the chelating agent must not be toxic. Oxalate is thus ruled out but citrate is safe within limits.

Fibrinolysis

Fibrinolysis is a continuous natural function which ensures the continuing fluidity of the circulating blood by bringing about the enzymatic degradation of fibrin. (*Figure 18.2*). This is important in the acute phase of haemostasis in preventing the formation of clots remote from the site of injury. In the longer term, dissolution of the clot is an important part of the healing process. The main component of the fibrinolytic system is plasminogen, an inactive precursor which can be converted into the proteolytic enzyme plasmin by a variety of endogenous activators. Plasmin acts on fibrin and fibrinogen to form a series of small peptide fragments, the fibrin/fibrinogen degradation products.

Several factors bring about the activation of plasminogen. Plasminogen activator is released from the vascular endothelium during vessel injury: kallikrein also directly

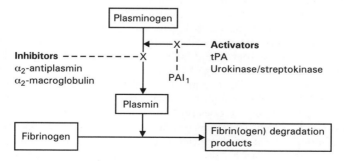

Figure 18.2 The fibrinolysis process

activates plasminogen. Urokinase is released from the urothelium and inhibits clot formation within the renal tract. Other activators have been obtained from bacteria, moulds, plants and now by genetic engineering using recombinant DNA technology.

Lysis of thrombus is possible with fibrinolytic agents. Therapeutic fibrinolysis reduces the morbidity and mortality after myocardial infarction and may be beneficial in peripheral arterial occlusion and acute pulmonary embolism. Therapeutic activators include streptokinase, anistreplase, recombinant tissue plasminogen activator (t-PA) and urokinase.

Streptokinase binds to and activates circulating plasminogen. As well as preferential fibrinolysis in the clot, there is systemic lysis causing reduction in fibrinogen, factors V and VIII. Allergic reactions are not uncommon and the formation of neutralizing antibody to streptokinase after therapy means that repeat treatment cannot be given for at least 2 years.

Anistreplase, an acylated plasminogen streptokinase activator complex (APSAC), has a longer half-life (about 90 minutes) and lytic potency than streptokinase alone but also induces antibody formation.

Recombinant tissue plasminogen activator (t-PA) binds preferentially to fibrin which aids localization to the clot and, through conformational change, converts plasminogen to plasmin leading to lysis of thrombus. Some systemic degradation of clotting factors occurs. It does not induce antibody formation.

Urokinase, a fibrinolytic activator found in urine, has been used extensively to treat deep-vein thrombosis, pulmonary embolism and peripheral arterial occlusion, but myocardial infarction is not currently an approved indication.

The major risk of thrombolytic agents is bleeding, whether it be from recent wounds or catastrophically into the brain. About 5 per cent of patients will have some bleeding problem and 1 per cent a severe haemorrhage. There is no routine monitoring laboratory test that is clinically useful; the prothrombin time, the activated partial thromboplastin time and fibrin degradation products all increase with therapy and the fibrinogen level falls. Patients must be clinically monitored for signs of bleeding and appropriate action taken, stopping therapy and initating transfusion if indicated. In view of the risks of bleeding, thrombolytic therapy is relatively contra-indicated in acute severe hypertension, within 6 weeks of surgery or trauma, and within six months of pericarditis or stroke.

Antifibrinolytic therapy

An important regulatory mechanism of intravascular clotting is the presence of inhibitors of proteolytic enzymes. In some pathological states, excessive production of these enzymes may result in the inhibitors being overwhelmed. Under these conditions the unrestrained activity of plasmin may cause not only excess fibrinolysis, but breakdown of other proteins such as factors V and VIII. Proteinase inhibition may thus be useful therapeutically. A naturally-occurring inhibitor, aprotinin, and a synthetic inhibitor, tranexamic acid, are available. They form a reversible complex with proteinases and are, therefore, competitive enzyme inhibitors. An effective inhibitor is one that has a much greater affinity for proteinase than does protein. This is so for aprotinin, but less marked for tranexamic acid, which therefore has to be given in large quantities. Natural proteinase inhibitors have a wide spectrum of action also, and inhibit many other enzymes. The main indications for proteinase inhibitor therapy are for the treatment of fibrinolysis and its prevention in high-risk cardiac surgery.

At least two syndromes of pathological bleeding are recognized as being due to imbalance between proteinases and their inhibitors, although unfortunately it is rarely possible to distinguish between these conditions quickly by clinical or laboratory methods. One such syndrome is hypofibrinogenaemia. This, it is suggested, arises when excess thromboplastic material from damaged tissue enters the circulation and causes widespread fibrin deposition. This causes over-activation of plasmin, which not only lyses the fibrin, but also attacks fibrinogen itself, converting them both into fibrinopeptides. This syndrome has also been called consumption coagulopathy, and is the likely pathology of excessive bleeding when tissues containing large amounts of thromboplastin are damaged. This occurs in many obstetric emergencies such as retroplacental haemorrhage, dead fetus and amniotic fluid embolism. Alternatively, the fibrinolytic system may be primarily activated, and this may occur as a result of severe stress and some shock states.

Therapy of these conditions with proteinase inhibitors is based on inhibition of both groups of activators. It is advisable to give fibrinogen concurrently, in case there has been excessive consumption of fibrin and fibrinogen.

Several other indications for fibrinolytic therapy have been suggested. In haemophilia, when there is deficient formation of fibrin, inhibition of fibrinolysis may permit adequate haemostasis, and treatment with tranexamic acid will reduce bleeding after extraction of teeth in haemophilia. (Desmopressin elevates factor VIII levels by a release mechanism and is also effective in haemophilia.)

Inhibition of fibrinolysis has been shown to reduce menstrual flow in menorrhagia; it will reduce the incidence of blood loss after prostatectomy, although it does not affect the incidence of thrombo-embolic complications unless heparin is given concurrently.

Aprotinin is best administered by continuous intravenous infusion after an initial dose of 50 000–100 000 kiu (kallikrein inactivator units). Because of a small risk of an allergic reaction, the first 5 ml of solution should be given slowly, over 5 minutes. To keep a constant level it is necessary to then give about 20 000 kiu per hour. In cardiac surgery, the inital dose is 200 000 kiu over 20 minutes followed by 50 000 kiu per hour. Aprotinin is excreted through the kidney in an inactive form. EACA is also best given as a continuous infusion of 3 g/h or may be given at a rate of 0.2 g/kg 1-hourly by mouth. The half-life in the plasma of a single intravenous injection is about 2 h and it is excreted unchanged almost entirely by the kidney within 12 h.

Oral anticoagulants

Dicoumarol was originally isolated from spoiled sweet clover hay, and found to prolong coagulation time and reduce the plasma prothrombin level. Since its introduction several other chemically related compounds have been produced which differ mainly in their duration of action. These compounds are of two chemical groupings, those related to dicoumarol and a newer group related to indanedione, the commonest being phenindione. In both cases they antagonize vitamin K which is required for the γ-carboxylation of factors II, VII, IX and X in the liver, an essential step in their production. In consequence the liver produces Proteins Induced by Vitamin K Antagonism (or absence) – PIVKAs.

The usage of phenindione is now much reduced due to the serious nature of some of the toxic effects that have been reported, particularly agranulocytosis. Severe allergic reactions involving the skin and kidney have also been reported. This drug should therefore be reserved for patients who have demonstrated sensitivity to other oral anticoagulants. The dose and other characteristics are given in *Table 18.2*.

Table 18.2 Duration of action and dosage of oral anticoagulants

Drug	Time of peak effect (h)	Duration after Discontinuing dose (days)	Initial dose (mg)	Maintenance dose (mg)
Warfarin	36–72	5–6	50	2–15
Ethyl biscoumacetate	18–36	2–3	1200 1st day, 600–900 2nd day	300–600
Dicoumarol	36–48	5–6	300 1st day, 200 2nd	25–150

Excessive doses of this group of drugs cause haemorrhages, particularly from mucous membranes, skin and the gastro-intestinal and genito-urinary tracts. Haematuria is probably the commonest manifestation, but uterine bleeding, ecchymosis and epistaxis can all occur and anaemia may be severe. It is important, therefore, that prothrombin levels should be estimated daily until they are stabilized. Overdose can be controlled by the administration of phytomenadione (vitamin K_1), 5–20 mg intravenously.

Interactions between oral anticoagulants and other drugs

A large number of commonly prescribed drugs can give rise to dangerous interactions during anticoagulant therapy by a variety of mechanisms.

Drugs that diminish the response

A wide variety of sedatives, tranquillizers and antidepressants stimulate the proliferation of liver microsomal enzymes, which are responsible for inactivating many other drugs, including the oral anticoagulants. Thus, a patient on one of these enzyme-inducing drugs will require a higher dose of anticoagulant to maintain the prothrombin time in the therapeutic range. If the sedative drug is stopped, there is an increase in anticoagulant effect and it may take weeks before the half-life of the anticoagulant returns to normal.

Diminution of effect would also be caused by the administration of vitamin K or by inhibition of absorption of the anticoagulant. Clofibrate and griseofulvin have been implicated in such a mechanism, but the clinical relevance is slight.

Drugs that enhance the response

Drugs of the coumarin–indanedione group are highly bound to plasma proteins and can be displaced by other highly protein-bound acidic drugs such as salicylates, indomethacin, nalidixic acid, sulphonamide, clofibrate and ethacrynic acid. Although this mechanism is well established, such enhancement is usually only very temporary. Displacement makes more drug available for biotransformation, the half-life is shortened and a new steady state is soon reached. However, serious haemorrhage has resulted when this possible complication has been overlooked.

Simultaneous interference with anticoagulant metabolism would, of course, make displacement from binding a much more serious problem; chloramphenicol, some monoamine oxidase inhibitors, and possibly other drugs may inhibit the hydroxylation of warfarin. Salicylates have an enhancing effect which may work through several mechanisms including the production of gastric erosions, inhibition of platelet function, and a hypo-prothrombinaemic effect. Broad-spectrum antibiotics or liquid paraffin may interfere with vitamin K absorption, but the effect is slight unless there is a deficient dietary intake of the vitamin.

There are many other miscellaneous interactions. Large doses of glucagon increase the effect of warfarin, although the mechanism has not been elucidated. Steroids can produce two opposing types of interaction: they cause enzyme induction but also compete for the same enzyme systems. In the case of the anabolic steroids, the predominant effect is to reduce warfarin requirements. Alcohol is also a potent enzyme inducer, but again a contrary effect has been reported, the suggestion being that either cholestasis leads to malabsorption of vitamin K or that defective secretion of bile salts inhibits the microsomal enzymes.

It is important, too, to remember that the initiation of anticoagulant therapy in a patient who is stabilized on some other chronic medication may lead to serious problems due to drug interactions. The coumarins inhibit the metabolism of tolbutamide, chlorpropamide and phenytoin, and may thus produce hypoglycaemia in diabetics or phenytoin intoxication in epileptics. Phenindione does not have this effect. A list of drugs that potentiate or antagonize coumarin anticoagulants, as well as drugs whose metabolism is affected by the anticoagulant, has been published by the Standing Advisory Committee for Haematology of the Royal College of Pathologists (1982).

Standing Advisory Committee for Haematology of the Royal College of Pathologists (1982) Drug interactions with coumarin derivative anticoagulants. *British Medical Journal*, **2**, 274

MONOGRAPHS

ANISTREPLASE

Anistreplase (rINN)

Anistreplase is also known as APSAC, an acronym for anisoylated plasminogen streptokinase activator complex. It is available in vials containing 30 u as a sterile powder. One unit is equivalent to 1 mg which contains about 36 000 iu of streptokinase. It can be reconstituted with water or saline and must then be used within 30 minutes.

Pharmacology

Anistreplase is an acylated complex of streptokinase with human *lys* plasminogen. Acylation protects that part of the complex that interacts with human plasminogen and thus the drug remains inactive until it is deacylated, a process which occurs in the circulation and at the interface between blood and clot. It has a half-life of about 90 minutes. In consequence it can be given as a single slow intravenous injection instead of by prolonged infusion. A second advantage is that by providing preformed plasminogen, the body's own plasminogen is not depleted. Finally, being in the *lys* form which is found in thrombus, as opposed to the *glu* form which is found in the circulation, there is more specific binding to the required site of action, namely the clot. Plasmin is thus formed and leads to fibrinolysis.

These theoretical advantages have been confirmed by clinical experience. Several trials have demonstrated both thrombolysis and reperfusion of coronary arteries when anistreplase has been given within a few hours of myocardial infarction, and some trials have demonstrated reductions in mortality.

Indications

Anistreplase is used for the treatment of acute coronary thrombosis, which is found in 80 per cent of all acute myocardial infarctions. It is more effective the earlier that it is given after the initial infarction. It is also on trial for the treatment of cerebral thrombosis.

Dosage and administration

Thirty units are administered by intravenous injection over 2–5 minutes. Thrombolysis usually occurs within 60 minutes. Heparinization is usually started some 2–24 h after signs of successful reperfusion.

Precautions

Arrhythmias are relatively common during reperfusion: therapy should therefore be undertaken with ECG monitoring in an environment which can treat acute arrhythmias promptly. The most common other side effect is bleeding, most of which is minor and does not require blood transfusion. Some allergic reactions have been reported.

DEXTRANS

Dextrans are plasma substitutes which are produced by the action of selected strains of *Leuconostoc mesenteroides* on sucrose. By controlling the hydrolysis, glucose chains of the desired average molecular weight can be selected. There is a range of different sized molecules in the preparation, those below the renal threshold (about 50 000 Da) being excreted by the kidneys quite quickly. The remainder leave the blood at a uniform rate of about one-third per day and enter the tissues and particularly the cells of the reticuloendothelial system. All the administered dextran molecules are believed to be metabolized eventually, but the precise route is not known.

Dextran 70 has an average molecular weight of 70 000 Da and is available in either 0.9 per cent saline or 5 per cent dextrose.

Dextran 40 has an average molecular weight of 40 000 Da and is available as a 10 per cent solution in either 0.9 per cent saline or 5 per cent dextrose. It was originally marketed with emphasis on the rheological benefits it was held to confer.

Antithrombotic properties

Both dextran 40 and dextran 70 have been used to prevent postoperative venous thrombosis. Dextran alters normal platelet function and tends to prevent platelet aggregation. It also alters the structure and chemical stability of fibrin and facilitates fibrinolysis by plasmin. Although dextran in doses of up to 1.5 g/kg body weight induces no measurable changes in the clotting mechanism, it does prolong the bleeding time and it should not be used in neurosurgery or other operations when this would be particularly undesirable. The antithrombotic effect is a property of the dextran molecule and unaffected by its molecular weight. Dextran 40 offers no advantages over dextran 70 for this purpose, as the average molecular weight of colloid remaining in the circulation 24 h after infusion of dextran 40 is 80 000 Da.

Dosage and administration

Before surgery starts, 500 ml of dextran 70 should be infused and the same volume repeated daily for 2–3 days postoperatively.

Precautions

Cross-matching of blood is affected by dextran and if there is any possibility of blood being needed, it is advisable to take the necessary sample from the patient for cross-matching before any dextran is given. It is advisable, because of its effect on clotting, to restrict the volume given to 1–1.5 litres. There are numerous reports linking the development of acute renal failure with the administration of dextran 40 and it should not be given when there is any reason to doubt renal function. Urine output should be maintained above 40 ml/h. The smaller molecules are rapidly excreted by the kidneys and concentrations as high as 40 g/100 ml of urine are seen, resulting in very viscous urine.

EPOPROSTENOL

Epoprostenol sodium (rINN)

Pharmacology

Epoprostenol (Flolan) is presented as 500 µg of a freeze-dried powder with 50 ml of sterile alkaline diluent (pH 10.5 ± 0.3) consisting of sodium chloride 0.147 per cent and glycine 0.188 per cent.

Epoprostenol (formerly known as prostacyclin) is one of the prostaglandins derived from arachidonic acid, and occurs naturally in the walls of blood vessels of all mammals. It may be given by continuous infusion intravenously or directly into the arterial inlet line to a haemofilter or haemodialyser. It is a powerful disaggregator of platelets and can be used alone to prevent clotting.

Some authorities recommend an initial bolus of heparin (500 u) when dialysis is started and a further increment if any clotting occurs in the bubble trap. Activated whole blood clotting time (AWBCT) should be kept at about 20 per cent of predialysis values by adjustment to the rate of administration.

Epoprostenol is also a potent vasodilator, and initial administration rates should be adjusted to maintain a systolic blood pressure above 100 mmHg (13 kPa).

Fate in the body   Epoprostenol is rapidly inactivated in the body by both enzymatic and hydrolytic mechanisms. It has a half-life in the circulation of less than 3 minutes and is cleared by many organs but not the lungs. Because it is a natural substance which may be actively generated during treatment, plasma concentration measurements have been found to be extremely variable. Furthermore, a similar therapeutic effect is exerted by its principal metabolite 6-oxo-PGF$_{1\alpha}$ which has a weaker effect but has a longer half-life of up to 30 minutes and may be present in much higher concentrations.

Dosage and administration

Initial recommended dose is 5 ng/kg/minute, i.e. 350 ng (0.35 μg) per minute for a 70 kg patient, which is roughly equivalent to 20 μg/h or 2 ml/h of the reconstituted Flolan solution. This should be given initially into a peripheral vein for 15–30 minutes and then transferred to the inlet of the dialysis machine. Dose rate should be adjusted by measuring the AWBCT. If given in conjunction with other anticoagulants, appropriate standard monitoring should also be employed. Epoprostenol prolongs the action of heparin and reduces its requirements. The combination of heparin 200–500 u/h with 2.5–5 ng/kg/h of epoprostenol provides adequate anticoagulation with minimal effect on the results of coagulation studies or on blood pressure.

Side effects

These are numerous and largely related to its vasodilating properties. The less severe include facial flushing, headache and local redness. More serious are hypotension and tachycardia, but these can be controlled by fluid administration. Occasionally, vagal attacks have occurred at high doses. Heart rate and blood pressure should be monitored regularly.

Precautions

The vasodilating effect will be augmented by other vasodilators: heparin is potentiated. Blood glucose may be elevated in diabetic patients. Care is needed in calculating doses if different dilutions are used, and precautions must be taken to avoid unintended bolus doses when flushing lines.

ETHAMSYLATE

Ethamsylate (rINN)

Pharmacology

Ethamsylate significantly reduces the bleeding time without any effect on the prothrombin time, clotting time or fibrinolysis. It acts principally on the capillary wall, causing a demonstrable increase in capillary strength. This is believed to be due to an enhanced resistance to the effect of bradykinin on the cement substance between capillary endothelial cells. It also seems to enhance platelet adhesiveness, thus maintaining the integrity of the capillary wall by platelet occlusion.

Indications

Ethamsylate has been recommended in a variety of situations in which capillary haemorrhage may be a problem. It has been shown to be effective in controlled trials in reducing haemorrhage associated with tonsillectomy and prostatectomy.

Dosage and administration

Ethamsylate is effective both orally and parenterally. Initial dosage should be between 0.75 and 1.0 g intravenously or intramuscularly. For prophylaxis or maintenance therapy, 500 mg should be given every 4–6 h.

Precautions and side effects

There are no known contra-indications, although there has been one report of an increase in experimentally detectable deep vein thrombosis. Transient falls in blood pressure have been reported after intravenous administration. Oral administration may cause nausea.

HEPARIN

Heparin (rINN) and Heparin sodium (BP)

Heparin is a mixture of naturally-occurring glycoaminoglycans extracted from bovine or porcine intestinal mucosa. In view of its heterogeneous composition and degree of sulphation, its molecular weight ranges between 15 000 and 25 000 Da. The BP preparation is the sodium salt and must contain at least 110 u/mg of anticoagulant activity. The USP preparation must contain 120 u/mg. A unit is that amount which will prevent 1.0 ml of citrated sheep plasma clotting for 1 h after addition of 0.2 ml of a 1:100 CaCl solution. Injection of heparin BP is a sterile solution in water for injections, pH 5–8.

Pharmacology

Heparin occurs widely throughout the body and is found in the granules of mast cells of connective tissue surrounding blood vessels. The physiological functions of heparin, if any, are a matter of debate. It is possible that its most important function is to bind amines such as 5-hydroxytryptamine, norepinephrine (noradrenaline) and histamine in mast cells, which it does exceedingly well by virtue of its negative charges. It is also a precursor of lipoprotein lipase, which appears to play a role in clearing lipid droplets from the blood, possibly by facilitating transport of triglyceride fatty acids through the vessel wall. It is released with histamine in anaphylactic and peptone shock.

The anticoagulant property of heparin probably depends on the fact that it has a strong electronegative charge. Its action can be antagonized by substances with a strong positive charge, such as protamine sulphate, or by a basic dye such as Toluidine Blue O (tolonium chloride – rINN). The mode of action is potentiation of the activity of antithrombin III, predominantly against the activated clotting factors IIa and Xa, but also against XIa and IXa. The plasma half-life of unfractionated heparin is about 1 h. Although clotting time is prolonged, bleeding time is unaffected. Bleeding from small abrasions is therefore not a hazard.

Fate in the body   After intravenous injection of large doses, the heparin concentration of plasma falls rapidly. Duration of effect is brief. A single dose will cause up to a five-fold increase in clotting time within 10 minutes and its effect lasts for 1–4 h. A portion is metabolized to an inactive material, uroheparin, by depolymerization; a little appears in the urine in an active form, and the remainder is destroyed in the body by the enzyme heparinase.

Indications

The chief uses of heparin are in the treatment of arterial and venous thrombosis and in vascular and cardiac surgery where an anticoagulant is required and when blood is circulating extracorporeally for any reason. Postoperatively it can be given by a low-dose subcutaneous regimen as a prophylaxis against deep vein thrombosis and embolism, but low molecular weight fractions are increasingly being preferred. Although it is not used as an anticoagulant for stored blood, it can be added to blood that has been anticoagulated with citrate–phosphate–dextrose (CPD). The calcium content can then be safely restored, thus eliminating at least one of the disadvantages associated with the transfusion of large quantities of stored blood. Heparin may be added to fat emulsion to reduce the liability to venous thrombosis and is the only drug that can be safely added to such preparations. It is also used at the start of treatment with oral anticoagulants, such as warfarin, and discontinued after 2–3 days when the slower acting drug has reached its full effect.

Dosage and administration

Owing to its rapid but transient action, heparin is usually administered by continuous intravenous infusion of 1000–2000 u/h after an intravenous bolus of 5000–10,000 u. The dose per hour infused is adjusted to keep the activated partial thromboplastin time (APTT) between 1.5 and 2.5 times the control. For prophylaxis in surgical patients, subcutaneous heparin is given in doses of 5000 u in 0.2 ml 8-hourly, the first dose being given immediately postoperatively. Heparin can be given intramuscularly, but larger doses are necessary and the response is slower. The injections are painful and haematomas may occur at the site of injection.

Precautions and side effects

Dilute solutions lose their stability if kept below pH 6, and should not be mixed with dextrose solutions which are usually acidic. Heparin is incompatible with drugs containing methyl groups such as streptomycin and cetrimide. It is also incompatible with hydrocortisone hemisuccinate, ristocetin and vancomycin. Heparin should therefore not be added to infusions containing these substances.

The main side effect of heparin is bleeding, but this risk can be minimized by closely monitoring the APTT. If the APTT is prolonged the heparin should be stopped and, because of the short half-life, this is usually sufficient to stop mild bleeding. If bleeding is severe, protamine sulphate can be given intravenously to neutralize the effects of heparin. The dose depends on the dose of heparin given and the time from injection. One milligram of protamine will neutralize 100 u of heparin given at the same time. One hour later only 50 per cent of the protamine dose will be required. Long-term heparin therapy may cause osteoporosis, which can be a particular problem in pregnancy.

In hypersensitive patients, allergic reactions have been observed. Heparin is contraindicated if a patient has a known tendency to bleed, in cases of subacute bacterial endocarditis, in peptic ulcer, in malignant disease, and in threatened abortion or advanced renal or hepatic disease.

Platelets should be monitored twice weekly in all patients receiving prolonged heparin therapy. There may be a mild reduction occurring in the first few days after heparin exposure which is transient and clinically insignificant. A severe and progressive reduction in platelet count may start after 5–7 days of heparin therapy and is a potentially fatal condition. Heparin-induced thrombocytopenia can be due to intravenous heparin, standard or low-dose subcutaneous heparin, heparin used to flush indwelling cannulae or low molecular weight heparin. The syndrome is due to an anti-heparin antibody that causes platelet aggregation. Most of the problems arise from the resulting arterial and venous thromboses which can form anywhere. Heparin must be stopped and an alternative anticoagulant such as the heparinoid danaparoid given.

Low molecular weight heparin

This is manufactured from unfractionated heparin using chemical or enzymatic methods. The average molecular weights range from 4000 to 6000 Da. Its mechanism of action is the same as unfractionated heparin, namely to potentiate antithrombin III but predominantly to inactivate factor Xa rather than factor IIa. Laboratory monitoring is not usually required. Low molecular weight heparin does not prolong the APTT. It has a high bioavailability from subcutaneous depots and a half life of 2–4 h and thus can be injected once or twice daily.

It is indicated for the prevention of deep-vein thrombosis in high risk situations such as orthopaedic surgery (Anon., 1998) and is as effective and as safe as unfractionated heparin in the treatment of this condition and has the potential advantage of being able to be given at home. Protamine does not reverse the effects of low molecular weight heparin. It cross-reacts with the antibodies in heparin-induced thrombocytopenia and therefore is not usually an option in this condition.

There is currently a controversy concerning the safety of prophylaxis with low molecular weight heparin and the use of spinal anaesthesia. Several cases of spinal haematomata have been reported in the USA, usually in patients with indwelling spinal catheters, shortly after their removal. This may be associated with higher doses than those used in Europe (Horlocker, 1998).

Anon (1998) Low molecular weight heparins for venous thrombosis. *Drug and Therapeutics Bulletin*, **36**, 25–9

Horlocker, T.T. (1998) Low-molecular-weight heparins. *New England Journal of Medicine*, **338**, 687

PROTAMINE

Protamine sulphate/sulfate injection (rINN)
Constitution: the sulphate of protamine, a protein from the sperm or mature testes of fish of the genera *Oncorhynchus, Salmo* or *Trutta*

Pharmacology

Protamine sulphate is a simple protein with basic properties manufactured from the sperm or mature testes of fish of the genera *Oncorhynchus, Salmo* or *Trutta*. Although it has anticoagulant properties, it is only used as an antagonist to heparin where its strongly positive charge can neutralize the negatively charged heparin molecule to form a complex which is rapidly deposited, probably on vascular endothelial cells.

Dosage and administration

It is given intravenously in a 1 per cent solution and should be administered slowly over a period of several minutes, otherwise a serious fall in blood pressure may be encountered.

The amount of protamine sulphate required is 1 mg for each 100 u of heparin injected. If more than 15 minutes has elapsed since the injection of the heparin, proportionately less is required, particularly as protamine sulphate is itself an anticoagulant. Not more than 50 mg should be injected at any one time. One hour after heparin administration, only 50 per cent of the protamine dose will be required. Protamine should be given slowly as it can cause bradycardia, hypotension and anaphylaxis.

TRANEXAMIC ACID

Tranexamic acid (rINN)

Pharmacology

Tranexamic acid is an antifibrinolytic agent that competitively inhibits the activation of plasminogen to plasmin. Approximately 90 per cent of an intravenous dose is excreted unchanged in the urine within 24 h. The plasma half-life is about 2 h.

Indications

Tranexamic acid can be used to treat excessive fibrinolysis. This may be localized fibrinolysis, e.g. after prostatectomy, or generalized, e.g. in certain cases of disseminated intravascular coagulation. It is also useful in reducing bleeding during surgery or dental extraction in patients with haemophilia. It can also be used to neutralize the action of thrombolytic drugs.

Dosage and administration

One gram of tranexamic acid is given intravenously over 10 minutes every 8 h. In moderate renal failure and in patients on haemofiltration, the dose should be halved.

Precautions

Tranexamic acid is contra-indicated in patients with a history of thrombo-embolic disease.

WARFARIN

Warfarin sodium (rINN)

Pharmacology

Warfarin antagonizes vitamin K, which is required for the γ-carboxylation, and hence function, of factors II, VII, IX and X and of proteins C and S. It is therefore not active *in vitro* and there is a delay in onset after administration of 12–24 h until the existing circulating clotting factors disappear.

Fate in the body Warfarin is readily and completely absorbed after oral administration and this is a most important advantage over other coumarin-type anticoagulants. It is 97 per cent bound to albumin and this contributes to its negligible urinary excretion and long half-life of about 36 h. Individual variation in half-life has been attributed to genetic factors. It is hydroxylated in the liver, the metabolites appearing in the urine. Warfarin crosses the placental barrier, anticoagulating the fetus, and may result in fatal intracranial haemorrhage. It is secreted in milk, but does not appear in the cerebrospinal fluid.

Indications

Warfarin is used in the treatment of thrombo-embolic disorders, particularly those of venous origin, and for prophylaxis against further thromboses and pulmonary embolism. After a considerable perid of popularity, the usage of coumarin anticoagulants in myocardial infarction has been progressively reduced. It is sometimes employed to minimize embolism associated with rheumatic heart disease.

Dosage and administration

The control of warfarin dosage is by the INR (international normalized ratio) which is a prothrombin time ratio corrected to an international standard thromboplastin. This allows continuous control of warfarin irrespective of which laboratory performs the monitoring. Target values of INR vary according to the reason for anticoagulation but fall in the range 2–4.5. Anticoagulation with warfarin is achieved by giving 2 days of a loading dose usually of 10 mg, followed by a maintenance dose usually between 3 and 9 mg, according to the INR. Smaller doses are advisable in the elderly. It takes 24–36 h after the first dose of oral anticoagulant before its effect can be assessed. The INR should therefore be measured on the morning before the third dose and then daily, adjusting the dose as required. When the patient is stabilized, the frequency of estimation can be reduced to once every few weeks.

Table 18.3 Recommendations by the British Society for Haematology for the management of warfarin overdose

Clinical state or haematology	Actions
Life threatening haemorrhage	Vit K_1 5 mg i.v. slowly + factor II, IX and X concentrate (with factor VII if possible). If unavailable, give 1 L fresh frozen plasma
Mild bleeding, e.g. haematuria epistaxis	Stop warfarin: for 1–2 days consider Vit K_1 0.5–2 mg i.v. slowly
INR>7 without haemorrhage	Stop warfarin: consider Vit K_1 0.5 mg i.v. slowly
INR 4.5–7	Stop warfarin for 1–2 days and review
Unexpected bleeding at therapeutic levels	Investigate for possible underlying cause, e.g. unsuspected renal or G.I. tract disease

INR: International Normalized Ratio.

If the patient has a prolonged INR the warfarin should be stopped. It is important to establish whether there is any evidence of bleeding and if so, the extent. *Table 18.3* summarizes guidelines on the management of warfarin overdose. It takes about 6 h after the administration of vitamin K before there is a significant demonstrable effect on the INR.

Surgery in the anticoagulated patient

For patients taking maintenance anticoagulation therapy having surgery, the type of surgery and thrombotic risk in the patient should be taken into account when planning anticoagulant control perioperatively. Certain types of surgery, such as neurosurgery, are particularly high risk for bleeding complications and a period without any anticoagulation may be necessary. Thrombotic risks of a mechanical mitral valve prosthesis are high.

Prior to surgery the INR should be reduced to less than 1.7 by adjusting the warfarin dose. This can be achieved by stopping warfarin at least 3 days preoperatively, monitoring the INR. If the underlying thrombotic risk is high (e.g. mechanical mitral valve prosthesis or venous thromboembolus within 1 month of surgery), i.v. heparin should be given when the INR is <3.0. Postoperatively, warfarin should be restarted as soon as possible, depending on the risk of postoperative haemorrhage. Heparin prophylaxis against venous thrombosis should be instituted for high–risk groups until the INR is in the therapeutic range.

Precautions

All coumarin-type anticoagulants can be the subject of numerous drug interactions (see page 462). Not only must changes in warfarin dose be monitored by INR estimations, therefore, but also all other drug regimen alterations. Warfarin is antagonized by phytomenadione (vitamin K_1); a dose of 10 mg is usually sufficient to reduce the prothrombin time to a safe level, but higher doses up to 150 mg may be required and are not toxic.

Cutaneous necrosis due to capillary thrombosis during induction of anticoagulation may occur in those patients heterozygous for protein C or S.

Dicoumarol was the earliest coumarin derivative but is now rarely employed in the United Kingdom. Absorption after oral administration is slower and more erratic than that of warfarin and the half-life is only 10–30 h, depending on dose. Apart from these differences, the mechanism of action, metabolism, toxic effects and precautions required are the same as for warfarin. It is susceptible to the same drug interactions. The recommended dose schedules for these and other similar compounds are given in *Table 18.2* (page 462). It is also teratogenic in the first trimester of pregnancy.

19

Antibiotics and other antimicrobial agents

History

Man's attempt to treat infection can be traced to the ancient Greek, Chinese and Middle Eastern physicians who were familiar with the therapeutic properties of mouldy bread, soyabean, wine and salt, but not with the idea of infection. They did, however, recognize the contagious character of some diseases. Fear of disease and the relatively vast distances between habitations ensured a certain degree of isolation and control of infection. With modern travel, these natural and geographical barriers against the spread of infectious diseases (and antibiotic-resistant microbes) have disappeared.

During the nineteenth century, the microbiological basis of infective diseases was established and the search for therapeutic agents began in earnest. Compounds containing arsenic or bismuth were tried for the treatment of syphilis (and their relative toxicity was observed), but the most significant steps in the treatment of infection were the discovery and use of sulphonamide in the 1930s, the description of the effect of penicillin in the 1940s, and the isolation of streptomycin in 1944. Antibiotics were once defined as substances, usually produced by micro-organisms, used to destroy or inhibit the growth of pathogenic microbes, but with the advent of synthetic antibiotics this description has become less definite.

Future medical historians will undoubtedly recognize that antibiotics were one of the most significant developments in this century, reducing mortality and morbidity and allowing expansion in many branches of medicine including previously undreamed of areas such as transplant surgery. However, despite an understanding of the mode of action of antibiotics and of selective toxicity, problems such as antibiotic resistance among recognized pathogens, the pathogenic role of organisms that were previously considered commensals, and the recognition of toxic effects of antibiotics on patients, have made antimicrobial therapy challenging. Furthermore, their widespread and indiscriminate use has exacerbated these problems. There is a need for less toxic and broader spectrum antibiotics, as well as for antibiotics with a narrow range of activity directed against specific pathogens.

General approach to the use of antibiotics

Rational antibacterial therapy is ideally based on microbiological culture from appropriate specimens. However, in life-threatening infections, empirical therapy must be started as soon as specimens have been collected but before the results of tests become available.

The choice of antibiotics must take into account the clinical state of the patient, the likely causative organism and a knowledge of the local sensitivity patterns of those pathogens and, increasingly, the cost of treatment.

It is preferable in theory to use narrow-spectrum rather than broad-spectrum antibiotics because of the impact of the latter on the normal flora. However, it is inadvisable to use a narrow-spectrum antibiotic unless the causative organism and its antibacterial susceptibility are known. Life-threatening infections will therefore initially necessitate the use of broad-spectrum agents. Unfortunately, all broad-spectrum regimens have microbiologically ineffective 'windows', so aside from the beneficial effects on the patient's disease that may or may not occur, they tend to destroy the patient's normal flora and to encourage the proliferation of resistant strains.

Combinations may be useful and justifiable in certain situations. The major indication for combinations of antibiotics is to broaden antibacterial cover in empirical therapy. However, combinations are sometimes used to achieve greater effectiveness against a known infectious organism. In most cases, the aim of antibiotic therapy is to 'conquer' the infection, and any remaining bacteria will be disposed of by the patient's endogenous defence systems, but in a few clinical circumstances the aim of treatment is eradication of the organism and in these cases combinations of antibiotics are the rule. Examples are infection with tuberculosis, and infection in immune-deficient patients. Advice or protocols from specialist medical microbiologists should be followed.

In cases of intermediate sensitivity, bactericidal drugs will be synergistic or additive in their action. Bacteriostatic drugs are generally additive, whereas combinations of bacteriostatic and bactericidal drugs can be antagonistic. In 'eradication therapy' this consideration is important, although very few combinations are contra-indicated (notably imipenem and ceftazidime, as the effect of imipenem on the bacterial cell wall renders ceftazidime ineffective at its site of action). Other combinations of antimicrobials are antagonistic because the presence of one affects the plasma concentration of another; for example, the combination of rifampicin and itraconazole is characterized by very low plasma levels of itraconazole.

Toxic effects of antibiotics are common. The aminoglycosides (gentamicin, amikacin, tobramicin, etc.) have well-known nephrotoxic and ototoxic side effects which may occur despite adequate monitoring of serum levels. The glycopeptides (vancomycin and teicoplanin) are also nephrotoxic. Aminoglycosides and glycopeptides are commonly given as a single daily dose, with plasma levels measured each day, and the dose being omitted if the plasma levels are above the maximal trough level.

Prophylaxis for surgery

Well-controlled, prospective, double-blind studies have outlined many areas in which antibiotic prophylaxis is beneficial. The following points should be considered when choosing a prophylactic antibiotic regimen: the nature of the surgical procedure, the likely range of organisms present, the route and timing of administration, and the dosage necessary to reach an effective tissue concentration.

Low surgical infection rates are best achieved by good surgical technique. In clean surgery, the indications for prophylactic antibiotics are limited to those involving implantation of a prosthetic foreign body. In other cases, the potential benefit is outweighed by the risk of harmful effects, which include toxic or allergic drug reactions, and bacterial and fungal superinfections. For surgery where there is a high probability of infection, prophylactic antibiotics are indicated. These include operations on the biliary tract, for which the standard prophylaxis is cefuroxime. For colonic surgery, metronidazole and cefuroxime are used because of the risk of contamination of the peritoneal cavity with anaerobes.

Surgery for ischaemic limbs also demands the administration of prophylactic antibiotics. The danger of gas gangrene exists in this situation and benzylpenicillin should be given immediately prior to surgery and then postoperatively for 5 days. Extensive trauma is similarly managed. Prophylactic use of antibiotic aerosols should be avoided because of the high risk of development of resistant strains. Antibiotic prophylaxis is not of value in the prevention of infection of urinary catheters or intravenous cannulae, but should be given before instrumenting a urinary tract that is known to be infected, to minimize the danger from the resulting severe bacteraemia. In burns, antibiotics are not routinely administered, but topical agents such as silver sulphadiazine are important adjuncts to treatment.

Prophylactic antibiotics should be given intravenously half an hour before surgery and maintained for 24 h only. Intravenous administration ensures reliable and rapid systemic entry with high concentrations in tissue fluids.

Active treatment of surgical infections

In the active treatment of surgical infections where there is preoperative contamination of a normally sterile tissue, the correct approach is prompt and adequate surgical inter-vention with simultaneous administration of antibiotics. The initial antibiotic regimen is chosen empirically, and during the next 48 h evidence of improvement or deterioration should be sought. If the patient's condition remains unchanged or deteriorates, consid-eration should be given to re-draining the focus of infection and to changing the anti-biotic regimen. At the earliest opportunity, the antibiotic regimen should be changed from broad spectrum and empirical to narrow spectrum and based on microbiological investigations such as culture of pus or blood.

Antibiotic policies

All hospitals should have a document, drawn up with the help of the microbiology department, containing antibiotic policies and guidelines tailored to local conditions. This will maximize the effectiveness of antibiotics and limit their misuse. For this to be effective, education should be given in parallel with guidance. Among the other contri-butions that this department can make is to monitor the local prevalence of resistant organisms, to advise on and monitor strategies to control cross-infection between patients, to ensure that the antibiotic policy is being adhered to and to advise on the need to isolate and barrier-nurse certain patients.

Mode of action of antibiotics

Antibiotics kill or inhibit the growth of bacteria by interfering with their synthetic pathways, their metabolic processes or their cell wall structure. There are many antibiotics that exert sufficient antibacterial toxicity compared with their side effects on the host to be considered effective therapeutic agents.

An antibiotic is bactericidal if it kills micro-organisms even in the absence of host defence mechanisms, whereas bacteriostatic antibiotics inhibit bacterial growth enabling the host's immune systems to dispose of the infective agent. In the absence of competent host immunity, the organism will start to grow again when such an agent is withdrawn. This distinction may disappear when the concentration of the antibiotic is increased or a different micro-organism is considered. For example, erythromycin is bactericidal only at high concentrations; chloramphenicol is bacteriostatic against *Streptococcus pneumoniae* and bactericidal against *Neisseria meningitidis*.

Site of action

Antibiotics act on micro-organisms by inhibiting the synthesis of the cell wall, altering the permeability of the cell membrane, or inhibiting the synthesis of protein or nucleic acid.

Inhibition of cell wall synthesis

Bacterial cell wall consists of polysaccharide, with *N*-acetyl glucosamine and acetyl muramic acid (specific to bacteria), and a highly cross-linked polypeptide. Pentapeptide chains are attached to the amino sugars. The rigidity of the bacterial cell wall is brought about by the cross-linking of the peptide chains.

Penicillins, cephalosporins, monobactams, carbapenems, vancomycin, bacitracin and cyclosporin each interfere with one of the many stages in cell wall synthesis.

Alteration of permeability of the cell membrane

The effectiveness of the selective permeability of cytoplasmic membrane, which controls the internal composition of the microbe, is vital to its survival. Substances that selectively disrupt the integrity of bacterial or fungal cytoplasmic membrane, in preference to animal cell membrane, thus have therapeutic value.

Polymyxins act like cationic detergents on the cytoplasmic membrane of Gram-negative bacteria, which are rich in negatively charged lipids. The cytoplasmic membrane in fungi contains sterols which are absent in bacterial cytoplasmic membrane although present in human cell membrane. The polyenes (amphotericin B and nystatin) interact with fungal sterols creating pores in the membrane leading to leakage of cytoplasmic components and death of the fungal cell. To a lesser extent, they also interact with human cell cytoplasmic membrane, leading to toxic manifestations. Imidazoles and triazoles also act at this level by inhibiting the synthesis of sterols.

Inhibition of protein synthesis

Human ribosomes are sufficiently different from bacterial ribosomes to tolerate the use of agents that selectively interfere with one of the stages in bacterial protein synthesis. Aminoglycosides, chloramphenicol, erythromycin, lincomycin, clindamycin and tetracyclines are some of the bacterial protein synthesis inhibitors.

Inhibition of nucleic acid synthesis

Several substances, such as actinomycin D and mitomycin C, inhibit the synthesis of nucleic acid in both bacterial and human cells without showing sufficient selectivity to be used as antimicrobial agents; they are therefore considered as cytotoxic. Others manifest their selectivity by interfering with the synthesis of purines and pyrimidines. They include the antivirals, e.g. idoxuridine; antifungals, e.g. fluocytosine; and antibacterials, e.g. rifampicin, nitrofurantoin, and quinolones including nalidixic acid, metronidazole and sulphonamides.

Mechanisms of antibiotic resistance

The existence of penicillin-resistant *Staphylococcus aureus* can be traced back to the period before the discovery of penicillin. When penicillin was first used, the incidence was less than 1 per cent. After five decades of use, leading to natural selection of resistant strains, the incidence of β-lactamase-producing *Staph. aureus* in some hospitals exceeds 90 per cent. The recent appearance and spread of methicillin-resistant *Staph. aureus* (MRSA) is another example of selection and the resilience of this most successful pathogen. Resistance to other antibiotics has also developed and generally the increase is proportional to the amount of antibiotics used. Frequent use of antibiotics, whether justified or not, leads to the emergence of resistant bacteria. This is well demonstrated by the appearance of different forms of resistance in different countries with different antibiotic policies. In the absence of antibiotics, bacteria gradually lose their resistance and revert back to their original sensitivity. There are a number of different mechanisms by which micro-organisms exhibit resistance to antimicrobials. These are described in the following paragraphs.

Enzymatic resistance

Some bacteria manifest their resistance to β-lactam antibiotics by the production of β-lactamase enzymes (penicillinases) which are either plasmid mediated or under chromosomal control. (Plasmids are pieces of DNA that exist and reproduce autonomously in the cytoplasm of bacteria.) They are proteins of different sizes with varying degree of activity against penicillins or cephalosporins. β-Lactamases produced by *Staph. aureus* are plasmid mediated and transferred from cell to cell. They are different in molecular size and mode of action from β-lactamases produced by Gram-negative bacteria which are also plasmid mediated and transferable to some other Gram-negative bacteria. The appearance and increase in the incidence of β-lactamase-producing *Neisseria gonorrhoeae* and *Haemophilus influenzae* is due to this transfer. A large number of β-lactamases, ranging from common to very rare, have been isolated from different Gram-negative bacteria, and have been characterized.

Enzymatic resistance of bacteria to aminoglycosides is mediated by one of the many enzymes involved with acetylation, adenylation or phosphorylation, modifying the antibiotic during its transport through the cytoplasmic membrane. They are found in Gram-positive cocci and Gram-negative bacilli. They have either low or high affinity to one or more of the aminoglycosides and therefore partially or totally modify their action. Selection of bacteria that produce enzymes active against aminoglycosides in a country or hospital is related to the type of aminoglycosides commonly used there.

Chloramphenicol acetyltransferase, a plasmid-mediated enzyme, confers resistance to both Gram-positive and Gram-negative bacteria. Erythromycin esterase, which hydrolyses erythromycin, is also plasmid mediated.

R-plasmids carrying the gene responsible for enzymatic resistance to sulphonamides are common in Gram-negative bacteria. Chromosomal and plasmid factors are responsible for enzymatic resistance to trimethoprim.

Alteration of permeability of bacterial membrane

Alteration of the permeability of bacterial membrane or interference with the transport of a drug across the membrane confers resistance on the organism, and these are features demonstrated against β-lactams, carbapenems, aminoglycosides, tetracyclines, and possibly vancomycin and teicoplanin. Since the structure of the membrane is different in

Gram-negative and Gram-positive bacteria, the mechanism of alteration of permeability is also different. It is suggested that, in the case of tetracycline, resistance is shown by active transport of the drug through the cytoplasmic membrane reducing its concentration within the bacterial cytoplasm.

Alteration of target sites

Several antibiotics, including tetracycline, aminoglycosides, chloramphenicol and erythromycin, attack the ribosomal binding sites to arrest protein synthesis and this eventually leads to cell death. Alteration in the binding sites or disruption of the process of binding will confer resistance on the organism. The determinant factors are located on either the bacterial plasmid or the chromosome.

Alteration of penicillin binding proteins (PBP) in the cytoplasmic membrane confers resistance against β-lactam antibiotics to *Strep. pneumoniae* and non-β-lactamase-producing *N. gonorrhoeae*. Induction of PBP is also responsible for the occurrence of MRSA, another example of a plasmid-mediated resistance.

In some Gram-negative bacteria, alteration of DNA gyrases is responsible for resistance to quinolones and nalidixic acid.

Alteration of metabolic pathways

This can occur through mutation and confers resistance to bacteria against trimethoprim.

Hypersensitivity

The most common and important side effect of the penicillins is hypersensitivity. It is seen more rarely with the use of other antibiotics. Clinically, hypersensitivity reactions may be described as immediate or late.

Immediate hypersensitivity reactions that occur within 1 h of administration manifest as anaphylaxis, hypotension, erythematous rash, angioneurotic oedema, gastro-intestinal upset and bronchospasm. Those occurring slightly later, but within the first 3 days of treatment, may display only bronchospasm or angioneurotic oedema. Late hypersensitivity reactions occur within 1–2 weeks of starting treatment and manifest as morbilliform rash, exfoliative dermatitis, neutropenia, haemolytic anaemia, thrombocytopenia, serum sickness, interstitial nephritis and Stevens–Johnson syndrome.

Although the incidence of anaphylactic shock is relatively low (1 in 50 000–100 000 for penicillin), epinephrine (adrenaline) should be readily available when antibiotics are administered parenterally. A history of allergy to any penicillin constitutes a contra-indication to all penicillins.

ANTIMICROBIAL AGENTS

Sulphonamides

The discovery of the sulphonamides in 1935 was one of the great milestones in antimicrobial chemotherapy. However, with increasing resistance and with the greater toxicity of sulphonamides compared with more recently discovered antibiotics, their use has greatly diminished. They are bacteriostatic drugs and their action is enhanced by the addition of trimethoprim. Co-trimoxazole, a combination of trimethoprim and sulfamethoxazole, is the only preparation in common use today.

Until recently, co-trimoxazole was used as a first-line treatment for urinary tract infections but recent work has shown that, in most cases, trimethoprim alone is as effective as the combination and has fewer unwanted effects. Co-trimoxazole is also used for chronic bronchitis, *Salmonella* infections and for the treatment of *Pneumocystis carinii* pneumonia (PCP). Sulphonamides cross the blood–brain barrier easily and were an important component of the treatment of meningitis for a long time. (Modern treatment of meningitis comprises cefotaxime or ceftriaxone with benzyl penicillin, but sulphonamides would be useful in the treatment of *Listeria* meningitis in a patient with allergy to penicillin.) The main drawbacks are crystalluria with crystal nephropathy, skin rashes (which may be severe, leading to the Stevens–Johnson syndrome), haemolytic anaemia and agranulocytosis. Sulphonamides are also useful in the treatment of *Nocardia* infection.

β-Lactam antibiotics

Since the isolation of benzyl penicillin in 1939, numerous other penicillins with different properties have been isolated or artificially synthesized. They all contain the basic three components of a thiazolidine ring, a β-lactam ring and a side chain. Cephalosporin C, the first of numerous cephalosporins available today, was discovered in 1948. It also has the three components of the β-lactams, but the side chain differs from the penicillins in having a dihydrothiazine ring. During the past two decades, carbapenems (imipenem and meropenem) and monobactams (aztreonam) have been added to the family of β-lactam antibiotics (*Figure 19.1*).

Penicillins

In patients who have a history of allergy to any penicillin, all penicillins are contraindicated.

Classification

All penicillins consist of a thiozolidine ring, the β-lactam ring and an amino side chain – variations in which confer the differences in antibacterial activity, absorption, excretion and protein binding. Currently available penicillins can be classified into four main

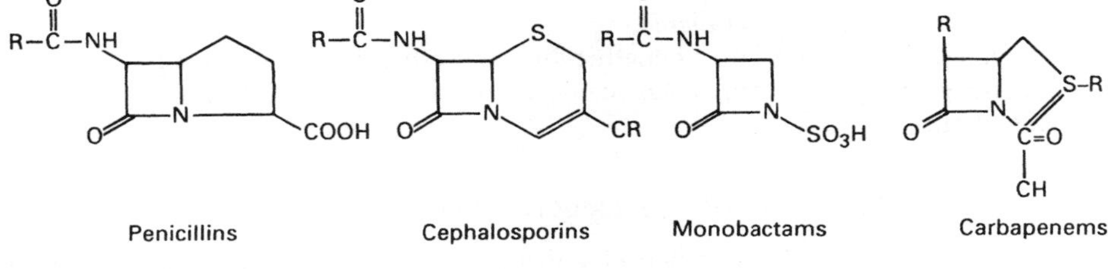

Penicillins   Cephalosporins   Monobactams   Carbapenems

Figure 19.1 β-Lactam antibiotics

groups on the basis of their antibacterial activity, although there is considerable overlap between them:

1. Standard or natural penicillins.
2. Anti-staphylococcal penicillins.
3. Penicillins which also have activity against Gram-negative bacilli ('broad-spectrum' penicillins).
4. Penicillins that are stable against Gram-negative β-lactamases.

Benzylpenicillin

Benzylpenicillin is susceptible to the action of β-lactamases (penicillinases), substances produced by many Gram-positive and Gram-negative bacteria which split the β-lactam ring while the enzyme amidase separates the side chain from the penicillin nucleus. It is active against *Streptococcus pneumoniae* with a few exceptions, other streptococci, *Neisseria meningitidis* (meningococci), *Corynebacterium diphtheriae*, *Clostridium perfringens*, *Treponema pallidum*, and gonococci and staphylococci which do not produce penicillinase. Some bacteria are developing resistance to penicillin by producing β-lactamase, whereas others, such as *Salmonella*, are intrinsically resistant, and can grow in the presence of penicillin without destroying it.

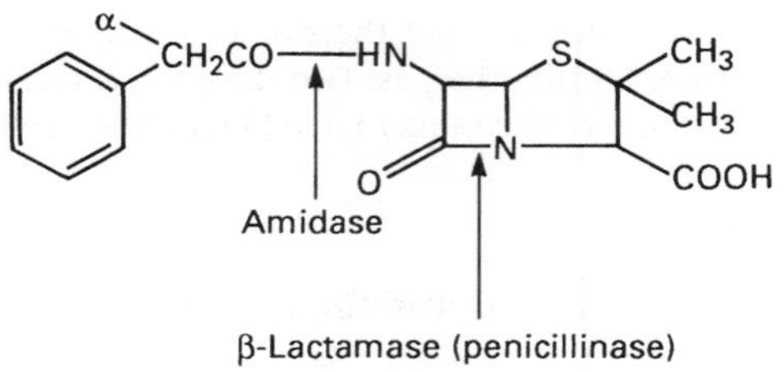

α CH₂CO — HN S CH₃ / CH₃ / O / N / COOH

Amidase

β-Lactamase (penicillinase)

Benzylpenicillin is inactivated by gastric acid and should therefore be given by intramuscular or intravenous injection. It is not toxic when given parenterally, even in large doses. It diffuses into many body cavities and crosses the placenta. Although the levels of benzylpenicillin in normal CSF are low, it crosses inflamed meninges more easily to reach adequate therapeutic levels. Penicillins should not be given by the intrathecal route.

The main clinical uses of benzylpenicillin are in upper respiratory tract infections due to *Strep. pyogenes*, lobar pneumonia due to *Strep. Pneumoniae*, meningococcal meningitis (in combination with cefotaxime), gonorrhoea, syphilis, diphtheria (together with antitoxin), carriers of *C. diphtheriae*, the treatment and prophylaxis of gas gangrene and other clostridial infections and the treatment of bacterial endocarditis due to Streptococci (sometimes together with gentamicin).

Phenoxymethyl-penicillin and phenethicillin are both acid-stable penicillins and can therefore be given by mouth. Their clinical applications are identical to those of benzylpenicillin.

Anti-staphylococcal penicillins

The removal of the side chain of benzylpenicillin to produce 6-aminopenicillanic acid was a major advance in therapy, providing a nucleus on which many new side chains could be substituted. Penicillinase-resistant penicillins that have long side chains include methicillin, cloxacillin and flucloxacillin.

The incidence of resistance to the above penicillins in staphylococci isolated in large hospitals is increasing at an alarming rate. Measures adopted to control the spread of infection in hospitals and attempts to reserve antibiotics for special use may have slowed down the spread of these organisms, but it is not infrequent to find a staphylococcal infection which is resistant to all commonly used antibiotics except the glycopeptides (vancomycin and teicoplanin), and resistance even to these has been reported.

Penicillins active against gram negative bacilli

AMPICILLIN AND AMOXYCILLIN

These are aminopenicillins. The substitution of an amino group on the α-carbon atom of the side chain of penicillin produces compounds that are active against a wide range of Gram-negative bacteria. Because the modification is on a side chain and not in the β-lactam ring, bacteria that produce penicillinase are resistant to aminopenicillins. Ampicillin has been associated with skin rashes more frequently than any other penicillin. This reaction is delayed, appearing 7–10 days after the start of therapy and almost 10 per cent of patients have been affected. In patients with glandular fever (infective mononucleosis), the incidence of rash is almost 100 per cent. It is likely that a mechanism different from true penicillin hypersensitivity is responsible for the rash in glandular fever. Ampicillin is very effective in urinary tract and respiratory tract infections. The antibacterial spectrum of amoxycillin is almost identical to that of ampicillin. It is somewhat better absorbed by mouth than ampicillin, and for this reason can be given 3 times a day (instead of 4 times for ampicillin). Amoxycillin is also presented in combination with a β-lactamase inhibitor, clavulanic acid. This combination is called co-amoxiclav. The clavulanic acid has no antibacterial effect, but confers 'stability' to Gram-negative β-lactamase to the amoxycillin component. It has activity against a wide range of Gram-negative and anaerobic bacteria, and is frequently used as perioperative prophylaxis against infection.

Other penicillins active against Gram-negative bacilli

These include carboxypenicillins, (e.g. carbenicillin and ticarcillin) ureidopenicillins (e.g. azlocillin and piperacillin), which are susceptible to β-lactamase, and temocillin, which is stable to it. Some are presented in combination with a β-lactamase inhibitor, e.g. ticarcillin with clavulanic acid, piperacillin with tazobactam.

Antibiotics in this group (particularly the ureidopenicillins) have activity against *Pseudomonas* spp. In this context there is useful synergy with the aminoglycosides. In order to limit the development of resistant strains, they should be reserved for bacteria resistant to less novel antibiotics.

Cephalosporins

These are based on a nucleus that is closely related to the basic nucleus of the penicillins – 7-aminocephalosporanic acid.

6-aminopenicillanic acid   7-aminocephalosporanic acid

These agents have been introduced for clinical use in three waves. First-generation cephalosporins included cefaloridine (which, because of its nephrotoxicity, is no longer used), cefazoline and cefradine. Second-generation cephalosporins included cefamandole, cefaclor, cefoxitin and cefuroxime. The third generation of cephalosporins consists of a large number of broad-spectrum cephalosporins that differ from each other according to their protein-binding ability or range of antibacterial activities. They include cefotaxime, ceftizoxime, ceftriaxone, moxalactam, ceftazidime and many other cephalosporins. They

Table 19.1 Classification of cephalosporins based upon chemical structure, antibacterial activity, β-lactamase stability and metabolic stability. Cephalosporins have a wide antibacterial activity but there are significant variations in the degree of activity against groups of bacteria

Group	Features	
I Oral group	Compounds that are very well absorbed after oral administration. Antibacterial activity relatively low compared with parenteral cephalosporins. Stable to Gram-positive β-lactamases and to some Gram-negative β-lactamases	Cephalexin Cephradine Cefaclor
II Gram-positive group	High activity against penicillinase-producing staphylococci and other Gram-positive bacteria. Activity against Gram-negative rods is relatively low; (a) is metabolically stable, (b) are desacetylated with loss of antibacterial activity	(a) Cephazolin (b) Cephalothin Cephacetrile
III Enterobacteria group	Compounds with high activity against many aerobia. Gram-negative rods and stability to many β-lactamases produced by these bacteria: (a) are metabolically stable, (b) is metabolically unstable	(a) Cephamandole Cefuroxime (b) Cefotaxine
IV Pseudomonas group	Compounds with high activity against *Pseudomonas* strains in addition to activity against enterobacteria. (a) Are more stable than (b) to plasmid-mediated β-lactamases	(a) Ceftazidime Cefsulodin (b) Cefoperazone Ceftriaxone
V Cephamycins (7-α-methoxycephalo-sporins)	Compounds with high stability to β-lactamases of aerobic and anaerobic bacteria	Cefoxitin Moxalactam Cefotetan

all have a broad range of activity and are of special value in treating Gram-negative infections. Some are active against *Pseudomonas* strains, e.g. ceftazidime; some are active against *Legionella pneumophila*, e.g. cefotaxime, whereas others such as moxalactam and cefoxitin are resistant to β-lactamases. Cefotaxime or ceftriaxone are useful in the 'blind' treatment of suspected meningococcal disease (infection with *Neisseria meningitidis*) in combination with benzylpenicillin. If there is meningitis caused by *Haemophilus influenzae* or another of the organisms linked with meningitis, it is likely to be sensitive to the cephalosporin. The benzylpenicillin extends the cover against Gram-positive organisms. If a penicillin-sensitive strain of *N. meningitidis* is isolated, the cephalosporin can then be stopped.

Some cephalosporins are available in oral form, e.g. cefaclor, and some in both oral and injectable forms, e.g. cephradine and cefuroxime. The broad-spectrum third-generation cephalosporins are available in an injectable form only. They have also been classified according to their range of antibacterial activities (*Table 19.1*).

Five to ten per cent of patients who have a history of allergy to a penicillin will have a similar reaction to a cephalosporin. Thus, in those patients in whom the reaction to a penicillin was life threatening, cephalosporins are also contra-indicated. The use of cephalosporins in intensive care is associated with pseudomembranous enterocolitis (infection with *Clostridium difficile*). Widespread use of these antibiotics has led to the selection of resistant organisms, including multiply-resistant strains, especially in hospitals.

IMIPENEM

This is a bicyclic β-lactam with a carbapenem nucleus, and has a very broad spectrum of activity. Since imipenem is extensively metabolized in the renal tubules by an enzyme which opens the lactam ring, cilastatin, an antagonist of the enzyme, can be added (in a ratio of 1:1) to maintain a reasonable degree of activity in the urinary tract. Higher concentrations of cilastatin lead to an increased level of imipenem in the urine, but also interfere with renal function. Imipenem is resistant to β-lactamases because of the unusual formation of its side chain, and can penetrate the bacterial cell wall of *Escherichia coli* faster than other β-lactam antibiotics because of the compactness of its structure. It can also penetrate through the cell wall of nearly all other Gram-negative bacteria. It acts by binding to the penicillin-binding proteins responsible for the elongation and lemon shape appearance of Gram-negative bacilli. It has been suggested that this 'fast kill' and the fact that there is less over-production of cell wall lipoprotein during bacterial death are advantageous to the patient.

Meropenem is a similar compound with a similar spectrum of activity, but it lacks the problem of metabolism in the renal tubules and therefore is presented alone, rather than in combination with cilastatin.

Of all the β-lactam antibiotics, imipenem and meropenem have the widest spectrum of activity against Gram-positive aerobic and anaerobic bacteria (with the exception of *Clostridium difficile*), and Gram-negative aerobic and anaerobic bacteria.

AZTREONAM

This is a synthetic β-lactam antibiotic with a range of activity limited to most of the aerobic Gram-negative bacteria. It has very little or no activity against anaerobic Gram-negative bacilli and Gram-positive bacteria. It is stable in the presence of a wide range of β-lactamases produced by Gram-negative bacilli. Although there is no report of cross-reactivity with penicillin or cephalosporin antibodies, the manufacturers advise caution in using aztreonam in β-lactam allergic patients. It is active against *Pseudomonas* spp. It is synergistic with amikacin, tobramycin, and with some of the β-lactam antibiotics, against some Gram-negative bacilli while showing antagonism against other β-lactams.

Aminoglycosides

Since Waksman's discovery of streptomycin in 1943, many more aminoglycosides have been described which are either less toxic or have different antibacterial activity. Amino-glycoside antibiotics include streptomycin, gentamicin, tobramycin, kanamycin, neomycin, netilmicin and sisomicin. They all have amino-sugars linked by glycosidic bonds to an aminocyclitol ring. (Spectinomycin, which is commonly included in this group, has neither the amino-sugar nor the glycosidic bond. 'Aminocyclitol antibiotics' has therefore been suggested as a better term to replace aminoglycoside.)

The selective action of aminoglycosides on bacteria is due to their active transport into the bacterial cell, a process that requires aerobic metabolic processes. These compounds therefore have no effect on anaerobic organisms; in conditions in which there is a reduced oxygen tension, their activity is greatly reduced. Aminoglycosides are bacterial antibiotics and, together with broad-spectrum β-lactams, are the mainstay of antimicrobial regimens in cases in which the causative agent has not been identified or for the treatment of Gram-negative infections. Aminoglycosides show synergistic activity when used in combination with other antibiotics such as penicillins for the treatment of streptococcal infections. Microbial resistance to aminoglycosides may be ribosomal, may be due to ineffective transport into the cells, or may be due to enzymatic resistance (see page 477).

Aminoglycosides are ototoxic and nephrotoxic to varying degrees. This toxicity is believed to be related to their blood level. Since aminoglycosides are excreted through the kidneys and the rate of excretion may vary even in people with normal renal function, monitoring of the serum levels is mandatory. They can be given in divided doses with measurement of peak and trough levels (for gentamicin, peak < 10 mg/litre, trough < 2 mg/litre), or by the more recently described single daily dosage regimen where a large dose is given once daily (e.g. 3 mg/kg of gentamicin), provided that serum levels have been checked and are below the trough level. Ototoxicity, manifesting as hearing loss or tinnitus, is seen in up to 5 per cent of patients and is due to selective destruction of the hair cells of the organ of Corti. Vestibular damage, manifesting as nausea, vomiting, vertigo and unsteady gait, is far less common and is seen in fewer than 0.5 per cent of patients treated with aminoglycosides. Prolonged or repeated aminoglycoside therapy increases the incidence of ototoxicity. Renal toxicity, defined as reduced glomerular filtration, is seen in 5–25 per cent of patients, and is related to advanced age, liver disease, high serum aminoglycoside levels and duration of therapy. Concomitant administration of cephalothin, cis-platinum, amphotericin or cyclosporin increases the incidence of renal toxicity.

A rare, but serious, toxic phenomenon of aminoglycoside therapy is neuromuscular paralysis. This is enhanced by the presence of non-depolarizing muscle relaxants, raised levels of magnesium and in patients suffering from botulism. This effect is mainly due to the inhibition of pre-synaptic release of acetylcholine, but there may also be some blockade of the post-synaptic acetylcholine receptors. It is more common in patients receiving intravenous boluses of aminoglycosides.

Streptomycin is still considered the aminoglycoside of choice for the treatment of *Mycobacterium tuberculosis*, *M. bovis*, *Francisella tolerances*, *Yersinia pestis*, *Brucella abortus* and *Br. melitensis*. It is not very effective against 'atypical' mycobacterial infections. Some still consider it the drug of choice, in combination with penicillin, for the treatment of *Streptococcus faecalis* (now called *Enterococcus* spp.) endocarditis.

GENTAMICIN

Gentamicin is comparatively inexpensive and is less toxic than streptomycin. It is commonly used for the treatment of serious infections, particularly Gram-negative infections and for the treatment of infections in which the organism is undiagnosed but treatment is urgent. The incidence of resistance among staphylococci and Gram-negative bacilli, especially *Pseudomonas aeruginosa*, is therefore increasing. There is evidence that control of gentamicin usage results in a fall in the incidence of resistance among microorganisms.

Tobramycin is, *in vitro*, slightly more active against *Ps. aeruginosa*, but this advantage has not been fully demonstrated clinically. The incidence of both ototoxicity and nephrotoxicity is claimed to be lower. Enzymatic resistance to tobramycin among Gram-negative bacilli is similar to gentamicin.

Amikacin has a clinical spectrum of action similar to that of other commonly used aminoglycosides, but its great advantage is its resistance to aminoglycoside inactivating enzymes. No doubt, with greater use, resistance among hospital strains will develop. Its use is mainly in the treatment of hospital-acquired Gram-negative infections.

Netilmicin has a similar antimicrobial activity and resistance profile to gentamicin and tobramycin, but causes less nephrotoxicity and ototoxicity.

Spectinomycin is an aminocyclitol antibiotic with antibacterial activity similar to that of the aminoglycosides, and acting by the inhibition of protein synthesis, but without their toxicity. Its use is limited to the treatment of *Neisseria gonorrhoea* infections, especially of strains resistant to penicillin.

Macrolides

ERYTHROMYCIN

Erythromycin, derived from *Streptomyces erythreus*, has a similar range of activity to benzylpenicillin and is active against Gram-positive cocci and bacilli and Gram-negative cocci. It is of special value in the treatment of *Legionella pneumophila*. It works by inhibiting bacterial protein synthesis. It is partly inactivated by the liver. There is an association between erythromycin estolate and abnormal liver function and jaundice. Apart from this, erythromycin is one of the safest drugs available, having little toxicity. It is often used as an alternative to benzylpenicillin for the treatment of patients who are sensitive to penicillin. All macrolides interact dangerously with cisapride (ventricular arrhythmias).

Other macrolides, **lincomycin** and **clindamycin**, are active against bacteroides and all Gram-positive cocci with the exception of *Streptococcus faecalis* (now called *Enterococcus* spp.). Side effects include abdominal pain and diarrhoea but, more importantly, pseudomembranous enterocolitis (infection with *Clostridium difficile*) has been reported. These two compounds are effective anti-staphylococcal agents, particularly for the treatment of staphylococcal osteomyelitis.

Erythromycin in combination with other antibiotics should be considered for blind therapy of community-acquired pneumonias because of the possibility of Legionnaires' disease.

Clarithromycin has a similar spectrum of activity to erythromycin, but has slightly greater tissue penetration.

Fusidic acid

This is highly active against staphylococci but, unfortunately, resistant strains appear quickly and therefore the drug should be used in combination with another agent such as penicillin. Use of topical fusidic acid, which encourages the appearance of resistant strains, should be avoided as far as possible. It is available in both oral and parenteral forms and is widely distributed throughout the body with the exception of the cerebrospinal fluid. Jaundice has been reported in association with fusidic acid therapy.

Tetracyclines

These are bacteriostatic antibiotics, interfering with protein synthesis. They have a broad spectrum of activity against Gram-positive and Gram-negative bacteria, spirochaetes, *Mycoplasma* spp., *Rickettsia* spp. and *Chlamydia* spp. Liver damage, staining of teeth and bones, nausea, diarrhoea and superadded infection are among the side-effects of these drugs. They are commonly used for the treatment of respiratory tract infections, especially with *Mycoplasma* spp., and for the treatment of chlamydial infections, rickettsial infections, brucellosis and trachoma.

Chloramphenicol

This broad-spectrum antibiotic can rarely cause bone marrow depression, and is used only as eye drops in infective conjunctivitis.

Quinolones

CIPROFLOXACIN

Ciprofloxacin is one of the synthetic quinolones distantly related chemically to nalidixic acid. It is marketed in both oral and parenteral forms. Ciprofloxacin is rapidly absorbed after oral administration, reaching its peak serum level within 1 h. Concomitant administration of antacids may interfere with absorption. The half-life of elimination from the serum after intravenous administration is between 3 and 4 hours; over a third of the dose can be recovered in active form from the urine. It is also excreted through the biliary system and, after oral administration, 30 per cent of the ciprofloxacin can be recovered from faeces. The remainder of the drug is inactivated and this inactive form can be recovered from the urine.

Ciprofloxacin has a wide range of activity and is active against both Gram-positive and Gram-negative bacteria and mycobacteria, but is inactive against bacteroides. Emergence of ciprofloxacin resistance has occurred with *Pseudomonas aeruginosa* and *Staphylococcus aureus*. In some cases, resistance has appeared while the patient has been on treatment.

Glycopeptides

VANCOMYCIN

This is a soluble polypeptide antibiotic with bactericidal action against Gram-positive organisms. It inhibits the synthesis of peptidoglycan polymers of the bacterial cell wall. It also alters the permeability of the cytoplasmic membrane and interferes with RNA synthesis. It is especially useful for the treatment of resistant forms of *Staphylococcus aureus*, particularly MRSA and *Staph. epidermidis*. Other Gram-positive organisms such as streptococci, corynebacteria and *Clostridium difficile* are highly susceptible.

Since vancomycin is potentially nephrotoxic and is eliminated by glomerular filtration, measurements of serum levels are essential (peak < 30 mg/litre, trough < 10 mg/litre). Ototoxicity is also possible. Like gentamicin, it can be given using a single daily-dose regimen. It must be given slowly (less than 10 mg/min) to avoid hypotension, flushing and wheeze (red man syndrome).

Teicoplanin has the same spectrum of activity as vancomicin, but has a longer duration of action and is usually given once daily. Assay of serum levels is advisable, but not mandatory. It can be given as a slow bolus rather than as an infusion.

Antimycobacterial agents

Infections by mycobacterial organisms usually respond to antibiotic therapy within a few weeks, but prevention of recurrent disease depends on many months of treatment. There is a high incidence of treatment failure because of poor motivation and failure to appreciate the importance of prolonged treatment. *Mycobacterium tuberculosis* is becoming more widespread at present in association with acquired immune deficiency syndrome. Other mycobacteria that infect man include *M. leprae*, which causes leprosy, and a host of mycobacteria commonly referred to as 'atypical', e.g. *M. Kansas* and *M. ulcerous*.

Antimycobacterial agents fall into three classes:

1. First-line and second-line antituberculous drugs.
2. Antileprotic agents.
3. Those acting on 'atypical' mycobacteria.

Antituberculous agents

First-line antituberculous drugs include isoniazid, rifampicin, streptomycin, ethambutol and pyrazinamide. Second-line agents are *p*-aminosalicylic acid, cycloserine, capreomycin, kanamycin and amikacin. The latter are either more toxic or less active than the first group and are only used in situations in which the first-line drugs have not been effective. Although *p*-aminosalicylic acid has been replaced by ethambutol as a first-line agent, it is still part of multi-drug regimens in the developing countries because of its low cost. In patients for whom enteral administration is impossible, preparations for parenteral administration are available for isoniazid, rifampicin, streptomycin and capreomycin. Hepatotoxicity is common among antituberculous drugs and regular liver function tests should be performed in patients on antituberculous therapy.

ISONIAZID

Isoniazid is a synthetic agent with bactericidal activity against replicating tubercle bacilli. Since some 1 per million of tubercle bacilli show a degree of tolerance, the use of isoniazid alone would result in the appearance of resistant infections within 3 months. It is well absorbed when given orally or intramuscularly, and well distributed throughout the body. The CSF level is about 20 per cent of the plasma level. It is metabolized in the liver, the rate being dependent on N-acetyl transferase, the effectiveness of which is genetically controlled and varies between ethnic groups. It is available as tablets and in injectable form. It can be given daily or as a larger dose twice weekly, which is useful in the context of enforced administration (which is sometimes necessary). The dosage must be modified in those with hepatic or renal impairment.

Hepatitis may occur and regular liver function tests should be performed. Peripheral neuropathy may occur, especially in patients with nutritional problems or with high dosage, and this can be prevented with pyridoxine. Isoniazid interacts with rifampicin, resulting in elevation of the levels of serum hepatic enzymes. It also enhances the neurotoxicity of phenytoin, especially in slow acetylators. Due to interference with acetylation, isoniazid levels will be abnormally high if it is administered together with p-aminosalicylic acid.

RIFAMPICIN

Rifampicin was first introduced as an antituberculous agent, but later was found to be useful in the treatment of leprosy, staphylococcal infections, brucellosis, and for chemoprophylaxis of meningococcal and *Haemophilus influenzae* infections. It is bactericidal against tubercle bacilli by inhibiting mycobacterial RNA polymerase. It is well absorbed when given orally and is well distributed throughout the body. In the presence of meningeal irritation, the cerebrospinal fluid levels can be as high as 50 per cent of the serum levels. It is metabolized in the liver into a more water-soluble but still active form and excreted into the bile, reaching the intestine where it is reabsorbed into the circulation. Concomitant administration of probenecid increases the serum level by inhibiting renal tubular secretion. More than half of the dose of rifampicin is eventually excreted in the faeces. Rifampicin is highly effective against tuberculosis, quickly achieving 'sputum conversion'. However, since *Mycobacterium tuberculosis* readily develops resistance to rifampicin, its use as a single antituberculous agent is to be discouraged. Its most striking clinical effect is that urine, saliva and other body secretions are coloured orange-red. It is contra-indicated in pregnancy. Regular liver function tests should be performed.

By increasing the activity of liver enzymes, it increases the hepatic metabolism of drugs such as methadone, disopyramide, mexiletine, quinidine, chloramphenicol, anticoagulants, oral hypoglycaemic agents, phenytoin, itraconazole, ketoconazole, haloperidol, propranolol, verapamil, corticosteroids, cyclosporin, contraceptive hormones, theophylline, thyroxine and H$_2$-blockers.

ETHAMBUTOL

Ethambutol is a synthetic antituberculous drug with bacteriostatic action and therefore it is given in combination with other antituberculous agents. It is well absorbed when given orally and is well distributed throughout the body, including the CSF when the meninges are inflamed. It is usually given in combination with isoniazid.

Since 80 per cent of the drug is excreted in the urine, the dosage must be carefully adjusted in patients with renal impairment. Toxic reactions include peripheral neuropathy, retrobulbar neuritis, visual impairment, blindness, hypersensitivity reactions and arthralgia.

Streptomycin is also an important antituberculous agent and is discussed under Aminoglycosides, above.

PYRAZINAMIDE

Pyrazinamide is a derivative of nicotinamide with bactericidal activity against *Mycobacterium tuberculosis*. It requires an acid environment and therefore it is active against intracellular bacilli. It is used in 'short course' treatment of *M. tuberculosis*. Pyrazinamide is not effective against *M. bovis* and has been used as one of the tests to distinguish between the two species. It is also ineffective against 'atypical' strains. Resistance develops very quickly, and it should therefore be used in combination with other agents.

Pyrazinamide is well absorbed when given orally in a single daily dose of 30–35 mg/kg body weight. It is well distributed throughout the body and crosses the inflamed meninges, reaching levels similar to those in the serum.

A small percentage of pyrazinamide is excreted in the urine in an active form, but most is metabolized in the liver. Pyrazinamide may also be concentrated and excreted in the bile. Hepatotoxicity has been reported in patients on high doses or for prolonged periods: regular liver function tests should be performed. Other side effects include arthralgia due to raised serum uric acid levels, anorexia, nausea, vomiting and, very rarely, cutaneous hypersensitivity reactions and photosensitivity.

p-Aminosalicylic acid

This synthetic antituberculous agent was one of the first-line drugs for many years. It has now been replaced by ethambutol, but due to its relatively low cost it remains one of the first-line drugs in developing countries. It is not active against 'atypical' mycobacteria. *p*-Aminosalicylic acid is well absorbed from the gastro-intestinal tract and distributed throughout the body. It does not cross the meninges. The usual dosage is 10–12 g/day and for children 200–300 mg/kg/day in divided doses.

Due to its gastro-intestinal side effects, it has very poor patient compliance. Its other side effects include hypersensitivity, lupus-like syndrome, lymphadenopathy, hepatosplenomegaly and hepatitis.

Cycloserine

This was first isolated from *Streptomyces* spp. and later synthesized. It interferes with cell wall synthesis and is active against *M. tuberculosis*, some 'atypical' mycobacteria, *Staphy-*

lococcus aureus, and some Gram-negative bacilli. Cycloserine is given orally, 250 mg twice daily. It is well absorbed and distributed throughout the body including the CSF. Neurotoxicity and psychotic disturbances are among its serious side effects. It can also be used for the treatment of infections by some atypical mycobacteria, e.g. *M. avium*.

Agents acting on 'atypical' mycobacteria

Other antimycobacterial agents used for the treatment of 'atypical' mycobacterial infections include amikacin, ethionamide, erythromycin, tetracyclines, sulphonamides, clofazimine, imipenem and ciprofloxacin.

Antileprotic agents

Antileprotic agents include rifampicin, dapsone, clofazimine, amithiozone and ethionamide .

Dapsone

Dapsone is one of the sulphone group of drugs and is bacteriostatic with good antileprotic activity. It is well absorbed when given orally and its metabolites are excreted in the urine. Treatment starts with 25 mg per week increasing gradually to reach the maximum of 100 mg/day. Side effects include fever, jaundice, lymphadenopathy and erythema nodosum.

Acedapsone, is a long-acting depot derivative of dapsone which can be given five times yearly.

Sulfoxone is another related antileprotic agent.

Antiprotozoal agents

Parasitic protozoa range from free-living to intracellular obligate forms challenging the human body with their complex life cycle and diverse metabolic processes adapted to their environment. Antiprotozoal agents are therefore aimed at protozoa of different classes but of one environment. For example, *Entamoeba histolytica*, *Giardia lamblia* and *Trichomonas vaginalis* infestation of the gastro-intestinal tract and the vagina can all be treated with metronidazole.

Emergence of malarial parasites resistant to antimalarial agents, the increasing ease of world-wide travel and parasitic infections secondary to HIV infections have all resulted in antiprotozoal treatment attracting greater attention. *Cryptosporidium* spp. and *Isospora belli* can cause diarrhoea and *Pneumocystis carinii* can cause pneumonia in AIDS patients. For a comprehensive description and discussion of antiparasitic agents, a major textbook should be consulted. This section is limited to a brief description of selected antiprotozoal agents.

Protozoa infecting the intestine and vagina include *E. histolytica*, *G. lamblia*, *Balantidium coli* and *Tr. vaginalis*. The antibiotic of choice for the treatment of the vegetative forms is metronidazole. Tinidazole, a similar but longer acting drug, is also effective. In chronic amoebiasis where only the cysts are found, diloxanide furoate is the drug of choice. In giardiasis, alternative treatment to metronidazole is either tinidazole or mepacrine hydrochloride.

METRONIDAZOLE

Metronidazole and related substances are potent drugs with selective toxicity against anaerobic and microaerophilic bacteria, and some protozoa. Its mode of action is believed to be due to its active metabolite which, besides acting as an 'electron sink', damages the helical structure of DNA and its template function.

When administered orally, up to 95 per cent of the dose is absorbed and the peak serum level is reached within 1 h. It is distributed throughout the body and to all tissues, abscesses, fluid compartments and bodily secretions. It is metabolized by the liver and most of the metabolites are excreted via the kidneys.

Dosage needs to be adjusted in liver dysfunction, but not for renal failure. Severe side effects are very rare. Gastro-intestinal side effects, including diarrhoea, vomiting, nausea and metallic taste, have been described. Headaches, dizziness, rash, urethral burning and oral and vaginal candidiasis have also been described. Very rare complications of sensory neuropathy or CNS involvement have been recorded. Although metronidazole is mutagenic for some bacteria, there is no evidence of increase in the prevalence of cancer in man. Since it is readily absorbed from the gastro-intestinal tract, there is little justification for administering it intravenously.

Malaria

One of the more important causes of morbidity and mortality in the world are the *Plasmodium* spp. Benign malaria is caused by *P. vivax*, *P. ovale* and *P. malaria*. Chloroquine is effective for the treatment of benign malaria, but the exoerythrocytic forms (within the liver cells) of *P. ovale* and *P. malaria* can be treated with primaquine.

Plasmodium falciparum, the cause of malignant malaria, is a more serious problem since it is associated with cerebral malaria, and chloroquine-resistant strains are encountered in many parts of the world. For prophylaxis and treatment, one needs to refer to the latest information from schools of tropical diseases or from Public Health doctors in Health Authorities. Quinine is effective for the treatment of chloroquine-resistant *P. falciparum*, and the erythrocytic forms of the other three species.

Other protozoa

Isospora belli, *Pneumocystis carinii* and *Cryptosporidium* spp., which hitherto were almost unheard of as pathogens, are now the cause of considerable morbidity and mortality in immunosuppressed patients, particularly those with AIDS. *Pneumocystis carinii* pneumonia ('PCP') is a recognized complication of AIDS. Co-trimoxazole is effective in the treatment of *Is. belli* and in high dosage for *Pn. carinii*. Pentamidine isethionate, which is a potentially toxic agent, has been used in patients in whom co-trimoxazole is contraindicated and in patients with severe pneumocystis pneumonia. Because of its toxicity, intravenous administration must be carefully monitored. Promising results have been reported for pentamidine given by aerosol, which is associated with a reduction in side effects. There is no known effective treatment for cryptosporidium infections.

Treatment of toxoplasmosis is indicated in immunosuppressed patients, with a combination of pyremethamine and a sulphonamide.

Antiviral agents

The search for effective antiviral agents has not been as fruitful as for antibacterial agents, partly because of the physiological dependence of viruses on the host cell for their replication. With the advent of transplant surgery, which requires a depressed immune state, and as a response to AIDS, the search for antiviral agents has gathered greater momentum and urgency. Apart from cryotherapy for the treatment of warts, physical agents have not been useful. Research has been concentrated on finding agents that will block the metabolic cycle of the virus during its development within the host, or prevent its attachment to the human cell without depressing or altering the immune response of the host and without having unacceptable toxic effects. Other areas of development include the provision of immune serum, interferon therapy, prophylaxis and prevention by immunization.

Development of resistance among viruses to antiviral agents may become as important as the challenge of antibiotic resistance among bacteria is today.

Interferons

Interferons are glycoproteins, synthesized by cells infected with viruses or other microorganisms. As result of recombinant DNA techniques, purified interferons are more easily available for studying their effect on the course of viral infections. There are three immunologically distinct classes of interferons: *a, b, x*. Interferon *x* is produced by T lymphocytes following mitogenic or antigenic stimulation, while *a* and *b* interferons are produced by other cells in viral infections. They have different spectra of activity, but together they show synergistic antiviral action. They also show synergism with some antiviral agents against herpes, influenza and some other viruses. Interferon *x*, because of its additional immunomodulation effects, is being investigated for the treatment of leprosy and HIV infections. However, all interferons can increase the cytotoxic effect of T lymphocytes by increasing HLA expression. Their usefulness is limited by their dose-related toxicity and their low potency.

Side effects of intravenous interferon therapy include bone marrow depression, neurotoxicity, cardiotoxicity, and other less serious manifestations such as vomiting, nausea, fever, headache and muscular pain. Intranasal administration avoids the serious side effects but can cause bleeding and ulceration of the nasal mucosa. Interferons have been used systemically in cytomegalovirus (CMV) infections, varicella zoster virus (VZV) infections in immunosuppressed patients, patients with chronic hepatitis (B and C), and topically for the treatment of herpes simplex infection of the eye and for protection against rhinovirus infections.

Interferon, in combination with other drugs like zidovudine or ribavirin, is undergoing clinical trials in patients with the acquired immunodeficiency syndrome.

Antiviral drugs

Idoxuridine, a thymidine analogue, inhibits replication of DNA viruses such as herpes simplex virus (HSV), VZV and cytomegalovirus. Its chief use is as a topical agent for the treatment of herpes virus simplex keratitis. Idoxuridine is available as 0.1 per cent ophthalmic solution and ointment. Occasionally it may cause corneal or eyelid inflammation, resulting in pain and pruritus. Five to 40 per cent idoxuridine dissolved in dimethyl sulphoxide (DMSO) has been used effectively in the treatment of herpes simplex and herpes zoster skin lesions.

Due to its toxicity and poor clinical response, idoxuridine is no longer used systemically. Experimentally it is teratogenic, mutagenic and immunosuppressive and is therefore contra-indicated during pregnancy.

Amantadine, a synthetic symmetrical tricyclic amine, inhibits multiplication of myxoviruses. Its virustatic effect is directed at RNA viruses, notably influenza A parainfluenza, rubella and respiratory syncytial virus, but it is not effective against influenza B or mumps. Its analogue, rimantadine, has been used extensively in the USSR for prophylaxis against outbreaks of influenza A. Amantadine prevents intracytoplasmic entry and replication of viruses by neutralizing acid vesicles within the cell. Oral administration of 100 mg twice daily has been used for prophylaxis in contacts of influenza A sufferers, with reduction in the incidence of cases reported. The dosage should be reduced for children and the elderly. It crosses into the CSF with values reaching 60 per cent of serum level. It is not metabolized and is excreted through the kidneys. Amantadine, given as an aerosol, has led to rapid clinical improvement but has not influenced virus shedding. The toxic effects of amantadine include anticholinergic side effects, psychosis and other effects resembling those of catecholamines in the nervous system. Experimentally it is teratogenic and is therefore not recommended for pregnant or lactating women. At the recommended dosage, it is relatively non-toxic. Its clinical antiviral use is limited to prevention and treatment of influenza A virus infections.

Cytosine arabinoside was originally developed as an antitumour agent, but was found to have anti-herpes virus activity. It is active against herpes simplex virus, varicella zoster virus and cytomegalovirus. Because of its toxic effects, which include bone marrow depression, its use is limited to topical treatment of herpes virus keratitis.

Adenine arabinoside is a purine analogue that has antiviral activity against herpes simplex virus, varicella zoster virus, Epstein–Barr virus, poxviruses, animal herpes viruses, rhabdoviruses and some RNA tumour viruses. It acts by selectively inhibiting the synthesis of viral DNA. It also inhibits the replication of acyclovir, or idoxuridine-resistant HSV, and of acyclovir-resistant VZV.

Adenine arabinoside is available as a 3 per cent eye ointment and in vials containing 200 mg/ml for intravenous use. It is used for the treatment of herpes virus encephalitis and other infections by HSV, and varicella zoster infections in immunocompromised patients. It also has been used in CMV infections, chronic hepatitis B and in Creutzfeldt–Jakob disease. It is as effective as idoxuridine for the local treatment of herpes virus ocular keratitis.

With increasing usage serious side effects have been recognized. These include gastrointestinal, haematological and neurological side effects, as well as thrombophlebitis at the intravenous site. Other local side effects have been reported with ophthalmic ointment.

ACYCLOVIR

Acyclovir is a guanosine analogue whose antiviral activity is limited to some herpes viruses. It also enhances the anti-HIV activity of zidovudine. It selectively inhibits viral DNA synthesis. Both *in vitro* and *in vivo* resistance to acyclovir have been reported.

Acyclovir is water soluble and can be given orally, intravenously and as ointment. Acyclovir is eliminated through the kidneys and 60 per cent can be recovered from the urine in active form. After intravenous therapy, it is distributed throughout the body and enters the CSF at 50 per cent of the serum level.

The antiherpetic activity of this compound has much interest. The mode of action appears to be very specifically related to virus metabolism, due to phosphorylation of acycloguanosine by thymidine kinase, which is concentrated in the virus-infected cells. The phosphorylated compound has an inhibitory effect on DNA polymerases of both type I and type II herpes virus hominis, and at higher concentrations on herpes zoster virus and Epstein–Barr virus. It potentiates the action of zidovudine and can be used parenterally for the treatment of disseminated herpes infection in man.

Ganciclovir is structurally similar to acyclovir, having an extra hydroxymethyl group on its side chain. It prevents the synthesis of viral DNA. The higher intracellular concentration of mono-, di- and triphosphate derivatives of ganciclovir may explain its greater effectiveness in inhibiting cytomegalovirus replication. It is also active against other herpes viruses. Ganciclovir is administered by intravenous infusion. Cerebrospinal fluid levels vary between 25 and 75 per cent of serum levels. It is excreted by the kidneys, and its elimination correlates very closely with creatinine clearance. Experimentally, ganciclovir is teratogenic and mutagenic, with side effects involving the male and female reproductive systems, gastro-intestinal tract, bone marrow and the CNS. Abnormal liver function tests, neutropenia, thrombocytopenia and anaemia have been reported. Thrombophlebitis at the site of infusion is a common problem.

Zidovudine is a thymidine analogue that has activity against HIV and other mammalian retroviruses. It inhibits the viral reverse transcriptase activity of HIV. It also inhibits the growth of some Gram-negative bacilli, as well as the protozoan, *Giardia lambdia*. It shows synergism with acyclovir but antagonism with ribavirin and thymidine.

Zidovudine is rapidly absorbed after oral administration and the peak serum level, of which approximately one-third is protein bound, is reached within 30–90 minutes. Its toxic effects include headache, nausea, muscular pain, severe neurological side effects and convulsion, anaemia, granulocytopenia and pancytopenia, requiring interruption of treatment.

Zidovudine is beneficial in reducing the incidence of HIV-associated neuropathy and improving CNS-related functions. Its usefulness in post-exposure prophylaxis is not yet proven.

Ribavirin is a synthetic nucleoside, an analogue of guanine, with activity against a variety of DNA and RNA viruses inhibiting their replication. Ribavirin triphosphate selectively inhibits influenza virus RNA polymerase activity and eventually inhibits viral protein synthesis. In high concentrations, it inhibits acute HIV infection of human lymphocytes but antagonizes the anti-HIV action of zidovudine. The combination of ribavirin with amantadine seems to be synergistic and has shown potential in the treatment of influenza. Ribavirin, given intravenously or as a small particle aerosol, has attracted great attention as a therapeutic agent against RSV, CMV and influenza virus infections. It is the drug of choice for the treatment of Lassa fever. Ribavirin is teratogenic, with dose-related toxic effect on the gastro-intestinal tract, CNS and the bone marrow.

Antifungal agents

Man's relative success in discovering and manufacturing newer, less toxic and broad-spectrum antibacterial agents has not been repeated with the antifungals. The increased incidence of fungal infections in immunocompromised patients, especially those undergoing bone marrow transplantation, and in patients with AIDS, together with the present difficulty in confirming the presumed diagnosis of such infections, has resulted in the widespread use of relatively toxic drugs.

Existing antifungal agents, some formidable for their toxicity, include: topical antifungals for cutaneous application only, the polyenes, fluocytosine, imidazoles, triazoles and griseofulvin.

Antifungal agents that are used as a cream, ointment, solution or powder include amphotericin B, compound benzoic acid ointment (Whitfield's ointment), clotrimazole, econazole, ketoconazole, miconazole, natamycin, nystatin, salicylic acid, tolnaftate and undeceonates.

The polyenes

The polyene group of antibiotics produced by a number of *Streptomyces* species includes nystatin, natamycin and amphotericin B. They are not water soluble and are not absorbed when given orally. The first two are so toxic that only topical preparations are available. Amphotericin B, although very toxic, is probably the most effective antifungal agent available for systemic use. Polyenes act by binding to the ergosterol of the cytoplasmic membrane of sensitive fungi, in preference to human sterol, increasing the permeability of the fungal membrane which eventually leads to cell lysis.

NYSTATIN

Nystatin, the first of the polyene antibiotics, was isolated from *Streptomyces noursei* in 1950. It is insoluble in water and too toxic for parenteral use. Although it has a wide range of activity against yeasts, yeast-like fungi and dimorphic fungi, its use is limited to topical applications and gut infections, since it is not absorbed from the gut. It is not useful for the treatment of ringworm.

Nystatin acts by binding to a specific sterol, only found in fungi, damaging the cytoplasmic membrane and making it more permeable. Nystatin has no side effects when applied topically, while large oral doses may lead to nausea and vomiting.

Clinical uses of nystatin are limited to candida skin infections, such as nappy rash, oral thrush (using nystatin suspension or lozenges), candida infections of the gastro-intestinal tract and vagina and in patients undergoing 'gut decontamination' to prevent candida overgrowth.

AMPHOTERICIN B

Amphotericin B, the most important of the polyene antibiotics available, was first isolated in 1956 from *Streptomyces nodosus*. It is not water soluble. The intravenous form is a colloidal complex of amphotericin B, desoxycholate and phosphate buffer in 5 per cent glucose.

The majority of *Candida albicans* strains, other candida species, *Cryptococcus neoformans*, dimorphic fungi and *Aspergillus* spp. are sensitive to amphotericin B. At high concentrations, amphotericin B is fungicidal, since it irreversibly alters the permeability of the cytoplasmic membrane leading to cell death. This may explain the synergistic action with rifampicin, fluocytosine and with tetracyclines which are normally inactive against amphotericin-sensitive fungi, by facilitating their penetration through the fungal cytoplasmic membrane. At low concentrations the action of amphotericin is fungistatic and is reversible. The mode of action of amphotericin on the cytoplasmic membrane may also explain its systemic toxicity.

Tolerance and acquired resistance, although uncommon, cannot be ruled out, especially in patients undergoing prolonged treatment. Side effects include nephrotoxicity and it should therefore be avoided in patients with renal failure. Intrathecal administration is associated with neurotoxicity. Cardiac arrest and other cardiovascular side effects may be associated with rapid infusion. Anaemia and other haematological problems associated with inhibition of erythropoietin production, headache, fever, nausea, vomiting, muscle and joint pain during intravenous infusion and, rarely, anaphylaxis have all been reported. Thrombophlebitis is a very common problem, which can be reduced by either changing the infusion site or using a central venous line. Many of the problems with toxicity have been overcome with the production of liposomal-associated amphotericin and similar preparations (see below) which can be given in higher doses with few problems apart from the great expense of the products available.

Amphotericin B is the antibiotic of choice for the treatment of systemic and opportunistic deep mycosis, since the two more common organisms, *Aspergillus* and *Candida* spp., are sensitive. Cryptococcal infections, particularly cryptococcal meningitis in immunocompromised patients (including those suffering from AIDS), may be successfully treated with amphotericin B. Its use has also been advocated in patients suffering from acute leukaemia since they are particularly vulnerable to aspergillus and candida infections.

Amphotericin B is available as tablets, suspensions, lozenges, ointments, cream, lotions and powder for reconstitution and liposomal-associated suspension. It is advisable to assess the patient's response to a test dose of 15mg given over 10–20 minutes.

Amphotericin is now available in a variety of lipid formulations which are given intravenously as treatment for systemic fungal infection. They are less toxic than intravenous amphotericin B, and are therefore given in higher doses, with a view to obtaining increased efficacy as well as a reduction in unwanted effects. The dose is different for the different preparations, but in general is in the order of 1 mg/kg on the first day, rising over several days to 3–5 mg/kg daily.

Fluocytosine (5-fluorocytosine), the fluorine analogue of cytosine, was first synthesized in 1957 as an antitumour drug but found to be more effective as an antifungal agent. It is thought to act by interfering with DNA synthesis. It is water soluble and can therefore be given orally as well as intravenously. Ninety per cent of the oral dose is absorbed and most of it is excreted via the kidneys in an active form. Fluocytosine is active against most of the strains of *Candida albicans* and other candida species, *Torulopsis glabrata* and *Cryptococcus neoformans*. Resistance may develop during treatment, particularly if it is interrupted. Because of the possibility of resistance, it is prudent to give it together with another antifungal agent such as amphotericin B. Fluocytosine is not active against *Aspergillus* spp. or *Histoplasma* spp.

At high concentrations, fluocytosine is fungicidal and at lower concentrations it is fungistatic. Side effects of fluocytosine include gastro-intestinal disturbances such as vomiting, abdominal pain and diarrhoea, bone marrow depression and hepatotoxicity. In the presence of renal impairment, serum levels of the drug must be closely monitored and should not exceed 80 mg/litre. The oral dose of 150–200 mg/kg/day is given 6 hourly. A 1 per cent intravenous preparation is available for infusion lasting 20–40 minutes, also given every 6 h.

Fluocytosine, in combination with amphotericin B, can be used for the treatment of systemic candidiasis of various forms, torulopsis, cryptococcosis and chromoblastomycosis.

Imidazoles

Clotrimazole was the first of the imidazoles to be synthesized. It was followed by miconazole and econazole, and by ketoconazole. These compounds are active against some of the fungi, protozoal parasites and some Gram-positive bacteria.

Clotrimazole has a wide range of antifungal activity. Cryptococci, *Candida albicans* and related species, and dimorphic and filamentous fungi, are highly sensitive.

It is only available for topical application and as vaginal tablets and cream, but is not recommended during the early stages of pregnancy. Its clinical use is limited to the treatment of cutaneous candida infections, trichomonas vaginitis and ringworm. The side effects of clotrimazole include gastro-intestinal disturbances, hepatotoxicity and neurotoxicity.

Miconazole, like clotrimazole, has a wide range of activity against fungi, some Gram-positive bacteria and some protozoa including *Plasmodium falciparum*, but not *Trichomonas vaginalis*.

Miconazole has been used to treat cryptococcal infections, systemic and superficial candida infections, torulopsis and amoebic meningoencephalitis. Its use as a systemic agent is very limited and it is now mainly used as a topical antifungal agent, as a 2 per cent cream, for the treatment of ringworm.

It shows antagonism with amphotericin B and rifampicin. It can be administered intravenously, with a total daily dose of 200–1200 mg, in 3 divided doses, and intrathecally for cryptococcal meningitis. Its side effects include gastro-intestinal disturbances, anaphylaxis, allergic rashes, thrombophlebitis, immunosuppression, cardiac arrest, neurotoxicity and a number of haematological manifestations.

Ketoconazole, the latest of the imidazoles, is active against a large variety of fungi and protozoa causing malaria, leishmaniasis and trypanosomiasis. The sensitivity of *Aspergillus fumigatus* is variable. There is evidence of antagonism when used with amphotericin B or with fluocytosine.

The mode of action of ketoconazole is very similar to the other imidazoles, inhibiting sterol synthesis in the susceptible fungal cytoplasmic membrane. Ketoconazole is given orally, 200–400 mg daily. It is best absorbed if taken just before or with a meal. It is metabolized in the liver and excreted as inactive metabolites in the bile and to a lesser extent in urine. Its absorption is altered in patients with serious gastrointestinal disorders and serum levels are affected in patients on H_2-receptor blocking agents, rifampicin, and possibly isoniazid. Other drugs that interact with ketoconazole include phenytoin, cyclosporin and oral anticoagulants.

Ketoconazole is used for the treatment of refractory dermatophyte infections of the skin where topical antifungal agents have failed, superficial and chronic candidiasis, coccidiomycosis and blastomycosis. Ketoconazole does not appear to be effective in the treatment of aspergillosis or cryptococcosis.

Side effects include nausea, vomiting, abdominal pain, allergic rash, depression of serum testosterone with gynaecomastia with loss of libido in men, menstrual irregularities in women which are reversible, and hepatitis. All patients on ketoconazole should have their liver function monitored and caution is advised when treating patients with pre-existing liver function abnormalities.

Triazoles

This group of antimycotic antibiotics, closely related to the imidazoles, includes terconazole, itraconazole and fluconazole.

Itraconazole has structural similarities to ketoconazole, but has a number of advantages over the latter. Like ketoconazole, over 90 per cent is protein bound. It is metabolized in the liver and thus renal impairment or dialysis have no influence on its level or removal.

Itraconazole is indicated for vaginal candidiasis and ringworm infections. It may prove to be effective in aspergillosis. It is available as 100 mg capsules, 1 or 2 to be taken daily. It is contra-indicated in those with liver dysfunction, pregnant women and breast-feeding mothers. There are reports of interaction with rifampicin and with cyclosporin. Itraconazole is also contra-indicated in patients with a history of hypersensitivity to imidazoles and triazoles.

Fluconazole has markedly different pharmacokinetic properties from the imidazoles and itraconazole. It is water soluble, and can be given orally or intravenously. It is excreted unchanged in the urine and crosses the meninges with a CSF level reaching 70 per cent of the serum level. It is indicated in superficial, mucosal and systemic *Candida albicans* candidiasis and cryptococcal infections including meningitis. Non-albicans *Candida* spp. can have resistance to fluconazole and in these infections, amphotericin B is more reliable.

Fluconazole is available as capsules and as an intravenous infusion.

One indication is in the treatment of patients with AIDS who should remain on maintenance dosage. The manufacturers report interactions with warfarin, sulphonylureas, hydrochlorthiazide and phenytoin. Gastro-intestinal side effects include nausea, diarrhoea and abdominal pain.

Griseofulvin, originally derived from *Penicillum griseofulvum*, is insoluble in water and supplied in the form of coarse or fine particles. It inhibits the growth of the dermatophytes by interfering with fungal microtubules and eventual impairment of cell wall synthesis, but it has little effect on *Candida* spp. and *Aspergillus* spp. It is well absorbed from the alimentary tract, and absorption is assisted by reducing its particle size and by a fatty diet. After absorption, it is deposited in keratin precursors, so that the antibiotic remains in the hair and nails and prevents the growth of fungi in these sites. It is metabolized in the liver.

Griseofulvin is available in 125 mg and 500 mg tablets (microsize particles), 0.5–1 g daily, and 330 mg tablets (ultramicrosize), 330–660 mg daily. Its use is limited to the treatment of dermatophyte infections given over a period of at least 4 weeks. Results depend upon the rate of keratinization and desquamation. Compared with other antimycotic agents, griseofulvin is relatively non-toxic. Its reported side effects are nausea, vomiting, diarrhoea, headache, peripheral neuritis, hypersensitivity including photosensitivity, rashes, leukopenia, neutropenia and disturbances of porphyrin metabolism. Drug interactions have been report with warfarin, barbiturates and oral contraceptives. It enhances the effect of alcohol.

Antimicrobial aerosols

The administration of antimicrobials in aerosol form may be beneficial when respiratory infections are caused by resistant micro-organisms requiring treatment with toxic antimicrobials, or are caused by persistent and recurrent infections involving prolonged or repeated treatment with potentially toxic drugs, or in cases of infection by sensitive pathogens in patients with accompanying systemic disease unable to receive parenteral therapy. Administration of antibiotics as aerosols, in conjunction with systemic antibiotic therapy, has been carried out with some success.

The frequency of delivery of drugs and the technical problems of the method, such as their concentration, particle size and stability, are being investigated and refined. Other factors that influence the effectiveness of the drug include the temperature and humidity, presence of thick mucopurulent sputum and the part of the respiratory tract the drug needs to reach. Since the administration of antimicrobial agents may lead to bronchospasm, they should be given together with bronchodilators.

Antibacterial aerosols have been successfully used in patients suffering from cystic fibrosis or severe bronchopulmonary infection by Gram-negative bacteria. Bacitracin, neomycin, polymyxin B, kanamycin, gentamicin and carbenicillin have been used for this purpose.

Antiviral aerosols. Amantadine aerosol has been more effective than the systemic form of the drug in experimental animals.

Antifungal aerosols. Both amphotericin B and nystatin aerosols have been used successfully for the treatment of pulmonary aspergillosis and candidiasis.

Antiprotozoal aerosols. Pentamidine isethionate aerosol has been effective in the prevention of *Pneumocystis carinii* pneumonia in patients suffering from AIDS.

20

Plasma substitutes

Fluids that have a colloid osmotic pressure similar to that of plasma can be used to replace plasma or whole blood within certain limits. They find their use in the treatment of hypovolaemic shock, plasma exchange, priming extracorporeal circuits, isolated organ perfusion and as a carrier solution for insulin. However, a recent meta-analysis of thirty-seven randomized controlled trials comparing colloid with crystalloids in critically ill patients, did not support the continued use of colloids in this situation (Schierhout and Roberts, 1998).

Human albumin has always been very expensive and three types of artificial preparation have been developed which can be used instead: the dextrans, the gelatins and hydroxyethyl starch (Hetastarch). In fact, the belief that these were inferior to the 'ideal' replacement qualities of albumin is now largely discredited (see below). Their actual behaviour is dependent on their physical properties and these are not easy to define. They are all solutions which contain macromolecules of varying sizes, in differing proportions. Unfortunately, the spread of sizes of molecules does not conform to a Gaussian distribution and no measure of central tendency fully describes the composition. Quoted are the mean molecular weight (M_w) and the mean of the number of particles at each molecular weight (M_n). If the solution contains a wide range of molecular sizes, M_w, is larger than M_n because the relatively fewer large molecules contribute more to the calculation of the average weight. The oncotic activity depends on the total number of particles and this can be adjusted to be either iso-oncotic or slightly hyperoncotic by the concentration of substance in the bottle as supplied. However, if there are many molecules below the renal threshold, the amount may be adjusted to take account of their rapid removal. This may then be marketed as an 'advantage' because it promotes urine flow. This is the case with the gelatins, which produce a marked diuresis.

The mode of removal varies: most of the molecules in the gelatins and hetastarch are excreted via the kidneys, although the large molecules have to be broken down to smaller fragments first: the smaller dextran molecules are excreted by the kidneys but the larger ones are taken up by the reticulo-endothelial system. They are eventually metabolized to carbon dioxide and water.

The preparations differ in their side effects. Much is made of these differences in promotional literature, but most of these differences are only of importance when large quantities are used. The most important is the ability of dextran to prevent platelet aggregation and alter the chemical stability of fibrin (see Chapter 18). These actions have encouraged its use for the prophylaxis of postoperative venous thrombosis, but it may increase surgical bleeding. Principally, however, it can interfere with cross-matching of blood. Hetastarch can increase partial thromboplastin time and reduce factor VIII activity, but this is likely

Table 20.1 Composition of plasma substitutes

	M_w	M_n	Concentration in bottle (g %)	Ca^{2+} contents (mmol/litre)	COP at 37°C* (cmH$_2$O)
Dextran 70 *BP*	70 000	35 200	6	–	26.8
Dextran 40 *BP*	40 000	Not stated	10	–	
Urea-linked gelatin: Haemaccel	35 000	24 500	3.5	6.25	35–39
Succinated gelatin: Gelofusine	30 000	22 600	4	< 0.4	46.5
Hetastarch: Hespan	450 000	70 000	6	–	28–30

* This information, provided by the various manufacturers, is difficult to interpret because there is no uniformity about the pore size of the dialysis membrane employed in the measurement.

to be significant only in patients with von Willebrand's disease. The other attribute which seems to influence choice of agent is the incidence of anaphylactoid responses. Dextran 70 has a lower incidence than Gelofusine and Hespan, although a higher proportion of those which do occur are severe: Haemaccel had a higher incidence. It is important to keep these observations, in proportion – one is talking about an incidence approaching 1 : 2000 overall. When given under anaesthesia and to replace lost volume, it is probably far lower. *Table 20.1* lists some of the differences between the available agents.

Schierhout, G. and Roberts, I. (1998) Fluid resuscitation with colloid or crystalloid solutions in critically ill patients: a systematic review of randomized trials. *British Medical Journal,* **316**, 961–4

Oxygen-carrying solutions

These can be divided into haemoglobin solutions and perfluorocarbon emulsions. When used intravenously, the most obvious application for these solutions is to make up for a low haemoglobin concentration secondary to blood loss. They may also have a place in improving oxygen uptake from the lung even in the presence of a normal red blood cell count and a normal haemoglobin concentration.

Perfluorocarbons have been used to achieve total liquid ventilation in experimental animals, and partial liquid ventilation in both animals and humans (see below).

Haemoglobin solutions

Haemoglobin molecules can be dissolved in an aqueous medium, and the resulting solution will bind oxygen to a similar degree to that of intracellular haemoglobin. This fact has been tantalizing researchers for some decades, but a clinically useful and acceptably safe product has yet to be developed.

Haemoglobin solutions hold great promise. They can be made to have colloid oncotic activity and viscosity comparable to human plasma while having oxygen-binding properties comparable to whole blood. They can be stored for prolonged periods and do not require to be typed or cross-matched prior to infusion. Furthermore, their ability to transport oxygen has been demonstrated repeatedly: the issues preventing clinical application are primarily ones of safety, not efficacy.

Haemoglobin in solution will bind oxygen but it has a very high affinity for oxygen (i.e. there is excessive 'left shift' of the dissociation curve). Generally, increasing the size of the haemoglobin moiety causes a 'right shift' of the haemoglobin–oxygen dissociation curve. Haemoglobinaemia secondary to haemolysis is well known to cause acute renal failure, but the whole haemoglobin moiety is responsible for very little of this; the normal α_2–β_2 tetramers consisting of two α-strands and two β-strands spontaneously dissociate into α β-dimers, and it is these smaller molecules which are associated with renal failure.

Both of these problems have been overcome by chemical or genetic modification of the haemoglobin molecule. The chemical modification starts with either out-of-date human donor blood or with bovine blood from which the haemoglobin is obtained. Larger molecules are then produced by a number of means including cross-linking with, for example, diaspirin to produce stable haemoglobin tetramers, polymerization by pyridoxylation (for example) typically to a molecular weight distribution of 128–400 kDa, modelling of haemoglobin by fixation of haem or haemopeptides to polymers, and filling of microcapsules of various polymers (including polylactic acid and polyisobutyl-cyano-acrylate) with haemoglobin solution. An alternative genetic approach has been to use recombinant nucleic acid technology to force bacteria (*Escherichia coli*) or plants (transgenic tobacco) to manufacture haemoglobins without the problem of dissociation into dimers (one example was an α_2–β_1 trimer).

Infusion of haemoglobin solution causes generalized vasoconstriction, although some workers have reported that this effect is less pronounced in the coronary and splanchnic vascular beds. The mechanism of this is thought to be 'scavenging' by haemoglobin of nitric oxide constitutively present in the vascular wall. This problem may be more pronounced with small haemoglobin molecules because there is extravasation into the vessel wall.

Solutions presented for therapeutic use typically contain 80–100 g/litre of haemoglobin. The intravascular half-life of the haemoglobin ranges between 6 and 18 h. Small molecules are eliminated through the kidney, but if the load is too great, renal failure will result. Larger molecules are not excreted renally and thus have somewhat longer half-lives, but are nevertheless rapidly cleared from the circulation.

Early attempts to produce haemoglobin solutions from bovine blood resulted in the prompt onset of a massive systemic inflammatory response. This has been largely overcome by removing cell debris to produce so-called 'stroma-free' solutions. With more

Table 20.2 Reported side effects of haemoglobin solutions administered to experimental animals or human subjects

1. Acute renal failure
2. Generalized vasoconstriction
3. Modification of the immune response (pro-inflammatory)
4. Modification of coagulation (pro-coagulant)
5. Methaemoglobinaemia (the free haemoglobin lacks the protective mechanisms present in red blood cells)
6. Heart rhythm disturbances, including direct negative chronotropism on the heart
7. Hepatotoxicity
8. Production of free radicals
9. Gastro-intestinal distress
10. Interference with colorimetric laboratory tests

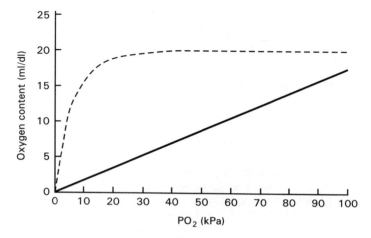

Figure 20.1 The relationship between partial pressure of oxygen and the resulting oxygen content, with flurocarbon emulsion contrasted with that of haemoglobin (——, fluorocarbon emulsion; -----, haemoglobin in cells or solution)

rigorous purification, the intravascular half-life becomes too short: some of the 'impurities' obviously serve to protect the haemoglobin molecule. These and other reported unwanted effects are listed in *Table 20.2.*

Despite the formidable list of safety concerns with haemoglobin solutions, there are some (e.g. the diaspirin cross-linked variety), the development of which has advanced to the stage of clinical trials.

Perfluorocarbons

Fluorocarbons are chemicals that display remarkable properties. They are inert, both chemically and biologically. Many have gas-dissolving actions. In general they have low surface tension and low viscosity. They are relatively insoluble both in water and in lipid. In most medical applications, the term perfluorocarbon is used: in this context the prefix 'per' implies a higher state of oxidation (as opposed to reduction) than would otherwise be the case.

There are several suggested applications for perfluorocarbons. Perfluorocarbon-in-water emulsion can function as an injectable oxygen-carrying fluid. Neat perfluorocarbon can be instilled into the trachea of ventilated patients as part of the treatment of acute respiratory failure by liquid ventilation or partial liquid ventilation. Perfluorocarbon-based or stabilized gas bubbles can be used as contrast agents for the assessment of heart function and detection of perfusion defects by ultrasound imaging. They can be infused (with dissolved oxygen) during percutaneous transluminal coronary angioplasty (PTCA) for high-risk patients. Their clinical evaluation is being pursued as an adjunct to cancer therapy and for treatment of myocardial infarction in conjunction with thrombolytic therapy.

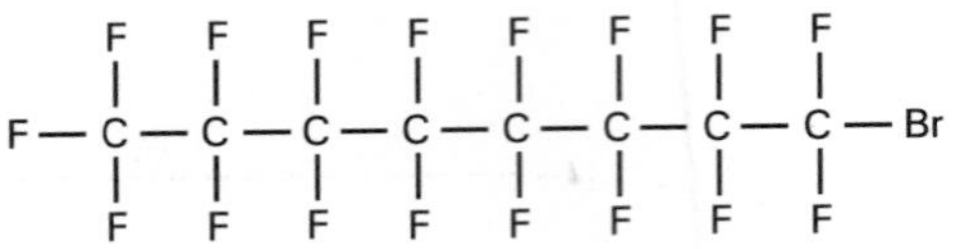

$$F-\overset{\overset{\displaystyle F}{|}}{\underset{\underset{\displaystyle F}{|}}{C}}-\overset{\overset{\displaystyle F}{|}}{\underset{\underset{\displaystyle F}{|}}{C}}-\overset{\overset{\displaystyle F}{|}}{\underset{\underset{\displaystyle F}{|}}{C}}-\overset{\overset{\displaystyle F}{|}}{\underset{\underset{\displaystyle F}{|}}{C}}-\overset{\overset{\displaystyle F}{|}}{\underset{\underset{\displaystyle F}{|}}{C}}-\overset{\overset{\displaystyle F}{|}}{\underset{\underset{\displaystyle F}{|}}{C}}-\overset{\overset{\displaystyle F}{|}}{\underset{\underset{\displaystyle F}{|}}{C}}-\overset{\overset{\displaystyle F}{|}}{\underset{\underset{\displaystyle F}{|}}{C}}-Br$$

Figure 20.2 The perflubron (*n*-perfluoro-octyl bromide) molecule

Intravenous perfluorocarbon emulsions

The oxygen-binding characteristics of perfluorocarbon emulsions is quite different from those of haemoglobin. The relationship between the partial pressure of oxygen and the quantity dissolved is linear (*Figure 20.1*).

The result of this is that 'loading' the fluid with a useful quantity of oxygen requires high inspired oxygen concentrations. The subsequent unloading of the oxygen into the tissues occurs readily, and indeed preferentially to the unloading of oxygen from native red cells.

The biological inertness means that they are unlikely to be degraded into toxic metabolites. Intravenous perfluorocarbon emulsions are cleared from the blood through a process involving phagocytosis of emulsion particles by reticulo-endothelial macrophages and ultimate elimination through the lung in expired air (the perfluorocarbons used are liquid at room temperature, but become vapours at body temperature).

This process causes stimulation of macrophages and subsequent release of intracellular products (particularly metabolites of the arachidonic acid cascade and cytokines) which are responsible for most of the biological effects associated with intravenous perfluorocarbon emulsions (i.e. myalgia, cutaneous flushing and fever at lower doses, and macrophage hypertrophy and recruitment at higher doses). Thrombocytopenia has also been reported.

A preparation trade-named Oxygent is currently undergoing clinical trials. It is a perfluorocarbon-in-water emulsion of which 60 per cent is perfluorocarbon; 58 per cent perfluoro-octyl bromide, termed perflubron (*Figure 20.2*), and 2 per cent perfluorodecyl bromide. The emulsifying agent is egg-yolk phospholipid, and the particle size is around 0.2 μm diameter (particles larger or smaller than this produce unwanted effects). It is typically given in a dose of around 1 ml/kg body weight.

Intratracheal perfluorocarbon instillation

Many experiments have demonstrated that air-breathing animals can be kept alive completely submersed in liquid perfluorocarbon with a high partial pressure of dissolved oxygen. In this context, the low viscosity and low surface tension of fluorocarbons assume particular importance.

While there is no obvious advantage to using total liquid ventilation in patients in intensive care, it has been suggested that partial liquid ventilation may be very beneficial in the management of respiratory failure.

In many pulmonary disease states, the gravitationally lowest part of the lung is not air filled, but filled with liquid, be this oedema fluid, secretions, pus or other fluids. This part of the lung produces true shunt: it allows passage of blood, but this blood undergoes no oxygenation. This liquid is either partially replaced by, or becomes mixed with, an oxygen-carrying liquid when perfluorocarbon is instilled into the tracheal tube.

If too much liquid is instilled, it starts to replace gaseous oxygen in some of the alveoli, and this will reduce oxygenation. In practice, therefore, the way it is used is to repeatedly instil aliquots of 10–20 ml of perfluorocarbon into the tracheal tube until the arterial saturation stops rising with each instillation. The perfluorocarbon gradually enters the gaseous phase to be eliminated in the exhaled gases, and as the effect wears off the process can be repeated.

As with the development of the intravenous application of perfluorocarbons, there is a preparation containing perflubron that has reached the stage of clinical trials.

MONOGRAPHS

DEXTRAN

Dextran is a plasma substitute which is produced by the action of selected strains of *Leuconostoc mesenteroides* on sucrose. By controlling the hydrolysis, glucose chains of the desired average molecular weight can be selected. There is a range of different sizes in the preparation, those below the renal threshold (about 50 000 Da) being excreted by the kidneys quite quickly. The remainder leave the blood at a uniform rate of about one-third per day and enter the tissues and particularly the cells of the reticulo-endothelial system. The most appropriate molecular weight for dextran as a plasma volume expander is therefore 70 000–110 000 Da. All the administered dextran molecules are believed to be metabolized eventually, but the precise route is not known.

Dextran 70 has an average molecular weight of 70 000 Da and is available in either 0.9 per cent saline or 5 per cent dextrose. There would seem to be no indication for giving the 5 per cent dextrose preparation if one is replacing plasma which contains 140 mmol/l of sodium. Dextran 70 is an effective substitute for whole blood or plasma and is as effective as stored blood in maintaining blood volume for up to 3 days after surgery.

Dextran 40 has an average molecular weight of 40 000 Da and is available as a 10 per cent solution in either 0.9 per cent saline or 5 per cent dextrose. It was originally marketed with emphasis on the rheological benefits it was held to confer. These are discussed in the accompanying Monograph on page 464. The current view is that it has no significant advantage over other plasma substitutes.

Precautions

Cross-matching of blood is affected by dextran and if there is any possibility of blood being needed it is advisable to take the necessary sample from the patient for cross-matching before any dextran is given. It is advisable, because of its effect on clotting, to restrict the volume given to 1–1.5 litres. There are numerous reports linking the development of acute renal failure with the administration of dextran 40. The smaller molecules are rapidly excreted by the kidneys and concentrations as high as 40 g/100 ml of urine are seen, resulting in very viscous urine. It should not be given when there is any reason to doubt renal function and urine output should be maintained above 40 ml/h.

GELATINS

Gelatin preparations are obtained from bovine collagen which is treated in different ways in order to obtain a fluid solution of gelatin. This has colloid osmotic activity and viscosity which make it a suitable plasma substitute. There are two preparations at present available in the UK: Gelofusine and Haemaccel. The molecular weights of all synthetic colloid solutions vary widely and for gelatin solutions the range is from 5000 to 50 000 Da. The molecular weights shown in *Table 20.1* are the average M_n of the products. Although the average molecular weights of the gelatins would lead one to expect very rapid renal excretion, the half-life in the circulation is claimed to be 4–6 h and there is extensive clinical experience of both products which shows them to be effective plasma substitutes.

Anaphylactoid reactions

Although at first it was claimed that gelatins were 'non-antigenic', there is now no doubt that they can cause anaphylactoid reactions. Gelofusine is a succinylated gelatin, whereas Haemaccel is urea-linked and their composition is different (*Table 20.3*). The balance of published reports at present favours the succinylated preparation as being very unlikely to cause serious anaphylactoid reactions, with a significantly lower incidence than is reported for dextran 70.

HUMAN ALBUMIN

Human albumin is prepared from pooled plasma by ethanol fractionation, sterilized by filtration and by heating to 60°C for 10 h to inactivate viruses. It is available as solutions of 4.5–5 per cent and 20 per cent. Both strengths contain sodium chloride sufficient to make them iso-osmotic: the 20 per cent solution is therefore relatively salt poor. Synthetic (genetically engineered) human albumin from yeast is under development.

Table 20.3 Constituents of the two preparations of gelatin at present available in the UK

	Gelofusine	*Haemaccel*
Synonyms	Succinylated gelatin Physiogel Modified fluid gelatin	Urea-linked gelatin Polygeline
Average molecular weight (M_n)	22 600	24 500
Gelatin	40 g/litre	35 g/litre
Sodium	154 mmol/litre	145 mmol/litre
Potassium	0.4 mmol/litre	5.1 mmol/litre
Magnesium	0.4 mmol/litre	–
Calcium	0.4 mmol/litre	6.26 mmol/litre
Carbonate	20–30 mmol/litre	–
Chloride	125 mmol/litre	145 mmol/litre

Pharmacology

Physiological concentrations of albumin account for 60–80 per cent of the normal plasma colloid osmotic pressure. The 5 per cent solution therefore has a similar colloid osmotic pressure to plasma, whereas the 20 per cent solution is hyper-oncotic. Human albumin was previously thought to approach the ideal colloid replacement solution for a number of reasons. Compared with synthetic colloidal solutions it is present naturally in blood and is therefore unlikely to be toxic or have toxic metabolites, it enhances protein-bound transport of drugs and endogenous chemicals, it has free-radical scavenging properties and it can be metabolized as a form of nutrition. Compared with other blood products it is a pasteurized product and is therefore less hazardous, it has a long shelf-life and it does not require refrigeration.

Despite these apparent advantages, the current thinking is that it should be used seldom if ever. The theoretical objection is based on the observation that with even a mild systemic inflammatory response there is an increase in the threshold of molecular weight at which substances can leak out of capillaries – the capillary leak threshold. In health, this threshold is just below the molecular weight of albumin, and when the threshold is raised, even slightly, albumin solution leaks out at the same rate as a crystalloid. Reservations about its use have been reinforced by clinical studies. Early studies showed that survival rates are not increased in intensive care with the use of albumin compared with gelatin. More recent studies have shown a reduction in survival rate with the use of albumin compared with crystalloids, with synthetic colloids and with other blood products in conditions as diverse as nephrotic syndrome, multiple organ failure and burns.

Indications and dosage

Most authorities now believe that there is currently no indication for the use of albumin. It has been compared with isotonic saline in trials which have shown, at least in younger patients, that there is surprisingly little difference between them in outcome terms. There is naturally concern that dilution with large volumes of crystalloid will lower oncotic pressure and lead to pulmonary oedema. What has been less appreciated is that albumin is also rapidly distributed across the capillary membrane and there is in fact a greater increase in lung water when albumin is used. The general guideline must be that when the primary deficit is of water, electrolytes or both, crystalloids should be given initially. If more than 2–3 litres are required, colloid should be added. Colloid may be beneficial in septic shock, ARDS and anaphylaxis, but crystalloids seem to be more beneficial in burns, despite the loss of protein in that condition.

Precautions

A recent meta-analysis (Cochrane Review, 1998) has concluded that albumin is associated with an increased mortality in critically ill patients. A commentary by Berger at the end of the paper suggests that albumin leakage from the capillaries is increased in severe shock states and overwhelms the ability of the lymphatic system to drain, particularly, the lungs.

The risks of transmitting disease are negligible. Concentrated albumin should be given cautiously if there is a risk of left ventricular failure. The product is much more expensive than other colloids: the advantages, if any, are hardly commensurate with the cost.

Cochrane Injuries Group Albumin Review. (1998) Human albumin administration in critically ill patients: systematic review of randomised controlled trials. *British Medical Journal*, **317**, 235–40

STARCH

Hetastarch

Hydroxyethyl starch (hetastarch) is available as a clear, pale yellow 6 per cent solution (Hespan) with NaCl 0.9 per cent with the pH adjusted to 5.6. The calculated osmolarity is 310 mosmol/litre. This product is derived from amylopectin by the introduction of hydroxyethyl ether groups into the glucose groups of the starch. The range of molecular weights is very wide so that the M_w is very high (450 000 Da). The solution is slightly hyperoncotic and therefore there is a slight increase in plasma volume over the volume infused. Approximately 40 per cent of the dose is lost via the kidney over the first 24 h; the remainder is broken down slowly over the next 2 weeks and excreted similarly.

Hetastarch increases the erythrocyte sedimentation rate. It should obviously be used with caution in the presence of renal failure. In common with other plasma substitutes it can produce dilutional effects and in large doses can cause clotting problems. It does not interfere with cross-matching. It can reduce Factor VIII levels, which can be of importance in von Willebrand's disease. The incidence of anaphylactoid reactions is acceptably low.

Pentastarch

Pentastarch is an artificial colloid derived from amylopectin. It has an average molecular weight of about 250 000 Da, with a range of 150 000–300 000 Da. It has a molar substitution of 0.45, which means that it has 45 hydroxyethyl groups for every 100 glucose units. It is available as a 10 per cent solution and has a calculated osmolality of approximately 320 mosmol/litre. The solution is slightly hypertonic and administration results in a 1.5 times greater volume expansion than Hetastarch. The volume expansion following pentastarch persists for about 18–24 h. Molecules less than 50 000 molecular weight are rapidly eliminated by renal excretion. About 70 per cent of a given dose is eliminated in the urine within 24 h and about 80 per cent within 1 week. Pentastarch causes an increase in erythrocyte sedimentation rate, but it does not interfere with blood clotting or cross-matching of blood.

It is used in conditions of hypovolaemia, but care must be taken in patients with renal failure not related to hypovolaemia and in those with congestive cardiac failure.

Appendix

Changes in the names of drugs

Following international agreement under the auspices of the World Health Organization, European law now lays down a requirement to replace existing national nomenclature with 'Recommended International Nonproprietary Names'. In conformity with this, the Medicines Control Agency (UK) is proposing a two-stage process. In the case of substances where there is a major change (e.g. using epinephrine for adrenaline), dual labelling will be used, with the rINN preceding the BAN (British Approved Name) on the label. This will continue for at least 5 years. There are 18 drugs in this category, of which 10 are of relevance to this textbook. They are listed in *Table A.I*, with the relevant ones in bold type.

Where the change is without significant hazard (e.g. using thiopental for thiopentone), the change will be immediate and brought in on a specified date by Statutory Instrument. The date is not known at the time of going to press. There are about 200 names on this list, many of which are no longer licensed. Some 50–60 are of possible relevance and again are printed in bold (Table A.II).

If a drug is not on either list, it is appropriate to continue to use the British (or USP) name. In most cases there is no difference, and these are now correctly described as rINN. In a few cases a change is proposed and the proposed name would be different. These are the subject of objection by the European Commission and so have the status of proposed name (pINN). For these substances the use of the BAN/BP name continues indefinitely. While we have tried to take account of this in the text, there is little point in reproducing the list.

Table A.I Major changes – use dual labelling

UK name (BAN/BANM/BP title)	Recommended INN/INNM	UK name (BAN/BANM/BP title)	Recommended INN/INNM
acrosoxacin	rosoxacin	**frusemide**	furosemide
adrenaline*	epinephrine	mitozantrone	mitoxantrone
amethocaine	tetracaine	*mustine≠*	*chlormethine*
bendrofluazide	bendroflumethiazide	**noradrenaline**	norepinephrine
benzhexol	trihexyphenidyl	oxpentifylline	pentoxifylline
chlorpheniramine	chlorphenamine	**procaine penicillin**	procaine benzylpenicillin
dicyclomine	dicycloverine	salcatonin	calcitonin (salmon)
dothiepin	dosulepin	thymoxamine	moxisylyte
eformoterol†	formoterol	**trimeprazine**	alimemazine
flurandrenolone	fludroxycortide		

* Entries in bold type in this table and in *Table A.II* are of relevance to anaesthetists.

† WHO is intending to change the INN *formoterol* to *eformoterol* – the requirement to dual label is therefore suspended.

≠ Entries in italic type in this table and in *Table A.II* are for non-marketed, discontinued or abandoned materials, although some may still be available on a 'named patient' basis.

Table A.II Minor changes – use new name*

UK name (BAN/BANM/BP title)	Recommended INN/INNM	UK name (BAN/BANM/BP title)	Recommended INN/INNM
acepifylline	*acefylline piperazine*	*buniodyl*	*bunamiodyl*
acinitrazole	*aminitrozole*	*bupropion*	*amfetbutamone*
actinomycin	*cactinomycin*	busulphan	busulfan
adenosine phosphate	*adenosine monophosphate*	*butamyrate*	*butamirate*
allyloestrenol	allylestrenol	butethamate	butetamate
aloxidone	*allomethadione*	*buthalitone sodium*	*buthalital sodium*
alphadolone	alfadolone	**butobarbitone**	butobarbital
alphaxalone	alfaxalone	*butoxamine*	*butaxamine*
amoxycillin	amoxicillin	*carbiphene*	*carbifene*
amphetamine	*amfetamine*	carbolonium bromide	hexcarbacholine bromide
amphomycin	*amfomycin*	carbophenthion	carbofenotion
amylobarbitone	amobarbital	*carphenazine*	*carfenazine*
amylobarbitone sodium	amobarbital sodium	cellacephate	cellacefate
azetepa	*azatepa*	**cephalexin**	cefalexin
balipramine	*depramine*	*cephaloglycin*	*cefaloglycin*
barbitone	*barbital*	*cephalonium*	*cefalonium*
beclomethasone	beclometasone	*cephaloram*	*cefaloram*
benorylate	benorilate	**cephaloridine**	*cefaloridine*
benzathine penicillin	benzathine benzylpenicillin	**cephalothin**	cefalotin
		cephamandole nefate	cefamandole nafate
benzphetamine	*benzfetamine*	cephazolin	cefazolin
benztropine	benzatropine	cephoxazole	cefoxazole
bethanidine	betanidine	cephradine	cefradine
bismuth glycollylarsanilate	*glycobiarsol*	*chlophedianol*	*clofedanol*
bromocyclen	*bromociclen*	chloral betaine	cloral betaine
bromodiphenhydramine	*bromazine*	chlorbutol	chlorobutanol

Table A.II *continued*

UK name (BAN/BANM/BP title)	Recommended INN/INNM	UK name (BAN/BANM/BP title)	Recommended INN/INNM
chlordantoin	clodantoin	ethacrynic acid	etacrynic acid
chlorfenvinphos	clofenvinfos	**ethamivan**	etamivan
chlorhexadol	chloralodol	ethamsylate	etamsylate
chlormethiazole	clomethiazole	ethebenecid	etebenecid
chlorthalidone	chlortalidone	ethenzamide	etenzamide
chlorthenoxazin	chlorthenoxazine	ethinyloestradiol	ethinylestradiol
cholecalciferol	colecalciferol	ethoglucid	etoglucid ethosalamide
cholestyramine	colestyramine	ethopropazine	profenamine
clamoxyquin	clamoxyquine	ethosalamide	etosalamide
clomiphene	clomifene	ethybenztropine	etybenzatropine
clorgyline	clorgiline	ethyloestrenol	ethylestrenol
clothiapine	clotiapine	ethynodiol	etynodiol
co-carboxylase	cocarboxylase	etifoxin	etifoxine
colistin sulphomethate sodium	colistimethate sodium	fanthridone	fantridone
		fenchlorphos	fenchlofos
corticotrophin	corticotropin	fenethylline	fenetylline
coumaphos	coumafos	fetoxylate	fetoxilate
cromoglycic acid	cromoglyicic acid	flumethasone	flumetasone
crotethamide	crotetamide	fluopromazine	triflupromazine
cumetharol	coumetarol	**flupenthixol**	flupentixol
cyacetazide	cyacetacide	flurothyl	flurotyl
cyclobarbitone calcium	cyclobarbital calcium	glycalox	glucalox
cycloprolol	cicloprolol	glycopyrronium bromide	glycopyrrolate
cystermine	mercaptamine	guaiphenesin	guaifenesin
danthron	dantron	halethazole	haletazole
deoxycortone	desoxycortone	halopyramine	chloropyramine
desoxymethasone	desoximetasone	heptabarbitone	heptabarb
dexamphetamine	dexamfetamine	hexachlorophane	hexachlorophene
diamphenethide	diamfenetide	hexamine hippurate	methenamine hippurate
diatrizoic acid	amidotrizoic acid	hexobarbitone	hexobarbital
diazinon	dimpylate	hydroxamethocaine	hydroxytetracaine
dichlorphenamide	diclofenamide	hydroxyamphetamine	hydroxyamfetamine
dienoestrol	dienestrol	hydroxyprogesterone hexanoate	hydroxyprogesterone caproate
dimethicone(s)	dimeticone		
dimethindine	dimetindine	hydroxyurea	hydroxycarbamide
dimethiscoquin	quinisocaine	**indomethacin**	indometacin
dimethothiazine	dimetotiazine	iodipamide	adipiodone
dimethyl sulphoxide	dimethyl sulfoxide	iophendylate	iofendylate
dioxathion	dioxation	iothalamic acid	iotalamic acid
dipenine bromide	diponium bromide	isobuzole	glysobuzole
diphenidol	difenidol	isoetharine	isoetarine
disulphamide	disulfamide	isometamidium	isometamidium chloride
doxybetasol	doxibetasol	ketobemidone	cetobemidone
doxycycline hydrochloride (hemihydrate hemiethanolate)	doxycycline hyclate	levamphetamine	levamfetamine
		lignocaine	lidocaine
		lynoestrenol	lynestrenol
		lysuride	lisuride
dyclocaine	dyclonine	malethamer	maletamer
epioestriol	epiestriol	meprothixol	meprotixol
epithiazide	epitizide	methadyl acetate	acetylmethadol

Table A.II *continued*

UK name (BAN/BANM/BP title)	Recommended INN/INNM	UK name (BAN/BANM/BP title)	Recommended INN/INNM
methallenoestrol	methallenestrol	phenyramidol	fenyramidol
methallibure	metallibure	phthalylsulphathiazole	phthalylsulfathiazole
methamphazone	metamfazone	pipazethate	pipazetate
metharbitone	metharbital	pipothiazine	pipotiazine
methenolone	metenolone	polyhexanide	polihexanide
methetoin	metetoin	**potassium clorazepate**	dipotassium clorazepate
methimazole	thiamazole	potassium	menadiol potassium
methindizate	metindizate	menaphthosulphate	sulfate
methisazone	metisazone	pramoxine	pramocaine
methixene	metixene	promethoestrol	methestrol
methohexitone	methohexital	promoxolan	promoxolane
methoin	mephenytoin	pronethalol	pronetalol
methotrimeprazine	levomepromazine	proquamezine	aminopromazine
methsuximide	mesuximide	prothionamide	protionamide
methyl cysteine	mecysteine	quinalbarbitone	secobarbital
methylene blue	methylthioninium chloride	riboflavine	riboflavin
methylphenobarbitone	methylphenobarbital	rolicypram	rolicyprine
metriphonate	metrifonate	salazosulphadimidine	salazosulfadimidine
metyzoline	metizoline	secbutobarbitone	secbutabarbital
monosulfiram	sulfiram	sissomicin	sisomicin
naphthalophos	naftalofos	**sodium calciumedatate**	sodium calcium edetate
nealbarbitone	nealbarbital	**sodium cromoglycate**	sodium cromoglicate
nicoumalone	acenocoumarol	sodium diatrizoate	sodium amidotrizoate
nitroxynil	nitroxinil	sodium ipodate	sodium iopodate
norbutrine	norbudrine	sodium ironedetate	sodium feredetate
norethynodrel	noretynodrel	sodium picosulphate	sodium picosulfate
noxiptyline	noxiptiline	sorbitan mono-oleate	sorbitan oleate
noxythiolin	noxytiolin	sorbitan monolaurate	sorbitan laurate
nylestriol	nilestriol	sorbitan monopalmitate	sorbitan palmitate
octacosactrin	tosactide	sorbitan monostearate	sorbitan stearate
octaphonium	octafonium chloride	stanolone	androstanolone
oestradiol	estradiol	stiboestrol	diethylstilbestrol
oestriol	estriol	streptonicozid	streptoniazid
oestriol sodium succinate	estriol sodium succinate	succinylsulphathiazole	succinylsulfathiazole
oestriol succinate	estriol succinate	sulglycotide	sulglicotide
oestrone	estrone	**sulphacetamide**	sulfacetamide
oxethazine	oxetacaine	sulphachlorpyridazine	sulfachlorpyridazine
oxyphenisatin	oxyphenisatine	**sulphadiazine**	sulfadiazine
oxypurinol	oxipurinol	sulphadimethoxine	sulfadimethoxine
pentaerythritol tetranitrate	pentaerithrityl tetranitrate	sulphadimidine	sulfadimidine
pentobarbitone	pentobarbital	sulphaethidole	sulfaethiodole
pentolinium tartrate	pentolonium tartrate	sulphaguanidine	sulfaguanidine
phanquone	phanquinone	sulphaloxic acid	sulfaloxic acid
phenbenicillin	fenbenicillin	sulphamethizole	sulfamethizole
phenbutrazate	fenbutrazate	sulphamethoxazole	sulfamethoxazole
phenethicillin	pheneticillin	sulphamethoxydiazine	sulfametoxydiazine
phenobarbitone	phenobarbital	sulphamethoxypyridazine	sulfamethoxypyridazine
phenoxypropazine	fenoxypropazine	sulphamoxole	sulfamoxole
phenyl aminosalicylate	fenamisal	sulphaphenazole	sulfaphenazole
		sulphaproxyline	sulfaproxyline

Table A.II *continued*

UK name (BAN/BANM/BP title)	Recommended INN/INNM	UK name (BAN/BANM/BP title)	Recommended INN/INNM
sulphasazine	sulfasalazine	thioguanine	tioguanine
sulphasomidine	*sulfisomidine*	*thiomesterone*	*tiomesterone*
sulphasomizole	*sulfasomizole*	**thiopentone**	thiopental
sulphathiazole	sulfathiazole	*thiothixene*	*tiotixene*
sulphathiourea	*sulfathioyrea*	*thioxolone*	*tioxolone*
sulphatolamide	*sulfatolamide*	**thyroxine**	levothyroxine
sulphaurea	sulfacarbamide	*triacetyloleandomycin*	*troleandomycin*
sulphinpyrazone	sulfinpyrazone	*trimustine*	*trichlormethine*
sulphomyxin sodium	*sulfomyxin sodium*	*troxidone*	*trimethadione*
sulthiame	sultiame	*tyformin*	*tiformin*
tetracosactrin	tetracosactide	urofollitrophin	urofollitropin
tetrahydrozoline	*tetryzoline*	*vinbarbitone*	*vinbarbital*
thiabendazole	tiabendazole	*vinylbitone*	*vinylbital*
thiacetazone	*thioacetazone*	*vipyrnium embonate*	*pyrvinium pamoate*
thialbarbitone	*thiabarbital*	**vitamin A**	retinol
thiazesim	*tiazesim*	*xanthinol nicotinate*	*xantinol nicotinate*
thiocarlide	*tiocarlide*	*xanthocillin*	*xantocillin*

Radicals and groups

besylate	besilate	isethionate	isetionate
camsylate	camsilate	mesylate	mesilate
closylate	closilate	methylsulphate	metilsulfate
edisylate	edisilate	napadisylate	napadisilate
enanthate	enantate	napsylate	napsilate
esylate	esilate	theoclate	teoclate
ethylsulphate	etilsulfate	tosylate	tosilate

* See footnotes * and ≠ in *Table A.I* concerning the use of bold and italic typefaces.

Index